Handbook of Experimental Pharmacology

Volume 194

Brendan J. Canning • Domenico Spina
Editors

Sensory Nerves

Contributors

R. Baron, S. Benemei, S.K. Bhangoo, L.A. Blackshaw, S.D. Brain, G. Burnstock, B.J. Canning, J.G. Capone, F. De Cesaris, D.N. Cortright, W.C. de Groat, R.J. Docherty, S.R. Eid, C.E. Farmer, E.S. Fernandes, P. Holzer, L.-W. Fu, P. Geppetti, T.D. Gover, N.G. Jones, H. Jung, J.C. Longhurst, F. Marchand, S.B. McMahon, R.J. Miller, T.H. Moreira, P. Nicoletti, A.J. Page, S.M. Schmidhuber, J.N. Sengupta, V.S. Seybold, D. Spina, C. Stein, D. Weinreich, F.A. White, N. Yoshimura, C. Zöllner

Springer

Editors
Dr. Brendan J. Canning
Johns Hopkins Asthma & Allergy Center
Dept. Medicine
5501 Hopkins Bayview Circle
Baltimore MD 21224
USA
bjc@jhmi.edu

Dr. Domenico Spina
King's College London
School of Biomedical & Health Sciences
Sackler Inst. Pulmonary
Pharmacology Guy's Campus
London
5th Floor, Hodkin Bldg.
United Kingdom SE1 9RT
domenico.spina@kcl.ac.uk

ISSN 0171-2004
ISBN 978-3-540-79089-1 e-ISBN 978-3-540-79090-7
DOI: 10.1007/978-3-540-79090-7

Springer Dordrecht Heidelberg London New York

Library of Congress Control Number: 2009926022

Cover design: SPi Publishers Services

Printed on acid-free paper

Springer-Verlag Berlin Heidelberg (www.springer.com)

Preface

The intention of this book is to provide a comprehensive and contemporary review of the biology of sensory nerves. In keeping with the theme of the *Handbook of Experimental Pharmacology* series, emphasis will be placed on the actions of drugs, transmitters and autacoids that initiate or inhibit sensory nerve activation (through actions on ion channels and receptors at their peripheral terminals) or modulate the release or actions of the transmitters released from the central terminals of sensory nerves. On the basis of extensive supportive evidence in the literature, it is our view that many diseases are characterized by alterations in sensory nerve function (e.g. pain, cardiovascular disease and migraine). It is our belief that this book will be unique, as it will comprehensively cover the role of sensory nerves across many therapeutic areas. To address directly one of the editorial board queries, this is not intended to be a book about the pharmacology of pain. That said, to most pharmacologists, pain is the most obvious indication for a role or sensory nerves in disease. We believe that the lessons learnt from the study of neuropathic pain will be invaluable for researchers in the other therapeutic areas covered in this volume. Since most interest has focused on the role of sensory nerves in neuropathic pain, we have added a number of chapters devoted to this subject.

The book is organized in three parts, covering the types and roles of sensory nerves in somatic and visceral disorders (Part I), specific targets on sensory nerves relevant to pain and visceral disorders (Part II) and a description of current and future therapeutic strategies for targeting sensory nerves (Part III).

The first two chapters in Part I are devoted to describing the clinical features of neuropathic pain and visceral pain. Our intention is for the authors to provide a clinical viewpoint on the features of these conditions and the advantages/disadvantages of current treatment modalities. The next five chapters in Part I focus on the role of sensory nerves in other pathological conditions. Several common themes will emerge in this part, including the mode of sensory nerve activation in various tissues and organs, the alterations in sensory nerve excitability associated with disease, and the importance of inflammation and inflammatory mediators in initiating altered sensory nerve function in disease.

Whilst the first part focuses on the clinical and/or systems physiology, Part II has its focus at the cell and molecular level. This part highlights the current understanding of proteins/ion channels/mediators that have created the most intense recent interest in the area of sensory nerve biology. Together, these chapters will give the reader important knowledge about how sensory nerve function can be altered pharmacologically. The last chapter in this part describes the processes that give rise to altered neural reflexes at the central level. The mechanisms described in these chapters reinforce the role of proteins/mediators highlighted in the preceding chapters. The role of these cellular, molecular and physiological processes in the diseases discussed in Part 1 are emphasized.

The aim of Part III is to highlight potential drug targets that might alter sensory nerve function. Most of the work has been devoted to the treatment of neuropathic pain and so this part heavily emphasizes this subject. However, as will be apparent from Part I, many of these targets could be utilized in other therapeutic areas that implicate sensory nerves in their pathophysiological processes. The focus of the chapters is on opioids and modulators of ion channels and then the final chapter is devoted to future treatment strategies for neuropathic pain.

Finally, we would like to thank all the contributors, including co-authors, who agreed to write chapters for this book and the publishers, especially Susanne Dathe, for their patience and assistance.

Baltimore *B.J. Canning*
London *D. Spina*

Contents

Contributors

Ralf Baron
Sektion Neurologische Schmerzforschung und Therapie, Klinik für Neurologie, Christian-Albrechts-Universität Kiel, Schittenhelmstr. 10, 24105 Kiel, Germany, r.baron@neurologie.uni-kiel.de

Silvia Benemei
Centre for the Study of Headache and Department of Preclinical and Clinical Pharmacology University of Florence, Florence, Italy

Sonia K. Bhangoo
Molecular Pharmacology and Structural Biochemistry, Northwestern University, Chicago, IL, USA

L. Ashley Blackshaw
Nerve Gut Research Laboratory, Level 1 Hanson Institute, Frome Road, Adelaide, SA 5000, Australia, ashley.blackshaw@adelaide.edu.au

Susan D. Brain
Cardiovascular Division, Franklin-Wilkins Building, Waterloo Campus, King's College London, London SE1 9NH, UK, sue.brain@kcl.ac.uk

Geoffrey Burnstock
Autonomic Neuroscience Centre, Royal Free and University College Medical School, Rowland Hill Street, London NW3 2PF, UK, g.burnstock@ucl.ac.uk

B.J. Canning
Johns Hopkins Asthma and Allergy Center, 5501 Hopkins Bayview Circle, Baltimore, MD 21224, USA, bjc@jhmi.edu

Jay G. Capone
Headache Center, University Hospital S.Anna, Ferrara, Italy

D.N. Cortright
Department of Biochemistry and Molecular Biology, Neurogen Corporation, 35 N.E. Industrial Road, Branford, CT, USA

Francesco De Cesaris
Centre for the Study of Headache and Department of Preclinical and Clinical Pharmacology University of Florence, Florence, Italy

William C. de Groat
Department of Pharmacology, West 1352 Starzl Biomedical Science Tower, University of Pittsburgh School of Medicine, Pittsburgh, PA 15261, USA, degroat@server.pharm.pitt.edu

Reginald J. Docherty
Neurorestoration Group, Wolfson CARD, King's College London, London SE1 9RT, UK, reginald.docherty@kcl.ac.uk

S.R. Eid
Department of Pain Research, Neuroscience Drug Discovery, Merck Research Laboratories, West Point, Philadelphia, USA, samer_eid@merck.com

Clare E. Farmer
Department of Molecular Neuroscience, Institute of Neurology, University College London, UK, c.farmer@ion.ucl.ac.uk

Elizabeth S. Fernandes
Cardiovascular Division, Franklin-Wilkins Building, Waterloo Campus, King's College London, London SE1 9NH, UK

Peter Holzer
Research Unit of Translational Neurogastroenterology, Institute of Experimental and Clinical Pharmacology, Medical University of Graz, Universitätsplatz 4, A-8010 Graz, Austria, peter.holzer@meduni-graz.at

Liang-Wu Fu
Department of Medicine, Susan Samueli Center for Integrative Medicine, School of Medicine, University of California, Irvine, CA 92697, USA

Pierangelo Geppetti
Centre for the Study of Headache and Department of Preclinical and Clinical Pharmacology University of Florence, Florence and Headache Center, Department of Neuroscience, Azienda Universita-Ospedale S. Anna, Ferrara, Italy, pierangelo.geppetti@unifi.it

T.D. Gover
Department of Pharmacology and Experimental Therapeutics, University of Maryland, School of Medicine, Baltimore, MD 21201-1559, USA

Nicholas G. Jones
King's College London, Neurorestoration, CARD Wolfson Wing, Hodgkin Building, Guy's Campus, London Bridge, London, SE1 1UL, UK

Hosung Jung
Molecular Pharmacology and Structural Biochemistry, Northwestern University, Chicago, IL, USA

John C. Longhurst
Department of Medicine, Department of Physiology and Biophysics, Susan Samueli Center for Integrative Medicine, School of Medicine, C240 Medical Sciences I, University of California, Irvine, CA 92697, USA, jcl@uci.edu

Fabien Marchand
King's College London, Neurorestoration, CARD Wolfson Wing, Hodgkin Building, Guy's Campus, London Bridge, London, SE1 1UL, UK

Stephen B. McMahon
King's College London, Neurorestoration, CARD Wolfson Wing, Hodgkin Building, Guy's Campus, London Bridge, London, SE1 1UL, UK, stephen.mcmahon@kcl.ac.uk

Richard J. Miller
Molecular Pharmacology and Structural Biochemistry, Northwestern University, Chicago, IL, USA, r-miller10@northwestern.edu

T.H. Moreira
Office of Science and Engineering Laboratories FDA/CDRH, 10903 New Hampshire Avenue, Building 62, Room 1229, Silver Spring, MD 20993-0002, USA

Amanda J. Page
Nerve Gut Research Laboratory, Level 1 Hanson Institute, Frome Road, Royal Adelaide Hospital, Discipline of Medicine and Discipline of Physiology, School of Molecular and Biomedical Sciences, University of Adelaide, Adelaide, SA 5000, Australia

Paola Nicoletti
Centre for the Study of Headache and Department of Preclinical and Clinical Pharmacology University of Florence, Florence, Italy

Sabine M. Schmidhuber
Cardiovascular Division, Franklin-Wilkins Building, Waterloo Campus, King's College London, London SE1 9NH, UK

V.S. Seybold
Department of Neuroscience, University of Minnesota, 6-145 Jackson Hall, 321 Church St., S.E., Minneapolis, MN 55455, USA, vseybold@umn.edu

Jyoti N. Sengupta
Division of Gastroenterology and Hepatology, Medical College of Wisconsin, 8701 Watertown Plank Road, Meilwaukee, WI 53051, USA, sengupta@mcw.edu

Domenico Spina
The Sackler Institute of Pulmonary Pharmacology, Division of Pharmaceutical Science, 5th Floor Hodgkin Building, King's College London, London SE1 1UL, UK, domenico.spina@kcl.ac.uk

Christoph Stein
Klinik für Anaesthesiologie und operative Intensivmedizin, Freie Universität Berlin, Charité – Campus Benjamin Franklin, 12200 Berlin, Germany, christoph.stein@charite.de

Daniel Weinreich
Department of Pharmacology and Experimental Therapeutics, University of Maryland, School of Medicine, Baltimore, MD 21201-1559, USA, dweinrei@umaryland.edu

Fletcher A. White
Cell Biology, Neurobiology & Anatomy, Anesthesiology, Loyola University, Chicago, Maywood, IL, USA

Naoki Yoshimura
Department of Urology, 700 Kaufman Building, University of Pittsburgh School of Medicine, Pittsburgh, PA 15261, USA

Christian Zöllner
Klinik für Anaesthesiologie und operative Intensivmedizin, Freie Universität Berlin, Charité – Campus Benjamin Franklin, 12200 Berlin, Germany

Part I
Role of Sensory Nerves in Disease

Neuropathic Pain: A Clinical Perspective

Ralf Baron

Contents

Abstract Neuropathic pain syndromes, i.e., pain after a lesion or disease of the peripheral or central nervous system, are clinically characterized by spontaneous pain (ongoing, paroxysms) and evoked types of pain (hyperalgesia, allodynia). A variety of distinct pathophysiological mechanisms in the peripheral and central nervous system operate in concert: In some patients the nerve lesion triggers

R. Baron
Sektion Neurologische Schmerzforschung und Therapie, Klinik für Neurologie, Christian-Albrechts-Universität Kiel, Schittenhelmstr. 10, 24105 Kiel, Germany
r.baron@neurologie.uni-kiel.de

B.J. Canning and D. Spina (eds.), *Sensory Nerves*,
Handbook of Experimental Pharmacology 194, DOI: 10.1007/978-3-540-79090-7_1,

molecular changes in nociceptive neurons that become abnormally sensitive and develop pathological spontaneous activity (upregulation of sodium channels and receptors, e.g., vanilloid TRPV1 receptors, menthol-sensitive TRPM8 receptors, or α-receptors). These phenomena may lead to spontaneous pain, shooting pain sensations, as well as heat hyperalgesia, cold hyperalgesia, and sympathetically maintained pain. Spontaneous activity in damaged large nonnociceptive A-fibers may lead to paresthesias. All these changes may also occur in uninjured neurons driven by substances released by adjacent dying cells and should receive more attention in the future. The hyperactivity in nociceptors in turn induces secondary changes (hyperexcitability) in processing neurons in the spinal cord and brain. This central sensitization causes input from mechanoreceptive A-fibers to be perceived as pain (mechanical allodynia). Neuroplastic changes in the central descending pain modulatory systems (inhibitory or facilitatory) may lead to further hyperexcitability. Neuropathic pain represents a major neurological problem and treatment of patients with such pain has been largely neglected by neurologists in the past. The medical management of neuropathic pain consists of five main classes of oral medication (antidepressants with reuptake blocking effect, anticonvulsants with sodium-blocking action, anticonvulsants with calcium-modulating actions, tramadol, and opioids) and several categories of topical medications for patients with cutaneous allodynia and hyperalgesia (capsaicin and local anesthetics). In many cases an early combination of compounds effecting different mechanisms is useful. At present existing trials only provide general pain relief values for specific causes, which in part may explain the failure to obtain complete pain relief in neuropathic pain conditions. In general, the treatment of neuropathic pain is still unsatisfactorily. Therefore, a new hypothetical concept was proposed in which pain is analyzed on the basis of underlying mechanisms. The increased knowledge of pain-generating mechanisms and their translation into symptoms and signs may in the future allow a dissection of the mechanisms that operate in each patient. If a systematic clinical examination of the neuropathic pain patient and a precise phenotypic characterization is combined with a selection of drugs acting against those particular mechanisms, it should ultimately be possible to design optimal treatments for the individual patient.

Keywords Neuropathy, Pathophysiology, Assessment, Treatment

1 Introduction and Definition of Neuropathic Pain

Modern research into the mechanisms of neuropathic pain has clearly demonstrated that a nerve lesion leads to dramatic changes in the sensory nervous system that makes it distinct from other chronic pain types in which the nociceptive system is intact (chronic nociceptive pain, e.g., osteoarthritis). The alterations include the appearance of novel receptor and channel proteins at the membrane of degenerating or regenerating neurons, changes in nociceptive signal processing in the peripheral nervous system (PNS) and the central nervous system (CNS), as well as anatomical rewiring of afferent connections. Therefore, also the drug targets differ in the lesioned nervous system and, hence, neuropathic pain states require different therapeutic approaches which are often not effective against nociceptive pain. For the clinician, it is, therefore, of utmost importance to know the specific medical history of neuropathic pain and have valid diagnostic tools that differentiate neuropathic from nociceptive pain or estimate the importance of the neuropathic pain component in combinations of different pain types. Both categories of pain are characterized by distinct clinical signs and symptoms that can be used to differentiate between them.

In 2007 a new definition for neuropathic pain was proposed by the Special Interest Group "Neuropathic pain" of the International Association for the Study of Pain (Treede et al. 2007). This proposal defines neuropathic pain as a "Pain arising as a direct consequence of a lesion or disease affecting the somatosensory system." The term "disease" refers to identifiable disease processes such as inflammatory, autoimmune conditions, or channelopathies, while "lesion" refers to macro- or microscopically identifiable damage. The restriction to the somatosensory system is necessary, because diseases and lesions of other parts of the nervous system may cause nociceptive pain. For example, lesions or diseases of the motor system may lead to spasticity or rigidity, and thus may indirectly cause muscle pain. The latter pain conditions are now explicitly excluded from the condition of neuropathic pain. If possible, neuropathic pain should be qualified as being of peripheral or central origin in terms of the location of the lesion or disease process. This distinction is important, as lesions or diseases of the CNS and PNS are distinct in terms of clinical manifestations and underlying pathophysiological mechanisms.

2 Classification

It is common clinical practice to classify neuropathic pain according to the underlying cause of the disorder and the anatomical location of the specific lesion (Jensen and Baron 2003). The majority of patients with lesions in the nervous system fall into four broad classes (Table 1): painful peripheral neuropathies (focal, multifocal, or generalized, e.g., traumatic, ischemic, inflammatory, toxic, metabolic, hereditary), central pain syndromes (e.g., stroke, multiple sclerosis, spinal cord injury), complex painful neuropathic disorders (complex regional pain syndromes, CRPS), and mixed-pain syndromes (combination of nociceptive and neuropathic pain, e.g., chronic low-back pain with radiculopathy).

The anatomical distribution pattern of the affected nerves provides valuable differential diagnostic clues as to possible underlying causes. Therefore, painful peripheral neuropathies are grouped into symmetrical generalized polyneuropathies (disease affecting many nerves simultaneously), and into asymmetrical neuropathies with a focal or multifocal distribution or processes affecting the brachial or lumbosacral plexuses.

Table 1 Disease/anatomy-based classification of painful peripheral neuropathies

Painful peripheral neuropathies
Focal, multifocal
Phantom pain, stump pain, nerve transection pain (partial or complete)
Neuroma (posttraumatic or postoperative)
Posttraumatic neuralgia
Entrapment syndromes
Mastectomy
Post thoracotomy
Morton's neuralgia
Painful scars
Herpes zoster and postherpetic neuralgia
Diabetic mononeuropathy, diabetic amyotrophy
Ischemic neuropathy
Borreliosis
Connective tissue disease (vasculitis)
Neuralgic amyotrophy
Peripheral nerve tumors
Radiation plexopathy
Plexus neuritis (idiopathic or hereditary)
Trigeminal or glossopharyngeal neuralgia
Vascular compression syndromes
Generalized (polyneuropathies)
Metabolic or nutritional
Diabetic, often "burning feet syndrome"
Alcoholic
Amyloid
Hypothyroidism
Beriberi, pellagra
Drugs
Antiretrovirals, cisplatin, disulfiram, ethambutol, isoniazid, nitrofurantoin, thalidomide, thiouracil
Vincristine, chloramphenicol, metronidazole, taxoids, gold
Toxins
Acrylamide, arsenic, clioquinol, dinitrophenol, ethylene oxide, pentachlorophenol, Thallium
Hereditary
Amyloid neuropathy
Fabry's disease
Charcot–Marie–Tooth disease type 5, type 2B
Hereditary sensory and autonomic neuropathy type 1, type 1B
Malignant
Carcinomatous (paraneoplastic), myeloma
Infective or postinfective, immune
Acute or inflammatory polyradiculoneuropathy (Guillain–Barré syndrome), borreliosis, HIV
Other polyneuropathies

(continued)

Table 1 (continued)

Erythromelalgia
Idiopathic small-fiber neuropathy
Trench foot (cold injury)
Central pain syndromes
Vascular lesions in the brain (especially brainstem and thalamus) and spinal cord:
Infarct
Hemorrhage
Vascular malformation
Multiple sclerosis
Traumatic spinal cord injury including iatrogenic cordotomy
Traumatic brain injury
Syringomyelia and syringobulbia
Tumors
Abscesses
Inflammatory diseases other than multiple sclerosis; myelitis caused by viruses, syphilis
Epilepsy
Parkinson's disease
Complex painful neuropathic disorders
Complex regional pain syndromes type I and II (reflex sympathetic dystrophy, causalgia)
Mixed-pain syndromes
Chronic low back pain with radiculopathy
Cancer pain with malignant plexus invasion
Complex regional pain syndromes

Central pain is defined as chronic pain following a lesion or disease of the CNS. The cause of pain is a primary process within the CNS. All lesions that cause central pain affect the somatosensory pathways. They may be located at any level of the neuraxis. Thus, lesions at the first synapse in the dorsal horn of the spinal cord or trigeminal nuclei, along the ascending pathways through the spinal cord and brainstem, in the thalamus, in the subcortical white matter, and in the cerebral cortex have all been reported (Leijon et al. 1989).

In addition to the classic neuropathic syndromes such as painful diabetic neuropathy, postherpetic neuralgia (PHN), or phantom limb pain, there are certain chronic painful conditions that share many clinical characteristics. These syndromes were formerly called reflex sympathetic dystrophy, Sudeck dystrophy, or causalgia and are now classified under the umbrella term "complex regional pain syndromes" (CRPS). CRPS are painful disorders that may develop as a disproportionate consequence of trauma typically affecting the limbs (Janig and Baron 2003; Baron and Janig 2004). CRPS type I usually develops after minor trauma with a small or no obvious nerve lesion at an extremity (e.g., bone fracture, sprains, bruises or skin lesions, surgeries). CRPS type II develops after trauma with a mostly large nerve lesion.

There is agreement that both nociceptive and neuropathic processes contribute to many chronic pain syndromes and that these different mechanisms may explain the qualitatively different symptoms and signs which patients experience (mixed-pain syndromes). In particular, patients with chronic low-back pain, cancer pain, and CRPS seem to fit into this theoretical construct (Baron and Binder 2004; Freynhagen et al. 2007).

3 Signs and Symptoms of Neuropathic Pain

Pain associated with nerve injury has several clinical characteristics (Baron 2006). If a mixed peripheral nerve with a cutaneous branch or a central somatosensory pathway is involved, there is almost always an area of abnormal sensation and the patient's maximum pain is coextensive with or within an area of sensory deficit. This is a key diagnostic feature for neuropathic pain. The sensory deficit is usually to noxious and thermal stimuli, indicating damage to small-diameter afferent fibers.

Beside these negative somatosensory signs (deficit in function), which are bothering but not painful, positive signs are also characteristic for neuropathic conditions. Paresthesias (ant crawling, tingling) are bothering but not painful. Painful positive signs are spontaneous (not stimulus-induced) ongoing pain and spontaneous shooting, electric-shock-like sensations. Many patients with neuropathic pain also have evoked types of pain (stimulus-induced pain, hypersensitivity) which are characterized by several sensory abnormalities. They may be adjacent to or intermingled with skin areas of sensory deficit. Most often, patients report mechanical hypersensitivity followed by hypersensitivity to heat and cold. Two types of hypersensitivity can be distinguished. First, allodynia is defined as pain in response to a nonnociceptive stimulus. In the case of mechanical allodynia, even gentle mechanical stimuli such as slight bending of hairs may evoke severe pain. Second, hyperalgesia is defined as an increased pain sensitivity to a nociceptive stimulus. Another evoked feature is summation, which is the progressive worsening of pain evoked by slow repetitive stimulation with mildly noxious stimuli, for example, pinprick. A small percentage of patients with peripheral nerve injury have a nearly pure hypersensitive syndrome in which no sensory deficit is demonstrable. The quality of the reported sensation may also be a clue; neuropathic pain commonly has a burning and/or shooting quality with unusual tingling, crawling, or electrical sensations (dysesthesiae). Although all these characteristics are neither universally present in nor absolutely diagnostic of neuropathic pain, when they are present the diagnosis of neuropathic pain is likely.

4 Pathophysiological Mechanisms and Drug Targets in Neuropathic Pain

Most of the present pathophysiological ideas are derived from experimental work with animal models for neuropathic pain (Fig. 1, Table 2). This work has delineated a series of partially independent pathophysiological mechanisms presumed to be

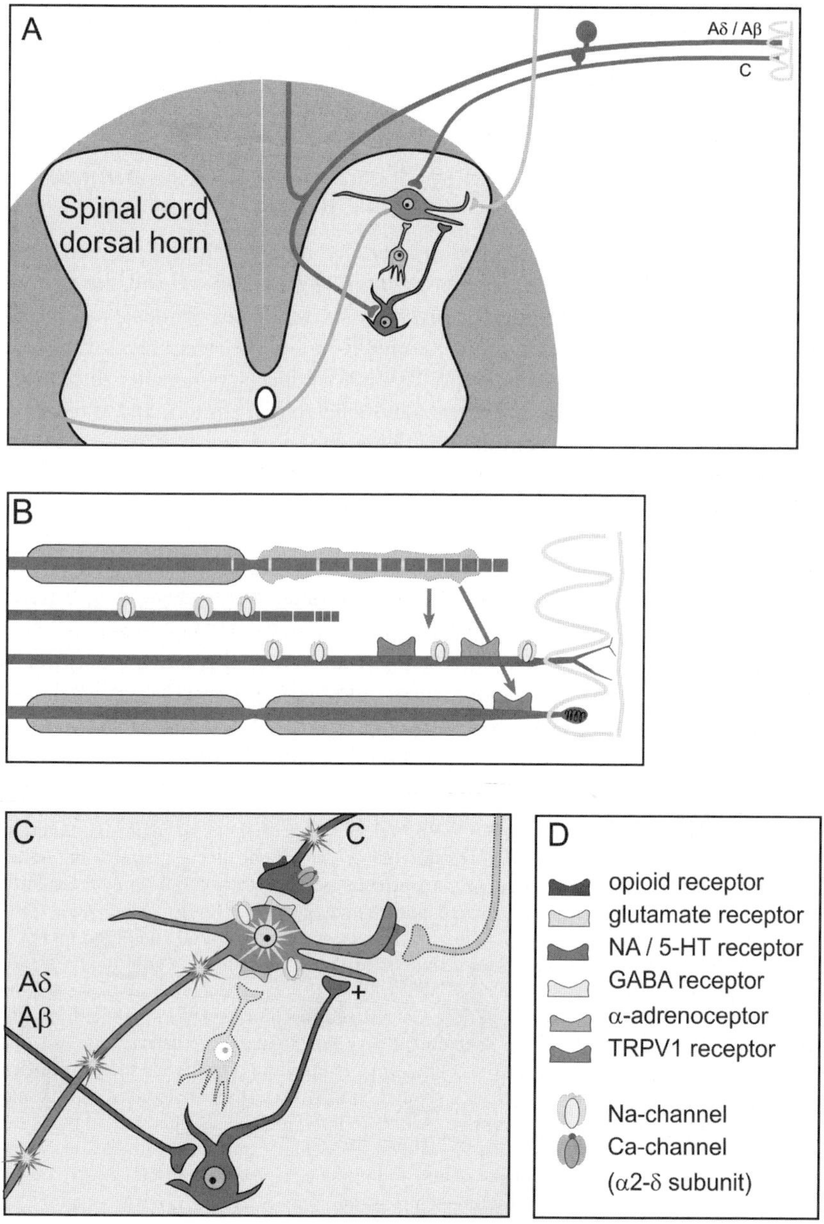

Fig. 1 Mechanisms of peripheral sensitization and central sensitization in neuropathic pain and relevant drug targets. **(a)** Primary afferent pathways and their connections in the spinal cord dorsal horn. Nociceptive C-fibers terminate at spinothalamic projection neurons in upper laminae whereas nonnociceptive myelinated A-fibers project to deeper laminae. The second-order projection neuron is of wide dynamic range (WDR) type, i.e., it receives direct synaptic input from nociceptive terminals and also multisynaptic input from myelinated A-fibers (innocuous information).

responsible for different types of neuropathic pain and different somatosensory abnormalities (Baron 2006):

4.1 Peripheral Sensitization of Primary Afferents in Animals

Pain sensations are normally elicited by activity in unmyelinated (C) and thinly myelinated (Aδ) primary afferent neurons. After peripheral nerve lesion, these neurons acquire an abnormal sensitization, i.e., *an increased responsiveness of primary nociceptors to stimulation of their receptive field.* The characteristic features of sensitized nociceptors are as follows: pathological spontaneous discharge, a lowered activation threshold for thermal and mechanical stimuli, and an enhanced discharge to suprathreshold stimulation (hyperalgesia).

A large number of dramatic molecular and cellular changes at the level of the primary afferent nociceptor that are triggered by the nerve lesion underlie these pathological changes.

Nerve injury is matched by increased expression of messenger RNA for voltage-gated sodium channels in primary afferent neurons. Two voltage-gated sodium channel genes ($Na_v1.8$ and $Na_v1.9$) are expressed selectively in nociceptive primary afferent neurons, and an embryonic channel ($Na_v1.3$) is also upregulated in damaged peripheral nerves and is associated with increased electrical excitability and spontaneous activity in neuropathic pain states. The accumulation of sodium

Fig. 1 (Continued) γ-Aminobutyric acid (GABA)-releasing interneurons normally exert inhibitory synaptic input on the WDR neuron. Furthermore descending modulatory systems synapse at the WDR neuron. **(b)** Peripheral changes at primary afferent neurons after partial nerve lesion leading to peripheral sensitization. Some axons are damaged and degenerate (*upper two axons*), whereas others (*lower two axons*) are still intact and connected with the peripheral end organ (skin). The lesion triggers the expression of sodium channels on damaged neurons. Furthermore, products such as nerve growth factor, which are associated with Wallerian degeneration, are released in the vicinity of spared fibers (*arrows*), triggering channel and receptor expression (sodium channels, TRPV1 receptors, adrenoceptors) on uninjured fibers. **(c)** Spontaneous activity in nociceptive C-fibers induces secondary changes in the central sensory processing by the action of glutamate on postsynaptic NMDA receptors. This leads to spinal cord hyperexcitability (central sensitization). This causes input from mechanoreceptive A-fibers (light touch and punctate stimuli) to be perceived as pain (dynamic and punctate mechanical allodynia; + indicates gating at the synapse). Several presynaptic (opioid receptors, calcium channels) and postsynaptic molecular structures (glutamate receptors, noradrenaline (adrenoceptors), serotonin receptors, GABA receptors, sodium channels) are involved in central sensitization. Inhibitory interneurons and descending modulatory control systems are dysfunctional after nerve lesions, leading to disinhibition or facilitation of spinal cord dorsal horn neurons and to further central sensitization. **(d)** Targets for drug therapy in neuropathic pain: opioid receptors – opioids; glutamate receptors – NMDA blocker (ketamine); noradrenaline (α-adrenoreceptors)/serotonin receptors – antidepressants, clonidine; GABA receptors – baclofen; α-adrenoreceptors – sympathetic blocks; TRPV1 receptor – capsaicin; sodium channel – lidocaine, carbamazepine, lamotrigine; calcium channel – gabapentin, pregabalin, ziconotide. (Modified from Baron 2006)

Table 2 Proposed model for the relationship between neuropathic pain mechanisms and clinical symptoms and signs, and possible targets for therapeutic interventions. 5-HT, 5-hydroxytryptamine (serotonin); ASIC, acid-sensing ion channel; GABA, γ-aminobutyric acid; NK1, neurokinin 1; NMDA, N-methyl-D-aspartate; TCA, tricyclic antidepressants

Compound / Intervention	Targets	Neuronal processes / Pathomechanisms	Sign / Symptom
		Peripheral nociceptor hyperexcitability	
Lidocaine, Carbamazepine, Lamotrigine	Na-channels	Ectopic impulse generation, oscillations in DRG	Spontaneous pain (ongoing) Spontaneous pain (shooting)
		Peripheral nociceptor sensitization	Spontaneous pain (ongoing)
Capsaicin	TRPV1-receptor TRPM8-receptor TRPA1-receptor ASIC-receptors	*Reduced activation threshold to:* heat cold mechanical stimuli	Heat hyperalgesia Cold hyperalgesia Static mechanical allodynia
Sympathetic blocks	α-receptor	noradrenaline	Sympathetically maintained pain
		Central dorsal horn hyperexcitability	
Opioids	*Presynaptic:* μ-receptors	*Central sensitization on spinal level* *Ongoing C-input induces increased synaptic transmission*	
Gabapentin, Pregabalin, Ziconotide	Ca-channels	Amplification of C-fiber-input	
Ketamine	*Postsynaptic:* NMDA-receptors NK-1-receptors Na-channels Intracellular cascades	Gating of A-fiber-input	Spontaneous pain (ongoing)
Baclofen	GABA-B receptors	*Intraspinal inhibitory interneurons* ↓ *(functional, degneration)* GABA-ergic	Dynamic and punctate mechanical allodynia
	Glicine-receptors	Glicine-ergic	
Antidepressants Amitriptyline, Venlafaxine, Duloxtine)	α-, 5-HT-receptors	*Changes of supraspinal descending modulation* inibitory control (NA, 5-HT) ↓	
Clonidine	α2-receptors		

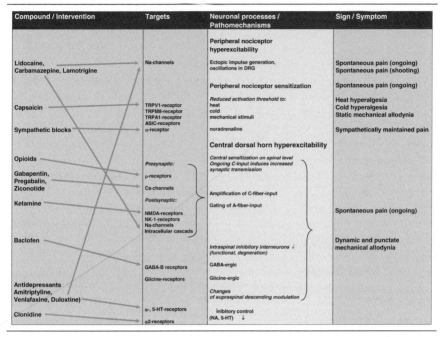

channels at sites of ectopic impulse generation (sodium-channel clusters) may be responsible for lowering the action potential threshold (Omana-Zapata et al. 1997; Lai et al. 2003). There is evidence that small primary afferent fibers may acquire a unique sodium-channel expression profile after nerve lesion (e.g., a specific relation of upregulation and downregulation of channel proteins), which makes them an interesting target (Wood et al. 2004).

After peripheral nerve damage, the accumulation of sodium-channel clusters does not only occur at the site of the nerve lesion but also proximally within the intact dorsal root ganglion. In the dorsal root ganglion a reciprocation between a phasically activating voltage-dependent, tetrodotoxin-sensitive sodium conductance and a passive, voltage-independent potassium leak generates characteristic membrane potential oscillations. Ectopic firing is triggered when the amplitude of oscillation sinusoids reaches the threshold (Amir et al. 2002). Pathological membrane properties within the dorsal root ganglion that occur after nerve lesion are of particular therapeutic interest since the dorsal root ganglion is spared of the blood-brain barrier and might be easily accessible for systemic therapies (Jacobs et al. 1976). In addition to sodium currents, impaired potassium conductances in myelinated fibers were demonstrated in experimental diabetes and may underlie hyperexcitability in these fibers.

Damage to peripheral primary nociceptors also induces upregulation of a variety of receptor proteins at the membrane, some of them only marginally expressed under physiological conditions. Vanilloid receptors (TRPV1) are located predominantly on nociceptive afferent fibers and can be activated by a constituent of hot chilli pepper (capsaicin). Physiologically, this receptor senses noxious heat (above 43°C) (Catarina et al. 2000). Accordingly, TRPV1-deficient knockout mice have obvious deficits in chemical and thermal heat nociception but normal reactions to noxious mechanical stimuli and to noxious cold stimuli.

After partial nerve injury and in streptozotocin-induced diabetic rats, the lesion triggers a TRPV1 downregulation on many damaged afferents but a novel expression of TRPV1 on uninjured C- and A-fibers (Fig. 1b; see below) (Hudson et al. 2001; Hong and Wiley 2005) which is likely involved in the development of C-nociceptor sensitization and the associated symptom of *heat hyperalgesia*. Recent studies also provide evidence for an upregulation of TRPV1 in medium and large injured dorsal root ganglion cells (Ma et al. 2005). However, TRPV1 does not appear to be the only transduction mechanism for heat sensitization after nerve injury. After partial sciatic nerve ligation, wild-type and TRPV1-null mice exhibited comparable persistent enhancement of mechanical and thermal nociceptive responses (Catarina et al. 2000). In this context, a recent study examined strain differences in the normal sensitivity to noxious heat in mice. These differences reflect differential responsiveness of primary afferent thermal nociceptors to heat stimuli due to a genetic variance in CGRP expression and sensitivity (Mogil et al. 2005).

In taxol-induced small-fiber painful polyneuropathy, TRPV4, which is normally activated by heat of more than 30°C, seems to play a crucial role in producing taxol-induced mechanical hyperalgesia (Alessandri-Haber et al. 2004).

Investigations into temperature-sensitive excitatory ion channels also identified several cold-sensing ion channels in peripheral neurons. The cold- and menthol-sensitive TRP channel (TRPM8) is activated within the range of 8–28°C (Patapoutian et al. 2003) and is sensitized by menthol. This receptor is expressed in around 10% of all afferent ganglion neurons of rats, primarily within small-diameter cells (McKemy et al. 2002). TRPA1 is activated at lower temperatures and its exogenous ligand is cinnamaldehyde, a constituent of cinnamon oil, mustard oil, and horseradish. Peripheral nerve lesions have been shown to upregulate the expression of cold-sensing ion channels in dorsal root ganglion cells of rats that developed cold hyperalgesia (Obata et al. 2005; Xing et al. 2007). Therefore, upregulation or gating of these channels after injury may lead to the peripheral sensitization of cold-sensitive C-nociceptors, resulting in the sensory phenomenon of cold hyperalgesia.

In addition to temperature-sensitive receptors, experimental nerve injury also triggers the expression of functional α_1- or α_2-adrenoceptors on cutaneous afferent fibers; these neurons develop adrenergic sensitivity (Fig. 2b). Intravenous adrenaline or physiological noradrenaline release after stimulation of sympathetic efferents that have regenerated into the neuroma can excite afferent nociceptors. After section and reanastomosis of peripheral nerves, electrical stimulation of the sympathetic trunk at physiological stimulus frequencies activates regenerated

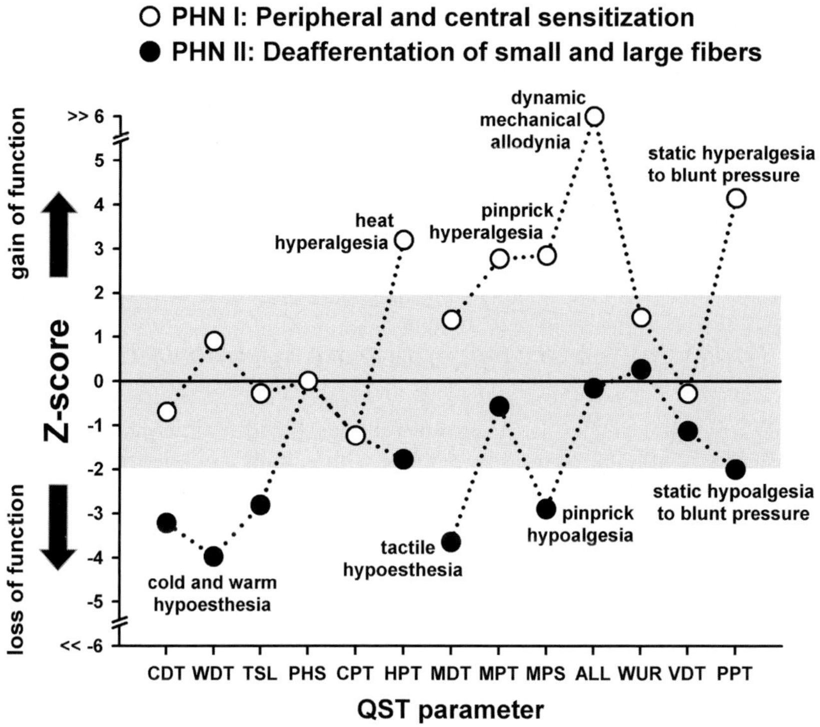

Fig. 2 *Z*-score sensory profiles of two patients suffering from postherpetic neuralgia (PHN). Patient PHN I (*open circles*) presents the QST profile of a 70-year-old woman suffering from PHN for 8 years. Ongoing pain was 80 on a 0–100 numerical rating scale. The profile shows a predominant gain of sensory function in terms of heat pain hyperalgesia (*HPT*), pinprick mechanical hyperalgesia (*MPS*), dynamic mechanical allodynia (*ALL*), and static hyperalgesia to blunt pressure (*PPT*) outside the 95% confidence interval of the distribution of healthy subjects (*gray zone*). This profile is consistent with a combination of peripheral and central sensitization. Patient PHN II (*filled circles*) shows the QST profile of a 71-year-old woman with pain for 8 months. Ongoing pain was 70 on a 0–100 numerical rating scale. The QST profile shows predominant loss of sensory function. Note the cold detection thresholds (*CDT*), warm detection thresholds (*WDT*), thermal sensory limen (*TSL*), heat pain thresholds (*HPT*), tactile detection thresholds (*MDT*), and mechanical pain thresholds to pinprick stimuli (*MPT*) outside the normal range as presented by the *gray zone*. This profile is consistent with a combined small and large fiber sensory deafferentation. The *Z* score is the number of standard deviations between patient data and the group-specific mean value. (After Rolke et al. 2006)

C-nociceptors through an α_1-adrenoceptor mechanism (Habler et al. 1987). Furthermore, sympathetic activity can sensitize identified intact nociceptors following damage to the nerve in which they run via an α_2-adrenoceptor mechanism (Sato and Perl 1991). The concept of a pathological coupling between sympathetic postganglionic fibers and afferent neurons via noradrenaline forms the conceptual framework for the therapeutic application of sympathetic blocks in certain pain syndromes, e.g., CRPS (Price et al. 1998; Baron et al. 1999b).

There is increasing evidence that *uninjured fibers* running in a partially lesioned nerve may also take part in pain signaling (Wasner et al. 2005). Uninjured fibers commingle with degenerating fibers in the same nerves. Products associated with Wallerian degeneration released in the vicinity of spared fibers (e.g., NGF) may be the trigger for channel and receptor expression and may alter the properties of uninjured afferents (Hudson et al. 2001; Wu et al. 2001). Expression of sodium channels, TRPV1 receptors, and adrenoreceptors and an increase of TNF-α sensitivity have been shown to play a role in uninjured fibers adjacent to lesioned axons.

4.2 Peripheral Sensitization of Primary Afferents in Patients

Microneurographic single-fiber recordings support the idea of peripheral sensitization of primary afferent neurons in patients with painful nerve lesions by demonstrating abnormal activity and reduced thresholds in cutaneous afferents. Abnormal ectopic activity of myelinated mechanosensitive fibers was found in traumatic nerve lesions, entrapment neuropathies, or radiculopathies. Since the ectopic nerve activity correlated in intensity and time course with the perceived *paresthesias*, it is likely that pathological activity in A-fibers is the underlying mechanism of positive nonpainful sensations.

Recordings from transected nerves in human amputees with phantom limb pain have demonstrated spontaneous ectopic activity as well as barrages of action potential firing in afferent A- and C-fibers projecting into the neuroma (Nystrom and Hagbarth 1981). Ectopic excitation occurred at multiple sites in damaged sensory neurons. Ongoing activity and mechanical sensitivity were recorded proximal to the nerve neuroma. Following local anesthetic blockade of the nerve distal to the recording site, impulses evoked by mechanical stimulation of the neuroma were abolished, but ongoing activity at the recording site continued, suggesting that this residual activity arose from the dorsal root ganglia. Since these patients suffered from *spontaneous burning pain* and *electric-shock-like sensations*, it is very likely that these symptoms are associated with ectopic firing in primary afferent C-fibers.

In a few patients with characteristic burning pain and heat hyperalgesia, microneurographic recordings have provided evidence for sensitized C-nociceptors. In patients with erythromelalgia, nociceptors displayed ongoing activity, which is normally not observed in nociceptors, and there was a sensitization of mechanically insensitive afferents to nonpainful tactile stimuli. These abnormalities were only present in nociceptive fibers, but not in the sympathetic unmyelinated fibers, as an indicator of a neuropathic process (Orstavik et al. 2003). In the autosomal dominantly inherited form of erythromelalgia, a mutation in SCN9A was found, a gene that encodes the $Na_v1.7$ sodium channel, leading to an altered firing pattern in afferent neurons (Dib-Hajj et al. 2005). Hence, erythromelalgia is the first channelopathy associated with chronic pain (Binder and Baron 2007). Interestingly, a different mutation in the $Na_v1.7$ sodium channel was found in families with congenital indifference to pain (Cox et al. 2006; Goldberg et al. 2007).

Several clinical observations also support the concept of sensitized nociceptors in PHN patients. About 30% of patients with PHN do not show any loss of sensory function in the affected extremity, indicating that in this particular group of patients loss of neurons is minimal or absent. Accordingly, thermal sensory thresholds in their region of greatest pain are either normal or even decreased (heat hyperalgesia) by up to 2–4°C (Rowbotham and Fields 1996; Pappagallo et al. 2000). The decrease of heat pain perception thresholds is a well-known phenomenon of peripheral nociceptor sensitization. With use of skin punch biopsy, it was shown that thermal sensitivity is directly correlated with the density of cutaneous innervation in the area of most severe pain (Rowbotham et al. 1996). Moreover, in PHN patients with heat hyperalgesia acute topical application of the vanilloid compound capsaicin (TRPV1 agonist) enhances pain, a sign which is indicative of an increased capsaicin sensitivity of nociceptors in the affected skin area and has been attributed to a sensitization of nociceptors as the driving element in some patients (Petersen et al. 2000). Furthermore, in a similar group of PHN patients cutaneous iontophoresis of histamine evoked a burning pain sensation, whereas only itch was elicited in normal skin. Again, this phenomenon indicates that nociceptive neurons in the affected skin are abnormally sensitive to histamine (Baron et al. 2001), probably owing to expression of a novel receptor pattern.

These observations suggest that *spontaneous burning pain and heat hyperalgesia* at least in part are associated with sensitization of primary afferent C-fibers to TRPV1 agonists and histamine or with an altered firing pattern in these fibers due to abnormal sodium channels.

Cutaneous hypersensitivity to cold, i.e., cold hyperalgesia, is particularly prominent in patients with posttraumatic neuralgias, some small-fiber polyneuropathies, and chronic CRPS. Another condition of acute cold intolerance occurs after systemic injection of the cancer chemotherapeutic agent oxaliplatin, which is associated with paresthesiae and painful hypersensitivity aggravated by cold. Psychophysical studies of human volunteers using the topical menthol model suggest that sensitization of cold-sensitive nociceptors can produce cold hyperalgesia in normal volunteers (Wasner et al. 2004). Peripheral sensitization also appears to occur in acute oxaliplatin-induced peripheral neuropathy (Lehky et al. 2004; Binder et al. 2007). Therefore, it is likely the *cold hyperalgesia* in some patients is induced by sensitization of primary afferent cold-sensitive nociceptors.

Several clinical observations support the idea that nociceptors acquire a sensitivity to catecholamines that permits an abnormal excitation by either noradrenaline or by circulating catecholamines. This chemical sensitization makes the nociceptors susceptible for noradrenaline released from efferent sympathetic fibers in the periphery. The consecutive pathological sympathetic–afferent coupling forms the conceptual framework for sympathetically maintained pain (SMP) states.

Noradrenergic sensitivity has been described in several human neuropathies and suggests that the ongoing pain can be caused or maintained by the sympathetic nervous system in selected patients: In amputees perineuromal administration of physiological doses of noradrenaline induces intense pain as compared with saline injections (Raja et al. 1998). Intraoperative stimulation of the sympathetic chain induces an increase of spontaneous pain in patients with causalgia (CRPS II) but not in patients with hyperhidrosis. In PHN, application of noradrenaline into a symptomatic skin area increased spontaneous pain and dynamic mechanical hyperalgesia (Choi and Rowbotham 1997). In CRPS II and posttraumatic neuralgias, intracutaneous noradrenaline rekindles pain and hyperalgesia that had been relieved by sympathetic blockade. Also intradermal noradrenaline, in physiologically relevant doses, was demonstrated to evoke greater pain in the affected regions of patients with SMP, than in the contralateral unaffected limb, and in control subjects (Ali et al. 2000). Because noradrenaline-induced pain occurs during a differential blockade of myelinated fibers, unmyelinated fibers appear to signal SMP (Torebjork et al. 1995; Schattschneider et al. 2007).

We performed a study in patients with CRPS I using physiological stimuli of the sympathetic nervous system (Baron et al. 2002). Cutaneous sympathetic vasoconstrictor outflow to the painful extremity was experimentally activated to the highest possible physiological degree by whole-body cooling. During the thermal challenge the affected extremity was clamped to 35°C to avoid thermal effects at the nociceptor level. The intensity as well as the area of spontaneous pain and mechanical hyperalgesia (dynamic and punctate) increased significantly in patients that had been classified as having SMP by positive sympathetic blocks but not in sympathetically independent *pain* patients. In summary, it is likely that SMP is a consequence of an adrenergic sensitization of C-nociceptors.

4.3 Pharmacological Approaches That Modify Peripheral Sensitization of Primary Afferents

4.3.1 Sodium-Channel Blockers

Local anesthetics block voltage-dependent sodium channels. Although the site of action of membrane-stabilizing drugs for relief of pain has not been proven in patients, in vitro studies have shown that ectopic impulses generated by damaged primary afferent nociceptors are abolished by concentrations of local anesthetics much lower than that required for blocking normal axonal conduction. Carbamazepine is very effective in trigeminal neuralgia. However, the strength of evidence is much lower for the benefit of these drugs in other types of neuropathic pain. Oxcarbazepine, which has fewer side effects and drug-drug interactions than carbamazepine, and also lamotrigine were not superior to a placebo in large trials on painful diabetic neuropathy. For lamotrigine there is evidence of efficacy for HIV sensory neuropathy and central poststroke pain. Lidocaine can also be applied topically on the affected painful skin areas. It is thought that the drug diffuses into the upper layers and soothes ectopic firing of afferent nerve endings. Studies report pain relief with topically applied special formulations of local anesthetic [lidocaine patches (5%)] in PHN and other neuropathies.

4.3.2 Topically Applied Capsaicin

Capsaicin is an agonist of the vanilloid receptor (TRPV1) which is present on the sensitive terminals of primary nociceptive afferents. On initial application it has an excitatory action and produces burning pain and hyperalgesia, but with repeated or prolonged application it inactivates the receptive terminals of nociceptors. Therefore, this approach is reasonable for those patients whose pain is maintained by anatomically intact sensitized nociceptors. Capsaicin has been reported to reduce the pain of PHN and painful diabetic neuropathy.

4.4 Central Sensitization in the Spinal Cord in Animals

As a consequence of peripheral nociceptor hyperactivity dramatic secondary changes in the spinal cord dorsal horn also occur. Peripheral nerve injury leads to an increase in the general excitability of nociceptive and multireceptive spinal cord neurons (multiple synaptic input from C-fibers as well as A fibers, wide-dynamic range neurons). This phenomenon is called "central sensitization" and is defined as an *increased responsiveness of nociceptive neurons in the CNS to their normal afferent input*. Central sensitization is manifested by at least three different modes: (1) increase of neuronal activity to noxious stimuli, (2) expansion of size of neuronal receptive fields, and (3) spread of spinal hyperexcitability to other segments.

Central sensitization is initiated and maintained by activity in pathologically sensitized C-fibers, which sensitize second-order spinal cord dorsal horn neurons by releasing glutamate acting on NMDA receptors and the neuropeptide substance P. Furthermore, central neuronal voltage-gated neural-type calcium channels located at the presynaptic sites on terminals of primary afferent nociceptors are involved in central sensitization by facilitation of the release of glutamate and substance P. This channel is overexpressed after peripheral nerve lesion and in rats with streptozotocin-induced diabetes (Luo et al. 2001). As a consequence of peripheral nerve lesion, the dorsal horn neurons abnormally express $Na_v1.3$ (Hains et al. 2004), also enhancing central sensitization. Several intracellular cascades contribute to central sensitization, in particular the mitogen-activated protein kinase system (Ji and Woolf 2001). If central sensitization is established, normally innocuous tactile stimuli become capable of activating spinal cord pain-signaling neurons via Aδ and Aß low-threshold mechanoreceptors (Tal and Bennett 1994). By this mechanism, light innocuous mechanical stimuli to the skin induce pain, i.e., punctuate and dynamic mechanical allodynia. Furthermore, vibratory stimuli can maintain the process of central sensitization (Kim et al. 2007). Beside these dramatic changes in the spinal cord, sensitized neurons were also found in the thalamus and primary somatosensory cortex after partial peripheral nerve injury (Guilbaud et al. 1992).

There is increasing evidence that neuropathic pain is in part mediated by an interaction of nonneural *spinal cord glia* and nociceptive neurons. In experimental pain states in animals, astrocytes and microglia are activated by neuronal signals, including substance P, glutamate, and fractalkine (Wieseler-Frank et al. 2005). Activation of glia by these substances in turn leads to the release of mediators that then act on other glia and also on central nociceptive neurons. These include proinflammatory cytokines and most likely also other neuroexcitatory compounds such as glutamate. By this interaction, central sensitization is augmented. While traditional therapies for pathological pain have focused on neuronal targets, glia might be new therapeutic targets.

Some patients with neuropathic pain, in particular patients with CRPS, characteristically report "extraterritorial" and/or "mirror"-image pain. The pain is experienced not only in the area of trauma but also in neighboring healthy tissues. In cases of mirror-image pain, the pain is perceived from the healthy, corresponding part on the opposite side of the body. New data suggest that communication of activated astrocytes via gap junctions may mediate such spread of pain.

4.5 Central Sensitization of the Spinal Cord in Patients

One hallmark of central sensitization of spinal cord neurons in animals is that activity in A-fiber mechanoreceptors is allowed to gain access to the nociceptive system and induce pain. These phenomena are called "mechanical allodynia" or "hyperalgesia."

Mechanical hypersensitivity is a common phenomenon in neuropathic pain states in patients. There are several lines of evidence that in patients central mechanisms also contribute to these sensory phenomena. Two distinct types have been described in patients: dynamic mechanical and pinprick mechanical hypersensitivity.

There is consensus that dynamic mechanical allodynia is signaled out of the skin by sensitive mechanoreceptors with large myelinated axons that normally encode nonpainful tactile stimuli: (1) reaction time measurements show dynamic mechanical allodynia in patients to be signaled by afferents with conduction velocities appropriate for large myelinated axons (Lindblom and Verrillo 1979; Campbell et al. 1988), (2) transcutaneous or intraneural stimulation of nerves innervating the allodynic skin can evoke pain at stimulus intensities which only produce tactile sensations in healthy skin (Gracely et al. 1992; Price et al. 1992), and (3) with use of differential nerve blocks dynamic allodynia is abolished at time points when tactile sensation is lost, but other modalities remain unaffected (Campbell et al. 1988; Ochoa and Yarnitsky 1993). Therefore, patients with *dynamic mechanical allodynia* would be expected to have central sensitization as the underlying mechanism.

Hyperalgesia to pinprick stimuli, typically elicited by probing of the skin with a stiff von Frey hair is distinct from dynamic mechanical allodynia because of its different spatial and temporal profile and the fact that it is signaled by nonsensitized, heat-insensitive, Aδ-nociceptors.

Notably, in many neuropathic pain patients the mechanically sensitive skin area expands widely into the secondary zone, i.e., the area not affected by the primary nerve lesion, which is also indicative for CNS mechanisms involved. Furthermore, the area of secondary mechanical hypersensitivity is a dynamic phenomenon. In PHN patients with signs of peripheral nociceptor sensitization (heat hyperalgesia, see above), cutaneous capsaicin application into the primary skin area leads to an increase of the allodynic zone into previously nonallodynic and nonpainful skin that had normal sensory function and cutaneous innervation. These observations support the hypothesis that allodynia in a subgroup of PHN patients is a form of chronic secondary hyperalgesia dynamically maintained by input from intact and possibly sensitized ("irritable") primary afferent nociceptors to a sensitized CNS (Fields et al. 1998; Petersen et al. 2000).

Since central sensitization involves the NMDA receptor, the fact that the NMDA receptor antagonist ketamine relieves some neuropathic pain disorders further supports the concept of central sensitization.

Beside these dramatic changes in the spinal cord there is now evidence that higher centers of the neuraxis demonstrate an increased excitability as well as fundamental changes in the somatosensory representation. MEG, PET, and functional MRI studies revealed cortical changes in patients with phantom limb pain, CRPS, and central pain syndromes (Flor et al. 1995; Pleger et al. 2004; Willoch et al. 2004; Maihofner et al. 2005) as well as experimental pain models (Baron et al. 1999a, 2000). Interestingly, these changes correlated with the intensity of the perceived pain and disappeared after successful treatment of the pain (Maihofner et al. 2004; Pleger et al. 2005).

4.6 Pharmacological Approaches That Modify Central Sensitization in the Spinal Cord

4.6.1 Calcium-Channel Modulators

The activation of neuronal calcium channels partly located at the presynaptic spinal terminals of primary afferent nociceptors is necessary for the release of excitatory amino acids and thus for central sensitization. Gabapentin and pregabalin bind to the $\alpha 2\delta$-subunit of these calcium channels. There have been extensive clinical trials of gabapentin for chronic neuropathic pain. These studies examined patients with PHN, diabetic peripheral neuropathy (DPN), mixed neuropathic pain syndromes, phantom limb pain, Guillain–Barré syndrome, and acute and chronic pain from spinal cord injury. Improvements in sleep, mood, and quality of life were also demonstrated. Pregabalin, the successor drug of gabapentin, was shown to be efficacious in PHN, DPN, and spinal cord injury. One advantage over gabapentin is its superior bioavailability, which makes it easier to use without the need for long titration periods. Gabapentin and pregabalin are generally well tolerated, safe, have few drug interactions and no negative impact on cardiac function. This advantage makes them a suitable option especially for the elderly, a population very often suffering from several comorbidities that need multiple-drug therapies.

Recently, a potent calcium-channel blocker, ziconotide, which was derived from a snail venom was shown to be effective for intrathecal treatment of otherwise intractable neuropathic pain.

4.6.2 Tramadol and Opioid Analgesics

Tramadol is a noradrenaline and serotonin reuptake inhibitor with a major metabolite that is a μ-opioid agonist. Sustained efficacy for several weeks has been demonstrated for orally administered tramadol in PHN, DPN, and in patients with painful polyneuropathy of various causes. Strong opioids are clearly effective in postoperative, inflammatory, and cancer pain. However, the use of narcotic analgesics for patients with chronic neuropathic pain was highly controversial, even among experts in the field of pain management. However, to date the findings of several positive trials of oral strong opioid analgesics in various neuropathic pain entities have been published. In an interesting three-period crossover study comparing treatment with opioid analgesics, tricyclic antidepressants (TCAs), and a placebo in patients with PHN, controlled-release morphine provided statistically significant benefits for pain and sleep but not for physical function and mood. In that trial, patients preferred treatment with opioid analgesics compared with TCAs and a placebo despite a greater incidence of adverse effects and more dropouts during opioid treatment (Raja et al. 2002). Our experience is that many patients with pain due to central and peripheral nerve injury can be successfully and safely treated on a chronic basis with stable doses of narcotic analgesics. However, the use of opioids requires caution in patients with a history of chemical dependence or pulmonary disease. We recommend using long-acting opioid analgesics (e.g., sustained-release preparation or transdermal applications) when alternative approaches to treatment have failed.

4.6.3 NMDA-Receptor Antagonists

These drugs block excitatory glutamate receptors in the CNS that are thought to be responsible for the increased central excitability (central sensitization) following noxious stimuli. Clinically available substances with NMDA-receptor blocking properties include ketamine, dextromethorphane, memantine, and amantadine. Studies of small cohorts have generally confirmed the analgesic effects of ketamine in patients suffering from PHN. However, studies with oral NMDA-antagonist formulations (e.g., dextromethorphane) showed positive results in DPN but the drug was without beneficial effect in PHN.

4.6.4 Cannabinoids

Type 1 cannabinoid receptors have been demonstrated in upper laminae of the spinal dorsal horn intimately concerned with the processing of nociceptive information as well as on the cell bodies of primary afferent neurons. Relief of central pain was found with the orally administered tetrahydocannabinol dronabinol in MS patients and for plexus avulsion pain, although in the latter case the primary outcome measure defined in the hypothesis failed. Cannabinoids were also effective in the treatment of mixed peripheral neuropathic pain.

4.7 Central Descending and Intraspinal Control Systems: Inhibition and Fascilitation in Animals and Patients

Physiologically, dorsal horn neurons receive a strong *intraspinal inhibitory control* by GABAergic interneurons. Partial peripheral nerve injury may promote a selective apoptotic loss of these GABAergic inhibitory neurons in the superficial dorsal horn of the spinal cord (Moore et al. 2002), a mechanism which would further increases central sensitization. Furthermore, there is a novel mechanism of disinhibition following peripheral nerve injury. This mechanism involves a transsynaptic reduction in the expression of the potassium chloride exporter KCC2 in lamina I nociceptive neurons. This induces a consequent disruption of the anion homeostasis in these dorsal horn neurons. The resulting shift in the transmembrane anion gradient causes normally inhibitory anionic synaptic currents to be excitatory. Owing to this mechanism, the release of GABA from normally inhibitory interneurons now exerts an excitatory action on lamina I neurons via $GABA_A$ receptors (Coull et al. 2003). The changes in lamina I neurons is induced by brain-derived neurotrophic factor released from activated spinal cord glia (Coull et al. 2005).

Dorsal horn neurons receive a powerful *descending modulating* control from supraspinal brainstem centers (inhibitory as well as facilitatory) (Vanegas and Schaible 2004) (Fig. 1a, c). It was hypothesized that a loss of function in the descending inhibitory serotonergic and noradrenergic pathway contributes to central sensitization and pain chronicity. This idea nicely explained the efficacy of serotonin and noradrenaline reuptake blocking antidepressants in neuropathic pain conditions. However, in animals, mechanical allodynia after peripheral nerve injury was dependent upon tonic activation of descending pathways that facilitate pain transmission, indicating that structures in the mesencephalic reticular formation – possibly the nucleus cuneiformis and the periaqueductal gray – are involved in central sensitization in neuropathic pain (Ossipov et al. 2000). Interestingly, exactly the same brainstem structures were shown to be active in humans with allodynia using advanced functional MRI techniques (Zambreanu et al. 2005). Because in most animal pain models descending facilitation and inhibition are triggered simultaneously, it will be important to elucidate why inhibition predominates in some neuronal pools and facilitation in others.

4.8 *Pharmacological Approaches That Modify Descending Control Systems*

The effectiveness of TCAs in neuropathic pain conditions may account for their broad range of pharmacological actions. These compounds are inhibitors of the reuptake of monoaminergic transmitters. They are believed to potentiate the effects of biogenic amines in central descending pain modulating pathways. In addition, they block voltage-dependent sodium channels and α-adrenergic receptors. Venlafaxine and duloxetine, which block both serotonin and noradrenaline reuptake, are efficacious in DPN. In a comparison of venlafaxine and imipramine in patients with painful polyneuropathy, both antidepressants demonstrated superior pain relief compared with a placebo but did not differ from each other. Selective serotonin reuptake inhibitors have fewer adverse effects and are generally better tolerated than TCAs; however, they have not shown convincing efficacy in neuropathic pain states.

5 Treatment Guidelines in Neuropathic Pain

The number of trials for peripheral neuropathic pain has expanded greatly in the last few years. These have been summarized in several recent meta-analyses that are referred to in the following: McQuay et al. (1995, 1996), Sindrup and Jensen (1999), Dworkin et al. (2003, 2007), Finnerup et al. (2005), Siddall and Middleton (2006), and Baron and Wasner (2006). For central neuropathic pain there are limited data. The treatments discussed above have all been demonstrated to provide statistically significant and clinically meaningful treatment benefits compared with a placebo in multiple randomized controlled trials (Table 3). However, the approval status is not addressed in this review and might differ from country to country. Nonmedical treatments, i.e., interventional procedures, neurostimulation techniques, neurosurgical destructive techniques, psychological therapy, as well as physiotherapy and occupational therapy, are not the focus of this review.

In summary, the recommended medical management of neuropathic pain consists of five main classes of oral medication (serotonin/noradrenaline-modulating antidepressants, sodium-blocker anticonvulsants, calcium-modulator anticonvulsants, tramadol, and opioids) and two categories of topical medications mainly for patients with cutaneous allodynia and hyperalgesia (capsaicin and local anesthetics).

A useful way to compare the efficacy of different treatments is the consultation of systematic reviews to determine the best available drugs (Sindrup and Jensen

Table 3 Pharmacological therapy of neuropathic pain syndromes (oral and dermal)

Compound	Evidence
Antidepressants	
Amitriptyline	PHN ⇑⇑, PNP ⇑⇑, PTN ⇑, STR ⇑
Venlafaxine	PNP ⇑⇑
Duloxetine	PNP ⇑⇑
Anticonvulsants (sodium channel)	
Carbamazepine	PNP ⇑, TGN ⇑⇑
Oxcarbazepine	PNP ⇔
Lamotrigine	HIV ⇑, PNP ⇔, STR ⇑
Anticonvulsants (calcium channel)	
Gabapentin	PHN ⇑⇑, PNP ⇑⇑, HIV ⇑, CRPS ⇑, PHAN ⇑, SCI ⇑, MIX ⇑, CANC ⇑
Pregabalin	PHN ⇑⇑, PNP ⇑⇑, SCI ⇑
Tramadol	PHN ⇑, PNP ⇑⇑
Long-acting strong opioids	
Morphine	PHN ⇑, PHAN ⇑
Oxycodone	PHN ⇑, PNP ⇑⇑
Cannabinoids	MS ⇑⇑, PA ⇔, MIX ⇑
Topical therapy	
Capsaicin cream	PHN ⇑, PNP ⇑, PTN ⇑
Lidocaine patch	PHN ⇑⇑, MIX ⇑

PHN postherpetic neuralgia, *PNP* polyneuropathy (mainly diabetic), *PTN* posttraumatic neuralgia, *STR* poststroke pain, *TGN* trigeminal neuralgia, *HIV* HIV neuropathy, *CRPS* complex regional pain syndrome, *PHAN* phantom pain, *SCI* spinal cord injury, *MIX* mixed neuropathic pain cohort, *CANC* neuropathic cancer pain, *MS* central neuropathic associated with MS, *PA* central neuropathic pain after plexus avulsion
Levels of evidence: ⇑⇑ several randomized controlled trials or meta-analyses,
⇑ at least one randomized controlled trial,
⇔ unclear
This does not reflect the approval status of drugs.

1999, 2000; Dworkin and Schmader 2003). Up to now the findings of more than 110 randomized controlled trials for the medical treatment of neuropathic pain have been published. In this respect the measure: "numbers needed to treat" (NNT) has been a useful measure. NNT is the number of patients needed to be treated with a certain drug to obtain one patient with a defined degree of pain relief. This method permits a comparison between different drugs and diseases and it allows generation of large numbers to provide reliable information about efficacy. Usually the NNT for more than 50% pain relief is used because it is easily understood and seems in many cases to be a relevant clinical effect. With this measure, for most of the available treatment strategies values between 2 and 6 have been calculated. This also clearly indicates, however, that 30–50% of the patients do not acquire clinically relevant pain relief – they are nonresponders.

Since more than one mechanism is at work in most patients, a combination of two or more analgesic agents to cover multiple types of mechanisms will generally produce greater pain relief and fewer side effects. Therefore, in most patients a stepwise process with a successive monotherapy is not appropriate. Early combination therapy of two or three compounds from different classes is the general practical approach. In fact, in a controlled four-period crossover trial, combined gabapentin and morphine achieved better analgesia at lower doses of each drug than did either as a single agent, with constipation, sedation, and dry mouth as the most frequent adverse effects.

Drug-related adverse effects are common in the treatment of neuropathic pain, not only because of the specific medications used, but also because many patients with this condition are older, take other medications, and have comorbid illnesses. Therefore, the drugs of first choice have to be judged on the basis of these data.

There are several exceptions from the above general treatment recommendations that should be emphasized: First, treatment guidelines for trigeminal neuralgia are distinct and include use of carbamazepine and baclofen. Second, the pharmacological therapy may be similar in CRPS, although controlled trials of first-line medications are lacking. However, it is very likely that antiinflammatory strategies in particular in the acute phase might be helpful. Third, chronic neuropathic back pain (i.e., cervical and lumbar radiculopathic pain) is probably the most prevalent pain syndrome to which neuropathic mechanisms contribute. It is likely that a combination of neuropathic, skeletal, and myofascial mechanisms account for this type of pain in many patients.

6 The Future: Diagnostic Tools To Dissect Individual Mechanisms and To Tailor Individual Treatment

Neuropathic pain represents heterogeneous conditions, which can be explained neither by one single cause or disease nor by a specific anatomical lesion, i.e., a disease- and anatomy-based classification is often insufficient. Probably owing to this notion, decades of rather discouraging systematic research on chronic pain therapy have revealed that a disease-based strategy is of no or little help for these patients and their pain.

These observations have raised the question of whether an entirely different strategy, in which pain is analyzed on the basis of underlying mechanisms (Jensen and Baron 2003), could provide an alternative approach for examining and classifying patients, with the ultimate aim of obtaining a better treatment outcome (Woolf et al. 1998; Baron 2006). Our increasing understanding of the mechanisms that underlie chronic pain, together with the discovery of new molecular therapy targets, has strengthened the demand for alternative concepts.

One theoretical possibility to identify pain mechanisms in patients is to assess differences in the somatosensory phenotype as precisely as possible. These specific patterns of signs and symptoms could be compared with the knowledge derived from animal experiments where the association of signs and symptoms and underlying mechanisms has been elucidated. This concept has led to the development of a symptom-oriented diagnostic approach to neuropathic pain conditions that supplements the cause-based classification scheme, which recognizes the fact that neuropathic pains are usually a composite of several pain symptoms. A symptom-oriented approach does not negate the fact that distinct neuropathies present differently clinically, and that some neuropathic disease states may predispose to certain constellations of pain symptoms (e.g., touch-evoked pain in PHN). Thus, a symptom-based approach to painful neuropathies can be useful for dissecting the underlying neural mechanisms, and this knowledge may eventually be harnessed for the development of novel analgesic drugs that differentially target these mechanisms. A very promising but still hypothetical approach is summarized in Table 2.

There are, however, some important caveats with such an approach. Recent clinical experimental studies indicate that it is not appropriate to link one single symptom with exactly one mechanism. It was shown that one specific symptom may be generated by several entire different underlying pathophysiological mechanisms. It became clear that only a specific symptom constellation, a symptom profile, i.e., a combination of negative and positive sensory phenomena, might be able to predict the mechanisms and not just one single symptom. To translate these ideas into the clinical framework of neuropathic pain, the most important approach is to characterize the somatosensory phenotype of the patients as precisely as possible.

For example, the standardized quantitative sensory testing (QST) methods can nicely distinguish between phenotypic subtypes of PHN patients with distinct sensory symptom constellations that are likely correlated with different underlying mechanisms (sensitization type, deafferentation type). Distinct pathophysiological changes in the excitability of peripheral and central neurons are likely involved in pain generation (for details see Fig. 2).

As attractive a subtype-classification based on the nociceptor function and evoked pain types might be, it should be emphasized that not all PHN patients fit exactly into one category or the other. It rather seems to be a continuum. Furthermore, the sensory patterns showed a variation over the time course of PHN. However, by classification of PHN patients due to sensory perception thresholds within the most painful skin area, it is possible to detect the predominant individual sensory profile and the most likely underlying pain-generating mechanism.

Another caveat addressing the predictive value of QST measurements for therapy was recently revealed by two independent studies. It was hypothesized that topically applied lidocaine, which is believed to act on ectopic discharges in nociceptive fibers, would be in particular beneficial for patients with sensitized peripheral nociceptors as compared with patients with a loss of dermal nociceptors. In contrast to the hypothesis, however, skin biopsies, QST, histamine test, as well nerve conduction studies could not identify lidocaine responders in painful neuropathies (Herrmann et al. 2006) and PHN (Wasner et al. 2005). Alternatively, it might be possible that surviving A-fibers in C-nociceptor-deprived skin may express sodium channels, develop ectopic firing, and might therefore be the target for lidocaine.

7 Conclusion

Neuropathic pain due to lesions or disease of the nervous system represents a major neurological challenge, and treatment of patients with neuropathic pain is a difficult. Existing trials only provide general pain relief values for specific causes, which might partially explain the failure to obtain complete pain relief in neuropathic pain conditions. Increased knowledge of pain-generating mechanisms and their translation into symptoms and signs in neuropathic pain patients should allow a dissection of the mechanisms that are at play in each patient. If a systematic clinical examination of the neuropathic pain patient and a precise phenotypic characterization is combined with a selection of drugs acting on those particular mechanisms, it should be possible in the future to design optimal treatments for individual patients.

Acknowledgements This work was supported by the Deutsche Forschungsgemeinschaft (DFG Ba 1921/1-2), the German Ministry of Research and Education within the German Research Network on Neuropathic Pain (BMBF, 01EM01/04), and an unrestricted educational grant from Pfizer (Germany).

References

Alessandri-Haber N, Dina OA, Yeh JJ, Parada CA, Reichling DB, Levine JD (2004) Transient receptor potential vanilloid 4 is essential in chemotherapy-induced neuropathic pain in the rat. J Neurosci 24:4444–4452

Ali Z, Raja SN, Wesselmann U, Fuchs P, Meyer RA, Campbell JN (2000) Intradermal injection of norepinephrine evokes pain in patients with sympathetically maintained pain. Pain 88:161–168

Amir R, Liu CN, Kocsis JD, Devor M (2002) Oscillatory mechanism in primary sensory neurones. Brain 125:421–435

Baron R (2006) Mechanisms of disease: neuropathic pain – a clinical perspective. Nat Clin Pract Neurol 2:95–106

Baron R, Binder A (2004) How neuropathic is sciatica? The mixed pain concept. Orthopade 33:568–575

Baron R, Janig W (2004) Complex regional pain syndromes – how do we escape the diagnostic trap? Lancet 364:1739–1741

Baron R, Wasner G (2006) Prevention and treatment of postherpetic neuralgia. Lancet 367:186–188

Baron R, Baron Y, Disbrow E, Roberts TPL (1999a) Brain processing of capsaicin-induced secondary hyperalgesia: a functional MRI study. Neurology 53:548–557

Baron R, Levine JD, Fields HL (1999b) Causalgia and reflex sympathetic dystrophy: does the sympathetic nervous system contribute to the generation of pain? Muscle Nerve 22:678–695

Baron R, Baron Y, Disbrow E, Roberts TPL (2000) Activation of the somatosensory cortex during Aß-fiber mediated hyperalgesia – a MSI study. Brain Res 871:75–82

Baron R, Schwarz K, Kleinert A, Schattschneider J, Wasner G (2001) Histamine-induced itch converts into pain in neuropathic hyperalgesia. Neuroreport 12:3475–3478

Baron R, Schattschneider J, Binder A, Siebrecht D, Wasner G (2002) Relation between sympathetic vasoconstrictor activity and pain and hyperalgesia in complex regional pain syndromes: a case-control study. Lancet 359:1655–1660

Binder A, Baron R (2007) Sodium channels in neuropathic pain – friend or foe? Nat Clin Pract Neurol 3:179

Binder A, Stengel M, Maag R, Wasner G, Schoch R, Moosig F, Schommer B, Baron R (2007) Pain in oxaliplatin-induced neuropathy – sensitisation in the peripheral and central nociceptive system. Eur J Cancer 43:2658–2663

Campbell JN, Raja SN, Meyer RA, Mackinnon SE (1988) Myelinated afferents signal the hyperalgesia associated with nerve injury. Pain 32:89–94

Catarina MJ, Leffler A, Malmberg AB, Martin WJ, Trafton J, Petersen-Zeitz KR, Koltzenburg M, Basbaum AI, Julius D (2000) Impaired nociception and pain sensation in mice lacking the capsaicin receptor. Science 288:306–313

Choi B, Rowbotham MC (1997) Effect of adrenergic receptor activation on post-herpetic neuralgia pain and sensory disturbances. Pain 69:55–63

Coull JA, Boudreau D, Bachand K, Prescott SA, Nault F, Sik A, De Koninck P, De Koninck Y (2003) Trans-synaptic shift in anion gradient in spinal lamina I neurons as a mechanism of neuropathic pain. Nature 424:938–942

Coull JA, Beggs S, Boudreau D, Boivin D, Tsuda M, Inoue K, Gravel C, Salter MW, De Koninck Y (2005) BDNF from microglia causes the shift in neuronal anion gradient underlying neuropathic pain. Nature 438:1017–1021

Cox JJ, Reimann F, Nicholas AK, Thornton G, Roberts E, Springell K, Karbani G, Jafri H, Mannan J, Raashid Y, Al-Gazali L, Hamamy H, Valente EM, Gorman S, Williams R, McHale DP, Wood JN, Gribble FM, Woods CG (2006) An SCN9A channelopathy causes congenital inability to experience pain. Nature 444:894–898

Dib-Hajj SD, Rush AM, Cummins TR, Hisama FM, Novella S, Tyrrell L, Marshall L, Waxman SG (2005) Gain-of-function mutation in Nav1.7 in familial erythromelalgia induces bursting of sensory neurons. Brain 128:1847–1854

Dworkin RH, Schmader KE (2003) Treatment and prevention of postherpetic neuralgia. Clin Infect Dis 36:877–882

Dworkin RH, Backonja M, Rowbotham MC, Allen RR, Argoff CR, Bennett GJ, Bushnell MC, Farrar JT, Galer BS, Haythornthwaite JA, Hewitt DJ, Loeser JD, Max MB, Saltarelli M, Schmader KE, Stein C, Thompson D, Turk DC, Wallace MS, Watkins LR, Weinstein SM (2003) Advances in neuropathic pain: diagnosis, mechanisms, and treatment recommendations. Arch Neurol 60:1524–1534

Dworkin RH, O'Connor AB, Backonja M, Farrar JT, Finnerup NB, Jensen TS, Kalso EA, Loeser JD, Miaskowski C, Nurmikko TJ, Portenoy RK, Rice AS, Stacey BR, Treede RD, Turk DC, Wallace MS (2007) Pharmacologic management of neuropathic pain: evidence-based recommendations. Pain 132:237–251

Fields HL, Rowbotham M, Baron R (1998) Postherpetic neuralgia: irritable nociceptors and deafferentation. Neurobiol Dis 5:209–227

Finnerup NB, Otto M, McQuay HJ, Jensen TS, Sindrup SH (2005) Algorithm for neuropathic pain treatment: an evidence based proposal. Pain 118:289–305

Flor H, Elbert T, Knecht S, Wienbruch C, Pantev C, Birbaumer N, Larbig W, Taub E (1995) Phantom-limb pain as a perceptual correlate of cortical reorganization following arm amputation. Nature 375:482–484

Freynhagen R, Rolke R, Baron R, Tolle TR, Rutjes AK, Schu S, Treede RD (2007) Pseudoradicular and radicular low-back pain – a disease continuum rather than different entities? Answers from quantitative sensory testing. Pain 135:65–74

Goldberg YP, MacFarlane J, MacDonald ML, Thompson J, Dube MP, Mattice M, Fraser R, Young C, Hossain S, Pape T, Payne B, Radomski C, Donaldson G, Ives E, Cox J, Younghusband HB, Green R, Duff A, Boltshauser E, Grinspan GA, Dimon JH, Sibley BG, Andria G, Toscano E,

Kerdraon J, Bowsher D, Pimstone SN, Samuels ME, Sherrington R, Hayden MR (2007) Loss-of-function mutations in the Nav1.7 gene underlie congenital indifference to pain in multiple human populations. Clin Genet 71:311–319

Gracely RH, Lynch SA, Bennett GJ (1992) Painful neuropathy: altered central processing maintained dynamically by peripheral input. Pain 51:175–194. Erratum (1993) Pain 52: 251–253

Guilbaud G, Benoist JM, Levante A, Gautron M, Willer JC (1992) Primary somatosensory cortex in rats with pain-related behaviours due to a peripheral mononeuropathy after moderate ligation of one sciatic nerve: neuronal responsivity to somatic stimulation. Exp Brain Res 92:227–245

Habler HJ, Janig W, Koltzenburg M (1987) Activation of unmyelinated afferents in chronically lesioned nerves by adrenaline and excitation of sympathetic efferents in the cat. Neurosci Lett 82:35–40

Hains BC, Saab CY, Klein JP, Craner MJ, Waxman SG (2004) Altered sodium channel expression in second-order spinal sensory neurons contributes to pain after peripheral nerve injury. J Neurosci 24:4832–4839

Herrmann DN, Pannoni V, Barbano RL, Pennella-Vaughan J, Dworkin RH (2006) Skin biopsy and quantitative sensory testing do not predict response to lidocaine patch in painful neuropathies. Muscle Nerve 33:42–48

Hong S, Wiley JW (2005) Early painful diabetic neuropathy is associated with differential changes in the expression and function of vanilloid receptor 1. J Biol Chem 280:618–627

Hudson LJ, Bevan S, Wotherspoon G, Gentry C, Fox A, Winter J (2001) VR1 protein expression increases in undamaged DRG neurons after partial nerve injury. Eur J Neurosci 13:2105–2114

Jacobs JM, Macfarlane RM, Cavanagh JB (1976) Vascular leakage in the dorsal root ganglia of the rat, studied with horseradish peroxidase. J Neurol Sci 29:95–107

Janig W, Baron R (2003) Complex regional pain syndrome: mystery explained? Lancet Neurol 2:687–697

Jensen TS, Baron R (2003) Translation of symptoms and signs into mechanisms in neuropathic pain. Pain 102:1–8

Ji RR, Woolf CJ (2001) Neuronal plasticity and signal transduction in nociceptive neurons: implications for the initiation and maintenance of pathological pain. Neurobiol Dis 8:1–10

Kim HK, Schattschneider J, Lee I, Chung K, Baron R, Chung JM (2007) Prolonged maintenance of capsaicin-induced hyperalgesia by brief daily vibration stimuli. Pain 129:93–101

Lai J, Hunter JC, Porreca F (2003) The role of voltage-gated sodium channels in neuropathic pain. Curr Opin Neurobiol 13:291–297

Lehky TJ, Leonard GD, Wilson RH, Grem JL, Floeter MK (2004) Oxaliplatin-induced neurotoxicity: acute hyperexcitability and chronic neuropathy. Muscle Nerve 29:387–392

Leijon G, Boivie J, Johansson I (1989) Central post-stroke pain – neurological symptoms and pain characteristics. Pain 36:13–25

Lindblom U, Verrillo RT (1979) Sensory functions in chronic neuralgia. J Neurol Neurosurg Psychiatr 42:422–435

Luo ZD, Chaplan SR, Higuera ES, Sorkin LS, Stauderman KA, Williams ME, Yaksh TL (2001) Upregulation of dorsal root ganglion (alpha)2(delta) calcium channel subunit and its correlation with allodynia in spinal nerve-injured rats. J Neurosci 21:1868–1875

Ma W, Zhang Y, Bantel C, Eisenach JC (2005) Medium and large injured dorsal root ganglion cells increase TRPV-1, accompanied by increased alpha2C-adrenoceptor co-expression and functional inhibition by clonidine. Pain 113:386–394

Maihofner C, Handwerker HO, Neundorfer B, Birklein F (2004) Cortical reorganization during recovery from complex regional pain syndrome. Neurology 63:693–701

Maihofner C, Forster C, Birklein F, Neundorfer B, Handwerker HO (2005) Brain processing during mechanical hyperalgesia in complex regional pain syndrome: a functional MRI study. Pain 114:93–103

McKemy DD, Neuhausser WM, Julius D (2002) Identification of a cold receptor reveals a general role for TRP channels in thermosensation. Nature 416:52–58

McQuay H, Carroll D, Jadad AR, Wiffen P, Moore A (1995) Anticonvulsant drugs for management of pain: a systematic review. BMJ 311:1047–1052

McQuay HJ, Tramer M, Nye BA, Carroll D, Wiffen PJ, Moore RA (1996) A systematic review of antidepressants in neuropathic pain. Pain 68:217–227

Mogil JS, Miermeister F, Seifert F, Strasburg K, Zimmermann K, Reinold H, Austin JS, Bernardini N, Chesler EJ, Hofmann HA, Hordo C, Messlinger K, Nemmani KV, Rankin AL, Ritchie J, Siegling A, Smith SB, Sotocinal S, Vater A, Lehto SG, Klussmann S, Quirion R, Michaelis M, Devor M, Reeh PW (2005) Variable sensitivity to noxious heat is mediated by differential expression of the CGRP gene. Proc Natl Acad Sci USA 102:12938–12943

Moore KA, Kohno T, Karchewski LA, Scholz J, Baba H, Woolf CJ (2002) Partial peripheral nerve injury promotes a selective loss of GABAergic inhibition in the superficial dorsal horn of the spinal cord. J Neurosci 22:6724–6731

Nystrom B, Hagbarth KE (1981) Microelectrode recordings from transected nerves in amputees with phantom limb pain. Neurosci Lett 27:211–216

Obata K, Katsura H, Mizushima T, Yamanaka H, Kobayashi K, Dai Y, Fukuoka T, Tokunaga A, Tominaga M, Noguchi K (2005) TRPA1 induced in sensory neurons contributes to cold hyperalgesia after inflammation and nerve injury. J Clin Invest 115:2393–2401

Ochoa JL, Yarnitsky D (1993) Mechanical hyperalgesias in neuropathic pain patients: dynamic and static subtypes. Ann Neurol 33:465–472

Omana-Zapata I, Khabbaz MA, Hunter JC, Clarke DE, Bley KR (1997) Tetrodotoxin inhibits neuropathic ectopic activity in neuromas, dorsal root ganglia and dorsal horn neurons. Pain 72:41–49

Orstavik K, Weidner C, Schmidt R, Schmelz M, Hilliges M, Jorum E, Handwerker H, Torebjork E (2003) Pathological C-fibres in patients with a chronic painful condition. Brain 126:567–578

Ossipov MH, Lai J, Malan TP Jr, Porreca F (2000) Spinal and supraspinal mechanisms of neuropathic pain. Ann N Y Acad Sci 909:12–24

Pappagallo M, Oaklander AL, Quatrano-Piacentini AL, Clark MR, Raja SN (2000) Heterogenous patterns of sensory dysfunction in postherpetic neuralgia suggest multiple pathophysiologic mechanisms. Anesthesiology 92:691–698

Patapoutian A, Peier AM, Story GM, Viswanath V (2003) ThermoTRP channels and beyond: mechanisms of temperature sensation. Nat Rev Neurosci 4:529–539

Petersen KL, Fields HL, Brennum J, Sandroni P, Rowbotham MC (2000) Capsaicin evoked pain and allodynia in post-herpetic neuralgia. Pain 88:125–133

Pleger B, Tegenthoff M, Schwenkreis P, Janssen F, Ragert P, Dinse HR, Volker B, Zenz M, Maier C (2004) Mean sustained pain levels are linked to hemispherical side-to-side differences of primary somatosensory cortex in the complex regional pain syndrome I. Exp Brain Res 155:115–119

Pleger B, Tegenthoff M, Ragert P, Forster AF, Dinse HR, Schwenkreis P, Nicolas V, Maier C (2005) Sensorimotor retuning [corrected] in complex regional pain syndrome parallels pain reduction. Ann Neurol 57:425–429

Price DD, Long S, Huitt C (1992) Sensory testing of pathophysiological mechanisms of pain in patients with reflex sympathetic dystrophy. Pain 49:163–173

Price DD, Long S, Wilsey B, Rafii A (1998) Analysis of peak magnitude and duration of analgesia produced by local anesthetics injected into sympathetic ganglia of complex regional pain syndrome patients. Clin J Pain 14:216–226

Raja SN, Abatzis V, Frank SM (1998) Role of a-adrenoceptors in neuroma pain in amputees. Anesthesiology 89:A1083

Raja SN, Haythornthwaite JA, Pappagallo M, Clark MR, Travison TG, Sabeen S, Royall RM, Max MB (2002) Opioids versus antidepressants in postherpetic neuralgia: a randomized, placebo-controlled trial. Neurology 59:1015–1021

Rolke R, Baron R, Maier C, Tolle TR, Treede RD, Beyer A, Binder A, Birbaumer N, Birklein F, Botefur IC, Braune S, Flor H, Huge V, Klug R, Landwehrmeyer GB, Magerl W, Maihofner C, Rolko C, Schaub C, Scherens A, Sprenger T, Valet M, Wasserka B (2006) Quantitative sensory testing in the German Research Network on Neuropathic Pain (DFNS): standardized protocol and reference values. Pain 123:231–43

Rowbotham MC, Fields HL (1996) The relationship of pain, allodynia and thermal sensation in post-herpetic neuralgia. Brain 119:347–354

Rowbotham MC, Yosipovitch G, Connolly MK, Finlay D, Forde G, Fields HL (1996) Cutaneous innervation density in the allodynic form of postherpetic neuralgia. Neurobiol Dis 3:205–214

Sato J, Perl ER (1991) Adrenergic excitation of cutaneous pain receptors induced by peripheral nerve injury. Science 251:1608–1610

Schattschneider J, Scarano M, Binder A, Wasner G, Baron R (2007) Modulation of sensitized C-fibers by adrenergic stimulation in human neuropathic pain. Eur J Pain 12:517–524

Siddall PJ, Middleton JW (2006) A proposed algorithm for the management of pain following spinal cord injury. Spinal Cord 44:67–77

Sindrup SH, Jensen TS (1999) Efficacy of pharmacological treatments of neuropathic pain: an update and effect related to mechanism of drug action. Pain 83:389–400

Sindrup SH, Jensen TS (2000) Pharmacologic treatment of pain in polyneuropathy. Neurology 55:915–920

Tal M, Bennett GJ (1994) Extra-territorial pain in rats with a peripheral mononeuropathy: mechano-hyperalgesia and mechano-allodynia in the territory of an uninjured nerve. Pain 57:375–382

Torebjork E, Wahren L, Wallin G, Hallin R, Koltzenburg M (1995) Noradrenaline-evoked pain in neuralgia. Pain 63:11–20

Treede RD, Jensen TS, Campbell JN, Cruccu G, Dostrovsky JO, Griffin JW, Hansson P, Hughes R, Nurmikko T, Serra J (2007) Neuropathic pain. Redefinition and a grading system for clinical and research purposes. Neurology 70:1630–1635

Vanegas H, Schaible HG (2004) Descending control of persistent pain: inhibitory or facilitatory? Brain Res Brain Res Rev 46:295–309

Wasner G, Schattschneider J, Binder A, Baron R (2004) Topical menthol – a human model for cold pain by activation and sensitization of C nociceptors. Brain 127:1159–1171

Wasner G, Kleinert A, Binder A, Schattschneider J, Baron R (2005) Postherpetic neuralgia: topical lidocaine is effective in nociceptor-deprived skin. J Neurol 252:677–686

Wieseler-Frank J, Maier SF, Watkins LR (2005) Immune-to-brain communication dynamically modulates pain: physiological and pathological consequences. Brain Behav Immun 19:104–111

Willoch F, Schindler F, Wester HJ, Empl M, Straube A, Schwaiger M, Conrad B, Tolle TR (2004) Central poststroke pain and reduced opioid receptor binding within pain processing circuitries: a [11C]diprenorphine PET study. Pain 108:213–220

Wood JN, Boorman JP, Okuse K, Baker MD (2004) Voltage-gated sodium channels and pain pathways. J Neurobiol 61:55–71

Woolf CJ, Bennett GJ, Doherty M, Dubner R, Kidd B, Koltzenburg M, Lipton R, Loeser JD, Payne R, Torebjork E (1998) Towards a mechanism-based classification of pain? Pain 77:227–229

Wu G, Ringkamp M, Hartke TV, Murinson BB, Campbell JN, Griffin JW, Meyer RA (2001) Early onset of spontaneous activity in uninjured C-fiber nociceptors after injury to neighboring nerve fibers. J Neurosci 21:RC140

Xing H, Chen M, Ling J, Tan W, Gu JG (2007) TRPM8 mechanism of cold allodynia after chronic nerve injury. J Neurosci 27:13680–13690

Zambreanu L, Wise RG, Brooks JC, Iannetti GD, Tracey I (2005) A role for the brainstem in central sensitisation in humans. Evidence from functional magnetic resonance imaging. Pain 114:397–407

Visceral Pain: The Neurophysiological Mechanism

Jyoti N. Sengupta

Contents

Abstract The mechanism of visceral pain is still less understood compared with that of somatic pain. This is primarily due to the diverse nature of visceral pain compounded by multiple factors such as sexual dimorphism, psychological stress, genetic trait, and the nature of predisposed disease. Due to multiple contributing factors there is an enormous challenge to develop animal models that ideally mimic the exact disease condition. In spite of that, it is well recognized that visceral hypersensitivity can occur due to (1) sensitization of primary sensory afferents innervating the viscera, (2) hyperexcitability of spinal ascending neurons (central sensitization) receiving synaptic input from the viscera, and (3) dysregulation of descending pathways that modulate spinal nociceptive transmission. Depending on the type of stimulus condition, different neural pathways are involved in chronic pain. In early-life psychological stress such as maternal separation, chronic pain occurs later in life due to dysregulation of the hypothalamic–pituitary–adrenal axis and significant increase in corticotrophin releasing factor (CRF) secretion. In

J.N. Sengupta
Division of Gastroenterology and Hepatology, Medical College of Wisconsin, 8701 Watertown Plank Road, Milwaukee, WI 53051, USA
sengupta@mcw.edu

B.J. Canning and D. Spina (eds.), *Sensory Nerves*,
Handbook of Experimental Pharmacology 194, DOI: 10.1007/978-3-540-79090-7_2,

contrast, in early-life inflammatory conditions such as colitis and cystitis, there is dysregulation of the descending opioidergic system that results excessive pain perception (i.e., visceral hyperalgesia). Functional bowel disorders and chronic pelvic pain represent unexplained pain that is not associated with identifiable organic diseases. Often pain overlaps between two organs and approximately 35% of patients with chronic pelvic pain showed significant improvement when treated for functional bowel disorders. Animal studies have documented that two main components such as (1) dichotomy of primary afferent fibers innervating two pelvic organs and (2) common convergence of two afferent fibers onto a spinal dorsal horn are contributing factors for organ-to-organ pain overlap. With reports emerging about the varieties of peptide molecules involved in the pathological conditions of visceral pain, it is expected that better therapy will be achieved relatively soon to manage chronic visceral pain.

Keywords Visceral pain, Visceral afferents, Spinal cord, Pelvic nerve, Splanchnic nerve, Colon, Urinary bladder, Gender difference, Sensitization

1 Introduction

Pain is inherent with any life that is linked with consciousness. It is a major concern in all aspects of human life. Although with the advances of medical science, the acute pain associated with infection and disease can be correctly diagnosed and treated, many chronic pain syndromes still remain a challenge for clinicians. Suffering from chronic pain can significantly deteriorate a person's quality of life and can often lead to disability. Such chronic pain in the viscera is observed in functional bowel disorders (e.g., noncardiac chest pain, chronic idiopathic dyspepsia, functional abdominal pain, irritable bowel syndrome; IBS) and chronic pelvic pain (e.g., chronic interstitial cystitis, painful bladder syndrome) that are multifaceted problems and still poorly understood. Functional bowel disorders and chronic pelvic pain represent unexplained symptoms that have no readily identifiable infectious, anatomical, or metabolic basis. The pain is diffuse and poorly localized and often it is confused as originating from other visceral organs. One example is noncardiac chest pain, where pain is very similar in nature to that of cardiac angina. About 15–30% of angiograms performed in chest pain patients are normal, and coronary artery disease rarely explains the symptoms (Richter et al. 2000). Among all functional bowel disorders, IBS is the most common and prevalent gastrointestinal (GI) disorder (about 18–20% of the patient population), having symptoms of cramping, abdominal pain, bloating, constipation, and/or diarrhea. Similarly, chronic pelvic pain affects approximately 15% of women. Interstitial cystitis and painful bladder syndrome are the most common. All functional bowel disorder and chronic pelvic pain patients exhibit one common symptom – lower abdominal pain. There are different factors that can cause or modify these disorders, such as persistent mental and social stress, a previous episode of infection or inflammation, genetic background, and early-life adverse events (e.g., abuse, trauma, and painful experience). Presumably in all functional disorders, patients develop excessive pain to painful stimuli (e.g., hyperalgesia) and may also experience pain to a nonpainful stimulus (e.g., allodynia). This was first documented in a very elegant physchophysical study in IBS patients where patients reported pain to nonpainful colonic distension and were compared with healthy subjects (Ritchie 1973). The general notion for visceral hypersensitivity is the presence of sensitization of the neural pathway (includes primary sensory afferents and spinal ascending neurons) involved in the transmission of visceral sensation to the supraspinal level and the dysregulation of descending pathways that modulate spinal signaling (Mayer and Gebhart 1994). Therefore, recent studies in several laboratories have focused on understanding the response characteristics of primary sensory afferents and spinal neurons to visceral stimuli and their sensitization. In addition, several laboratories are evaluating the cortical processing to painful signal by employing positron emission tomography or field magnetic resonance imaging techniques, which is critical in understanding the ultimate processing mechanism in sensing pain.

Considering the vastness of the subject, this chapter will be restricted to our current knowledge regarding different animal models for evaluating visceral pain, the contribution of different types of visceral sensory afferents, sensitization, and cross-sensitization of visceral afferents in pathological conditions and pharmacological modulation of visceral pain. The chapter will focus only on visceral pain originating from the abdominal viscera and spinal processing will only be mentioned in the context of the sensory afferent's projection and pain modulation.

2 Behavioral Studies for Visceral Pain in Laboratory Animals

Considering the diverse nature of the disease, it is extremely difficult to design a model of visceral pain in laboratory animals that can exactly mimic all the characteristics of functional visceral pain. The majority of animal models of visceral hyperalgesia have been developed in rats and mice. Pain can be assessed by distending the hollow viscera and recording the somatic muscle reflex (visual observation of abdominal contraction or EMG recordings from the abdominal musculature) or autonomic responses (change in systemic blood pressure and heart rate). These methods have been employed to assess visceral pain from the stomach (Ozaki et al. 2002), colon (Ness and Gebhart 1988, 1990), gall bladder (Cervero 1982), ureter (Olivar and Laird 1999; Giamberardino et al. 1995), urinary bladder (Castroman and Ness 2001; Ness et al. 2001; Cruz and Downie 2006; DeBerry et al. 2007; Su et al. 2008), and uterus (Berkley et al. 1995). To produce hyperalgesia, the viscera are either inflamed with chemicals or the animals are subjected to stress in early life.

2.1 *Inflammatory Model*

The most commonly used inflammatory models are produced by injecting inflammatory agents into the viscera [e.g., 2,4,6-trinitrobenzene sulfonic acid (TNBS) or zymosan induced colitis, acid-infused esophagitis, cyclophosphamide, or zymosan-induced cystitis]. Although in a strict sense, these inflammatory models cannot be considered as true models for nonpathological functional visceral pain, hyperalgesia manifested by the animals may closely resemble the nature of pain observed in patients.

Instillation of haptens such as TNBS, dinitrobenzene sulfonic acid, or dichlorobenzene sulfonic acid into the colon produces ulcerative colitis-like symptoms in rats (Morris et al. 1989; Rachmilewitz et al. 1989; Elson et al. 1995; Wallace et al. 1995). The inflammation peaks in 4-5 days following the injection and persists for about 1 month (Miampamba and Sharkey 1998). Rats exhibit significant hyperalgesia to colon distension after TNBS-induced inflammation (Morteau et al. 1994a; Fargeas et al. 1995; Sengupta et al. 1999; Friedrich and Gebhart 2000, 2003; Diop et al. 2002; Delafoy et al. 2003; Lamb et al. 2006; Miranda et al. 2007). It has recently been shown that about 24% of the rats treated with TNBS exhibit visceral hyperalgesia for up to 16 weeks following complete remission of the inflammation (Zhou et al. 2008). It appears that these rats behave very similarly to the subset of patients having postinfectious IBS, where pain persists despite the resolution of inflammation. Like TNBS, zymosan, an insoluble carbohydrate from the yeast cell wall, has also been used to induce colon inflammation (Coutinho et al. 1996, 2000; Traub et al. 1999; Jones et al. 2007). However, the severity of inflammation is much less compared with that caused by TNBS and generally does not produce mucosal ulceration.

Urinary bladder inflammation is commonly induced by intravesicular injection of 0.2% acetic acid (Cruz and Downie 2006), zymosan (Randich et al. 2006a, b; DeBerry et al. 2007), or acrolein (Bjorling et al. 2007). Earlier studies used intraperitoneal injection of cyclophosphamide, an antitumoral agent, to produce bladder inflammation (Boucher et al. 2000) and visceral pain. Although the drug produces selective cystitis via its metabolite, acrolein, in the bladder, it has a severe toxic effect in other organs that can complicate the evaluation of bladder pain.

2.2 *Neonatal Maternal-Separation-Induced Stress Model*

The early neonatal period is a critical time for the development of the nociceptive neural pathways, which require use-dependent activity for normal development. However, abnormal stimuli such as stress, sustained pain, or inflammation in the neonatal period may adversely affect the development and subsequently lead to lower thresholds for pain in later life (Anand 1998; Anand et al. 1999; Lidow et al. 2001; Pattinson and Fitzerald 2004; Fitzerald 2005). The objective of developing the neonatal maternal-separation (MS)-induced stress model was to evaluate the effects of stress early in life on visceral sensitivity in the absence of visceral inflammation. The model possibly mimics the subset of IBS patient having a history of traumatic experiences, including physical, sexual, and emotional abuse and a life-threatening situation in early life (Chitkara et al. 2008). In rats, the neonatal period from postnatal day 2 (P2) to postnatal day 14 (P14) is extremely critical for neurological development. There is a large body of literature suggesting that neonatal MS leads to dysregulation of the hypothalamic–pituitary–adrenal axis resulting in long-term changes in neuroendocrine and neuropeptide secretion (Liu et al. 1997; Caldji et al. 1998; Plotsky et al. 2005; Barreau et al. 2004a, b, 2007; Chung et al. 2007a, b; Ren et al. 2007). Plotsky et al. (2005) have demonstrated that brief (15 min) or prolong (180 min) MS of rat pups at P2 to P14 results in significant elevation of corticotrophin-releasing factor (CRF) messenger RNA (mRNA) and the CRF1 receptor immunoreactivity in the paraventricular nucleus, amygdala, and locus ceruleus. Subsequent studies have shown that MS for 180 min (MS180) results in visceral hyperalgesia to colon distension (Coutinho et al. 2002). The hyperalgesia in MS180 rats is exacerbated following 1 h of water-avoidance stress, and this can be prevented by preemptive administration of a selective CRF1 antagonist, suggesting that CRF indeed may play a critical role in the development of visceral hyperalgesia (Schewtz et al. 2005). The manifestation of visceral hyperalgesia in MS rats is possibly a global pain hyperresponsiveness and may not be somatotopically restricted. In a recent study, it was shown that orogastric suction for 30–45 s in Long-Evans rats during P2 to P14 results in visceral hyperalgesia to colon distension when tested at their adult age (postnatal day 60) (Smith et al. 2007). This result is similar to that reported by a retrospective clinical study that frequent gastric suction in newly born babies has a potential risk for functional disorders in later life (Anand et al. 2004). An animal study has also shown that pretreatment with CRF1 receptor antagonist 10 min prior to orogastric suction averted the visceral hyperalgesia to colon distension (Smith et al. 2007). It is very likely that the stress in early life induces functional changes in the central neurons affecting the descending modulatory system that may contribute to hyperalgesia. For example, in neonatal MS rats there is significantly higher c-fos expression in the cingulate cortex and superficial (I and II) and deeper (V–VI) laminae of the spinal cord to colon distension compared with c-fos expression in naïve non-handled rats (Chung et al. 2007a; Ren et al. 2007). The notion that early-life stress or a noxious stimulus affects the descending modulatory system is also evident in recent behavioral studies where naloxone, a nonselective opioid antagonist, failed to facilitate the visceromotor response (VMR) to colonic distension in MS compared with naïve non-MS rats (Coutinho et al. 2002; DeBerry et al. 2007).

Although the initial concept was that MS-induced stress triggers central sensitization leading to visceral hyperalgesia, later studies showed that stress also affects the immune system of the viscera and subsequent visceral inflammation. It is now well established that mast cells play a critical role in stressed-induced gut inflammation (Barreau et al. 2007). In rats, MS enhances mast cell density and degranulation in the GI tract, resulting in disruption of the mucosal barrier and luminal bacterial translocation into the tissue (Barreau et al. 2004a, 2007; Gareau et al. 2006). Recent studies indicate that peripheral CRF triggers mast cell degranulation via the activation of CRF1 receptors of the cell, leading to the release of serotonin (5-HT), nerve growth factor (NGF), proteases, and proinflammatory cytokines in the gut to trigger the inflammation. NGF released from mast cells possibly enhances tissue permeability and excitation of sensory neurons to produce visceral hypersensitivity, since anti-NGF antibody treatment abolishes these effects (Barreau et al. 2004a, 2007).

2.3 Neonatal Noxious-Stimulus-Induced Visceral Hyperalgesia Model

Population-based studies have demonstrated that approximately 8% of children experience functional recurrent abdominal pain and about 18–61% of these children continue to report abdominal pain or IBS-like symptoms in their adulthood (Chitkara et al. 2005). Similar to MS-induced stress, a neonatal noxious stimulus can lead to visceral hyperalgesia later in life. Recent studies have shown that visceral or somatic noxious stimulation in the early stage of life (P2–P28) can result in chronic hyperalgesia in rats. In all of these studies, the hyperalgesia was present in the absence of persistent inflammation (Al-Chaer et al. 2000; Miranda et al. 2006; Randich et al. 2006a, b; DeBerry et al. 2007). Repetitive noxious colon distension (60 mmHg, two distensions 30 min apart) during postnatal day 8–21 or repetitive instillation of mustard oil (0.2 ml of a 5% solution) results in visceral allodynia in adulthood. In addition, the lumbosacral spinal neurons and colonic afferents in adult rats were shown to be highly sensitized to colon distension and somatic stimuli compared with those of saline-treated pups (Al-Chaer et al. 2000; Lin and Al-Chaer 2003). It is possible that the spinal neuron sensitization observed in Al-Chaer's study is contributed by sensitization of primary sensory neurons. Interestingly, if the same stimuli are given at a later stage in life (postnatal day 21 or 45), animals do not develop visceral hypersensitivity (Al-Chaer et al. 2000).

Randich et al. (2006a, b) have shown that cystitis induced in early life by intravesicle injection of zymosan (1%) during postnatal days 14–16 in female rats results in visceral hyperalgesia to bladder distension. These rats exhibited higher micturition frequency (i.e., bladder hyperreflexia) as adults and when these rats were rechallenged with zymosan they exhibited significantly higher response to bladder distension and augmented inflammatory response compared with neonatally saline-injected rats. Following a similar experimental protocol, we have observed that neonatally zymosan-treated rats also exhibit visceral hyperalgesia to colon distension in later life (A. Miranda and J.N. Sengupta, unpublished observation). Although a similar finding has been reported in adult rats where cyclophosphamide-induced cystitis exhibits hyperalgesia to colon distension, it is not known whether the effect is long term (Bielefeldt et al. 2006). Such overlap of sensitization may suggest two possible mechanisms: (1) sensitization of dichotomized (i.e., peripheral axon collaterals) primary sensory neurons innervating two visceral organs (see Fig. 1a; Malykhina et al. 2006; Christianson et al. 2007) and/or (2) sensitization of spinal horn neurons having synaptic input from two organs (i.e., viscerovisceral convergence, see Fig. 1b; McMahon and Morrison 1982; Qin et al. 2004). This is discussed in more detail in Sect. 3.3.

Manifestation of hyperalgesia to colon distension is not only observed after noxious stimulation of the bladder, but also occurs following a noxious stimulus to

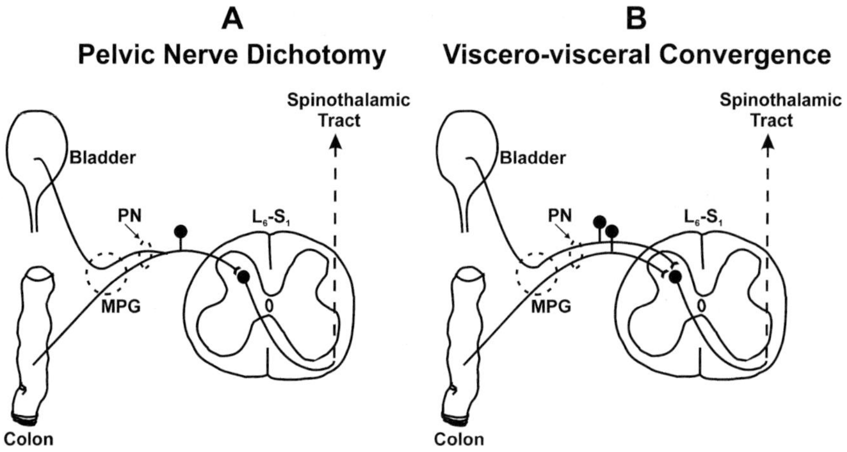

Fig. 1 Illustrates the pelvic nerve dichotomy (**A**) and viscero-visceral convergence of colon and bladder afferent fibers on to spinal dorsal horn neuron (**B**). **A:** Although the primary sensory neurons are pseudounipolar cells, retrograde labeling of bladder and colon shows colabeling of dorsal root ganglion (DRG) soma in the lumbosacral spinal cord, suggesting that there are two axon collaterals innervating two pelvic structures. Therefore, sensitization of a spinal neuron by inflammation of one organ may influence the sensitivity of the noninflamed organ innervated by the axon collateral. **B:** Common convergence of two primary sensory afferents from two organs a spinal dorsal neuron is another neural pathway which can exhibit cross-organ sensitization. It has been documented that a small proportion of colorectal distension-sensitive neurons are also sensitive to urinary bladder distension and most of these neurons are in the deeper laminae of the spinal cord.

the somatic referral site in neonatal rats (Miranda et al. 2006). This phenomenon is due to somatovisceral convergence in the spinal cord and the sensitization occurs at the spinal level, since an ipsilateral noxious stimulus to the hind limb results in contralateral mechanical hyperalgesia. However, there is a distinct difference between rats that received a noxious somatic stimulus in adulthood and rats that received a similar stimulus in their early postnatal (P4–14) life. In adult rats, repetitive low-pH saline injection in the gastrocnemius muscle significantly augments the VMR to colon distension that persists about 2 weeks (Miranda et al. 2004, 2006). In contrast, the adult rats that received low-pH saline injection during postnatal days 8–12 exhibited visceral hyperalgesia lasting up to 5 weeks (Miranda et al. 2006). Although the resultant effect is the same for neonatal stress and a neonatal noxious stimulus, it may or may not share the same neural pathways, neurotransmitters, and neuroendocrine systems. In addition, there could be differential cognitive processing in the brain for different experiences, which is still poorly understood.

3 Contribution of Sensory Afferents in Visceral Pain

3.1 Anatomical Distribution of Visceral Afferents

We have come a long way in our understanding of the existence and contribution of visceral sensory afferents in regards to visceral sensation. Historically, there was a misconception that the visceral organs did not receive any sensory innervation and therefore could not perceive any sensation when the viscera were cut, pinched, or pricked (Von Haller 1755; Lennander 1901). Later, the sensory innervation was recognized, but a notion was formed that visceral dysfunction could only lead to somatic pain since, clinically, muscle tenderness and pain was evident during visceral dysfunction (Mackenzie 1893). It took many years to understand that true visceral pain did exist and that somatic tenderness observed during visceral dysfunction was due to convergence of visceral and somatic sensory afferents in the spinal cord, a phenomenon commonly known as "referred pain" (Bloomfield and Polland 1931; Lewis and Kellgren 1939; Ruch 1946, 1961; Doran 1967).

The majority of thoracic and abdominal visceral organs, except the pancreas, are dually innervated by parasympathetic (craniosacral) and sympathetic (thoracolumbar) outflows. Thoracic viscera and upper abdominal viscera are primarily innervated by the vagus (cranial nerve X) and spinal thoracolumbar outflows. The lower abdominal viscera, including the small and the large intestine and the urogenital organs, are innervated by thoracolumbar (i.e., lumbar splanchnic nerve, LSN, and hypogastric nerve, HGN) and sacral (i.e., pelvic nerve, PN) outflows. For a detailed description of the anatomical organization of visceral afferents, see Jänig and McLachlan (1987) and Sengupta and Gebhart (1994c,1998). The primary sensory afferents are pseudounipolar cells having central and peripheral axonal processes. The peripheral process innervating the visceral organ may have specialized end-organ-like pacinian corpuscles or intraganglionic laminar endings or free nerve endings with multiple parallel branches known as "intramuscular array fiber" (Berthoud et al. 1997; Fox et al. 2000; Phillips and Powley 2000; Zagorodnyuk et al. 2000, 2001, 2003, 2005; Lynn et al. 2003, 2005). The central processes enter the spinal cord via the dorsal root and project primarily to superficial lamina I and deeper laminae V–VII (Cervero 1983; Cervero and Tattersall 1986).

3.2 Response Characteristics of Visceral Afferents

Sensory afferents innervating the visceral organs are not just a homogeneous group of afferents signaling visceral pain to the CNS. It is now a general notion that pain is primarily signaled by spinal afferents, while vagal afferents signal nonpainful sensations such as hunger, satiety, fullness, and nausea. Studies in the esophagus have shown that the response characteristics of vagal afferent fibers to mechanical and chemical stimuli are distinctly different from those of the spinal afferents (for a detailed review, see Sengupta 2006). The vagal afferents may not signal pain, but several human and animal studies have documented that vagal nerve stimulation attenuates somatic and visceral pain. The analgesic effect by vagal activation could be related to its descending inhibitory influence on responses of spinal dorsal horn neurons or via the release of catecholamines from the adrenal medullae (Multon and Schoenen 2005; Sedan et al. 2005; Kirchner et al. 2000; Ness et al. 2000; Jänig et al. 2000; Thurston and Randich 1992; Ren et al. 1991, 1993). Recent studies have also revealed that even the spinal afferents running via the thoracolumbar (LSN) and sacral (PN) pathways are not functionally a homogeneous group of afferents (Brierley et al. 2004, 2005a) and transmit different qualities of signals to the spinal cord (Traub et al. 1992; Wang et al. 2005). In addition, it has been shown that the PN afferents counterbalance the activities of thoracolumbar spinal neurons via the supraspinal descending loop (Wang et al. 2007). Since visceral pain is primarily transmitted via spinal afferents, the following subsections will mainly focus on the functional characteristics of spinal afferents resulting from various types of stimulus.

3.2.1 Visceral Afferents in the Gastrointestinal Tract

In the GI tract, according to the location of the receptive endings in the gut, spinal afferents are classified as mucosal, muscle or tension-sensitive, muscle/mucosal (also known as "tension/mucosal"), serosal, and mesenteric afferents. There is a differential distribution of these afferents in the LSN and PN of mice (Brierley et al. 2004). For example, mesenteric afferents are only identified in the LSN, but not in the PN. Conversely, muscle/mucosal afferents are only found in the PN, but not in the LSN. Although the serosal, muscle, and mucosal afferents are commonly found in both nerves, the population of mucosal (4%) and muscle (10%) afferents in the LSN is much less than the population of those afferents in the PN (23 and 21%, respectively). It is not known whether this differential anatomical distribution of the LSN and the PN holds true in other species.

The majority of mucosal, muscle, muscle/mucosal, serosal, and mesenteric afferents are mechanosensitive, having typical characteristics of response to a mechanical stimulus. Apart from these mechanosensitive afferents, a small group of afferents have been found in the colon mucosa that responded exclusively to chemicals (Lynn et al. 1999). The mucosal mechanosensitive afferents are mostly located in or below the mucosal epithelium. These afferents were previously studied in the vagus nerve, with a major focus on its ability to sense pH and nutrients in the lumen (for review see Mei 1985; Grundy and Scratchard 1989; Sengupta and Gebhart 1994c). Recently, mucosal afferents have been identified and characterized in the LSN and PN afferents (Lynn and Blackshaw 1999; Berthoud et al. 2001; Brierley et al. 2004, 2005a). Under normal conditions, these afferents are either silent or have very low spontaneous firing (< 1 impulse s^{-1}). They exhibit extremely dynamic firing to discrete probing of the mucosal receptive spot, but rarely respond to luminal distension or stretch. It is thought that the mucosal afferents monitor the dynamic events of mechanical positioning of the gut and passage of a bolus through the lumen. The majority of these mucosal mechanosensitive afferents are also chemosensitive and respond to a hyperosmolar solution, acid, bile, 5-HT, ATP, and capsaicin (Lynn and Blackshaw 1999; Berthoud et al. 2001; Brierley et al. 2004, 2005a ; Hicks et al. 2002). Although there is no direct experimental evidence on how spinal mucosal afferent are involved in visceral pain, considering their multimodal character, it can be speculated that these afferents are possibly the first line of the neural pathway that signal pain and discomfort due to a change in the luminal chemical environment, mucosal damage, or inflammation.

The mechanosensitive muscle afferents in the LSN and the PN have been studied extensively in different laboratory animals (Bahns et al. 1987; Blumberg et al. 1983; Clerc and Mei 1983; Haupt et al. 1983; Janig and Koltzenburg 1990, 1991; Sengupta et al. 1990, 1992, 2002; Sengupta and Gebhart 1994a, b; Lynn and Blackshaw 1999; Ozaki and Gebhart 2001; Lynn et al. 2003; Zagorodnyuk et al. 2005). These afferents respond to distension and stretch of the hollow viscera; therefore, they are also known as “distension-sensitive receptors” or “tension receptors.” Typically, muscle afferents demonstrate slow adaptation to tonic distension and the frequency of firing is directly related to tension developed in the smooth muscle. The majority (70–85%) of muscle mechanosensitive afferents have a low threshold for response to luminal distension. However, a small population (15–20%) of afferents exhibit a high threshold (more than 30 mmHg) for response, which could be evidence for their role in visceral nociception (Jänig and Koltzenburg 1990, 1991; Cervero and Jänig 1992; Sengupta et al. 1990, 1992; Sengupta and Gebhart 1994a; Ozaki and Gebhart 2001). Like mucosal afferents, muscle mechanosensitive afferents are also multimodal in character. The effect of the algogenic peptide bradykinin (BK) has been tested in several studies (Haupt et al. 1983; Cervero and Sharkey 1988; Sengupta et al. 1992; Sengupta and Gebhart 1994a; Brierley et al. 2005b). BK excites muscle afferents via the activation of B_2 receptors, since the effect is blocked by the selective B_2 receptor antagonist, HOE140 (Sengupta et al. 1992; Sengupta and Gebhart 1994a; Brierley et al. 2005b). Interestingly, in the opossum esophagus, muscle afferents in the vagus and splanchnic nerves responded differentially to BK (Sengupta et al. 1992). The splanchnic afferents exhibited greater sensitivity to BK compared with those from the vagus nerve. Activation of vagal afferent fibers by BK was primarily associated with strong smooth muscle contraction, which was attenuated after muscle paralysis. In contrast, the effect of BK on splanchnic afferent fibers was found to be a result of direct action on the nerve endings, since the excitation resulting from exposure to BK was unaffected after paralysis of the smooth muscle (Sengupta et al. 1992). Similar findings were also reported in other areas of the GI tract (Haupt et al. 1983; Cervero and Sharkey 1988; Sengupta and Gebhart 1994a). Studies have also shown that spinal afferents are also sensitive to hot and cold temperatures (Zamiyatina 1954; Su and Gebhart 1998; Ozaki and Gebhart 2001); however, the exact mechanism of the thermosensitivity of these afferents is still not known. It is very likely that the hot and cold sensations are mediated via the activation of TRPV1-

2 and TRPM8 channels, respectively. The existence of muscle/mucosal (tension/mucosal) afferents is a relatively new finding in in vitro studies (Page and Blackshaw 1998; Lynn et al. 1999; Brierley et al. 2004, 2005a). The morphological structure of this small subset of afferents is not known. However, from the typical response to muscle tension and mucosal probing, it can be speculated that these afferents have axonal collaterals innervating the muscle layers and mucosa. Alternatively, these afferents can terminate in the submucosal layer and respond to distension and mucosal probing (Paintal 1954). The exact functional role of these afferents has not been suggested, but it is possible that sensitization of the mucosal endings by luminal toxin or chemicals may cross-sensitize the muscular endings, resulting in sensitization of response to distension.

The serosal layer of the GI tract and its adjacent mesentery are innervated by C- and Aδ-afferents. These afferents are commonly found in both the LSN and the PN. One mechanosensitive serosal afferent often has multiple receptive points along the mesenteric blood vessels and at the branching points of the capillary blood vessels supplying the serosal surface (Bessou and Perl 1966; Morrison 1973; Ranieri et al. 1973; Crousillat and Ranieri 1980; Blumberg et al. 1983; Floyd and Morrison 1974; Floyd et al. 1976; Lew and Longhurst 1986; Longhurst and Dittman 1987; Longhurst et al. 1984; Berthoud et al. 2001; Brierley et al. 2004, 2005a, b; Haupt et al. 1983). The majority of serosal afferents have spontaneous firing that does not correlate with movement of the bowel or with changes in intraluminal pressure. Since their receptive fields are close to blood vessels, it can be speculated that serosal afferents possibly sense the serosal blood flow by mechanical sensing of the capillary diameter (Gammon and Bronk 1935). These afferents may also signal an ischemic state of the gut, since occlusion of the descending aorta or mesenteric artery excites these afferents (Sheehan 1932; Haupt et al. 1983; Longhurst and Dittman 1987). Excessive distension due to obstruction may cause blanching of the viscera and excitation of the serosal afferents to signal pain. Serosal mechanosensitive afferents are highly sensitive to several endogenously released substances, such BK, substance P (SP), and 5-HT (Cervero and Sharkey 1988; Haupt et al. 1983; Lew and Longhurst 1986; Longhurst and Dittman 1987; Longhurst et al. 1984). Approximately 65% of serosal mechanosensitive afferents that are sensitive to ischemia are also simulated by BK and prostanoids. It is very likely that the excitation of the serosal afferents during ischemia is due to the release of prostanoids, since treatment with the cyclooxygenase inhibitors aspirin and indomethacin prior to ischemia attenuates excitation (Longhurst et al. 1991).

3.2.2 Visceral Afferents in the Urinary Tract

Under the normal physiological condition, the main function of the urinary bladder is to store and periodically empty (i.e., micturition) urine. This is a reflex process coordinated by three sets of nerves that innervate the lower urinary tract; the PN, the HGN branch of the LSN, and the pudendal nerve (sacral somatic nerves mostly control the external urethral sphincter). There are a large numbers of sensations associated with the process of storage and micturition that range from fullness to urgency, pubic discomfort, and pain. These sensations are transmitted to the CNS via LSN and PN afferents. In the rat, retrograde tracer transport studies have revealed that the LSN bladder afferents enter the spinal cord via L1 and L2 dorsal roots, while PN afferents enter via the L6 and S1 roots (Applebaum et al. 1980; Vera and Nadelhaft 1990, 1992; Nadelhaft and Vera 1991; Pascual et al. 1989, 1993). However, in the cat, LSN afferents run via L2 to L5 dorsal roots, while PN afferents run via S1 to S4 dorsal roots (Applebaum et al. 1980). The variation of segmental distribution has also been observed between females and males and between strains of rats. For example, in female Sprague-Dawley rats, 84% of PN afferents enter the spinal cord via the L6 dorsal root (Vera and Nadelhaft 1990), whereas in male Wistar rats bladder afferents run via the S1 dorsal root (Pascual et al. 1989, 1993). The PN appears to be the major pathway for sensation from the lower urinary tract, because morphological studies in different species of animals clearly indicate that the PN carries a much greater number of afferents than the LSN and selective sacral (S3) nerve denervation in human alleviates bladder pain and urgency (Baron et al. 1985a, b; Hulseboch and Coggeshall 1982; Nadelhaft and Booth 1984; Nadelhaft et al. 1983; Jänig and McLachlan 1987; Schnitzlein et al. 1960; Torrens and Hald 1979). The patterns of innervation of PN and LSN afferents have been studied in the cat bladder by using a selective ganglionectomy induced nerve degenerative technique (Uemura et al. 1973, 1974, 1975). According to these studies, the PN afferents are more abundant in the muscle than in the suburothelium and are widely distributed throughout the bladder, including the dome, body, and trigone area of the bladder. In contrast, LSN afferent innervation is more restricted in the dorsal trigone and neck regions and the nerve terminals are predominantly found in the suburothelium. This strategic innervation by the LSN and the PN may discriminate the mode of sensations arising from the bladder. For example, distension of the bladder can induce sensations in the suprapubic and perineal area, including the perineum and penis. The midline suprapubic sensation associated with bladder overdistension is very likely mediated via LSN afferents entering the thoracolumbar spinal cord, because these segments of the spinal cord innervate the suprapubic dermatomes and myotomes (Morrison 1987). Perineal sensations are thought to be mediated via the PN afferents which enter the sacral spinal segments having a dermatomal distribution in the perineal area.

Until recently, most electrophysiology studies characterized the response of bladder afferents in intact animals by employing intravesicle fluid distension or by punctate probing of the serosal surface, which demonstrated the presence of distension and/or stretch-sensitive afferents (Evans 1936; Talaat 1937; Iggo 1955; Floyd et al. 1976, 1977; Winter 1971; Clifton et al. 1976; Bahns et al. 1986; Häbler et al. 1988a, 1990; Jänig and Koltzenburg 1990; Sengupta and Gebhart 1994b; Su et al. 1997a, b; Dmitrieva and McMahon 1996; Shea et al. 2000; Roppolo et al. 2005). Recently, bladder afferents in the LSN and the PN have been characterized by using an in vitro electrophysiology recording technique from isolated bladders of rats, mice, and guinea pigs (Namasivayam et al. 1999; Rong et al. 2002; Zagorodnyuk et al. 2007; Daly et al. 2007; Xu and Gebhart 2008). These studies revealed different classes of afferents, which are quite similar to the types found in the GI tract. Xu and Gebhart (2008) demonstrated four classes of afferents from the LSN and the PN: serosal, muscle, muscle/urothelial, and urothelial. Interestingly, in the LSN, serosal afferents are predominant (67%) and devoid of urothelial afferents, whereas in the PN, muscle afferents are predominant (63%) compared with serosal afferents (14%). The distribution of receptive fields of LSN and PN afferents in mice is very similar to that reported in cats, where LSN receptive fields, irrespective of class of afferents, are mostly located at the base of the bladder and PN afferents are widely distributed throughout the whole organ (Xu and Gebhart 2008). The only difference between cats and mice is that in cats the LSN afferents innervate urothelium, whereas such innervation is absent in mice (Uemura et al. 1973, 1974, 1975; Xu and Gebhart 2008). Species difference is also evident in the guinea pig, where serosal afferents are nonexistent (Zagorodnyuk et al. 2007). The recordings in this study were done from the nerve trunks in close proximity to the bladder and therefore the pathway of the recorded afferents was not known. Unlike colon mechanosensitive afferents in the LSN and the PN of mice that exhibit differential mechanosensitivity (see Sect. 3.2.1; Brierley et al. 2004, 2005a), bladder mechanosensitive afferents in the LSN and the PN of mice do not exhibit any difference in mechanosensitivity (Xu and Gebhart 2008). However, multiunit recordings from HGN and PN afferents have demonstrated that HGN afferents are sensitive to intravesicle KCl, while PN afferents rarely (1/15 units) responded (Moss et al. 1997).

In addition to the four classes of mechanosensitive afferents, there is a subset of afferents that are unresponsive to a noxious mechanical stimulus (Häbler et al. 1990). These afferents, commonly known as “silent nociceptors,” have been identified by electrical stimulation of the PN trunk (Häbler et al. 1990) or by chemical stimulation with α,β-methylene ATP in the isolated bladder (Rong et al. 2002). Interestingly, instillation of irritant substances such as mustard oil or turpentine oil into the bladder sensitizes these afferents to become mechanosensitive. Due to technical limitation and lack of knowledge of adequate natural stimuli, these afferents have not been studied systematically. It is still not known whether these afferents are exclusively chemospecific and how they become mechanosensitive following chemical sensitization. It is generally thought that these afferents participate in pain signaling following tissue inflammation.

In the PN, muscle afferents exhibit ongoing resting firing when the bladder is empty (Evans 1936; Talaat 1937; Sengupta and Gebhart 1994b; Su et al. 1997a, b; Shea et al. 2000). The spontaneous firing of the muscle afferents has also been reported in in vitro experiments from isolated bladder of mice (Rong et al. 2002; Daly et al. 2007). This is in contrast to some studies in the cat where PN afferent fibers did not exhibit spontaneous firing (Bahns et al. 1987; Häbler et al. 1990, 1993; Iggo 1955). The muscle afferents respond to passive distension of the bladder and the majority of them exhibit a linear increasing response to a graded increase in intravesicle pressure (see the example in Fig. 2) (Sengupta and Gebhart 1994b; Shea et al. 2000; Roppolo et al. 2005) or muscular stretch (Zagorodnyuk et al. 2007; Xu and Gebhart 2008). However, some afferent fibers, mostly those innervating the

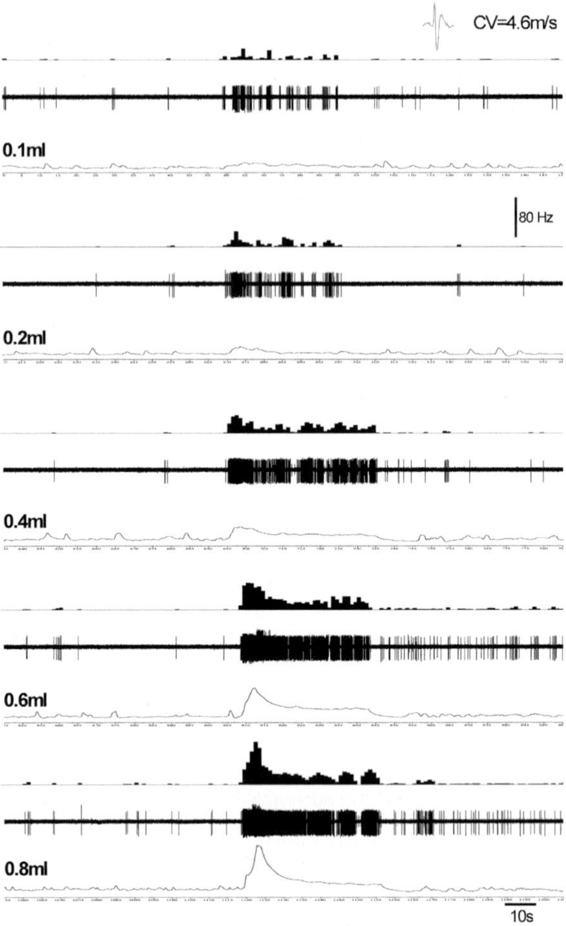

Fig. 2 Illustrates response characteristics of a thinly myelinated (conduction velocity 4.6 ms^{-1}) pelvic nerve afferent fiber to isovolumic distension. The fiber exhibited low ongoing spontaneous firing when the bladder was empty. With increasing volume of distension (0.1–0.8 ml), the firing frequency of the fibers progressively increased and with higher volume (0.6 and 0.8 ml) it developed a post-stimulus increase in spontaneous firing even when the bladder was empty. In each panel, the *top trace* represents the frequency histogram (1s binwidth), the *middle trace* shows nerve action potentials, and the *bottom trace* shows the isovolumic distension of the bladder. (unpublished data of Sengupta JN)

body of the bladder, do not exhibit a linear relationship with increasing intravesicle pressure (Shea et al. 2000; Daly et al. 2007). These fibers exhibit peak firing at lower pressure and reach a plateau or a decline in firing when the intravesicle pressure reaches the maximum. Although it has been reported that bladder afferents in the cat HGN have a high threshold for response to distension (Evans 1936), their existence in the urinary bladder and GI tract was questioned by investigators (Jänig and Morrison 1986; Morrison 1987). Often it was thought that afferents exhibiting a high threshold for response were not adequately stimulated, as their receptive fields were away from the site of the stimulus. It has now been well documented in several studies, including in vitro studies where the stimulus can be applied to the organ more precisely, that there is a large proportion (approximately 75%) of afferents having a low threshold for response and a small proportion (approximately 25%) of fibers having a high threshold for response (Häbler et al. 1990, 1991, 1993; Sengupta and Gebhart 1994b; Shea et al. 2000; Rong et al. 2002; Daly et al. 2007; Xu and Gebhart 2008). In humans, a sensation of bladder fullness generally occurs at an intravesicle pressure of 5–15 mmHg. A sense of urgency to void occurs when the intravesicle pressure reaches 20–25 mmHg and a pressure exceeding 30 mmHg gives rise to a sense of discomfort and suprapubic pain (Morrison 1987). In rats, the majority of low-threshold afferents respond to an intravesicle pressure below 15 mmHg, while high-threshold afferents start to respond at a pressure above 25 mmHg (Fig. 3). Since low-threshold afferents respond to small increments of intraluminal pressure, they exhibit a change in firing rate during the spontaneous contraction of the detrusor muscle, suggesting that they constantly monitor bladder filling to signal the urgency of micturition. On the other hand, high-threshold afferents do not respond until the intravesicle pressure reaches a certain degree, which signals the sense of discomfort and pain (Fig. 4). A recent report indicates

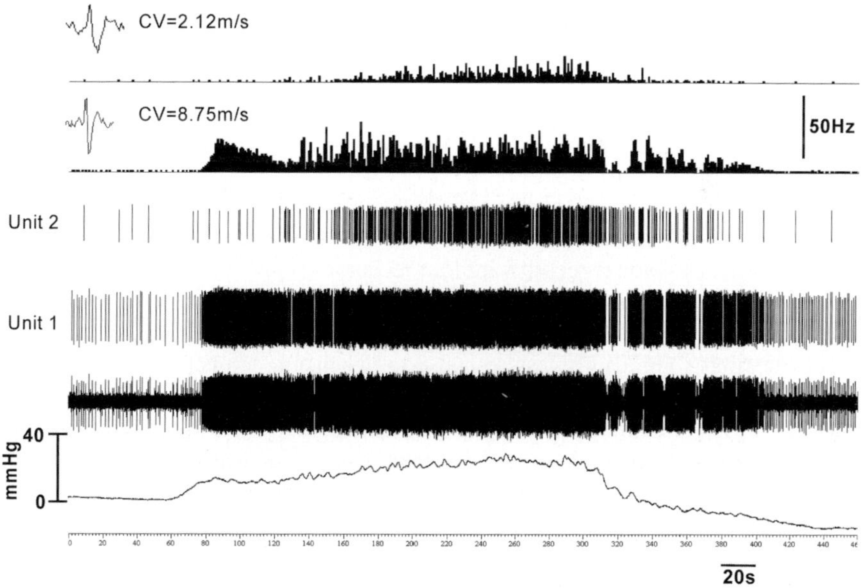

Fig. 3 In rats, majority of low-threshold afferent fibers respond to intravesicle pressure < 15 mmHg, while a small proportion of high-threshold afferent fibers respond at a pressure > 25 mmHg. This figure illustrates examples of two pelvic nerve afferent fibers in a multiunit recording. Unit 1 having conduction velocity 8.75 ms^{-1} exhibited a low threshold for response (approximately 17 mmHg), whereas unit 2 (conduction velocity 2.12 ms^{-1}) began to respond at about 32 mmHg. The low-threshold afferent (unit 1) had relatively higher spontaneous firing compared with the high-threshold afferent (unit 2). (unpublished data of Sengupta JN)

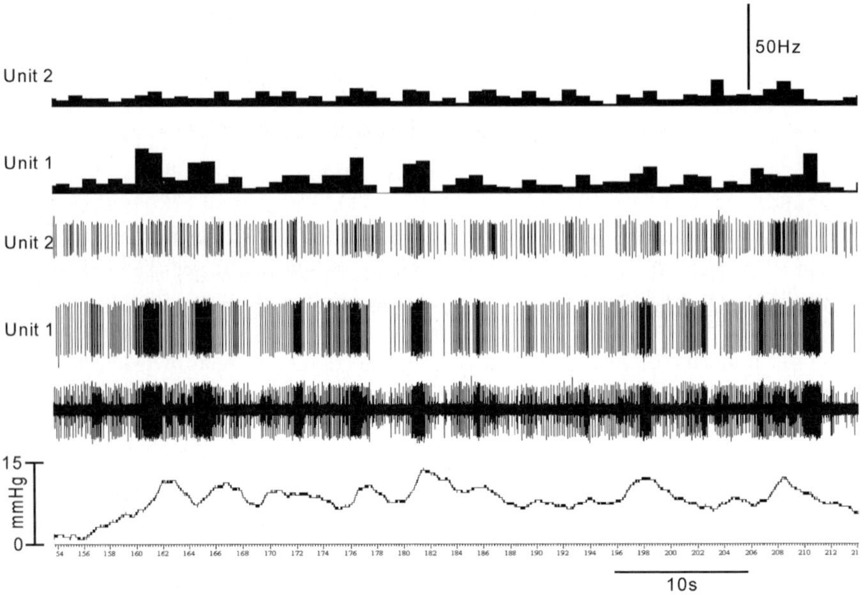

Fig. 4 Illustrates response characteristics of the same two units shown in figure 3 during intravesicle pressure change when the bladder is empty. Low-threshold afferent fiber (unit 1) responds to small increments of intravesicle pressure and exhibits a change in firing rate during the spontaneous contraction of the detrusor muscle. Therefore, these afferents can constantly monitor bladder filling to signal the urgency of micturition. On the other hand, high-threshold afferent fiber (unit 2) does not respond until the intravesicle pressure reaches a certain degree to signal the sense of discomfort and pain. (unpublished data of Sengupta JN)

that the excitability of low-threshold, but not high-threshold, afferents is associated with transient receptor potential vanilloid receptor 1 (TRPV1) (Daly et al. 2007). The mechanotransduction of low-threshold afferents can be attenuated by the TRPV1 antagonist capsazepine in wild-type mice. Similarly, muscle afferents from TRPV$^{-/-}$ mice exhibit significantly less response to distension compared with wild-type littermates. Therefore, it is concluded that TRPV1 channels may play an important role in normal bladder function. The mechanosensitive muscle afferents are also sensitive to several chemical stimuli, including hypertonic NaCl, KCl, 50 mM HCl, capsaicin, BK, 5-HT, and histamine. In addition, endogenous substances such as ATP, NGF, and prostaglandins are released by the bladder afferents, the urothelium, and by inflammatory cells, which leads to excitation and sensitization of response bladder afferents to a mechanical stimulus (Chuang et al. 2001; Rong et al. 2002; Yu and de Groat 2008). It appears that the urothelial layer play a critical role in the bladder sensory mechanism and disruption of the urothelial barrier by protamine sulfate may sensitize responses of mechanosensitive bladder afferents to a mechanical (Fig. 5) and a chemical (Fig. 6) stimulus. The effect of ATP and the $P2X_3$ agonist α,β-methylene ATP has been widely tested on bladder afferents and they are known to excite the bladder afferents and sensitize their response to distension

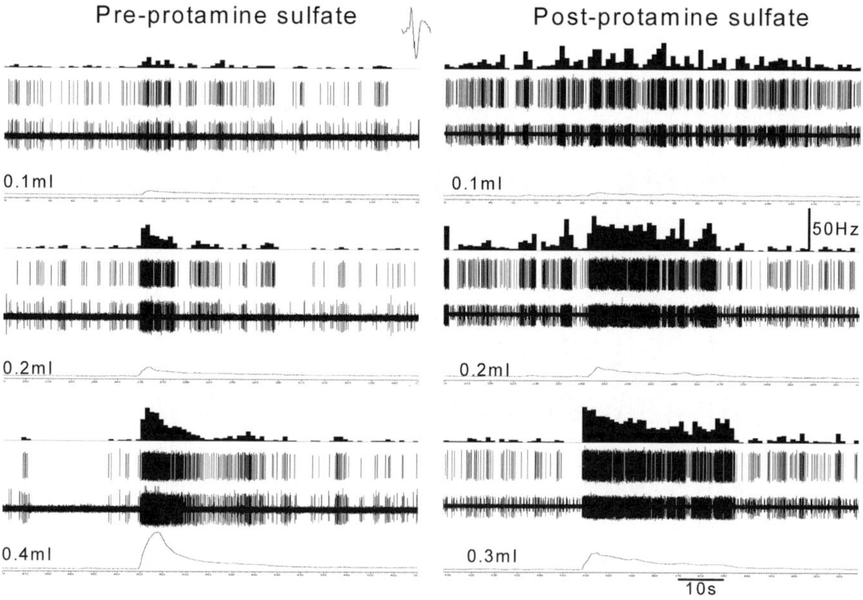

Fig. 5 Instillation of protamine sulfate in to the bladder can sensitize mechanosensitive afferent fiber to urinary bladder distension (UBD). The *left column* illustrates responses of a pelvic nerve afferent fiber to 0.1, 0.2, and 0.4 ml of distension, respectively. Thirty minutes following the instillation of protamine sulfate (1 mgml^{-1}) the fiber exhibited greater response (*right column*) to UBD. Note that the fibers exhibited markedly higher response at lower volume (0.3 ml) of distension

(Namasivayam et al. 1999; Rong et al. 2002; Zagorodnyuk et al. 2007; Yu and de Groat 2008). The sensitization by ATP and α,β-methylene ATP is most likely via the activation of $P2X_3$ receptors, since the selective P2X antagonist trinitrophenyl ATP blocks the effect (Rong et al. 2002).

Clinical studies have shown that rapid filling of the bladder with ice-cold water causes immediate detrusor muscle contraction in paraplegic patients. This is known as the "bladder cooling reflex" (Bors and Blinn 1957). During ice-cold-water infusion, patients report a cold sensation in the urethra or in the suprapubic regions. Patients with painful bladder syndrome report significantly higher pain in the suprapubic area following ice-water instillation compared with the same volume (100 ml) of distension with saline at room temperature, suggesting that cold temperature elicits a painful signal (Mukerji et al. 2006b). Experimental studies in the cat and humans have indicated that cold-saline-induced bladder cooling reflex is not initiated by activation of bladder-distension-sensitive afferents, since the reflex occurs at a volume and pressure that is much less than the threshold intensity to activate bladder afferents. This observation suggests that the cold temperature possibly excites thermospecific afferents (Fall et al. 1990; Lindström and Mazieres 1991; Giersson et al. 1993, 1999). Thermospecific afferents could be located in the urothelium, since immunoreactivity of cold- and menthol-sensitive

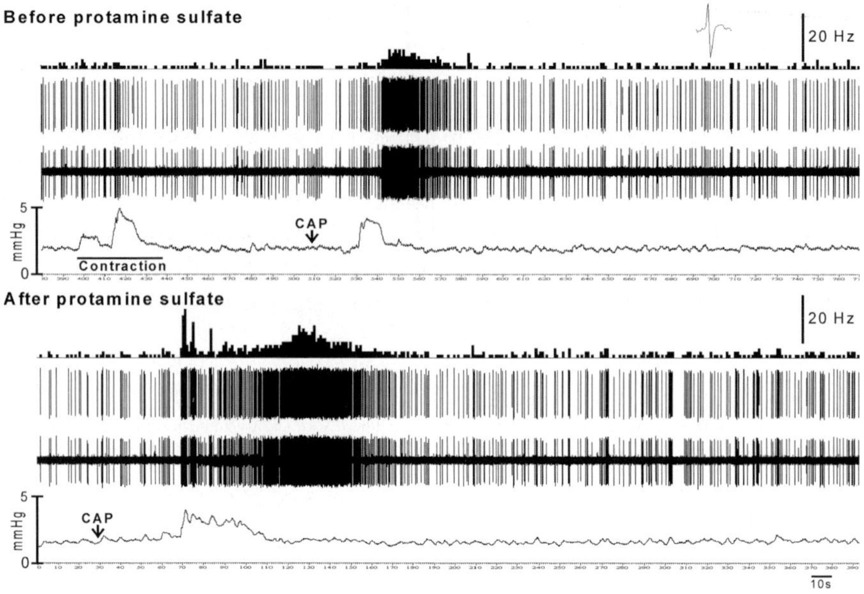

Fig. 6 Sensitization of a bladder afferent fiber to chemical stimulus following protamine sulfate treatment. Before protamine sulfate application, intravesicular injection of capsaicin (10 μl of 1 mgml^{-1}) produced detrusor muscle contraction and an increase in firing of the fiber. However, the firing was not associated with the detrusor muscle contraction, suggesting that capsaicin (CAP) directly stimulated the fiber. Following protamine sulfate treatment, the fiber exhibited markedly greater response to the same dose of CAP. The initial dynamic increase in firing was possibly associated with muscle contraction. However, a prolonged increase in firing was maintained after the intravesicle pressure returned to the baseline. (unpublished data of Sengupta JN)

TRPM8 channels has been detected in nerve fibers scattered in the suburothelium of human bladder tissue (Mukerji et al. 2006a). Alternatively, it is possible that urothelial mechanosensitive afferents are multimodal in character and sensitive to temperature, but this is yet to be documented. A recent study has shown that saline (38°C) containing menthol (0.6 mM) decreases the voiding threshold in guinea pigs and menthol pretreatment significantly enhances cold-saline-induced bladder cooling reflex (Tsukimi et al. 2005). The existence of cold- and menthol-sensitive bladder afferents in the PN of the cat has been previously documented (Jiang et al. 2002). All the afferents responding to cold temperature are unmyelinated C-fibers unresponsive to bladder distension and their response characteristics resemble those of cutaneous cold receptors. However, the exact location of these afferents in the bladder is not known. The notion that cold-sensitive afferents are unmyelinated C-fibers has been supported by an immunohistochemistry study showing that TRPM8 expression is predominantly in small-diameter neurons in the S1 sacral dorsal root ganglion (DRG) of the guinea pig (Tsukimi et al. 2005). The exact functional role of cold-sensitive afferents in the bladder is not known. However, there are indications that these afferents may participate in nociception. For example, the density of TRPM8 immunoreactivity in suburothelium nerve fibers is significantly higher in patients with painful bladder syndrome and idiopathic detrusor overactivity (Mukerji et al. 2006a). The functional role of cold-sensitive afferents under pathological conditions is difficult to understand because it is not known what the endogenous ligand is for the TRPM8 channel.

Pain is the only conscious sensation arising from the ureter. Afferents from the ureter are mostly found in the L2-L3 and S1-S2 DRGs in the guinea pig (Semenenko and Cervero 1992). Interestingly, retrograde injection of a dye in one ureter revealed a large number of labeled cells in the DRGs of the contralateral side, suggesting that pain originating from one ureter can spread bilaterally to a wide referral site. The majority of labeled neurons were small-diameter neurons containing SP or calcitonin gene-related peptide (CGRP) and about 65% of them exhibited colocalization of SP and CGRP. This result is in agreement with a subsequent study in chickens showing that the ureter is primarily innervated by afferents rich in SP and CGRP (Sann et al. 1997). Electrophysiology recordings from the ureter nerve of chickens and guinea pigs have revealed a large proportion (64–90%) of afferents having a high threshold (range 25–40 mmHg) for response to intraluminal distension, with about 10–30% of afferents having a low threshold (range 7–10 mmHg) for response (Hammer et al. 1993; Sann et al. 1997; Sann 1998). Both low- and high-threshold ureter afferents in the guinea pig were sensitive to algogenic substances such as ATP, α,β-methylene ATP, BK, capsaicin, and KCl, with the exception for SP, that selectively excited high-threshold afferents (Rong et al. 2004; Sann 1998; San et al. 1997). Similar to bladder afferents, both high- and low-threshold ureteric afferents exhibit sensitization of response to distension following intraluminal infusion of ATP or α,β-methylene ATP (Rong et al. 2004). Recordings from the thoracolumbar (T12-L1) spinal dorsal horn neurons have documented that all excitatory neurons respond to distending pressures > than 20 mmHg (Laird et al. 1996), thus suggesting that ureter afferents are largely involved in signaling a painful stimulus.

3.2.3 Visceral Afferents in the Female Reproductive Organs

Like the colon, bladder, and ureter, the female internal reproductive organs, including the uterus, cervix, and vaginal canal, are dually innervated by the HGN branch of the LSN and the PN. Retrograde labeling has revealed a topographical organization of innervation of the vagina, cervix, and uterine horns (Berkley et al. 1993). In rats, afferents from the vaginal canal predominantly enter the spinal cord via the lumbosacral (L6-S1) dorsal roots, while the projections from the mid portion of the uterine cervix are equally distributed in lumbosacral (L6-S1) and the first two lumbar (L1-L2) roots. Projections from the uterine horn run through the lumbar (L1-L2) roots. The majority of afferents innervating the reproductive organs are multimodal in character and respond to both mechanical (uterine distension, punctuate probing, stretching) and chemical (BK, KCl, 5-HT, NaCN, and capsaicin) stimuli (Berkley et al. 1988, 1990, 1993; Hong et al. 1993). Similar to colonic afferents of the HGN and PN afferents in mice, the uterine afferents in these two pathways differ in their sensitivity to a mechanical stimulus. PN afferents are more sensitive to mechanical stimulation compared with HGN afferents (Berkley et al. 1993). HGN afferents mostly respond to discrete probing of the surface of the uterine horn and respond only to a high intensity of uterine distension. This response characteristic is very similar to that of LSN serosal afferents in the colon. In contrast, PN afferents respond best to vaginal and cervical distension and often to probing the internal surface of the cervix (Berkley et al. 1990). Unlike colonic afferents in mice, where PN afferents are less sensitive to BK, uterine PN afferents in rats are more sensitive to BK and other chemicals (5-HT and NaCN) than their HGN counterparts. This difference is not thought to be influenced by the estrous cycle (Berkley et al. 1990). Considering the pattern of innervation and response to mechanical and chemical stimuli, it appears that PN and HGN afferents signal different types of sensations from the reproductive organs. The intensity of pain sensation is variable at different stages of the estrous cycle and is primarily influenced by estrogen (Berkley et al. 1995). It has been shown that both the PN and HGN afferents in rats are more sensitive, including an expanded receptive field, in the proestrous stage compared with diestrous/metestrous stages (Berkley et al. 1988, 1990; Robbins et al. 1990, 1992).

3.3 Sensitization and Cross-Sensitization of Visceral Afferents

Behavioral studies (see Sect. 2) in laboratory animals indicate that inflammation-induced hyperalgesia requires hyperexcitability of afferents to initiate the central (spinal and supraspinal) sensitization. In several studies, acute sensitization of spinal visceral afferents was achieved following application of irritants (mustard oil, turpentine), algogenic substances (BK, capsaicin, ATP, NGF), an inflammatory cocktail (5-HT, histamine, BK, prostaglandin), and inflammogens (zymosan) (Häbler et al. 1993; Dmitrieva and McMahon 1996; Coutinho et al. 2000; Ozaki and Gebhart 2001; Rong and Burnstock 2004; Rong et al. 2002; Xu and Gebhart 2008; Mitsui et al. 2001; Wynn et al. 2004). It is not known how long the afferent sensitization lasts following chemical application and whether the sensitization is always associated with the tissue inflammation. Another important question is whether a long-term ongoing sensitization of afferents is required to maintain the visceral hyperalgesia. There is a dearth of systematic studies that have addressed these questions and the available results are conflicting and incomplete. Sensitization of afferents and its duration could be variable depending on several factors, including the time required for a particular chemical to produce inflammation, the number of applications of a certain chemical, the duration of inflammation, and the stages of life (neonate or adult) during which the stimulus is applied. For example, single intracolonic application of zymosan in adult Sprague-Dawley rats maximally sensitized low- and high-threshold and mechanically unresponsive afferents to colon distension 30 min after injection, but normal sensitization was achieved within 1 h. However, when the VMR response to colon distension is tested at different time periods (1, 2, 3, 4, 5, 6, and 24 h), rats exhibit progressive hyperalgesia (Coutinho et al. 2000). This result suggests that the hyperalgesia outlasts the sensitization of PN afferents and sustained sensitization of afferents is not required to maintain the hyperalgesia. This should be regarded as acute hyperalgesia, since zymosan-induced visceral hyperalgesia generally normalizes by 48 h (Randich et al. 2006a, b). In dextran sulfate sodium induced small intestinal inflammation, mesenteric afferents exhibit significantly higher responses to 5-HT and capsaicin during acute inflammation and after recovery from the inflammation (21 days), but not to mechanical stimulation (Coldwell et al. 2007). Thus, from these two studies, it appears that depending on the type of chemical and the duration of inflammation, visceral afferents exhibit a differential sensitization to mechanical and chemical stimuli in adult rats. In contrast to these reports in adult rats, afferents in neonatally challenged rats behave completely differently to mechanical stimulation. In neonatal rats (postnatal days 8–12) that received repetitive (three times) colonic irritation with mustard oil or noxious distension, PN afferents exhibited a long-term sensitization of response to colon distension when the rats were tested during adulthood when there is complete absence of inflammation (Lin and Al-Chaer 2003). Therefore, it appears that noxious insult during the neonatal period resulted in a long-term phenotypic change of the colonic afferents. Such long-term sensitization of afferents in neonatally challenged rats could be due to sustained upregulation of several receptor molecules, including TRPV1 and P2X purine receptors in the DRGs (Winston et al. 2007; Xu et al. 2008). This is different from adult rats, where a high expression of TRPV1 and SP in DRGs was associated with tissue inflammation (Miranda et al. 2007; Banerjee et al. 2007). In adult rats, premptive treatment with a selective TRPV1 antagonist prevented the development of colonic inflammation and normalized TRPV1 expression in DRGs and hypersensitivity to colon distension, whereas in nontreated rats hypersensitivity was still observed even though TRPV1 expression following inflammation was no different from that of noninflamed naïve rats (Miranda et al. 2007). This difference in duration of overexpression of TRPV1 in the DRGs between neonatally inflamed and adult-inflamed rats may explain the short- and long-term sensitization of afferents observed in electrophysiology studies (Coutinho et al. 2000; Lin and Al-Chaer 2003; Coldwell et al. 2007). However, more systematic study is needed to establish the fact that neonatal noxious insult produces chronic peripheral sensitization.

There are several clinical reports documenting an overlap between IBS and chronic pelvic pain (Longstreth 1994; Longstreth and Drossman 2002; Talley et al. 2003). Approximately 35% of patients with chronic pelvic pain showed significant improvement when treated for IBS (Williams et al. 2004, 2005). In recent years, it has been documented in rats that there is an organ-to-organ cross-sensitization of pelvic viscera, including colon, bladder, and female reproductive organs, which may contribute to the overlap of lower abdominal pain (Pezzone et al. 2005; Malykhina 2007; Ustinova et al. 2006; Qin et al. 2004, 2005; Winnard et al. 2006). At the peripheral and spinal level, there are two potential pathways involved in such cross-sensitization: (1) axonal dichotomy of visceral sensory afferents (Fig. 1A) and (2) convergence of two visceral afferents from two organs on spinal neurons (Fig. 1B). Injections of two different retrograde tracers in the bladder and colon, respectively, have revealed approximately 7–14% colabeled soma in the lumbosacral and thoracolumbar DRGs, suggesting an axonal dichotomy in the pelvic viscera (Malykhina et al. 2006; Christianson et al. 2007). VMR recordings in anesthetized rats demonstrated that bladder irritation with protamine sulfate and KCl significantly increased the VMR to colon distension. In a similar fashion, TNBS-induced colon inflammation induces bladder hyperreflexia (Pezzone et al. 2005) and sensitized responses of bladder afferents to bladder distension (Ustinova et al. 2006, 2007). It has been suggested that such cross-organ sensitization is due to initiation of axon reflex of dichotomized afferents innervating the urinary bladder to produce neurogenic inflammation and an increase in mast cell density in the bladder (Ustinova et al. 2007; Liang et al. 2007). Another recent study has shown that inflammation of the colon or uterus can produce significant inflammation of the bladder. Interestingly, there is no such cross-organ inflammation between the colon and the uterus, suggesting that the bladder is more vulnerable to cross-organ inflammation (Winnard et al. 2006). This study also documented that following HGN sectioning (with intact PN) there is a significant reduction of bladder inflammation, indicating that the HGN plays a major role in cross-organ sensitization in the pelvic viscera. However, this result does not fit well with retrograde tracing data, which have shown a greater number of colabeled cells in the sacral S1 DRG (20%) compared with lumbar L1 DRG (7%) (Malykhina et al. 2006). The cross-sensitization of response to bladder distension has been observed in lumbosacral spinal neurons following inflammation of the colon (Qin et al. 2005). The sensitization of spinal neurons observed in this study could involve viscerovisceral convergence of afferents from two sensitized organs or synaptic input from dichotomized sensory afferents. In addition to the roles of dichotomized afferents and viscerovisceral convergence in the spinal cord, there could be another potential mechanism that can explain organ-to-organ cross-sensitization. This involves axon collaterals of visceral afferents synapsing on secreto/motor (S/M) neurons at the prevertebral ganglia (Aldskogius et al. 1986; Matthews et al. 1987). If these S/M neurons from the prevertebral ganglia (e.g., major pelvic ganglion) innervate different pelvic viscera, then it will be logical to think that the sensitization of afferents can excite the S/M resulting in altered function of the innervated viscera.

It is well recognized that visceral pain can influence the sensitivity of somatic structures, including the skin and muscle (i.e., viscerosomatic hypersensitivity). For example, IBS patients often experience somatic and cutaneous hyperalgesia, which is thought to be the result of central sensitization (Verne et al. 2001, 2003; Verne and Price 2002; Price et al. 2006). These clinical observations have been confirmed in a recent study of experimental cystitis, where mice exhibited cutaneous thermal hyperalgesia (Bielefeldt et al. 2006). Similar to viscerovisceral hypersensitivity, chronic somatic pain can also influence the sensitivity of the visceral organs. Approximately 64% of patients with somatic pain syndromes such as fibromyalgia have frequent abdominal pain and a large proportion of these patients (30–70%) have IBS-like symptoms (Veale et al. 1991; Sperber et al. 1999; Triadafilopolous et al. 1991; Caldarella et al. 2006). Recent studies have documented that a chronic painful stimulus in the somatic referral site alters visceral sensitivity in rats (Miranda et al. 2004; Bielefeldt et al. 2006; Cameron et al. 2007). Miranda et al. (2004) first documented that somatic pain, in the form of low-pH (4.0) saline injections in the gastrocnemius muscle of rat, results in somatic and colonic hypersensitivity. The somatic hyperalgesia in these rats was also observed on the contralateral hind limb, suggesting that this was a result of central sensitization. In a subsequent electrophysiology study, it was documented that spinal neurons responsive to colon distension exhibit sensitization of response to distension following acute low pH saline injection in the gastrocnemius muscle. The sensitized response of these neurons was unaffected by cervical spinal transection, confirming that the sensitization occurs at the spinal level. Since it was an acute experiment, it could be also secondary to hyperexcited primary sensory afferent input. The study documented that the sensitization was primarily driven by glutamates as *N*-methyl-D-aspartate (NMDA) and α-amino-3-hydroxy-5-methyl-4-isoxazolepropionate (AMPA) antagonists significantly attenuated the sensitization (Peles et al. 2004). These behavioral and electrophysiology studies suggest that colonic hypersensitivity following noxious somatic stimulation is due to somatovisceral convergence in the spinal cord and is unlikely due to axonal dichotomy, since the existence of somatovisceral dichotomized afferents is very rare (Häbler et al. 1988b).

3.4 Pharmacological Modulation of Visceral Afferents and Visceral Pain

Considering the fact that afferent nerve sensitization initiates visceral hypersensitivity, attempts have been made to pharmacologically modulate the excitability of the afferents to alleviate visceral sensitivity. The advantage of targeting visceral afferents with a peripherally restricted drug is to avoid unnecessary CNS complications. Among many target receptors, κ-opioid receptors (KOR), P2X purine receptors, $5\text{-}HT_3$ and $5\text{-}HT_4$ seretonin receptors, NMDA receptors (NMDAr), tachykinin (NK1, NK2, and NK3) receptors, TRPV1, and $GABA_B$ receptors have been documented to have modulating effects on responses of sensory afferents and spinal processing of pain.

3.4.1 κ-Opioid Receptor

Behavioral studies in rats have shown that unlike μ- and δ-opioid receptor agonists, KOR agonists have no effect when injected spinally, but exhibit significant antinociceptive effects to noxious colon distension when injected systemically (Danzebrink and Gebhart 1995; Sengupta et al. 1999). Thus, this suggests that the effect of KOR agonists is either peripherally or supraspinally mediated. In subsequent studies, it was shown that the majority of arylacetamide KOR agonists such as U50,488, U69,488, EMD 61,753, and IC204,488 dose-dependently attenuate the responses of colonic and bladder mechanosensitive PN afferents to noxious distension (Sengupta et al. 1996, 1999; Su et al. 1997a, b). Interestingly, the inhibitory effects of these KOR agonists were not blocked by the selective KOR antagonist nor-binaltorphimine (nor-BNI) or the nonselective antagonist naloxone. Further evaluation revealed that similar to the local anesthetic arylacetamide, KOR agonists attenuate the mechanotransduction of visceral afferents by blocking the tetrodotoxin-sensitive and tetrodotoxin-resistant Na^+ channels of sensory afferents (Joshi et al. 2000, 2003; Su et al. 2002).

3.4.2 P2X Purine Receptors

Among different subtypes of P2X receptors, $P2X_2$ and $P2X_3$ receptors are thought to be involved in mechano- and chemosensory transduction and these two receptors are primarily expressed in small-diameter sensory neurons in DRGs. It is well recognized that ATP and P2X receptors play important roles in bladder pain associated with the inflammation (Burnstock 2002, 2006). Studies in rodents and humans have documented that both $P2X_2$ and $P2X_3$ receptor expression is upregulated in cystitis and possibly contribute to bladder hyperreflexia and pain (Tempest et al. 2004; Nazif et al. 2007; Dang et al. 2008). Exogenous application of ATP and the P2X-selective agonist α,β-methylene ATP sensitizes the responses of afferents to distension. These responses can be attenuated by the nonselective P2X receptor blockers trinitrophenyl ATP and pyridoxal phosphate 6-azophenyl-2′,4′-disulfonic acid (Rong and Burnstock 2004; Rong et al. 2002; Wynn et al. 2003). Therefore, selective antagonists for $P2X_2$ and $P2X_3$ receptors could be useful in the modulation of bladder pain.

3.4.3 5-HT$_3$ and 5-HT$_4$ Seretonin Receptors

The GI tract is the largest source of seretonin (5-HT), located primarily in the enterochromaffin and mast cells. The presence of toxins in the gut triggers the release of 5-HT from these cells, resulting in altered gut motility, nausea, vomiting, and abdominal pain. It is now well recognized from human and animal studies that 5-HT$_3$ and 5-HT$_4$ receptors play critical roles in visceral hypersensitivity in IBS (Gershon and Liu 2007; Spiller 2007; Greenwood-van Meerveld 2007). Behavioral studies in rats have documented that both 5-HT$_3$ antagonists and 5-HT$_4$

agonists have antinociceptive effects resulting from noxious colon distension and this effect is thought to be peripherally mediated (Morteau et al. 1994b; Kozlowski et al. 2000; Greenwood-van Meerveld et al. 2006). Immunohistochemical studies have revealed the existence of 5-HT_3 receptors in LSN and PN afferents, indicating that these receptors are involved in peripheral 5-HT-mediated signaling to the brain. This was confirmed in electrophysiology recordings from the LSN where serosal, muscle, and mucosal afferents responded to 5-HT and a selective 5-HT_3 agonist. The effects of 5-HT and 5-HT_3 agonist were blocked by alosetron, suggesting that the 5-HT effect in GI sensory afferents is mediated via 5-HT_3 receptors (Hicks et al. 2002; Coldwell et al. 2007). These studies showed that 5-HT_3 receptors are not involved in mechanotransduction of LSN afferents, since alosetron did not affect the responses to mechanical stimulation. Therefore, the question arises how 5-HT_3 antagonists produced antinociceptive effects in behavioral studies where mechanical distension was employed to stimulate the colonic mechanosensitive afferents (Morteau et al. 1994b; Kozlowski et al. 2000). It has recently been documented that alosetron significantly attenuates intracolonic glycerol-induced visceral hyperalgesia, but not to colonic distension (Mori et al. 2004). It is possible that intraluminal injection of glycerol produces visceral pain by releasing 5-HT from the enterochromaffin cells to stimulate the sensory afferents and this activation of afferents by 5-HT can be blocked by alosetron. In addition to its peripheral effect to modulate the chemically induced hyperalgesia, it may also be possible that the antinociceptive effect of 5-HT_3 antagonist is partly a central effect. Recent studies have shown that intrathecal injection of alosetron into the lumbosacral spinal cord attenuates VMR to colon distension in sensitized rats (Miranda et al. 2006; Bradesi et al. 2007). The 5-HT_4 agonists are more known for their prokinetic effect in the GI tract by enhancing motility and water and electrolyte secretion. However, in recent years, it has been documented that the 5-HT_4 agonist tegaserod has antinociceptive effects in the viscera (Greenwood-van Meerveld et al. 2006). The effects of 5-HT_4 agonists is possibly peripherally mediated, since the antinociceptive effects were observed only when the agonists were injected systemically (intraperitoneal), but not when they were injected centrally into the ventricular space (Greenwood-van Meerveld et al. 2006). However, recent study in our laboratory indicates that antinociceptive effect of tegaserod is via the activation supraspinal 5-HT4 receptors linked with opioidergic descending inhibitory pathway. Intracerebroventricular (icv) injection of tegaserod produces visceral analgesia, which can be blocked by selective 5-HT4 receptor antagonist GR113808 and non-selective opioid receptor antagonist naloxone. The drug fails to attenuate the mechanotransduction of colonic mechanosensitive afferents. In addition, our immunohistochemistry study indicates that in LSN (T13 and L1 DRGs) and PN (L6 and S1 DRGs) nerves mostly large and medium diameter cells are 5-HT4 positive. None of the isolectin B4 (IB4) positive small diameter cells and very few SP-containing DRG cells are 5-HT4 positive. Therefore, it is very unlikely that 5-HT4 has any role in peripheral nociceptive transmission. On the other hand, we have found that endorphin or enkephalin containing neurons in the rostroventral medulla (RVM) are 5-HT4 positive. We believe that 5-HT4 agonist tegaserod activates opiodergic neurons in the RVM to release endogenous opioids to produce descending inhibition of spinal neurons and that results in visceral analgesia.

3.4.4 *N*-Methyl-D-aspartate Receptor (NMDAr)

Glutamate is the major excitatory neurotransmitter that plays a critical role in the development of visceral hyperalgesia. Animal and human studies have documented that ionotropic glutamate NMDAr antagonists can modulate visceral pain (Olivar and Laird 1999; Zhai and Traub 1999; McRoberts et al. 2001; Castroman and Ness 2002; Gaudreau and Plourde 2004; Ji and Traub 2001; Strigo et al. 2005; Willert et al. 2004, 2007). In the human esophagus, acid-induced secondary hyperalgesia is significantly attenuated by the NMDA channel blocker ketamine (Willert 2004). This drug has been found to be more effective in attenuating visceral pain than somatic pain (Willert 2004, 2007; Strigo et al. 2005). Animal studies have provided substantial evidence that NMDA antagonists modulate visceral pain by attenuating responses of spinal neurons to noxious colon distension (Kohlekar and Gebhart 1994, 1996; Zhai and Traub 1999; Ji and Traub 2001; Traub et al. 2002; Peles et al. 2004). The excitation of central terminals of sensory afferents leads to the release of glutamate to activate the postsynaptic NMDAr and induce spinal neuron sensitization. In addition, glutamate released at the synaptic junction also activates presynaptic NMDAr to regulate the release of SP from the afferent terminals (Marvizon et al. 1997). Although NMDAr are ubiquitously present in the CNS, their presence in spinal visceral afferents has been documented in rats. It has also been shown that colonic inflammation upregulates and phosphorylates the NR1 subunit of the receptor, resulting a functional change (Marvizon et al. 2002; Li et al. 2006). Therefore, other than its effect in the spinal cord, NMDAr antagonist may also attenuate responses of spinal afferents. Olivar and Laird (1999) reported that vasopressor response induced by ureter distension in rats was significantly inhibited by the NMDA channel blockers memantine and ketamine as well as by the NR1 glycine-B site modulator MRZ 2/576. Similarly, memantine attenuated the visceral sensitivity to colon distension when it was injected intravenously, but not intrathecally. Since memantine dose-dependently attenuated the responses of PN afferents to colon distension, the analgesic effect of the drug was thought to be via peripheral NMDAr (McRoberts et al. 2001). Recent studies have documented that the female gonadal hormone estrogen influences the function of NMDAr, which is possibly one of the reasons for the fluctuation of pain sensitivity observed at different phases of the menstrual cycle (Tang et al. 2008; McRoberts et al. 2007). A behavioral study showed that intrathecal injection of an NMDAr antagonist attenuates the VMR response more effectively in overectomized rats compared with overectomized rats supplemented with estradiol, indicating that estradiol modulates the function of the NMDAr channel. In addition, estrogen receptors α and NMDArs coexist in spinal neurons and activation of estrogen receptors α enhances pain signaling by increasing the NR1 subunit expression and phosphorylation of the subunit (Tang et al. 2008). Similarly, in dissociated DRG cells, the average current density of NMDAr was 2.8-fold greater in cells from female rats than in those from male rats. Further, exogenous application of estradiol enhances the current significantly more in female DRGs (55%) than that in male DRGs (19%) (McRoberts et al. 2007). Thus, this suggests that female sex hormones influence the intensity of pain by modulating the function of the receptor molecules, which could be one of the factors accounting for sexual dimorphism in pain sensation.

3.4.5 Tachykinin Receptors: NK1, NK2, and NK3

Three tachykinins SP such as, neurokinin A, and neurokinin B are constitutively present in small-diameter sensory neurons. Although SP is the preferred ligand for NK1, neurokinin A for NK2, and neurokinin B for NK3, all three ligands bind to all three receptors with different affinities. It is well recognized that SP is one of the major neurotransmitters involved in visceral pain and deletion of the NK1 gene in mice significantly affects visceral pain (Laird et al. 2000, 2001a, b). However, regarding the effects of neurokinin receptor antagonists in alleviating visceral pain, reports are conflicting. This is largely due to several factors, including the selection of animal models, lack of selectivity and affinity of the antagonists, bioavailability, and the lack of receptor homology among the species. For the same reasons, many compounds designed for human neurokinin receptors failed to exhibit any analgesic effect in animal studies. Regardless, several animal studies have documented that selective antagonists for all three receptors (NK1, NK2, and NK3) attenuate visceral pain in several animal species, including mice, rats, rabbits, guinea pigs and gerbils (Gardeau and Plourde 2003; Julia et al. 1994, 1999; Laird et al. 2001a, b; Kamp et al. 2001; Fioramonti et al. 2003; Birder et al. 2003; Greenwood-van Meerveld et al. 2003; Bradesi et al. 2003; Okano et al. 2002; Kakol-Palm et al. 2008). Although in many of these studies, the sites of action of the antagonists were not well characterized, presumably most of the antagonists modulate spinal processing by blocking presynaptic and/or postsynaptic neurokinin receptors in the spinal cord. Similarly, there are a few reports of the evaluation of the peripheral effects of these drugs. Two reports have documented the inhibitory effects of NK2 and NK3 receptor antagonists on colonic PN afferents (Julia et al. 1999; Birder et al. 2003).

3.4.6 Transient Receptor Potential Vanilloid 1

The TRPV1 receptor is a ligand-gated, nonselective cation channel sensitive to many natural stimuli, including noxious heat (42–53°C), acidic pH (5.0–6.0), lipid derivatives, anandamide, and H_2S (Caterina et al. 1999; Caterina and Julius 2001;

Olah et al. 2001; Trevisani et al. 2005). Traditionally, it was thought that TRPV1 was associated with somatic thermal hyperalgesia in tissue inflammation (Caterina and Julius 2001); however, recent studies suggest that the TRPV1 channel plays a significant role in visceral hyperalgesia associated with tissue inflammation (Apostolidis et al. 2005; Dinis et al. 2004; Fujino et al. 2004, 2006; Matthews et al. 2004; Schicho et al. 2004; Yiangou et al. 2001). In inflammatory bowel disease and esophagitis, the expression of TRPV1 receptors in the lamina propria markedly increases, suggesting that the channel is closely associated with inflammatory process of the GI tract (Matthews et al. 2004; Yiangou et al. 2001). In immunohistochemical examination of tissues from rectosigmoid biopsies, it has been reported that the TRPV1 immunoreactivity was significantly higher (3.5-fold) in the nerve fibers from IBS patients compared with controls. The high TRPV1 immunoreactivity was associated with significantly high SP immunoreactivity in the nerve fibers, mast cells, and lymphocytes in the tissues in the IBS group. This study also reported that high TRPV1 immunoreactive fibers and tissue mast cells closely correlated with the abdominal pain score in patients. Increased TRPV1 immunoreactive nerve fibers were observed in IBS together with a low-grade inflammatory response (Akbar et al. 2008). Similarly, the expression of TRPV1 significantly increases in the DRGs of rats following exposure of the esophagus and stomach to acid (Schicho et al. 2004; Banerjee et al. 2007). In a rat model of cystitis, TRPV1 plays an important role in bladder hyperreflexia, which can be significantly attenuated by blocking the TRPV1 channels (Dinis et al. 2004). It has been shown that hyperreflexia in cystitis is associated with activation of the TRPV1 channel through inflammation-induced release of anandamide, an endogenous ligand for TRPV1 channels (Dinis et al. 2004). It appears that the TRPV1 channel functions via positive feedback during the inflammatory process and visceral sensitivity. For example, the activation of the channel in sensory neurons leads to neurogenic inflammation by release of SP and CGRP. Once the inflammation of the tissue has set in, inflammatory products, including cycloxygenase derivatives of arachidonic acid and other inflammatory cytokines, activate the channel to further enhance the inflammatory process. As indicated in Sect. 3.2.2, TRPV1 plays an important role in mechanotransduction properties of muscle afferents and for that reason visceral sensitivity to mechanical distension of the colon was found to be significantly reduced in TRPV1 knockout mice (Daly et al. 2007; Jones et al. 2005). Therefore, it is very likely that blocking the TRPV1 channel may reduce visceral pain. This has been confirmed in recent studies documenting that pretreatment or posttreatment of a selective TRPV1 antagonist significantly improves colonic inflammation and attenuates the visceral hypersensitivity (Fujino et al. 2004; Miranda et al. 2007; Winston et al. 2007).

3.4.7 GABA$_B$ Receptor

γ-Aminobutyric acid (GABA), a major inhibitory neurotransmitter, plays an important role in antinociception. The effect is largely mediated by GABA$_B$ receptors, which are ubiquitously present in the brain and spinal cord. Baclofen, a $GABA_B$ receptor agonist, produces antinociception in the rat model of visceral pain (Abelli et al. 1989; Hara et al. 1999). It has been shown that in conscious rats subcutaneous injection of baclofen prevents the behavioral responses of pain produced by instilling xylene into the urinary bladder (Abelli et al. 1989). Similarly, intrathecal injection of baclofen increases the threshold for VMR to colon distension (Hara et al. 1999). The c-fos expression in the lumbosacral spinal cord from intracolonic mustard oil induced inflammation was markedly reduced by intraperitoneal injection of baclofen (Lu and Westlund 2001). The effect was primarily via the activation of presynaptic $GABA_B$ receptors that regulate the release of SP from the afferent terminals in the spinal cord (Barber et al. 1978; Malcangio and Bowery 1996; Marvizon et al. 1999; Riley et al. 2001). Electrophysiology studies have documented that $GABA_B$ receptor agonists modulate responses of vagal mucosal and muscle afferents innervating the esophagus and proximal stomach, suggesting the presence of functional $GABA_B$ receptors at the receptive terminals of the vagal afferent fibers (Page and Blackshaw 1999; Partosoedarso et al. 2001; Smid et al. 2001). The existence of $GABA_B$ receptor and receptor mRNA has been documented in DRGs (Towers et al. 2000). $GABA_B$ receptor mRNA is highly expressed in both small- and large-diameter DRG cells. A recent electrophysiology study showed that baclofen dose-dependently attenuates responses of mechanosensitive PN afferents to noxious colon distension, providing direct evidence that $GABA_B$ receptor agonist can modulate visceral pain by acting at the peripheral site (Sengupta et al. 2002). Since $GABA_B$ receptor agonist other than its antinociceptive effect has multiple undesirable CNS effects, including sedation, tolerance, respiratory depression, and motor deficiency, its therapeutic use for visceral pain could be seriously limited. However, $GABA_B$ is a unique G protein coupled receptor, which requires dimerization of two subunits ($GABA_{B1}$ and $GABA_{B2}$) to form a functional receptor. A number of splice variants of the $GABA_{B1}$ subunit ($GABA_{1a}$, $GABA_{1b}$, $GABA_{1c}$, and $GABA_{1d}$) have been identified in the rat and human, which are differentially expressed in different tissues (Isomoto et al. 1998). For example, the $GABA_{B1}$ subunit is ubiquitously present in the CNS and nonneuronal tissues, whereas the $GABA_{B2}$ subunit is present only in the neurons of the brain and spinal cord (Bolser et al. 1994). Therefore, a peripherally restricted agonist targeting for the $GABA_{B2}$ splice variant may be a useful to modulate the visceral pain.

4 Conclusion

Despite the large number of reports emerging, the mechanism of visceral pain is still less understood than that of somatic pain. This is primarily due to the diverse nature of visceral pain compounded by multiple factors such as sexual dimorphism, psychological stress, genetic trait, and the nature of predisposed disease. Sensitization of primary sensory afferents is an important underlying mechanism for visceral hypersensitivity and hyperalgesia and the duration of sensitization is possibly the determinant of the chronic nature of the pain. In short-term sensitization, excitation of afferent fibers lasting 1–2 h may lead to a widespread increase in cell responsiveness in the CNS owing to enhanced synaptic strength, whereas in long-term sensitization there could be morphological changes of neurons (e.g., sprouting), central synaptic connectivity, expression of receptor molecules, an altered descending modulatory system, and cortical processing. Findings in animal studies have indicated that the mechanism of neonatal stress-induced visceral hyperalgesia could be different from that in adults. Stress and a noxious stimulus early in life permanently alter the hypothalamic–pituitary–adrenal axis, the descending pain modulatory system, and the expression profile of receptor molecules, and these animals exhibit chronic hyperalgesia later in their life. Such a pain mechanism is possibly different from that observed in postinfectious, diarrhea- or constipation-predominant IBS or in painful bladder syndrome. Similarly, sexual dimorphism plays a critical role in differential pain sensation. Considering this diverse mechanism of visceral pain, the treatment strategy and therapeutic intervention will depend on the disease symptoms.

Acknowledgements The author acknowledges the support of NIH (RO1 DK062312-A2) to obtain unpublished data reported in this chapter. The author also acknowledges Adrian Miranda and Bidyut K. Medda for their comments and suggestions.

References

Abelli L, Conte B, Somma V, Maggi CA, Giulaini S, Meli A (1989) A method of studying pain arising from the urinary bladder in conscious, freely-moving rats. J Urol 141:148–151

Akbar A, Yiangou Y, Facer P, Walters JR, Anand P, Ghosh S (2008) Increased capsaicin receptor TRPV1 expressing sensory fibres in irritable bowel syndrome and their correlation with abdominal pain. Gut 57(7):923–929

Al-Chaer ED, Kawasaki M, Pasricha PJ (2000) A new model of chronic visceral hypersensitivity in adult rats induced by colon irritation during postnatal development. Gastroenterology 119:1276–1285

Aldskogius H, Elfvin LG, Forsman CA (1986) Primary sensory afferents in the inferior mesenteric ganglion and related nerves of the guinea pig. An experimental study with anterogradely transported wheat germ agglutinin-horseradish peroxidase conjugate. J Auton Nerv Syst 15:179–190

Anand KJ (1998) Clinical importance of pain and stress in preterm neonates. Biol Neonate 73:1–9

Anand KJ, Coskun V, Thirvikraman KV, Nemeroff CB, Plotsky PM (1999) Long-term behavioral effects of repetitive pain in neonatal rat pups. Physiol Behav 66:627–637

Anand KJ, Runeson B, Jacobson B (2004) Gastric suction at birth associated with long-term risk for functional intestinal disorders in later life. J Pedatr 144:449–454

Apostolidis A, Brady CM, Yiangou Y, Davis J, Fowler CJ, Anand P (2005) Capsaicin receptor TRPV1 in urothelium of neurogenic human bladders and effect of intravesical resiniferatoxin. Urology 65:400–405

Applebaum AE, Vance WH, Coggeshall RE (1980) Segmental localization of sensory cell that innervate the bladder. J Comp Neurol 192:203–209

Bahns E, Ernsberger U, Jänig W, Nelke A (1986) Functional characteristics of lumbar visceral afferent from the urinary bladder and urethra in the cat. Pflügers Arch 407:510–518

Bahns E, Halsband U, Jänig W (1987) Responses of visceral afferents from the lower urinary tract, colon and anus to mechanical stimulation. Pflugers Arch 410:296–303

Banerjee B, Medda BK, Lazarova Z, Bansal N, Shaker R, Sengupta JN (2007) Effect of reflux-induced inflammation on transient receptor potential vanilloid one (TRPV1) expression in primary sensory neurons innervating the oesophagus of rats. Neurogastroenterol Motil 19: 681–691

Barber RP, Vaughn JE, Saito K, McLaughlin BJ, Roberts E (1978) GABAergic terminals are presynaptic to primary afferent terminals in the substantia gelatinosa of the rat spinal cord. Brain Res 141:35–55

Baron R, Jänig W, McLachlan EM (1985a) The afferent and sympathetic components of the lumbar spinal outflow to the colon and pelvic organs in the cat. I. The hypogastric nerve. J Comp Neurol 238:135–146

Baron R, Jänig W, McLachlan EM (1985b) The afferent and sympathetic components of the lumbar spinal outflow to the colon and pelvic organs in the cat. II. The lumbar splanchnic nerves. J Comp Neurol 238:147–157

Barreau F, Cartier C, Ferrier L, Fioramonti J, Bueno L (2004a) Nerve growth factor mediates alterations of colonic sensitivity and mucosal barrier induced by neonatal stress in rats. Gastroenterology 127:524–534

Barreau F, Ferrier L, Fioramonti J, Bueno L (2004b) Neonatal maternal deprivation triggers long term alterations in colonic epithelial barrier and mucosal immunity in rats. Gut 53:501–506

Barreau F, Ferrier L, Fioramonti J, Bueno L (2007) New insight in the etiology and pathophysiology of irritable bowel syndrome: contribution of neonatal stress models. Pediatr Res 62:240–245

Berkley KJ, Robbins A, Sato Y (1988) Afferent fibers supplying the uterus in the rat. J Neurophysiol 59:142–163

Berkley KJ, Hotta H, Robbins A, Sato Y (1990) Functional properties of afferent fibers supplying reproductive and other pelvic organs in pelvic nerve of female rat. J Neurophysiol 63(2): 256–272

Berkley KJ, Robbins A, Sato Y (1993) Functional differences between afferent fibers in the hypogastric and pelvic nerves innervating female reproductive organs in the rat. J Neurophysiol 69:533–544

Berkley KJ, Wood E, Scofield SL, Little M (1995) Behavioral responses to uterine or vaginal distension in the rat. Pain 61:121–31

Berthoud HR, Patterson LM, Neumann F, Neuhuber WL (1997) Distribution and structure of vagal afferent intraganglionic laminar endings (IGLEs) in the rat gastrointestinal tract. Anat Embryol 195:183–1891

Berthoud HR, Lynn PA, Blackshaw LA (2001) Vagal and spinal mechanosensors in the rat stomach and colon have multiple receptive fields. Am J Physiol 280:R1371–R1381

Bessou P, Perl ER (1966) A movement receptor of the small intestine. J Physiol Lond 182:404–426

Bielefeldt K, Lamb K, Gebhart GF (2006) Convergence of sensory pathways in the development of somatic and visceral hypersensitivity. Am J Physiol Gastrointest Liver Physiol 291: G658–G665

Birder LA, Kiss S, de Groat WC, Lecci A, Maggi CA (2003) Effect of nepadutant, a neurokinin 2 tachykinin receptor antagonist, on immediate-early gene expression after trinitrobenzene sulfonic acid-induced colitis in the rat. J Pharmacol Exp Ther 304:272–276

Bjorling DE, Elkahwaji JE, Bushman W, Janda LM, Boldon K, Hopkins WJ, Wang ZY (2007) Acute acrolein-induced cystitis in mice. BJU Int 99:1523–1529

Bloomfield AL, Polland WS (1931) Experimental referred pain from the gastrointestinal tract. Part II. Stomach, duodenum and colon. J Clin Invest 10:453–473

Blumberg H, Haupt P, Jänig W, Kohler W (1983) Encoding of visceral noxious stimuli in the discharge patterns of visceral afferent fibers from the colon. Pflugers Arch 398:33–40

Bolser DC, DeGennaro FC, O'Reilly S, Chapman RW, Kreutner W, Egan RW, Hey JA (1994) Peripheral and central site of action of GABA-B agonists to inhibit the cough reflex in the cat and guineapig. Br J Pharmacol 113:1344–1348

Bors EH, Blinn KA (1957) Spinal reflex activity from the vesical mucosa in paraplegic patients. AMA Arch Neurol Psychiatry 78:339–354

Boucher M, Meen M, Codron JP, Coudore F, Kemeny JL, Eschalier A (2000) Cyclophosphamide-induced cystitis in freely-moving conscious rats: behavioral approach to a new model of visceral pain. J Urol 164:203–208

Bradesi S, Eutamene H, Garcia-Villar R, Fioramonti J, Bueno L (2003) Stress-induced visceral hypersensitivity in female rats is estrogen-dependent and involves tachykinin NK1 receptors. Pain 102:227–234

Bradesi S, Lao L, McLean PG, Winchester WJ, Lee K, Hicks GA, Mayer EA (2007) Dual role of 5-HT3 receptors in a rat model of delayed stress-induced visceral hyperalgesia. Pain 130:56–65

Brierley SM, Jones RCW, Gebhart GF, Blackshaw LA (2004) Splanchnic and pelvic mechanosensory afferents signal different qualities of colonic stimuli in mice. Gastroenterology 127:166–178

Brierley SM, Carter R, Jones W 3rd, Xu L, Robinson DR, Hicks GA, Gebhart GF, Blackshaw LA (2005a) Differential chemosensory function and receptor expression of splanchnic and pelvic colonic afferents in mice. J Physiol 567:267–281

Brierley SM, Jones RC 3rd, Xu L, Gebhart GF, Blackshaw LA (2005b) Activation of splanchnic and pelvic colonic afferents by bradykinin in mice. Neurogastroenterol Motil 17:854–862

Burnstock G (2002) Potential therapeutic targets in the rapidly expanding field of purinergic signalling. Clin Med 2:45–53

Burnstock G (2006) Purinergic P2 receptors as targets for novel analgesics. Pharmacol Ther 110:433–454

Caldarella MP, Giamberardino MA, Sacco F, Affaitati G, Milano A, Lerza R, Balatsinou C, Laterza F, Pierdomenico SD, Cuccurullo F, Neri M (2006) Sensitivity disturbances in patients with irritable bowel syndrome and fibromyalgia. Am J Gastroenterol 101:2782–2789

Caldji C, Tannenbaum B, Sharma S, Francis D, Plotsky PM, Meaney MJ (1998) Maternal care during infancy regulates the development of neural systems mediating the expression of fearfulness in the rat. Proc Natl Acad Sci USA 95:5335–5340

Cameron DM, Brennan TJ, Gebhart GF (2007) Hind paw incision in the rat produces long-lasting colon hypersensitivity. J Pain 9:246–253

Castroman P, Ness TJ (2001) Vigor of visceromotor responses to urinary bladder distension in rats increases with repeated trials and stimulus intensity. Neurosci Lett 306:97–100

Castroman PJ, Ness TJ (2002) Ketamine, an N-methyl-D-aspartate receptor antagonist, inhibits the spinal neuronal responses to distension of the rat urinary bladder. Anesthesiology 96: 1410–1419

Caterina MJ, Julius D (2001) The vanilloid receptor: a molecular gateway to the pain pathway. Ann Rev Neurosci 24:487–517

Caterina MJ, Rosen TA, Tominaga M, Brake AJ, Julius D (1999) A capsaicin-receptor homologue with a high threshold for noxious heat. Nature 398:436–441

Cervero F (1982) Afferent activity evoked by natural stimulation of the biliary system in the ferret. Pain 13:137–151

Cervero F (1983) Somatic and visceral inputs to the thoracic spinal of the cat. J Physiol 337:51–67

Cervero F, Jänig W (1992) Visceral nociceptor: a new world order? Trends Neurosci 15:374–378

Cervero F, Sharkey KA (1988) An electrophysiological and anatomical study of intestinal afferent fibers in the rat. J Physiol Lond 401:381–397

Cervero F, Tattersall JEH (1986) Somatic and visceral sensory integration in the thoracic spinal cord. Prog Brain Res 67:189–205

Chitkara DK, Rawat DJ, Talley NJ (2005) The epidemiology of childhood recurrent abdominal pain in Western countries: a systematic review. Am J Gastrol 100:1868–1875

Chitkara DK, van Tilburg MA, Blois-Martin N, Whitehead WE (2008) Early life risk factors that contribute to irritable bowel syndrome in adults: a systematic review. Am J Gastrol 103:765–774

Christianson JA, Liang R, Ustinova EE, Davis BM, Fraser MO, Pezzone MA (2007) Convergence of bladder and colon sensory innervation occurs at the primary afferent level. Pain 128:235–243

Chuang YC, Fraser MO, Yu Y, Chancellor MB, de Groat WC, Yoshimura N (2001) The role of bladder afferent pathways in bladder hyperactivity induced by the intravesical administration of nerve growth factor. J Urol 165:975–979

Chung EKY, Zhang X, Li Z, Zhang H, Xu HX, Bian ZX (2007a) Neonatal maternal separation enhances central sensitivity to noxious colorectal distension in rat. Brain Res 1153:68–77

Chung EKY, Zhang XJ, Li Z, Xu HX, Sung JJY, Bian ZX (2007b) Visceral hyperalgesia induced by neonatal maternal separation is associated with nerve growth factor-mediated central neural plasticity in rat spinal cord. Neuroscience 149:685–695

Clerc N, Mei N (1983) Thoracic esophageal mechanoreceptor connected with fibers following sympathetic pathways. Brain Res Bull 10:1–7

Clifton GL, Coggeshall RE, Vance WH, Willis WD (1976) Receptive fields of unmyelinated ventral root afferent fibers. J Physiol Lond 256:573–600

Coldwell JR, Phillis BD, Sutherland K, Howarth GS, Blackshaw LA (2007) Increased responsiveness of rat colonic splanchnic afferents to 5-HT after inflammation and recovery. J Physiol 579:203–213

Coutinho SV, Meller ST, Gebhart GF (1996) Intracolonic zymosan produces visceral hyperalgesia in the rat that is mediated by spinal NMDA and non-NMDA receptors. Brain Res 736:7–15

Coutinho SV, Su X, Sengupta JN, Gebhart GF (2000) Role of sensitized pelvic nerve afferents from the inflamed rat colon in the maintenance of visceral hyperalgesia. Prog Brain Res 129:375–387

Coutinho SV, Plotsky PM, Sablad M, Miller JC, Zhou H, Bayati AI, McRoberts JA, Mayer EA (2002) Neonatal maternal separation alters stress-induced responses to viscerosomatic nociceptive stimuli in rat. Am J Physiol 282:G307–G316

Crousillat J, Ranieri F (1980) Mecanorecepteurs splanchniques de la voie biliaire et dedon peritoine. Exp Brain Res 40:146–153

Cruz Y, Downie JW (2006) Abdominal muscle activity during voiding in female rats with normal or irritated bladder. Am J Physiol 290:R1436–R1445

Daly D, Rong W, Chess-Williams R, Chapple C, Grundy D (2007) Bladder afferent sensitivity in wild-type and TRPV1 knockout mice. J Physiol 583:663–674

Dang K, Lamb K, Cohen M, Bielefeldt K, Gebhart GF (2008) Cyclophosphamide-induced bladder inflammation sensitizes and enhances P2X receptor function in rat bladder sensory neurons. J Neurophysiol 99:49–59

Danzebrink RM, Green SA, Gebhart GF (1995) Spinal mu and delta, but not kappa, opioid-receptor agonists attenuate responses to noxious colorectal distension in the rat. Pain 63:39–47

DeBerry J, Ness TJ, Robbins MT, Alan R (2007) Inflammation-induced enhancement of the visceromotor reflex to urinary bladder distension: modulation of endogenous opioids and the effects of early-in-life experience with bladder inflammation. J Pain 8:914–923

Delafoy L, Raymond F, Doherty AM, Eschalier A, Diop L (2003) Role of nerve growth factor in the trinitrobenzene sulfonic acid-induced colonic hypersensitivity. Pain 105:489–497

Dinis P, Charrua A, Avelino A, Yaqoob M, Bevan S, Nagy I, Cruz F (2004) Anandamide-evoked activation of vanilloid receptor 1 contributes to the development of bladder hyperreflexia and nociceptive transmission to spinal dorsal horn neurons in cystitis. J Neurosci 24:11253–11263

Diop L, Raymond F, Fargeau H, Petoux F, Chovet M, Doherty AM (2002) Pregabalin (CI-1008) inhibits the trinitrobenzene sulfonic acid-induced chronic colonic allodynia in the rat. J Pharmacol Exp Ther 302:1013–1022

Dmitrieva N, McMahon SB (1996) Sensitisation of visceral afferents by nerve growth factor in the adult rat. Pain 66:87–97

Doran FSA (1967) The site to which pain is referred from the common bile duct in man and implication for the theory of referred pain. Br J Surg 54:599–606
Elson CO, Sartor BR, Tennyson GS, Riddel RH (1995) Experimental models of inflammatory bowel disease. Gastroenterology 109:1344–1367
Evans JP (1936) Observations on the nerves of supply to the bladder and urethra of the cat, with a study of their action potentials. J Physiol 86:396–414
Fall M, Lindström S, Mazières L (1990) A bladder-to-bladder cooling reflex in the cat. J Physiol 427:281–300
Fargeas MJ, Theodorou V, More J, Wal JM, Fioramonti J, Bueno L (1995) Boosted systemic immune and local responsiveness after intestinal inflammation in orally sensitized guinea pigs. Gastroenterology 109:53–62
Fioramonti J, Gaultier E, Toulouse M, Sanger GJ, Bueno L (2003) Intestinal anti-nociceptive behaviour of NK3 receptor antagonism in conscious rats: evidence to support a peripheral mechanism of action. Neurogastroenterol Motil 15:363–369
Fitzerald M (2005) The development of nociceptive circuits. Nat Neurosci 6:507–520
Floyd K, Morrison JFB (1974) Splanchnic mechanoreceptor in the dog. Q J Exp Physiol Cogn Med Sci 59:361–366
Floyd K, Hick EV, Morrison JFB (1976) Mechanosensitive afferent units in the hypogastric nerve of the cat. J Physiol Lond 259:457–471
Floyd K, Hick EV, Koley J, Morrison JFB (1977) The effect of bradykinin on afferent units in intra-abdominal sympathetic nerve trunks. Q J Exp Physiol Cogn Med Sci 62:19–25
Fox EA, Phillips RJ, Martinson FA, Baronowsky EA, Powley TL (2000) Vagal afferent innervation of smooth muscle in the stomach and duodenum of the mouse: morphology and topography. J Comp Neurol 428:558–576
Friedrich AE, Gebhart GF (2000) Effects of spinal cholecystokinin receptor antagonists on morphine antinociception in a model of visceral pain in the rat. J Pharmacol Exp Ther 292:538–544
Friedrich AE, Gebhart GF (2003) Modulation of visceral hyperalgesia by morphine and cholecystokinin from the rat rostroventral medial medulla. Pain 104:93–101
Fujino K, Takami Y, Sebastian G, de la Fuente, Ludwig KA, Christopher R, Mantyh MD (2004) Inhibition of the vanilloid receptor subtype-1 attenuates TNBS-colitis. J Gastrointest Surg 8:842–847
Fujino K, de la Fuente SG, Takami Y, Takahashi T, Mantyh CR (2006) Attenuation of acid-induced oesophagitis in VR-1 deficient mice. Gut 55:34–40
Gammon GD, Bronk DW (1935) The discharges of impulses from pacinian corpuscles in the mesentery and its relation to vascular changes. Am J Physiol 114:77–84
Gareau MG, Jury J, Yang PC, MacQueen G, Perdue MH (2006) Neonatal maternal separation causes colonic dysfunction in rat pups including impaired host resistance. Pediatr Res 59: 83–88
Gaudreau GA, Plourde V (2003) Role of tachykinin NK1, NK2 and NK3 receptors in the modulation of visceral hypersensitivity in the rat. Neurosci Lett 351:59–62
Gaudreau GA, Plourde V (2004) Involvement of N-methyl-D-aspartate (NMDA) receptors in a rat model of visceral hypersensitivity. Behav Brain Res 150:185–189
Geirsson G, Lindström S, Fall M (1993) The bladder cooling reflex in man – characteristics and sensitivity to temperature. Br J Urol 71:675–680
Geirsson G, Lindström S, Fall M (1999) The bladder cooling reflex and the use of cooling as stimulus to the lower urinary tract. J Urol 162:1890–1896
Gershon MD, Liu MT (2007) Serotonin and neuroprotection in functional bowel disorders. Neurogastroenterol Motil 19(Suppl 2):19–24
Giamberardino MA, Valente R, de Bigontina P, Vecchiet L (1995) Artificial ureteral calculosis in rats: behavioural characterization of visceral pain episodes and their relationship with referred lumbar muscle hyperalgesia. Pain 61:459–469

Greenwood-Van Meerveld B (2007) Importance of 5-hydroxytryptamine receptors on intestinal afferents in the regulation of visceral sensitivity. Neurogastroenterol Motil 19(Suppl 2):13–18

Greenwood-Van Meerveld B, Gibson MS, Johnson AC, Venkova K, Sutkowski-Markmann D (2003) NK1 receptor-mediated mechanisms regulate colonic hypersensitivity in the guinea pig. Pharmacol Biochem Behav 74:1005–1013

Greenwood-Van Meerveld B, Venkova K, Hicks G, Dennis E, Crowell MD (2006) Activation of peripheral 5-HT receptors attenuates colonic sensitivity to intraluminal distension. Neurogastroenterol Motil 18(1):76–86

Grundy D, Scratcherd T (1989) Sensory afferents from the gastrointestinal tract. In: Handbook of physiology; gastrointestinal system, vol 1. American Physiological Society, Bethesda, pp 593–620

Häbler J, Jänig W, Koltzenburg M (1988a) A novel type of unmyelinated chemosensitive nociceptor in the acutely inflamed urinary bladder. Agent Act 25:219–212

Häbler HJ, Jänig W, Koltzenburg M (1988b) Dichotomizing unmyelinated afferents supplying pelvic viscera and perineum are rare in the sacral segments of the cat. Neurosci Lett 94:119–124

Häbler J, Jänig W, Koltzenburg M (1990) Activation of unmyelinated afferent fibers by mechanical stimuli and inflammation of the urinary bladder of the cat. J Physiol Lond 425:545–562

Häbler J, Jänig W, Koltzenburg M (1991) Spinal cord integration of colon function: Afferent and efferent pathways. In: Y Tache, D Wingate (eds) Brain–gut interactions. CRC, Boca Raton, pp 147–160

Häbler HJ, Jänig W, Koltzenburg M (1993) Myelinated primary afferents of the sacral spinal cord responding to slow filling and distension of the cat urinary bladder. J Physiol 463:449–460

Hammer K, Sann H, Pierau FK (1993) Functional properties of mechanosensitive units from the chicken ureter in vitro. Pflugers Arch 425:353–361

Hara K, Saito Y, Kirihara Y, Yamada Y, Sakura S, Kosaka Y (1999) The interaction of antinociceptive effects of morphine and GABA receptor agonists within the rat spinal cord. Anesth Analg 89:422–427

Haupt P, Jänig W, Kohler W (1983) Response patterns of visceral afferent fibers, supplying the colon, upon chemical and mechanical stimuli. Pflugers Arch 398:41–47

Hicks GA, Coldwell JR, Schindler M, Ward PA, Jenkins D, Lynn PA, Humphrey PP, Blackshaw LA (2002) Excitation of rat colonic afferent fibres by 5-HT(3) receptors. J Physiol 544:861–869

Hong SK, Han HC, Yoon YW, Chung JM (1993) Response properties of hypogastric afferent fibers supplying the uterus in the cat. Brain Res 622(1–2):215–225

Hulsebosch CE, Coggeshall RE (1982) An analysis of the axon populations in the nerve to the pelvic viscera in the rat. J Comp Neurol 211:1–10

Iggo A (1955) Tension receptors in the stomach and urinary bladder. J Physiol Lond 128:593–607

Isomoto S, Kaibara M, Sakurai-Yamashita Y, Nagayama Y, Uenzo Y, Yano K, Taniyama K (1998) Cloning and tissue distribution of novel splice variants of the rat $GABA_B$ receptor. Biochem Biophys Res Comm 253:10–15

Jänig W, Koltzenburg M (1990) On the function of spinal primary afferent fibers supplying colon and urinary bladder. J Auton Nerv Syst 30:S89–S96

Jänig W, Koltzenburg M (1991) Receptive properties of sacral primary afferent neurons supplying the colon. J Neurophysiol 65:1067–1077

Jänig W, McLachlan EM (1987) Organization of lumbar spinal outflow to distal colon and pelvic organs. Physiol Rev 67:1332–1404

Jänig W, Morrison JFB (1986) Functional properties of spinal visceral afferents supplying abdominal and pelvic organs, with special emphasis on visceral nociception. In: Visceral sensation. Progress in brain research, vol 67. Elsevier, Amsterdam, pp 87–114

Jänig W, Khasar SG, Levine JD, Miao FJ (2000) The role of vagal visceral afferents in the control of nociception. Prog Brain Res 122:273–287

Ji Y, Traub RJ (2001) Spinal NMDA receptors contribute to neuronal processing of acute noxious and nonnoxious colorectal stimulation in the rat. J Neurophysiol 86:1783–1791

Jiang CH, Mazieres L, Lindström S (2002) Cold- and menthol-sensitive C afferents of cat urinary bladder. J Physiol 543:211–220

Jones RC III, Xu L, Gebhart GF (2005) The mechanosensitivity of mouse colon afferent fibers and their sensitization by inflammatory mediators require transient receptor potential vanilloid 1 and acid-sensing ion channel 3. J Neurosci 25:10981–10989

Jones RCIII, Otsuka E, Wagstrom E, Jensen CS, Price MP, Gebhart GF (2007) Short-term sensitization of colon mechanoreceptors is associated with long-term hypersensitivity to colon distention in the mouse. Gastroenterology 133:184–194

Joshi SK, Su X, Porreca F, Gebhart GF (2000) Kappa-opioid receptor agonists modulate visceral nociception at a novel, peripheral site of action. J Neurosci 20:5874–5879

Joshi SK, Lamb K, Bielefeldt K, Gebhart GF (2003) Arylacetamide kappa-opioid receptor agonists produce a tonic- and use-dependent block of tetrodotoxin-sensitive and -resistant sodium currents in colon sensory neurons. J Pharmacol Exp Ther 307:367–372

Julia V, Morteau O, Buéno L (1994) Involvement of neurokinin 1 and 2 receptors in viscerosensitive response to rectal distension in rats. Gastroenterology 107:94–102

Julia V, Su X, Buéno L, Gebhart GF (1999) Role of neurokinin 3 receptors on responses to colorectal distention in the rat: electrophysiological and behavioral studies. Gastroenterology 116:1124–1131

Kakol-Palm D, Brusberg M, Sand E, Larsson H, Martinez V, Johansson A, von Mentzer B, Påhlman I, Lindström E (2008) Role of tachykinin NK(1) and NK(2) receptors in colonic sensitivity and stress-induced defecation in gerbils. Eur J Pharmacol 582:123–131

Kamp EH, Beck DR, Gebhart GF (2001) Combinations of neurokinin receptor antagonists reduce visceral hyperalgesia. J Pharmacol Exp Ther 299:105–113

Kirchner A, Birklein F, Stefan H, Handwerker HO (2000) Left vagus nerve stimulation suppresses experimentally induced pain. Neurology 55(8):1167–1171

Kolhekar R, Gebhart GF (1994) NMDA and quisqualate modulation of visceral nociception in the rat. Brain Res 651:215–226

Kolhekar R, Gebhart GF (1996) Modulation of spinal visceral nociceptive transmission by NMDA receptor activation in the rat. J Neurophysiol 75:2344–2353

Kozlowski CM, Green A, Grundy D, Boissonade FM, Bountra C (2000) The 5-HT(3) receptor antagonist alosetron inhibits the colorectal distention induced depressor response and spinal c-fos expression in the anaesthetized rat. Gut 46:474–480

Laird JM, Roza C, Cervero F (1996) Spinal dorsal horn neurons responding to noxious distension of the ureter in anesthetized rats. J Neurophysiol 5:3239–3248

Laird JM, Olivar T, Roza C, De Felipe C, Hunt SP, Cervero F (2000) Deficits in visceral pain and hyperalgesia of mice with a disruption of the tachykinin NK1 receptor gene. Neuroscience 98:345–352

Laird JM, Roza C, De Felipe C, Hunt SP, Cervero F (2001a) Role of central and peripheral tachykinin NK1 receptors in capsaicin-induced pain and hyperalgesia in mice. Pain 90:97–103

Laird JM, Olivar T, Lopez-Garcia JA, Maggi CA, Cervero F (2001b) Responses of rat spinal neurons to distension of inflamed colon: role of tachykinin NK2 receptors. Neuropharmacology 40:696–701

Lamb K, Zhong F, Gebhart GF, Bielefeldt K (2006) Experimental colitis in mice and sensitization of converging visceral and somatic afferent pathways. Am J Physiol 290:G451–G457

Lennander KB (1901) Ueber die sensibilität der bauchhohle und ueber lokale und allgemeine anasthesie bei bruch und bauchoperationen. Zentralbl Chir 28:200–223

Lew WYW, Longhurst JC (1986) Substance-P, 5-hydroxytryptamine, and bradykinin stimulate abdominal visceral afferent fiber endings in cats. Am J Physiol 250:R465–R473

Lewis T, Kellgren JH (1939) Observation related to referred pain, viscerosomatic reflexes and other associated phenomena. Clin Sci 4:47–71

Li J, McRoberts JA, Ennes HS, Trevisani M, Nicoletti P, Mittal Y, Mayer EA (2006) Experimental colitis modulates the functional properties of NMDA receptors in dorsal root ganglia neurons. Am J Physiol 291:G219–G228

Liang R, Ustinova EE, Patnam R, Fraser MO, Gutkin DW, Pezzone MA (2007) Enhanced expression of mast cell growth factor and mast cell activation in the bladder following the resolution of trinitrobenzene sulfonic acid (TNBS) colitis in female rats. Neurourol Urodyn 226:887–893

Lidow MS, Song ZM, Ren K (2001) Long-term effects of short-lasting early local inflammatory insult. Neuroreport 12:399–403

Lin C, Al-Chaer ED (2003) Long-term sensitization of primary afferents in adult rats exposed to neonatal colon pain. Brain Res 971:73–82

Lindström S, Mazières L (1991) Effect of menthol on the bladder cooling reflex in the cat. Acta Physiol Scand 141:1–10

Liu D, Diorio J, Tannenbaum B, Caldji C, Francis D, Freedman A, Sharma S, Pearson D, Plotsky PM, Meaney MJ (1997) Maternal care, hippocampal glucocorticoid receptors, and hypothalamic–pituitary–adrenal responses to stress. Science 277:1659–1662

Longhurst JC, Dittman LE (1987) Hypoxia, bradykinin and prostaglandins stimulate ischemically sensitive visceral afferents. Am J Physiol 253:H556–H567

Longhurst JC, Kaufman MP, Ordway GA, Musch TI (1984) Effects of bradykinin and capsaicin on endings of afferent fibers from abdominal visceral organs. Am J Physiol 247:R552–R559

Longhurst JC, Rotto DM, Kaufman MP, Stahl GL (1991) Ischemically sensitive abdominal visceral afferents: response to cyclooxygenase blockade. Am J Physiol 261:H2075–H2081

Longstreth GF (1994) Irritable bowel syndrome and chronic pelvic pain. Obstet Gynecol Surv 49:505–507

Longstreth GF, Drossman DA (2002) New developments in the diagnosis and treatment of irritable bowel syndrome. Curr Gastroenterol Rep 4:427–434

Lu Y, Westlund KN (2001) Effects of baclofen on colon inflammation-induced Fos, CGRP and SP expression in spinal cord and brainstem. Brain Res 889:118–130

Lynn PA, Blackshaw LA (1999) In vitro recordings of afferent fibres with receptive fields in the serosa, muscle and mucosa of rat colon. J Physiol 518:271–282

Lynn PA, Olsson C, Zagorodnyuk V, Costa M, Brookes SJ (2003) Rectal intraganglionic laminar endings are transduction sites of extrinsic mechanoreceptors in the guinea pig rectum. Gastroenterology 125:786–794

Lynn P, Zagorodnyuk V, Hennig G, Costa M, Brookes S (2005) Mechanical activation of rectal intraganglionic laminar endings in the guinea pig distal gut. J Physiol 564:589–601

Mackenzie, J (1893) Some points bearing on the association of sensory disorders and visceral disease. Brain 16:321–353

Malcangio M, Bowery NG (1996) GABA and its receptors in the spinal cord. Trends Pharmacol Sci 17:457–462

Malykhina AP (2007) Neural mechanisms of pelvic organ cross-sensitization. Neuroscience 149:660–672

Malykhina AP, Qin C, Greenwood-van Meerveld B, Foreman RD, Lupu F, Akbarali HI (2006) Hyperexcitability of convergent colon and bladder dorsal root ganglion neurons after colonic inflammation: mechanism for pelvic organ cross-talk. Neurogastroenterol Motil 18:936–948

Marvizón JC, Martínez V, Grady EF, Bunnett NW, Mayer EA (1997) Neurokinin 1 receptor internalization in spinal cord slices induced by dorsal root stimulation is mediated by NMDA receptors. J Neuroscience 17:8129–8136

Marvizon JC, Grady EF, Stefani E, Bunnett NW, Mayer EA (1999) Substance P release in the dorsal horn assessed by receptor internalization: NMDA receptors counteract a tonic inhibition by GABAB receptors. Eur J Neurosci 11:417–426

Marvizón JC, McRoberts JA, Ennes HS, Song B, Wang X, Jinton L, Corneliussen B, Mayer EA (2002) Two N-methyl-D-aspartate receptors in rat dorsal root ganglia with different subunit composition and localization. J Comp Neurol 446:325–341

Matthews MR, Connaughton M, Cuello AC (1987) Ultrastructure and distribution of substance P-immunoreactive sensory collaterals in the guinea pig prevertebral sympathetic ganglia. J Comp Neurol 258:28–51

Matthews PJ, Aziz Q, Facer P, Davis JB, Thompson DG, Anand P (2004) Increase Capsaicin Receptor TRPV1 nerve fibers in the inflamed human oesophagus. Eur J Gastroenterol Hepatol 16:897–902

Mayer EA, Gebhart GF (1994) Basic and clinical aspects of visceral hyperalgesia. Gastroenterology 107:271–293

McMahon SB, Morrison JF (1982) Two group of spinal interneurones that respond to stimulation of the abdominal viscera of the cat. J Physiol 322:21–34

McRoberts JA, Coutinho SV, Marvizón JC, Grady EF, Tognetto M, Sengupta JN, Ennes HS, Chaban VV, Amadesi S, Creminon C, Lanthorn T, Geppetti P, Bunnett NW, Mayer EA (2001) Role of peripheral N-methyl-D-aspartate (NMDA) receptors in visceral nociception in rats. Gastroenterology 120:1737–1748

McRoberts JA, Li J, Ennes HS, Mayer EA (2007) Sex-dependent differences in the activity and modulation of N-methyl-D-aspartic acid receptors in rat dorsal root ganglia neurons. Neuroscience 148(4):1015–20

Mei N (1985) Intestinal chemosensitivity. Physiol Rev 65:211–237

Miampamba M, Sharkey K (1998) Distribution of calcitonin gene-related peptide, somatostatin, substance P and vasoactive intestinal polypeptide in experimental colitis in rats. Neurogastroenterol Motil 10:315–329

Miranda A, Peles S, Rudolph C, Shaker R, Sengupta JN (2004) Altered visceral sensation in response to somatic pain in the rat. Gastroenterology 126:1082–1089

Miranda A, Peles S, Shaker R, Rudolph C, Sengupta JN (2006) Neonatal nociceptive somatic stimulation differentially modifies the activity of spinal neurons in rats and results in altered somatic and visceral sensation. J Physiol 572:775–785

Miranda A, Nordstrom E, Smith C, Sengupta JN (2007) The Role of TRPV1 in Mechanical and Chemical Visceral Hyperalgesia Following Experimental Colitis. Neuroscience 148: 1021–1032

Mitsui T, Kakizaki H, Matsuura S, Ameda K, Yoshioka M, Koyanagi T (2001) Afferent fibers of the hypogastric nerves are involved in the facilitating effects of chemical bladder irritation in rats. J Neurophysiol 86:2276–2284

Mori T, Kawano K, Shishikura T (2004) 5-HT3-receptor antagonist inhibits visceral pain differently in chemical and mechanical stimuli in rats. J Pharmacol Sci 94:73–76

Morris GP, Beck PL, Herridge MS, Depew WT, Szewczuk MR, Wallace JL (1989) Hapten-induced model of chronic inflammation and ulceration in the rat colon. Gastroenterology 96:795–803

Morrison JFB (1973) Splanchnic slowly adapting mechanoreceptor with punctate receptive fields in the mesentery and gastrointestinal tract of the cat. J Physiol Lond 233:340–361

Morrison JFB (1987) Sensation arising from the lower urinary tract. In: Torrens M, Morrison JFB (eds) Physiology of the lower urinary tract. Springer, New York, pp 89–131

Morteau O, Hachet T, Caussette M, Bueno L (1994a) Experimental colitis alters visceromotor response to colorectal distension in awake rats. Dig Dis Sci 39:1239–1248

Morteau O, Julia V, Eeckhout C, Bueno L (1994b) Influence of 5-HT3 receptor antagonists in visceromotor and nociceptive responses to rectal distension before and during experimental colitis in rats. Fundam Clin Pharmacol 8:553–562

Moss NG, Harrington WW, Tucker MS (1997) Pressure, volume, and chemosensitivity in afferent innervation of urinary bladder in rats. Am J Physiol 272:R695–R703

Mukerji G, Yiangou Y, Corcoran SL, Selmer IS, Smith GD, Benham CD, Bountra C, Agarwal SK, Anand P (2006a) Cool and menthol receptor TRPM8 in human urinary bladder disorders and clinical correlations. BMC Urol 6:6–13

Mukerji G, Waters J, Chessell IP, Bountra C, Agarwal SK, Anand P (2006b) Pain during ice water test distinguishes clinical bladder hypersensitivity from overactivity disorders. BMC Urol 6:31–42

Multon S, Schoenen J (2005) Pain control by vagus nerve stimulation: from animal to man ... and back. Acta Neurol Belg 105(2):62–67

Nadelhaft I, Booth AM (1984) The location and morphology of preganglionic neurons and the distribution the distribution of the visceral afferents from the rat pelvic nerve: a horseradish peroxidase study. J Comp Neurol 226:238–245
Nadelhaft I, Vera PL (1991) Neurons labelled after the application of tracer to the distal stump of the transected hypogastric nerve in the rat. J Auton Nerv Syst 36:87–96
Nadelhaft I, Roppolo C, Morgan C, De Groat WC (1983) Parasympathetic preganglionic neurons and visceral primary afferents in monkey sacral spinal cord revealed following application of horseradish peroxidase to pelvic nerve. J Comp Neurol 216:36–52
Namasivayam S, Eardley I, Morrison JF (1999) Purinergic sensory neurotransmission in the urinary bladder: an in vitro study in the rat. Br J Urol 854-860
Nazif O, Teichman JM, Gebhart GF (2007) Neural upregulation in interstitial cystitis. Urology 69:24–33
Ness TJ, Gebhart GF (1988) Colorectal distension as a noxious visceral stimulus: physiologic and pharmacologic characterization of pseudaffective reflexes in the rat. Brain Res 450:153–169
Ness TJ, Gebhart GF (1990) Visceral pain: a review of experimental studies. Pain 41:167–234
Ness TJ, Metcalf AM, Gebhart GF (1990) A psychophysical study in humans using phasic colonic distension as a noxious visceral stimulus. Pain 43:377–386
Ness TJ, Fillingim RB, Randich A, Backensto EM, Faught E (2000) Low intensity vagal nerve stimulation lowers human thermal pain thresholds. Pain 86:81–85
Ness TJ, Lewis-Sides A, Castroman P (2001) Characterization of pressor and visceromotor reflex responses to bladder distention in rats: sources of variability and effect of analgesics. J Urol 165:968–975
Okano S, Ikeura Y, Inatomi N (2002) Effects of tachykinin NK1 receptor antagonists on the viscerosensory response caused by colorectal distention in rabbits. J Pharmacol Exp Ther 300:925–931
Olah Z, Karai L, Iadarola MJ (2001) Anandamide activates vanilloid receptor 1 (VR1) at acidic *p*H in dorsal root ganglia neurons and cells ectopically expressing VR1. J Biol Chem 276:31163–31170
Olivar T, Laird JM (1999) Differential effects of N-methyl-D-aspartate receptor blockade on nociceptive somatic and visceral reflexes. Pain 79:67–73
Ozaki N, Gebhart GF (2001) Characterization of mechanosensitive splanchnic nerve afferent fibers innervating the rat stomach. Am J Physiol 281:G1449–G1459
Ozaki N, Bielefeldt K, Sengupta JN, Gebhart GF (2002) Models of gastric visceral hyperalgesia. Am J Physiol 283:G666–G676
Page AJ, Blackshaw AL (1998) An in vitro study of the properties of vagal afferent fibres innervating the ferret oesophagus and stomach. J Physiol 512:907–916
Page AJ, Blackshaw AL (1999) $GABA_B$ receptors inhibit mechanosensitivity of primary afferent endings. J Neurosci 19:8597–8602
Paintal AS (1954) A method of location of the receptors of visceral afferent fibers. J Physiol Lond 124:166–172
Partosoedarso ER, Young RL, Blackshaw AL (2001) GABAB receptors on vagal afferent pathways: peripheral and central inhibition. Am J Physiol Gastrointest Liver Physiol 280: G658–G668
Pascual JI, Insausti R, Gonzalo LM (1989) The pelvic innervation in the rat: different spinal origin and projections in Sprague-Dawley and Wistar rats. Brain Res 480:397–402
Pascual JI, Insausti R, Gonzalo LM (1993) Urinary bladder innervation in male rat: termination of primary afferents in the spinal cord as determined by transganglionic transport of WGA-HRP. J Urol 150:500–504
Pattinson D, Fitzerald M (2004) The neurobiology of infant pain: development of excitatory and inhibitory neurotransmission in the spinal dorsal horn. Reg Anes Pain Med 29:36–44
Peles S, Miranda A, Shaker R, Sengupta JN (2004) Acute nociceptive somatic stimulus sensitizes neurons in the spinal cord to colonic distension in the rat. J Physiol 560:291–302

Pezzone MA, Liang R, Fraser MO (2005) A model of neural cross-talk and irritation in the pelvis: implications for the overlap of chronic pelvic pain disorders. Gastroenterology 128:1953–1964

Phillips RJ, Powley TL (2000) Tension and stretch receptors in gastrointestinal smooth muscle: re-evaluating vagal mechanoreceptor electrophysiology. Brain Res Brain Res Rev 34:1–26

Plotsky PM, Thrivikraman KV, Nemeroff CB, Caldji C, Sharma S, Meaney MJ (2005) Long-term consequences of neonatal rearing on central corticotropin-releasing factor systems in adult male rat offspring. Neuropsychopharmacology 30:2192–204

Price DD, Zhou Q, Moshiree B, Robinson ME, Nicholas Verne G (2006) Peripheral and central contributions to hyperalgesia in irritable bowel syndrome. J Pain 7:529–535

Qin C, Foreman RD (2004) Viscerovisceral convergence of urinary bladder and colorectal inputs to lumbosacral spinal neurons in rats. Neuroreport 15:467–471

Qin C, Malykhina AP, Akbarali HI, Foreman RD (2005) Cross-organ sensitization of lumbosacral spinal neurons receiving urinary bladder input in rats with inflamed colon. Gastroenterology 129:1967–1978

Rachmilewitz D, Simon PL, Schwartz LW, Griswold DE, Fondacaro JD, Wasserman MA (1989) Inflammatory mediators of experimental colitis in rats. Gastroenterology 97:326–337

Randich A, Uzzell T, Cannon R, Ness TJ (2006a) Inflammation and enhanced nociceptive responses to bladder distension produced by intravesical zymosan in the rat. BMC Urol 6:2–8

Randich A, Uzzell T, DeBerry JJ, Cannon R, Ness TJ (2006b) Neonatal urinary bladder inflammation produces adult bladder hypersensitivity. J Pain 7:468–479

Ranieri F, Mei N, Crousillat, J (1973) Splanchnic afferent arising from gastrointestinal and peritoneal mechanoreceptor. Exp Brain Res 16:276–290

Ren K, Randich A, Gebhart GF (1991) Effects of electrical stimulation of vagal afferents on spinothalamic tract cells in the rat. Pain 44:311–319

Ren K, Zhuo M, Randich A, Gebhart GF (1993) Vagal afferent stimulation-produced effects on nociception in capsaicin-treated rats. J Neurophysiol 69(5):1530–1540

Ren TH, Wu J, Yew D, Ziea E, Lao L, Leung WK, Berman B, Hu PJ, Sung JJ (2007) Effects of neonatal maternal separation on neurochemical and sensory response to colonic distension in a rat model of irritable bowel syndrome. Am J Physiol 292:G849–G856

Richter JE, Heading RC, Janssens J, Wilson J (2000) Functional esophageal disorders. In: Drossman DA (ed) Rome II; the functional gastrointestinal disorders, 2nd edn. Degnon, McLean, chap 5

Riley RC, Trafton JA, Chi SI, Basbaum AL (2001) Presynaptic regulation of spinal cord tachykinin signaling via $GABA_B$ but not $GABA_A$ receptor activation. Neuroscience 103:725–737

Ritchie J (1973) Pain from the pelvic colon by inflating a balloon in the irritable colon syndrome. Gut 14:125–132

Robbins A, Sato Y, Hotta H, Berkley KJ (1990) Responses of hypogastric nerve afferent fibers to uterine distension in estrous or metestrous rats. Neurosci Lett 110:82–85

Robbins A, Berkley KJ, Sato Y (1992) Estrous cycle variation of afferent fibers supplying reproductive organs in the female rat. Brain Res 596:353–356

Rong W, Burnstock G (2004) Activation of ureter nociceptor by exogenous and endogenous ATP in guinea pig. Neuropharmacology 47:1093–1101

Rong W, Spyer KM, Burnstock G (2002) Activation and sensitisation of low and high threshold afferent fibres mediated by P2X receptors in the mouse urinary bladder. J Physiol 541:591–600

Roppolo JR, Tai C, Booth AM, Buffington CA, de Groat WC, Birder LA (2005) Bladder Adelta afferent nerve activity in normal cats and cats with feline interstitial cystitis. J Urol 173(3):1011–1015

Ruch TC (1946) Visceral sensation and referred pain. In: Fulton JF (ed) Howell's textbook of physiology, 15th edn. Saunders, Philadelphia, pp 385–401

Ruch TC (1961) Pathophysiology of pain. In: Ruch TC, Patton JD, Woodbury JW, Towe AL (eds) Medical physiology and biophysics, 9th edn. Saunders, Philadelphia, pp 350–368

Sann H (1998) Chemosensitivity of nociceptive, mechanosensitive afferent nerve fibres in the guinea-pig ureter. Eur J Neurosci 10:1300–1311

Sann H, Hammer K, Hildesheim IF, Pierau FK (1997) Neurons in the chicken ureter are innervated by substance P- and calcitonin gene-related peptide-containing nerve fibres: immunohistochemical and electrophysiological evidence. J Comp Neurol 380:105–118

Schicho R, Waltraud F, Liebmann I, Holzer P, Lippe IT (2004) Increased expression of TRPV1 receptor in dorsal root ganglia by acid insult of the rat gastric mucosa. Eur J Neurosci 19:1811–1818

Schnitzlein HN, Hoffman HH, Tucker CC, Quigley MB (1960) The pelvic splanchnic nerves of the male Rheusus monkey. J Comp Neurol 114:51–65

Schwetz I, McRoberts JA, Coutinho SV, Bradesi S, Gale G, Fanselow M, Million M, Ohning G, Taché Y, Plotsky PM, Mayer EA (2005) Corticotropin-releasing factor receptor 1 mediates acute and delayed stress-induced visceral hyperalgesia in maternally separated Long-Evans rats. Am J Physiol 289:G704–G712

Sedan O, Sprecher E, Yarnitsky D (2005) Vagal stomach afferents inhibit somatic pain perception. Pain 113:354–359

Semenenko FM, Cervero F (1992) Afferent fibres from the guinea-pig ureter: size and peptide content of the dorsal root ganglion cells of origin. Neuroscience 47:197–201

Sengupta JN (2006) Esophageal sensory physiology. In: GI motility online. Nature, New York

Sengupta JN, Gebhart GF (1994a) Characterization of mechanosensitive pelvic nerve afferent fibers innervating the colon of the rat. J Neurophysiol 71:2046–2060

Sengupta JN, Gebhart GF (1994b) Mechanosensitive properties of pelvic nerve afferent fibers innervating the urinary bladder of the rat. J Neurophysiol 72:2420–30

Sengupta JN, Gebhart GF (1994c) Gastrointestinal afferent fibers and visceral sensations. In: Johnson LRet-al (eds) Physiology of the gastrointestinal tract. Raven, New York, pp 483–519

Sengupta JN, Gebhart GF (1998) The sensory innervation of the colon and its modulation. Curr Opin Gastrol 14:15–20

Sengupta JN, Saha JK, Goyal RK (1990) Stimulus-response function studies of esophageal mechanosensitive nociceptor in sympathetic afferents of opossum. J Neurophysiol 64:796–812

Sengupta JN, Saha JK, Goyal RK (1992) Differential sensitivity of bradykinin to esophageal distension-sensitive mechanoreceptor in vagal and sympathetic afferents of the opossum. J Neurophysiol 68:1053–1067

Sengupta JN, Su X, Gebhart GF (1996) Kappa, but not mu or delta, opioids attenuate responses to distention of afferent fibers innervating the rat colon. Gastroenterology 111:968–980

Sengupta JN, Snider A, Su X, Gebhart GF (1999) Effects of kappa opioids in the inflamed rat colon. Pain 79:175–185

Sengupta JN, Medda BK, Shaker R (2002) Effect of GABA(B) receptor agonist on distension-sensitive pelvic nerve afferent fibers innervating rat colon. Am J Physiol 283:G1343–G1351

Shea VK, Cai R, Crepps B, Mason JL, Perl ER (2000) Sensory fibers of the pelvic nerve innervating the Rat's urinary bladder. J Neurophysiol 84:1924–1933

Sheehan D (1932) The afferent nerve supply of the mesentery and significance in the causation of abdominal pain. J Anat 67:233–249

Smid SD, Young RL, Cooper NJ, Blackshaw AL (2001) $GABA_BR$ expressed on vagal afferent neurons inhibit gastric mechanosensitivity in ferret proximal stomach. Am J Physiol Gastrointest Liver Physiol 281:G1494–G1501

Smith C, Nordstrom E, Sengupta JN, Miranda A (2007) Neonatal gastric suctioning results in chronic somatic and visceral hyperalgesia: role of corticotropin releasing factor. Neurogastroenterol Motil 19:692–699

Sperber AD, Atzmon Y, Neumann L, Weisberg I, Shalit Y, Abu-Shakrah M, Fich A, Buskila D (1999) Fibromyalgia in the irritable bowel syndrome: studies of prevalence and clinical implications. Am J Gastroenterol 94:3541–3546

Spiller R (2007) Recent advances in understanding the role of serotonin in gastrointestinal motility in functional bowel disorders: alterations in 5-HT signalling and metabolism in human disease. Neurogastroenterol Motil 19(Suppl 2):25–31

Strigo IA, Duncan GH, Bushnell MC, Boivin M, Wainer I, Rodriguez Rosas ME, Persson J (2005) The effects of racemic ketamine on painful stimulation of skin and viscera in human subjects. Pain 113:255–264

Su X, Gebhart GF (1998) Mechanosensitive pelvic nerve afferent fibers innervating the colon of the rat polymodal in character. J Neurophysiol 80:2632–2644

Su X, Sengupta JN, Gebhart GF (1997a) Effects of opioids on mechanosensitive pelvic nerve afferent fibers innervating the urinary bladder of the rat. J Neurophysiol 77:1566–1580

Su X, Sengupta JN, Gebhart GF (1997b) Effects of kappa opioid receptor-selective agonists on responses of pelvic nerve afferents to noxious colorectal distension. J Neurophysiol 78:1003–1012

Su X, Joshi SK, Kardos S, Gebhart GF (2002) Sodium channel blocking actions of the kappa-opioid receptor agonist U50,488 contribute to its visceral antinociceptive effects. J Neurophysiol 87:1271–1279

Su X, Riedel ES, Leon LA, Laping NJ (2008) Pharmacologic evaluation of pressor and visceromotor reflex responses to bladder distension. Neurourol Urodyn 27:249–253

Talaat M (1937) Afferent impulses in the nerves supplying the urinary bladder. J Physiol Lond 89:1–13

Talley NJ, Dennis EH, Schettler-Duncan VA, Lacy BE, Olden KW, Crowell MD (2003) Overlapping upper and lower gastrointestinal symptoms in irritable bowel syndrome patients with constipation or diarrhea. Am J Gastroenterol 98:2454–2459

Tang B, Ji Y, Traub RJ (2008) Estrogen alters spinal NMDA receptor activity via a PKA signaling pathway in a visceral pain model in the rat. Pain 137:540–549

Tempest HV, Dixon AK, Turner WH, Elneil S, Sellers LA, Ferguson DR (2004) P2X and P2X receptor expression in human bladder urothelium and changes in interstitial cystitis. BJU Int 93:1344–1348

Thurston CL, Randich A (1992) Electrical stimulation of the subdiaphragmatic vagus in rats: inhibition of heat-evoked responses of spinal dorsal horn neurons and central substrates mediating inhibition of the nociceptive tail flick reflex. Pain 51:349–365

Torrens M, Hald T (1979) Bladder denervation procedures. Urol Clin North Am 6:283–293

Towers S, Princivalle A, Billinton A, Edmunds M, Bettler B, Urban L, Castro-Lopes J, Bowery NG (2000) GABAB receptor protein and mRNA distribution in rat spinal cord and dorsal root ganglia. Eur J Neurosci 12:3201–3210

Traub RJ, Pechman P, Iadarola MJ, Gebhart GF (1992) Fos-like proteins in the lumbosacral spinal cord following noxious and non-noxious colorectal distention in the rat. Pain 49:393–403

Traub RJ, Hutchcroft K, Gebhart GF (1999) The peptide content of colonic afferents decreases following colonic inflammation. Peptides 20:267–273

Traub RJ, Zhai Q, Ji Y, Kovalenko M (2002) NMDA receptor antagonists attenuate noxious and nonnoxious colorectal distention-induced Fos expression in the spinal cord and the visceromotor reflex. Neuroscience 113:205–211

Trevisani M, Patacchini R, Nicoletti P, Gatti R, Gazzieri D, Lissi N, Zagli G, Creminon C, Geppetti P, Harrison S (2005) Hydrogen sulfide causes vanilloid receptor 1-mediated neurogenic inflammation in the airways. Br J Pharmacol 145:1123–1131

Triadafilopoulos G, Simms RW, Goldenberg DL (1991) Bowel dysfunction in fibromyalgia syndrome. Dig Dis Sci 36:59–64

Tsukimi Y, Mizuyachi K, Yamasaki T, Niki T, Hayashi F (2005) Cold response of the bladder in guinea pig: involvement of transient receptor potential channel, TRPM8. Urology 65:406–410

Uemura E, Fletcher TF, Dirks VA, Bradley WE (1973) Distribution of sacral afferent axons in cat urinary bladder. Am J Anat 136:305–313

Uemura E, Fletcher TF, Bradley WE (1974) Distribution of lumbar afferent axons in muscle in muscle coat of cat urinary bladder. Am J Anat 139:389–398

Uemura E, Fletcher TF, Bradley WE (1975) Distribution of lumbar and sacral afferent axons in submucosa of cat urinary bladder. Anat Rec 183:579–587

Ustinova EE, Fraser MO, Pezzone MA (2006) Colonic irritation in the rat sensitizes urinary bladder afferents to mechanical and chemical stimuli: an afferent origin of pelvic organ cross-sensitization. Am J Physiol 290:F1478–F1487

Ustinova EE, Gutkin DW, Pezzone MA (2007) Sensitization of pelvic nerve afferents and mast cell infiltration in the urinary bladder following chronic colonic irritation is mediated by neuropeptides. Am J Physiol 292:F123–F130

Veale D, Kavanagh G, Fielding JF, Fitzeral O (1991) Primary fibromyalgia and the irritable bowel syndrome: different expressions of a common pathogenic process. Br J Rheumatol 30:220–222

Vera PL, Nadelhaft I (1990) Conduction velocity distribution of afferent fibers innervating the rat urinary bladder. Brain Res 520:83–89

Vera PL, Nadelhaft I (1992) Afferent and sympathetic innervation of the dome and the base of the urinary bladder of the female rat. Brain Res 29:651–658

Verne GN, Price DD (2002) Irritable bowel syndrome as a common precipitant of central sensitization. Curr Rheumatol Rep 4:322–328

Verne GN, Robinson ME, Price DD (2001) Hypersensitivity to visceral and cutaneous pain in the irritable bowel syndrome. Pain 93:7–14

Verne GN, Himes NC, Robinson ME, Gopinath KS, Briggs RW, Crosson B, Price DD (2003) Central representation of visceral and cutaneous hypersensitivity in the irritable bowel syndrome. Pain 103:99–110

Von Haller A (1755) A dissertation of the sensible and irritable parts of animals. Nourse, London

Wallace JL, Le T, Carter L, Appleyard CB, Beck P (1995) Hapten-induced colitis in the rat: alternatives to trinitrobenzene sulfonic acid. J Pharmacol Toxicol Methods 33:237–239

Wang G, Tang B, Traub RJ (2005) Differential processing of noxious colonic input by thoraco-lumbar and lumbosacral dorsal horn neurons in the rat. J Neurophysiol 94:3788–3794

Wang G, Tang B, Traub RJ (2007) Pelvic nerve input mediates descending modulation of homovisceral processing in the thoracolumbar spinal cord of the rat. Gastroenterology 133:1544–1553

Willert RP, Woolf CJ, Hobson AR, Delaney C, Thompson DG, Aziz Q (2004) The development and maintenance of human visceral pain hypersensitivity is dependent on the N-methyl-D-aspartate receptor. Gastroenterology 126:683–692

Willert RP, Delaney C, Kelly K, Sharma A, Aziz Q, Hobson AR (2007) Exploring the neurophysiological basis of chest wall allodynia induced by experimental oesophageal acidification – evidence of central sensitization. Neurogastroenterol Motil 19:270–278

Williams RE, Hartmann KE, Sandler RS, Miller WC, Steege JF (2004) Prevalence and characteristics of irritable bowel syndrome among women with chronic pelvic pain. Obstet Gynecol 104:452–458

Williams RE, Hartmann KE, Sandler RS, Miller WC, Savitz LA, Steege JF (2005) Recognition and treatment of irritable bowel syndrome among women with chronic pelvic pain. Am J Obstet Gynecol 192:761–767

Winnard KP, Dmitrieva N, Berkley KJ (2006) Cross-organ interactions between reproductive, gastrointestinal, and urinary tracts: modulation by estrous stage and involvement of the hypogastric nerve. Am J Physiol 291(6):R1592–R1601

Winston J, Shenoy M, Medley D, Naniwadekar A, Pasricha PJ (2007) The vanilloid receptor initiates and maintains colonic hypersensitivity induced by neonatal colon irritation in rats. Gastroenterology 132:615–627

Winter DL (1971) Receptor characteristics and conduction velocites in bladder afferents. J Psychiatr Res 8:225–235

Wynn G, Ma B, Ruan HZ, Burnstock G (2004) Purinergic component of mechanosensory transduction is increased in a rat model of colitis. Am J Physiol 287:G647–G657

Xu L, Gebhart GF (2008) Characterization of mouse lumbar splanchnic and pelvic nerve urinary bladder mechanosensory afferents. J Neurophysiol 99:244–253

Xu GY, Shenoy M, Winston JH, Mittal S, Pasricha PJ (2008) P2X receptor-mediated visceral hyperalgesia in a rat model of chronic visceral hypersensitivity. Gut 57(9):1230–1237
Yiangou Y, Facer P, Dyer NHC, Chan CLH, Knowles C, Williams NS, Anand P (2001) Vanilloid receptor 1 immunoreactivity in inflamed human bowel. Lancet 357:1338–1339
Yu Y, de Groat WC (2008) Sensitization of pelvic afferent nerves in the in vitro rat urinary bladder-pelvic nerve preparation by purinergic agonists and cyclophosphamide pretreatment. Am J Physiol Renal Physiol 294:F1146–F1156
Zagorodnyuk VP, Brookes SJH (2000) Transduction sites of vagal mechanoreceptors in the guinea-pig esophagus. J Neurosci 20:6249–6255
Zagorodnyuk VP, Chen BN, Brookes SJ (2001) Intraganglionic laminar endings are mechano-transduction sites of vagal tension receptors in the guinea-pig stomach. J Physiol 534:255–268
Zagorodnyuk VP, Chen BN, Costa M, Brookes SJH (2003) Mechanotransduction by intraganglionic laminar endings of vagal tension receptors in the guinea-pig oesophagus. J Physiol 553:575–587
Zagorodnyuk VP, Lynn P, Costa M, Brookes SJ (2005) Mechanisms of mechanotransduction by specialized low-threshold mechanoreceptors in the guinea pig rectum. Am J Physiol 289: G397–G406
Zagorodnyuk VP, Gibbins IL, Costa M, Brookes SJ, Gregory SJ (2007) Properties of the major classes of mechanoreceptors in the guinea pig bladder. J Physiol 585:147–163
Zamyatina ON (1954) Electrophysiological characteristics and functional significance of afferent impulses originating in the intestinal wall. Transaction of I.P. Pavlov Institute of Physiology 3:193–208
Zhai QZ, Traub RJ (1999) The NMDA receptor antagonist MK-801 attenuates c-Fos expression in the lumbosacral spinal cord following repetitive noxious and non-noxious colorectal distention. Pain 83(2):321–329
Zhou Q, Price DD, Caudle RM, Verne N (2008) Visceral and somatic hypersensitivity in a subset of rats following TNBS-induced colitis. Pain 134:9–15

Migraine

Silvia Benemei, Paola Nicoletti, Jay G. Capone, Francesco De Cesaris and Pierangelo Geppetti

Contents

Abstract Migraine is a neurovascular disorder which affects one fifth of the general population. Disability due to migraine is severe and involves patients from infancy through senescence and it is aggravated by the fact there is no complete cure. However, various drugs for the symptomatic or prophylactic treatment of the disease are available. Recently, better knowledge of the neurobiological and pharmacological aspects of a subset of trigeminal primary sensory neurons has provided key information for the development of effective molecules that specifically target the activation of the trigeminovascular system and may represent a significant advancement in the treatment of the disease. These novel antagonists block the receptor for the sensory neuropeptide calcitonin gene-related peptide (CGRP), which upon release from peripheral terminals of trigeminal perivascular neurons dilates cranial arterial vessels. Whether neurogenic vasodilatation is the major contributing factor to generate the pain and the associated symptoms of the migraine attack or whether other sites of action of CGRP receptor antagonists

P. Geppetti (✉)
Centre for the Study of Headache and Department of Preclinical and Clinical Pharmacology, University of Florence, Florence, Italy, and Headache Center, University Hospital S. Anna, Ferrara, Italy

B.J. Canning and D. Spina (eds.), *Sensory Nerves*,
Handbook of Experimental Pharmacology 194, DOI: 10.1007/978-3-540-79090-7_3,

are responsible for the antimigraine effect of these compounds is the subject of current and intense research.

Keywords Neurogenic vadodilatation, Calcitonin gene-related peptide, Primary sensory neurons, CGRP receptor

1 Introduction

More than 70 years ago, Sir Thomas Lewis postulated that one portion of a widely branching sensory fiber responds to the injury, and that action potentials generated by this event are carried, antidromically, to other branches of the fiber, where they release a chemical substance that causes the flare and increases the sensitivity of other sensory axons responsible for pain (Lewis 1937). The neurons that mediate these responses have been proposed to belong to a previously unrecognized subgroup and termed "nocifensors" because of their dual function. The first function is to sense injurious stimuli and the second function is to promote a first line of defense by a neurovascular response which encompasses arterial vasodilatation, plasma protein extravasation, and other responses. Decades after these pioneering observations, the concept that a neurogenic component of inflammation exists has been generally recognized (Geppetti and Holzer 1996; Szolcsanyi 1977). Despite the fact that in experimental animals neurogenic inflammation has been well documented and has been proven in the majority of tissues and organs, and its role has been robustly established in relevant models of human diseases, the demonstration that neurogenic inflammation has a significant contribution to human diseases, and particularly in migraine, is still a matter of debate. However, very recent clinical trials (Doods et al. 2007) have given support to the hypothesis originating from a number of neurochemical and pharmacological data that neurogenic inflammation plays a key role in the mechanism of migraine (Markowitz et al. 1987).

The major somatosensory innervation to the extracranial tissues is supplied by the trigeminal nerve, which has a smaller, but important, intracranial component that provides a sensory innervation to the cranial meninges (Penfield and McNaughton 1940). This latter component has attracted most attention in the pathophysiology of migraine following the neurosurgical observation that direct stimulation of the meninges, particularly at vascular sites, could evoke painful, headache-like sensations (Fay 1935; Feindel et al. 1960; Ray and Wolff 1940). Intracranial sensory innervation supplies both the major cerebral arteries (as the middle cerebral arteries) and the dural venous sinuses. The arterial nerve supply and pain sensation does not extend to the brain itself, as the sensory innervation is restricted to the meningeal covering around the outside of the brain. Although it cannot be excluded that the nerve supply to extracranial arterial vessels plays a significant role, it has been postulated that meningeal sensory innervation has a major contribution to the migraine headache. Thus, the present chapter will focus of the neurochemical and functional features of the subset of sensory neurons which mediate neurogenic inflammation in the cranial district, and particularly in the meninges.

2 A Subset of Sensory (Nocifensor) Neurons Exerts a Dual Afferent and Efferent Function and Mediates Neurogenic Inflammation

The stimulation of peripheral terminals of a subset of primary sensory neurons is not only associated with the transmission of nociceptive, or pain, signals, but also results in a series of proinflammatory responses collectively referred to as "neurogenic inflammation" (Geppetti and Holzer 1996). The neurons which mediate neurogenic inflammation have Aδ- and C-fibers, are defined as polymodal nociceptors because they sense thermal, chemical, and high-threshold mechanical stimuli, and are characterized by their content in neuropeptides, namely, the calcitonin gene-related peptide (CGRP) and the tachykinins substance P (SP) and neurokinin A (NKA). Finally, this subset of sensory neurons is uniquely sensitive to capsaicin, the pungent principle contained in plants of the genus *Capsicum*. Sensitivity to capsaicin is given by the expression on the plasma membrane of the neuron of a protein which belongs to the superfamily of the transient receptor potential (TRP) ion channels. TRP channels, in mammals, currently encompasses 28 proteins belonging to six different families, which transduce a variety of sensations produced by both chemical and physical stimuli (Nilius et al. 2007).

TRPV1 (*V* indicates the sensitivity to vanilloid molecules), also termed the "capsaicin receptor," was cloned 10 years ago (Caterina et al. 1997) and it was soon recognized as an integrator of various sensory stimuli, including noxious heat, low extracellular pH, various lipid derivatives, including anandamide, *N*-arachidonoyl dopamine, and eicosanoids, and other stimuli (Caterina et al. 1997; Huang et al. 2002; Hwang et al. 2000; Tominaga et al. 1998; Zygmunt et al. 1999). Capsaicin, by stimulating TRPV1, produces a burning sensation and releases sensory neuropeptides, which causes neurogenic inflammation. In addition, exposure to high concentrations/doses of capsaicin for a prolonged time, after an initial excitatory phase, and in a time- and concentration/dose-dependent manner, desensitizes sensory neurons or nerve endings, an effect that ultimately results in the inability of the nerve fibers to evoke pain and neurogenic inflammation (Szallasi and Blumberg 1999; Szolcsanyi 1977). This specific feature of capsaicin and TRPV1 has been of great value for the current understanding of the multiple functions of sensory neurons, as well as of their role in models of human diseases. In addition, because after capsaicin application the desensitized tissue becomes irresponsive to a series of painful stimuli, this procedure has been used to successfully treat various painful conditions (Knotkova et al. 2008). In addition to TRPV1 (Caterina et al. 1997), other TRP channels are expressed by C-fiber nociceptors, including TRPV2, TRPV3, and TRPV4 (gated by warm, nonnoxious and noxious temperatures and small reductions in tonicity) and TRPM8 (activated by menthol and moderately low temperature) (Alessandri-Haber et al. 2003; Bautista et al. 2007; Caterina et al. 1999; Liedtke et al. 2000; McKemy et al. 2002; Peier et al. 2002). TRPA1 is a recently identified channel, almost entirely coexpressed with TRPV1 on sensory neurons (Nagata et al. 2005; Story et al. 2003) and activated by isothiocyanates, thiosulfinate, or cinnamaldehyde compounds, which are the pungent ingredients found in mustard, garlic, and cinnamon, respectively (Bandell et al. 2004; Bautista et al. 2006; Jordt et al. 2004; Macpherson et al. 2005). Thus, all these channels and their appropriate stimuli are potentially implicated in the activation of neurogenic inflammatory responses.

Biological effects produced by either tachykinins or CGRP account for all the responses mediated by stimulation of capsaicin-sensitive sensory nerves, and, accordingly, the three neuropeptides (SP, NKA, and CGRP) are considered the mediators of neurogenic inflammation. SP or NKA activates with diverse affinities three different heterotrimeric G protein coupled receptors, NK1, NK2, and NK3, which are associated with $G_{q/11}$ proteins and mobilization of Ca^{2+} ions in the cytosol. Stimulation of NK1 receptors on endothelial cells of postcapillary venules activates intracellular contractile elements and opens tight gap junctions between these cells, thus allowing the passage of macromolecules, including albumin, into the interstitial space and by this mechanism produces inflammatory plasma protein extravasation. NK1 receptor activation also mediates leukocyte adhesion to the venular endothelium (Baluk et al. 1995). Less evident is the receptor subtype involved in mast cell degranulation and inflammatory mediator release evoked by SP. However, apart from arterial vasodilatation, the vascular and cellular inflammatory responses produced by capsaicin and other selective stimulants of capsaicin-sensitive sensory nerves are entirely mediated by tachykinin NK1 receptors. The observation that the plasma protein extravasation that follows trigeminal nerve stimulation occurs not only in the extracranial tissue but also in the meninges of rodents suggested that this mechanism could be important for the mechanism of migraine (Markowitz et al. 1987). Additional findings that drugs effective for the acute treatment of the migraine attack such as ergotamine or triptans markedly inhibited meningeal neurogenic plasma extravasation further supported this hypothesis (Moskowitz and Buzzi 1991). In those same years the discovery of the first nonpeptidic NK1 receptor antagonist was reported (Snider et al. 1991) and it was soon followed by the identification of a series of nonpeptidic, high-affinity and selective NK1 receptor antagonists, which boosted the clinical scrutiny of these compounds as novel antimigraine medicines. Unfortunately, none of these drugs proved to be efficacious in reducing the pain and the allied symptoms of the migraine attack because in various randomized clinical trials different NK1 receptor antagonists, including RPR100893 (Diener 2003), GR205171 (Connor et al. 1998), and lanepitant (Goldstein et al. 1997), failed to show efficacy. Pharmacokinetic issues or other reasons might have been of importance for the failure of these drugs, but it is also possible that neurogenic, NK1-receptor-mediated plasma extravasation does not play any role in this disease.

Although there is little doubt that SP/NKA and NK1 receptors mediate neurogenic plasma extravasation in rodents, the certainty that a similar mechanism exists in man is far from clear. For example, capsaicin administration to the human skin causes a remarkable erythema and arteriolar vasodilation (Simone and Ochoa 1991), but there are no reports that capsaicin causes plasma extravasation in the human skin. SP and NKA potently contract human bronchi and the urinary bladder in vitro, indicating that NK2 and NK1 receptors are expressed in the smooth muscle of these human tissues. However, there is no report that capsaicin produces any contractile responses in isolated human bronchi or bladder. Thus, it is possible that in man either there is no anatomofunctional vicinity between the sensory nerve terminal and the tachykinin receptor expressing effector cell or an insufficient amount of tachykinins is released from sensory nerve terminals. Failure to detect a measurable amount of SP/NKA following exposure of human sensory nerve terminals to capsaicin in vitro (Geppetti et al. 1992) strengthens this latter proposal. In conclusion, in man neurogenic inflammation does not seem to include plasma protein extravasation as a major feature of this type of inflammatory response.

It is a common experience, and scientifically well documented, that capsaicin application to the human skin produces a neurogenic flare response (Brain et al. 1985; Simone and Ochoa 1991), which is most likely mediated by CGRP, and there is also direct neurochemical or indirect pharmacological evidence that capsaicin or other TRPV1-dependent or TRPV1-indepedent stimuli release CGRP from human tissues in vitro (Franco-Cereceda 1991; Gazzieri et al. 2007; Geppetti et al. 1992). Thus, it is possible to propose that in human somatic and presumably visceral tissues, neurogenic inflammation exists and its main, if not sole component, is the arterial vasodilatation mediated by the unknown substance, hypothesized by Sir Thomas Lewis in 1936, and that, at present, we can identify with CGRP.

3 CGRP, Its Receptor, and Receptor Antagonists

The alternative processing of RNA transcripts from the calcitonin gene results in the production of two distinct messenger RNAs (mRNAs), one of them encoding calcitonin and the other a 37-amino acid neuropeptide: CGRP (Amara et al. 1985). In contrast with the expression of mRNA for calcitonin in the thyroid, CGRP mRNA is predominantly expressed in the nervous system and particularly in primary sensory neurons of the dorsal root, trigeminal, and vagal ganglia (Quirion et al. 1992). CGRP belongs to a family of peptides that includes adrenomedullin and amylin (Cooper et al. 1987; Kitamura et al. 1993), which affect glucose metabolism and exert other biological functions. Of the two isoforms of CGRP, αCGRP and βCGRP (Amara et al. 1985; Morris et al. 1984), βCGRP, which differs from αCGRP by three amino acids, is mostly located within enteric nerves (Mudderry et al. 1988) and the pituitary gland (Petermann et al. 1987). The half-life of CGRP in the circulation is approximately 7–10 min in human plasma (Struthers et al. 1986), and there is no evidence for a specific proteolytic pathway involved in CGRP metabolism, although mast cell tryptase in the skin (Brain and Williams 1989) and matrix metalloproteinase II have the ability to metabolize CGRP and remove its vasodilator activity (Fernandez-Patron et al. 2000).

The existence of two distinct receptors for CGRP (CGRP1 and CGRP2) was postulated on a pure pharmacological basis because $CGRP_{8-37}$, a 30 amino acid fragment of CGRP, behaves as an antagonist with a relative selectivity for the CGRP1 receptor (Chiba et al. 1989). Rat and human calcitonin receptor-like (CL) receptor (Fluhmann et al. 1995; Njuki et al. 1993) surprisingly did not bind CGRP in the cells studied and therefore it was, at first, considered an orphan receptor. Only if the CL receptor complementary DNA was expressed in cells coexpressing the receptor-activity-modifying protein (RAMP), a single transmembrane domain protein with 148 amino acids necessarily required to be associated with CL, did the "mature" receptor acquire activity (McLatchie et al. 1998). It is now accepted that RAMP1 associates with CL to produce the CGRP receptor (CGRP1) that is antagonized by $CGRP_{8-37}$ and other antagonists.

The discovery of BIBN4096BS (olcegepant), 1-piperidinecarboxamide, *N*-[2-[[5-amino-1-[[4-(4-pyridinyl)-1-piperazinyl]carbonyl]pentyl]amino]-1-[(3,5-dibromo-4-hydroxyphenyl)-methyl]-2-oxoethyl]-4-(1,4-dihydro-2-oxo-3(2*H*)-quinazolinyl) a competitive nonpeptide potent (K_i, 14.4 ± 6.3 pM) antagonist at the human CGRP1 receptor (Doods et al. 2000) has boosted research in the area of CGRP in relation to the trigeminovascular system and migraine. Additional molecules with affinities lower than that of olcegepant, such as compound 1, (4-(2-oxo-2,3-dihydro-benzoimidazol-1-yl)-piperidine-1-carboxylic acid [1-3,5-dibromo-4-hydroxy-benzyl)-2-oxo-2-(4-phenyl-piperazin-1-yl)-ethyl]-amide) and SB-273779 [*N*-methyl-*N*-(2-methylphenyl)-3-nitro-4-(2-thiazolylsulfinyl)-nitrobenzanilide] have been reported. Compound 1 showed a pK_i of 7.8 in binding experiments on SK-N-MC as compared with 8.9 for $CGRP_{8-37}$ (Aiyar et al. 2001; Edvinsson et al. 2001). Subsequently, other peptide antagonists have been developed (Boeglin et al. 2007; Taylor et al. 2006). However, a major breakthrough was the report of the first, nonpeptide, orally available and high-affinity CGRP receptor antagonist, MK-0974 [*N*-[(3*R*,6*S*)-6-(2,3-difluorophenyl)-2-oxo-1-(2,2,2-trifluoroethyl)azepan-3-yl]-4-(2-oxo-2,3-dihydro-1*H*-imidazo[4,5-*b*]pyridin-1-yl)piperidine-1-carbox amide] (Paone et al. 2007; Salvatore et al. 2008).

4 CGRP Release and CGRP-Mediated Responses

CGRP release from nerve terminals of nociceptors is finely tuned by a series of prejunctional receptors and channels expressed on the plasma membrane of these neurons and these receptors/channels represent a therapeutic opportunity for migraine treatment. However, only a few of them seem to contribute to the pathophysiological changes accompanying migraine because most of these receptor/channel agonists and antagonists have failed to significantly affect the migraine attack. TRPV1 and other excitatory channels and receptors enhance CGRP release, and in contrast ergot derivatives and triptans reduce sensory neuropeptide release from trigeminal perivascular endings. TRPV1 undergoes marked plasticity by neurotrophic factors or by several proinflammatory mediators (Chuang et al. 2001;

Premkumar and Ahern 2000), which may play a role in migraine. In particular, the observations that low extracellular pH, which is easily encountered at the site of inflammation, and ethanol (a known trigger of migraine attack) stimulate TRPV1 (Bevan and Geppetti 1994; Tominaga et al. 1998; Trevisani et al. 2002) and by this mechanism release sensory neuropeptides from the dura mater (Fanciullacci et al. 1991) or produce a CGRP-dependent vasodilatation of dural blood vessels (Nicoletti et al. 2008), suggesting that TRPV1 might be involved in the initiation of the process that ultimately results in the migraine attack.

CGRP shows a potency as a vasodilator substance approximately tenfold greater than the prostaglandins and 2–3 orders of magnitude greater than that of other classic vasodilators, including acetylcholine, adenosine, serotonin, and SP. This effect of CGRP is particularly relevant in small vessels. In the venous tissue, which is also densely innervated by CGRP-containing nerves, the role of the peptide is less clear. Generally, CGRP induces an endothelium-independent relaxation, apart from in some vessels, including the rat aorta and the human internal mammary artery, where the relaxation to CGRP depends on the presence of an intact endothelium and is attenuated by inhibitors of NO synthase, implying an NO-dependent mechanism (Brain et al. 1985; Gray and Marshall 1992; Raddino et al. 1997).

5 Sensory Neurons and Migraine

The precise mechanism of migraine is still unknown. Hitherto undetermined, but probable, genetic abnormalities should initiate the alteration of the response threshold to migraine-specific triggers in the brain (Goadsby et al. 2002a). The common observation reported by Lance (1969) that alcohol and other vasodilators are well recognized as inducers of migraine or cluster headache and vasoconstrictors are instrumental in ending them accompanies the pioneering finding by Wolff and colleagues (Wolff 1948) that stimulation of cerebral and meningeal arteries caused headache. These and other data contributed to the widespread belief that vasodilatation of intracranial blood vessels is the underlying mechanism for migraine headache (Ferrari and Saxena 1993). Although positron emission tomography has shown increased blood flow (an index of neuronal activity) during spontaneous migraine attacks in the cerebral hemispheres (Welch 2003), more recent evidence (Schoonman et al. 2008) obtained with 3-T magnetic resonance angiography negated any vasodilatation occurring in cerebral and meningeal arteries during the headache phase of the migraine attack induced by nitroglycerine. It is worth noting that vasodilator substances such as nitroglycerine (Thomsen et al. 1993) and CGRP (Lassen et al. 2002) can trigger migraine in susceptible subjects, although migraine arises a few hours after the occurrence of the relatively short lived vasodilating response caused by these agents. Also, extracranial vessels may contribute to the pain of the migraine attack as suggested by Graham and Wolff (1938), who observed that ergotamine decreased migraine headache along with the pulse amplitude measured over the temporal artery. However, both ergotamine and dihydroergotamine may affect vessel caliber in a different manner depending on the state of the artery during the migraine attack (Brazil and Friedman 1957). Another way by which ergot derivatives may affect vessel caliber is through inhibition of CGRP release from perivascular trigeminal nerve endings by stimulating the inhibitory serotonin 5-HT$_{1B/D}$ receptor. Although this neuronal effect of ergots and triptans has been more extensively studied with respect to SP-mediated plasma protein extravasation (Markowitz et al. 1987; Moskowitz and Buzzi 1991), there is also evidence that by the same mechanism the 5-HT$_{1B/D}$ receptor inhibits CGRP-mediated vasodilatation. This seems to be the case for ergotamine and triptans, which in addition to contracting dilated cranial blood vessels and carotid arteriovenous anastomoses (Tfelt-Hansen et al. 2000) reduce CGRP release from perivascular trigeminal nerve endings and inhibit nociceptive transmission on peripheral and central endings of trigeminal sensory nerves (Goadsby et al. 2002a, b; Williamson et al. 2001). Human trigeminal ganglia and sensory nerve fibers express 5-HT$_{1B/1D}$ receptors (Smith et al. 2002), thus supporting the role of presynaptic inhibitory effects on the antimigraine effect of triptans (Edvinsson 2004). Reduction of neuropeptide release from sensory nerve endings by stimulation of presynaptic receptors has been proposed for drugs different from triptans. GR79236 (*N*-[(2-methylphenyl)methyl]adenosine (metrifudil), 2-(phenylamino)adenosine), an agonist of the inhibitory adenosine A1 receptor, has been found to reduce neurogenic vasodilatation in rats (Humphrey et al. 2001), trigeminal nociception and CGRP release in cats (Goadsby et al. 2002a, b), and trigeminal nociception in humans (Giffin et al. 2003). The promising clinical studies that reported that GR79236 has an antimigraine action, probably due to an inhibitory effect on nociceptive trigeminal neurons (Humphrey et al. 2001), have been, however, hampered by concerns regarding the cardiovascular safety of this drug.

The concept that antimigraine activity of triptans is mainly, if not solely, due to their inhibitory action on primary sensory neuron discharge rather than to a mere vasoconstrictor activity has boosted further research on selective neuronal versus vascular 5-HT$_1$ receptor agonists, with the aim of maintaining antimigraine activity with fewer cardiovascular side effects. Selective agonists of the 5-HT$_{1D}$ receptor, such as PNU-109291 ([(*S*)-3,4-dihydro-1-ethyl]-*N*-methyl-1*H*-2-benzopyran-6-carboximide) (Ennis et al. 1998), or the 5-HT$_{1F}$ receptor, such as LY334370 (4-fluoro-*N*-[3-(1-methyl-4-piperidinyl)-1*H*-indol-5-yl]-benzamide) (Ramadan et al. 2003), have been developed following this hypothesis. However, failure of PNU-142633 (Gomez-Mancilla et al. 2001) and efficacy of LY334370 only at doses which may interact with 5-HT$_{1B}$ receptors (Goldstein et al. 1999; Ramadan et al. 2003) did not give clinical support to this view.

6 CGRP Antagonists in Migraine

Trigeminal sensory nerve fibers expressing abundant CGRP-like immunoreactivity are well represented in the intracranial and extracranial circulation (Williamson et al. 2001). CGRP but not SP release has been demonstrated from human tissues innervated by nontrigeminal (Franco-Cereceda 1991) or trigeminal (Geppetti et al. 1992) sensory nerve endings. In addition, plasma concentrations of CGRP, but not of SP, were found to be elevated during spontaneous or nitroglycerine-provoked attacks of migraine (Goadsby et al. 1990) and cluster headache (Fanciullacci et al. 1995). More importantly, intravenous infusion of CGRP produced a migraine-like headache (Lassen et al. 2002), and intravenous infusion of NO evoked a migraine-like headache with an associated increase in plasma CGRP levels (Juhasz et al. 2003). Baseline CGRP plasma levels were more elevated in migraine patients, and changes in plasma CGRP levels during migraine attacks significantly correlated with the headache intensity (Juhasz et al. 2003). All these findings suggested that CGRP could contribute to the migraine mechanism and that inhibition of the CGRP receptor could be beneficial in the treatment of the migraine attack. Thus, when high-affinity and selective antagonists of the CGRP receptor become available they will have to be quickly subjected to clinical scrutiny in migraine patients.

$CGRP_{8-37}$, the first peptide CGRP receptor antagonist, was found to be ineffective in migraine (Durham 2004), most likely because of its low potency and very short half-life (Chiba et al. 1989). A novel selective CGRP receptor antagonist, olcegepant (BIBN4096BS), showed the following relevant features: reduction of the vasodilatation induced by trigeminal stimulation in marmosets (Doods 2001), inhibition of the vasodilator responses induced by capsaicin in porcine carotid, including carotid arteriovenous anastomotic dilatation and decreased CGRP-induced porcine carotid vasodilatation, and arterial-jugular venous oxygen saturation difference (Kapoor et al. 2003). Furthermore, although its peptoid nature requires a parenteral route of administration, the unique high affinity for the human CGRP receptor (Doods et al. 2000) suggested that olcegepant could be developed as an antimigraine medicine. Indeed, olcegepant is effective in the acute treatment of migraine without significant side effects (Olesen et al. 2004) or intrinsic vasoconstrictor effects (Petersen et al. 2005). Already at a dose of 2.5 mg it reduced migraine headache by 66% as compared with 27% for a placebo. Olcegepant also showed significant superiority over a placebo in improving the nausea, photophobia, phonophobia, functional capacity, and the time to meaningful relief (Olesen et al. 2004). The most frequent adverse effect was paresthesia and overall side effects were 25% with olcegepant compared with 12% with the placebo. Of interest is the finding that intracranial and extracranial vessel caliber and systemic hemodynamics were not affected by olcegepant, suggesting that, under basal conditions, circulating CGRP does exert a tonic vasodilatory activity and CGRP receptor antagonists should not provoke cerebral or systemic vasospasm (Petersen et al. 2005).

Another breakthrough in the development of novel CGRP antagonists was obtained with the discovery of MK-0974, an orally available drug which originated from a (3*R*)-amino-(6*S*)-phenylcaprolactam core (Paone et al. 2007). High affinity (approximately nanomolar) for the human and the rhesus monkey CGRP receptor compared with the canine and the rat CGRP receptor and the ability of the orally administered drug to inhibit dermal vasodilatation evoked by capsaicin application into the rhesus monkey skin (Salvatore et al. 2008) indicated MK-0974 as a suitable drug for clinical testing in migraine patients. Indeed, apart from the oral dose of 400 mg, the other two doses of 300 and 600 mg showed a better headache response at 2-h (68.1 and 76.5%, respectively, vs. the placebo 46.3%; $p < 0.015$). In the same study the response to rizatriptan was 69.5% (Ho et al. 2007). Adverse events did not appear to be augmented with increasing doses of the drug and MK-0974 was generally well tolerated (Ho et al. 2007). Two recent review articles summarized results of these early clinical studies showing that both olcegepant and MK-0974, in addition to causing a better headache response, produced a significantly better pain-free state at 2 h and a better recurrence rate (olcegepant) or sustained pain-free condition (MK-0974) as compared with a placebo (Doods et al. 2007). Of interest is the report (Knotkova et al. 2008) that the sustained pain-free rate at 24 h after MK-0974 administration showed a tendency to be superior to that of rizatriptan (Ho et al. 2007), and that after olcegepant administration it was also apparently better than that produced in a study with sumatriptan (Ferrari et al. 2001). Obviously, further studies and in particular phase III randomized and placebo controlled trials are need to confirm these early results and to show a highly desirable superiority of CGRP antagonists, in terms of safety and duration of action, over current antimigraine medicines.

7 Conclusions

The recent clinical data obtained with chemically different CGRP antagonists point to this neuropepeptide, selectively released from a subset of nociceptive TRPV1-expressing trigeminal nerve fibers, as an important contributing molecule in the mechanism of migraine. This implies that whatever the initiating factor, primary sensory neurons of cranial nerve V play a key role in migraine. The most parsimonious hypothesis to explain the beneficial effect of CGRP receptor blockade in migraine suggests that olcegepant or MK-0974 inhibits the receptor expressed on vascular smooth muscle cells and the subsequent vasodilatation provoked by CGRP within the cranial microcirculation, which somehow is associated with the headache phase of the migraine attack. This hypothesis conflicts with some evidence that vasodilatation is not always present or may be only an epiphenomenon in migraine. On the other hand, the hypothesis that the beneficial effect of olcegepant is due to a central mode of action is challenged by the finding that this peptoid molecule does not very effectively antagonize CGRP-mediated vasodilatation of intracerebral vessels (Petersen et al. 2005), and therefore is assumed not to cross the blood-brain barrier readily. A recent detailed investigation on the distribution of immunoreactivity for the CL receptor, RAMP-1, or CGRP in the rat trigeminovascular system (Lennerz et al. 2008) identified individual components of the CGRP pathway in peripheral and central cells and did not exclude the possibility that a central site of action is involved in migraine mechanism. However, "complete" and therefore functional receptors were only observed in arterial smooth muscle cells and possibly in inflammatory cells of the macrophage lineage and in Schwann cells (Lennerz et al. 2008). Thus, the absence of "mature" receptors in neurons of the spinal trigeminal nucleus or of autoreceptors in sensory nerve endings cannot exclude, but strongly argues against, the hypothesis that antimigraine CGRP-receptor antagonists act at a central site of action. During the last 5 years, major progress has been accomplished in the perspective of a better therapy of migraine. This advancement also has an enormous impact on the understanding of the mechanism of the disease, and further confirms that better knowledge of the pathophysiological and pharmacological aspects of trigeminal primary sensory neurons can be one of the main strategies to fight against migraine and other primary headaches.

During the completion of the present chapter a report of a phase III study has been published (Ho TW, Ferrari MD, Dodick DW, Galet V, Kost J, Fan X, Leibensperger H, Froman S, Assaid C, Lines C, Koppen H, Winner PK (2008) Efficacy and tolerability of MK-0974 (telcagepant), a new oral antagonist of calcitonin gene-related peptide receptor, compared with zolmitriptan for acute migraine: a randomised, placebo-controlled, parallel-treatment trial (2008) Lancet 372:2115–23). Results show that the orally active CGRP receptor antagonist, telgacepant (300 mg), is more effective than placebo and as effective as zolmitroptan (5 mg) in reducing the headache and other symptoms of migraine attacks, with fewer adverse effects than the triptan.

Acknowledgements The paper was supported in part by grants from Consorzio Ferrara Ricerche, Ferrara, and by Fondazione DEI-Onlus, Florence, Italy.

References

Aiyar N, Daines RA, Disa J et al (2001) Pharmacology of SB-273779, a nonpeptide calcitonin gene-related peptide 1 receptor antagonist. J Pharmacol Exp Ther 296:768–775

Alessandri-Haber N, Yeh JJ, Boyd AE et al (2003) Hypotonicity induces TRPV4-mediated nociception in rat. Neuron 39:497–511

Amara SG, Arriza JL, Leff SE et al (1985) Expression in brain of a messenger RNA encoding a novel neuropeptide homologous to calcitonin gene-related peptide. Science 229:1094–1097

Baluk P, Bertrand C, Geppetti P et al (1995) NK1 receptors mediate leukocyte adhesion in neurogenic inflammation in the rat trachea. Am J Physiol 268:L263–L269

Bandell M, Story GM, Hwang SW et al (2004) Noxious cold ion channel TRPA1 is activated by pungent compounds and bradykinin. Neuron 41:849–857

Bautista DM, Jordt SE, Nikai T et al (2006) TRPA1 mediates the inflammatory actions of environmental irritants and proalgesic agents. Cell 124:1269–1282

Bautista DM, Siemens J, Glazer JM et al (2007) The menthol receptor TRPM8 is the principal detector of environmental cold. Nature 448:204–208

Bevan S, Geppetti P (1994) Protons: small stimulants of capsaicin-sensitive sensory nerves. Trends Neurosci 17:509–512

Boeglin D, Hamdan FF, Melendez RE et al (2007) Calcitonin gene-related peptide analogues with aza and indolizidinone amino acid residues reveal conformational requirements for antagonist activity at the human calcitonin gene-related peptide 1 receptor. J Med Chem 50:1401–1408

Brain SD, Williams TJ (1989) Interactions between the tachykinins and calcitonin gene-related peptide lead to the modulation of oedema formation and blood flow in rat skin. Br J Pharmacol 97:77–82

Brain SD, Williams TJ, Tippins JR et al (1985) Calcitonin gene-related peptide is a potent vasodilator. Nature 313:54–56

Brazil P, Friedman A (1957) Further observations in craniovascular studies. Neurology 7:52–55

Caterina MJ, Schumacher MA, Tominaga M et al (1997) The capsaicin receptor: a heat-activated ion channel in the pain pathway. Nature 389:816–824

Caterina MJ, Rosen TA, Tominaga M et al (1999) A capsaicin-receptor homologue with a high threshold for noxious heat. Nature 398:436–441

Chiba T, Yamaguchi A, Yamatani T et al (1989) Calcitonin gene-related peptide receptor antagonist human CGRP-(8–37). Am J Physiol Endocrinol Metab 256:E331–E335

Chuang HH, Prescott ED, Kong H et al (2001) Bradykinin and nerve growth factor release the capsaicin receptor from PtdIns(4,5)P2-mediated inhibition. Nature 411:957–962

Connor H, Bertin L, Gillies S et al (1998) The GR205171 clinical study group. Clinical evaluation of a novel, potent, CNS penetrating NK1 receptor antagonist in the acute treatment of migraine. Cephalalgia 18:392

Cooper GJS, Willis AC, Clark A et al (1987) Purification and characterization of a peptide from amyloid-rich pancreases of type 2 diabetic patients. Proc Natl Acad Sci USA 84:8628–8632

Diener HC (2003) RPR100893, a substance-P antagonist, is not effective in the treatment of migraine attacks. Cephalalgia 23:183–185

Doods H (2001) Development of CGRP antagonists for the treatment of migraine. Curr Opin Investig Drugs 2:1261–1268

Doods H, Hallermayer G, Wu D et al (2000) Pharmacological profile of BIBN4096BS, the first selective small molecule CGRP antagonist. Br J Pharmacol 129:420–423

Doods H, Arndt K, Rudolf K et al (2007) CGRP antagonists: unravelling the role of CGRP in migraine. Trends Pharmacol Sci 28:580–587

Durham PL (2004) CGRP-receptor antagonists – a fresh approach to migraine therapy? New Engl J Med 350:1073–1075

Edvinsson L (2004) Blockade of CGRP receptors in the intracranial vasculature: a new target in the treatment of headache. Cephalalgia 24:611–622

Edvinsson L, Sams A, Jansen-Olesen I et al (2001) Characterisation of the effects of a non-peptide CGRP receptor antagonist in SK-N-MC cells and isolated human cerebral arteries. Eur J Pharmacol 415:39–44

Ennis MD, Ghazal NB, Hoffman RL et al (1998) Isochroman-6-carboxamides as highly selective 5-HT1D agonists: potential new treatment for migraine without cardiovascular side effects. J Med Chem 41:2180–2183

Fanciullacci M, Tramontana M, Bianco ED et al (1991) Low pH medium induces calcium dependent release of CGRP from sensory nerves of guinea-pig dural venous sinuses. Life Sci 49:PL27–PL30

Fanciullacci M, Alessandri M, Figini M et al (1995) Increase in plasma calcitonin gene-related peptide from the extracerebral circulation during nitroglycerin-induced cluster headache attack. Pain 60:119–123

Fay T (1935) The mechanism of headache. Trans Am Neurol Assoc 62:74–77

Feindel W, Penfield W, Mc NF (1960) The tentorial nerves and localization of intracranial pain in man. Neurology 10:555–563

Fernandez-Patron C, Stewart KG, Zhang Y et al (2000) Vascular matrix metalloproteinase-2-dependent cleavage of calcitonin gene-related peptide promotes vasoconstriction. Circ Res 87:670–676

Ferrari MD, Saxena PR (1993) On serotonin and migraine: a clinical and pharmacological review. Cephalalgia 13:151–165

Ferrari MD, Roon KI, Lipton RB et al (2001) Oral triptans (serotonin 5-HT(1B/1D) agonists) in acute migraine treatment: a meta-analysis of 53 trials. Lancet 358:1668–1675

Fluhmann B, Muff R, Hunziker W et al (1995) A human orphan calcitonin receptor-like structure. Biochem Biophys Res Commun 206:341–347
Franco-Cereceda A (1991) Calcitonin gene-related peptide and human epicardial coronary arteries: presence, release and vasodilator effects. Br J Pharmacol 102:506–510
Gazzieri D, Trevisani M, Springer J et al (2007) Substance P released by TRPV1-expressing neurons produces reactive oxygen species that mediate ethanol-induced gastric injury. Free Radic Biol Med. 43:581–589
Geppetti P, Holzer P (1996) Neurogenic inflammation. CRC, Boca Raton
Geppetti P, Del Bianco E, Cecconi R et al (1992) Capsaicin releases calcitonin gene-related peptide from the human iris and ciliary body in vitro. Regul Pept 41:83–92
Giffin NJ, Kowacs F, Libri V et al (2003) Effect of the adenosine A1 receptor agonist GR79236 on trigeminal nociception with blink reflex recordings in healthy human subjects. Cephalalgia 23:287–292
Goadsby PJ, Edvinsson L, Ekman R (1990) Vasoactive peptide release in the extracerebral circulation of humans during migraine headache. Ann Neurol 28:183–187
Goadsby PJ, Lipton RB, Ferrari MD (2002a) Migraine – current understanding and treatment. New Engl J Med 346:257–270
Goadsby PJ, Hoskin KL, Storer RJ et al (2002b) Adenosine A1 receptor agonists inhibit trigeminovascular nociceptive transmission. Brain 125:1392–1401
Goldstein DJ, Wang O, Saper JR et al (1997) Ineffectiveness of neurokinin-1 antagonist in acute migraine: a crossover study. Cephalalgia 17:785–790
Goldstein J, Roon I, Offen W et al (1999) Migraine treatment with selective with 5-ht1F receptor agonist (SSOFRA) LY334370. Cephalalgia 19:318
Gomez-Mancilla B, Cutler N, Leibowitz M et al (2001) Safety and efficacy of PNU-142633, a selective 5-HT1D agonist, in patients with acute migraine. Cephalalgia 21:727–732
Graham J, Wolff H (1938) Mechanism of migraine headache and action of ergotamine tartrate. Arch Neurol Psychiatry 39:737–763
Gray DW, Marshall I (1992) Human alpha-calcitonin gene-related peptide stimulates adenylate cyclase and guanylate cyclase and relaxes rat thoracic aorta by releasing nitric oxide. Br J Pharmacol 107:691–696
Ho TW, Mannix LK, Fan X et al (2007) Randomized controlled trial of an oral CGRP antagonist, MK-0974, in acute treatment of migraine. Neurology 70:1304–1312
Huang SM, Bisogno T, Trevisani M et al (2002) An endogenous capsaicin-like substance with high potency at recombinant and native vanilloid VR1 receptors. Proc Natl Acad Sci USA 99:8400–8405
Humphrey PP, Bland-Ward PA, Carruthers AM et al (2001) Inhibition of trigemnial nociceptive afferents by adenosine A1 receptor activation: a novel approach towards the design of new anti-migraine compounds. Cephalalgia 21:268–269
Hwang SW, Cho H, Kwak J et al (2000) Direct activation of capsaicin receptors by products of lipoxygenases: endogenous capsaicin-like substances. Proc Natl Acad Sci USA 97:6155–6156
Jordt SE, Bautista DM, Chuang HH et al (2004) Mustard oils and cannabinoids excite sensory nerve fibres through the TRP channel ANKTM1. Nature 427:260–265
Juhasz G, Zsombok T, Modos EA et al (2003) NO-induced migraine attack: strong increase in plasma calcitonin gene-related peptide (CGRP) concentration and negative correlation with platelet serotonin release. Pain 106:461–470
Kapoor K, Arulmani U, Heiligers JPC et al (2003) Effects of the CGRP receptor antagonist BIBN4096BS on capsaicin-induced carotid haemodynamic changes in anaesthetised pigs. Br J Pharmacol 140:329–338
Kitamura K, Kangawa K, Kawamoto M et al (1993) Adrenomedullin: a novel hypotensive peptide isolated from human pheochromocytoma. Biochem Biophys Res Commun 192:553–560
Knotkova H, Pappagallo M, Szallasi A (2008) Capsaicin (TRPV1 Agonist) therapy for pain relief: farewell or revival? Clin J Pain 24:142–154
Lance J (1969) Mechanism and management of headache. Butterworths, New York

Lassen LH, Haderslev PA, Jacobsen VB et al (2002) CGRP may play a causative role in migraine. Cephalalgia 22:54–61

Lennerz JK, Ruhle V, Ceppa EP et al (2008) Calcitonin receptor-like receptor (CLR), receptor activity-modifying protein 1 (RAMP1), and calcitonin gene-related peptide (CGRP) immunoreactivity in the rat trigeminovascular system: differences between peripheral and central CGRP receptor distribution. J Comp Neurol 507:1277–1299

Lewis T (1937) The nocifensor system of nerves and its reactions. Br Med J 194:431–435

Liedtke W, Choe Y, Marti-Renom MA et al (2000) Vanilloid receptor-related osmotically activated channel (VR-OAC), a candidate vertebrate osmoreceptor. Cell 103:525–535

Macpherson LJ, Geierstanger BH, Viswanath V et al (2005) The pungency of garlic: activation of TRPA1 and TRPV1 in response to allicin. Curr Biol 15:929–934

Markowitz S, Saito K, Moskowitz MA (1987) Neurogenically mediated leakage of plasma protein occurs from blood vessels in dura mater but not brain. J Neurosci 7:4129–4136

McKemy DD, Neuhausser WM, Julius D (2002) Identification of a cold receptor reveals a general role for TRP channels in thermosensation. Nature 416:52–58

McLatchie LM, Fraser NJ, Main MJ et al (1998) RAMPs regulate the transport and ligand specificity of the calcitonin-receptor-like receptor. Nature 393:333–339

Morris HR, Panico M, Etienne T et al (1984) Isolation and characterization of human calcitonin gene-related peptide. Nature 308:746–748

Moskowitz MA, Buzzi MG (1991) Neuroeffector functions of sensory fibres: implications for headache mechanisms and drug actions. J Neurol 238:S18–S22

Mudderry PK, Ghatei MA, Spokes RA et al (1988) Differential expression of [alpha]-CGRP and [beta]-CGRP by primary sensory neurons and enteric autonomic neurons of the rat. Neuroscience 25:195–205

Nagata K, Duggan A, Kumar G et al (2005) Nociceptor and hair cell transducer properties of TRPA1, a channel for pain and hearing. J Neurosci 25:4052–4061

Nicoletti P, Trevisani M, Manconi M et al (2008) Ethanol causes neurogenic vasodilation by TRPV1 activation and CGRP release in the trigeminovascular system of the guinea pig. Cephalalgia 28:9–17

Nilius B, Owsianik G, Voets T et al (2007) Transient receptor potential cation channels in disease. Physiol Rev 87:165–217

Njuki F, Nicholl CG, Howard A et al (1993) A new calcitonin-receptor-like sequence in rat pulmonary blood vessels. Clin Sci (Lond) 85:385–388

Olesen J, Diener HC, Husstedt IW et al (2004) Calcitonin gene-related peptide receptor antagonist BIBN 4096 BS for the acute treatment of migraine. N Engl J Med 350:1104–1110

Paone DV, Shaw AW, Nguyen DN et al (2007) Potent, orally bioavailable calcitonin gene-related peptide receptor antagonists for the treatment of migraine: discovery of *N*-[(3*R*,6*S*)-6-(2,3-difluorophenyl)-2-oxo-1-(2,2,2-trifluoroethyl)azepan-3-yl]-4-(2-oxo-2,3-dihydro-1*H*-imidazo [4,5-b]pyridin-1-yl)piperidine-1-carboxamide (MK-0974). J Med Chem 50:5564–5567

Peier AM, Moqrich A, Hergarden AC et al (2002) A TRP channel that senses cold stimuli and menthol. Cell 108:705–715

Penfield W, McNaughton M (1940) Dural headache and the innervation of the dura mater. Arch Neurol Psychiatr 44:43–75

Petermann J, Born W, Chang J et al (1987) Identification in the human central nervous system, pituitary, and thyroid of a novel calcitonin gene-related peptide, and partial amino acid sequence in the spinal cord. J Biol Chem 262:542–545

Petersen K, Birk S, Lassen L et al (2005) The CGRP-antagonist, BIBN4096BS does not affect cerebral or systemic haemodynamics in healthy volunteers. Cephalalgia 25:139–147

Premkumar LS, Ahern GP (2000) Induction of vanilloid receptor channel activity by protein kinase C. Nature 408:985–990

Quirion R, D Van Rossum, Dumont Y et al (1992) Characterization of CGRP1 and CGRP2 receptor subtypes. Ann N Y Acad Sci 657:88–105

Raddino R, Pela G, Manca C et al (1997) Mechanism of action of human calcitonin gene-related peptide in rabbit heart and in human mammary arteries. J Cardiovasc Pharmacol 29:463–470
Ramadan NM, Skljarevski V, Phebus LA et al (2003) 5-HT1F receptor agonists in acute migraine treatment: a hypothesis. Cephalalgia 23:776–785
Ray B, Wolff H (1940) Experimental studies on headache: pain-sensitive structures of the head and their significance in headache. Arch Surg 41:813–856
Salvatore CA, Hershey JC, Corcoran HA et al (2008) Pharmacological characterization of MK-0974 [*N*-[(3*R*,6*S*)-6-(2,3-difluorophenyl)-2-oxo-1-(2,2,2-trifluoroethyl)azepan-3-yl]-4-(2-oxo-2,3-dihydro-1*H*-imidazo[4,5-b]pyridin-1-yl)piperidine-1-carbox amide], a potent and orally active calcitonin gene-related peptide receptor antagonist for the treatment of migraine. J Pharmacol Exp Ther 324:416–421
Schoonman GG, van der Grond J, Kortmann C et al (2008) Migraine headache is not associated with cerebral or meningeal vasodilatation – a 3T magnetic resonance angiography study. Brain 131:2192–2200
Simone DA, Ochoa J (1991) Early and late effects of prolonged topical capsaicin on cutaneous sensibility and neurogenic vasodilatation in humans. Pain 47:285–294
Smith D, Hill RG, Edvinsson L et al (2002) An immunocytochemical investigation of human trigeminal nucleus caudalis: CGRP, substance P and 5-HT1D-receptor immunoreactivities are expressed by trigeminal sensory fibres. Cephalalgia 22:424–431
Snider RM, Constantine JW, Lowe JA 3rd et al (1991) A potent nonpeptide antagonist of the substance P (NK1) receptor. Science 251:435–437
Story GM, Peier AM, Reeve AJ et al (2003) ANKTM1, a TRP-like channel expressed in nociceptive neurons, is activated by cold temperatures. Cell 112:819–829
Struthers AD, Brown MJ, Macdonald DW et al (1986) Human calcitonin gene related peptide: a potent endogenous vasodilator in man. Clin Sci (Lond) 70:389–393
Szallasi A, Blumberg PM (1999) Vanilloid (capsaicin) receptors and mechanisms. Pharmacol Rev 51:159–212
Szolcsanyi J (1977) A pharmacological approach to elucidation of the role of different nerve fibres and receptor endings in mediation of pain. J Physiol 73:251–259
Taylor CK, Smith DD, Hulce M et al (2006) Pharmacological characterization of novel alpha-calcitonin gene-related peptide (CGRP) receptor peptide antagonists that are selective for human CGRP receptors. J Pharmacol Exp Ther 319:749–757
Tfelt-Hansen P, De Vries P, Saxena PR (2000) Triptans in migraine: a comparative review of pharmacology, pharmacokinetics and efficacy. Drugs 60:1259–1287
Thomsen LL, Iversen HK, Brinck TA et al (1993) Arterial supersensitivity to nitric oxide (nitroglycerin) in migraine sufferers. Cephalalgia 13:395–399
Tominaga M, Caterina MJ, Malmberg AB et al (1998) The cloned capsaicin receptor integrates multiple pain-producing stimuli. Neuron 21:531–543
Trevisani M, Smart D, Gunthorpe MJ et al (2002) Ethanol elicits and potentiates nociceptor responses via the vanilloid receptor-1. Nat Neurosci 5:546–551
Welch KMA (2003) Concepts of migraine headache pathogenesis: insights into mechanisms of chronicity and new drug targets. Neurol Sci 24:S149–S153
Williamson DJ, Hill RG, Shepheard SL et al (2001) The anti-migraine 5-HT(1B/1D) agonist rizatriptan inhibits neurogenic dural vasodilation in anaesthetized guinea-pigs. Br J Pharmacol 133:1029–1034
Wolff H (1948) Headache and other head pain. Oxford University Press, New York, pp 59–97
Zygmunt PM, Petersson J, Andersson DA et al (1999) Vanilloid receptors on sensory nerves mediate the vasodilator action of anandamide. Nature 400:452–457

Afferent Nerve Regulation of Bladder Function in Health and Disease

William C. de Groat and Naoki Yoshimura

Contents

W.C. de Groat (✉)
Department of Pharmacology, West 1352 Starzl Biomedical Science Tower, University of Pittsburgh School of Medicine, Pittsburgh, PA 15261, USA
degroat@server.pharm.pitt.edu

B.J. Canning and D. Spina (eds.), *Sensory Nerves*,
Handbook of Experimental Pharmacology 194, DOI: 10.1007/978-3-540-79090-7_4,

Abstract The afferent innervation of the urinary bladder consists primarily of small myelinated (Aδ) and unmyelinated (C-fiber) axons that respond to chemical and mechanical stimuli. Immunochemical studies indicate that bladder afferent neurons synthesize several putative neurotransmitters, including neuropeptides, glutamic acid, aspartic acid, and nitric oxide. The afferent neurons also express various types of receptors and ion channels, including transient receptor potential channels, purinergic, muscarinic, endothelin, neurotrophic factor, and estrogen receptors. Patch-clamp recordings in dissociated bladder afferent neurons and recordings of bladder afferent nerve activity have revealed that activation of many of these receptors enhances neuronal excitability. Afferent nerves can respond to chemicals present in urine as well as chemicals released in the bladder wall from nerves, smooth muscle, inflammatory cells, and epithelial cells lining the bladder lumen. Pathological conditions alter the chemical and electrical properties of bladder afferent pathways, leading to urinary urgency, increased voiding frequency, nocturia, urinary incontinence, and pain. Neurotrophic factors have been implicated in the pathophysiological mechanisms underlying the sensitization of bladder afferent nerves. Neurotoxins such as capsaicin, resiniferatoxin, and botulinum neurotoxin that target sensory nerves are useful in treating disorders of the lower urinary tract.

Keywords Cystitis, Neurotrophic factors, Overactive bladder, Spinal cord injury, Neuroplasticity.

1 Anatomy and Innervation of the Lower Urinary Tract

The storage and periodic elimination of urine are dependent upon the activity of two functional units in the lower urinary tract: (1) a reservoir (the urinary bladder) and (2) an outlet consisting of the bladder neck, urethra, and striated muscles of the external urethral sphincter (EUS) (Fig. 1) (Fowler et al. 2008; Morrison et al. 2005). These structures are in turn regulated by three sets of peripheral nerves: sacral parasympathetic (pelvic nerves), thoracolumbar sympathetic (hypogastric nerves and sympathetic chain), and somatic nerves (pudendal nerves) distributed bilaterally (Fig. 1) (de Groat 1986; Morrison et al. 2005). The nerves consist of efferent and afferent axons originating at thoracolumbar and sacral spinal levels. Parasympathetic efferent nerves contract the bladder and relax the urethra. Sympathetic efferent nerves relax the bladder and contract the urethra. Somatic efferent nerves contract the EUS.

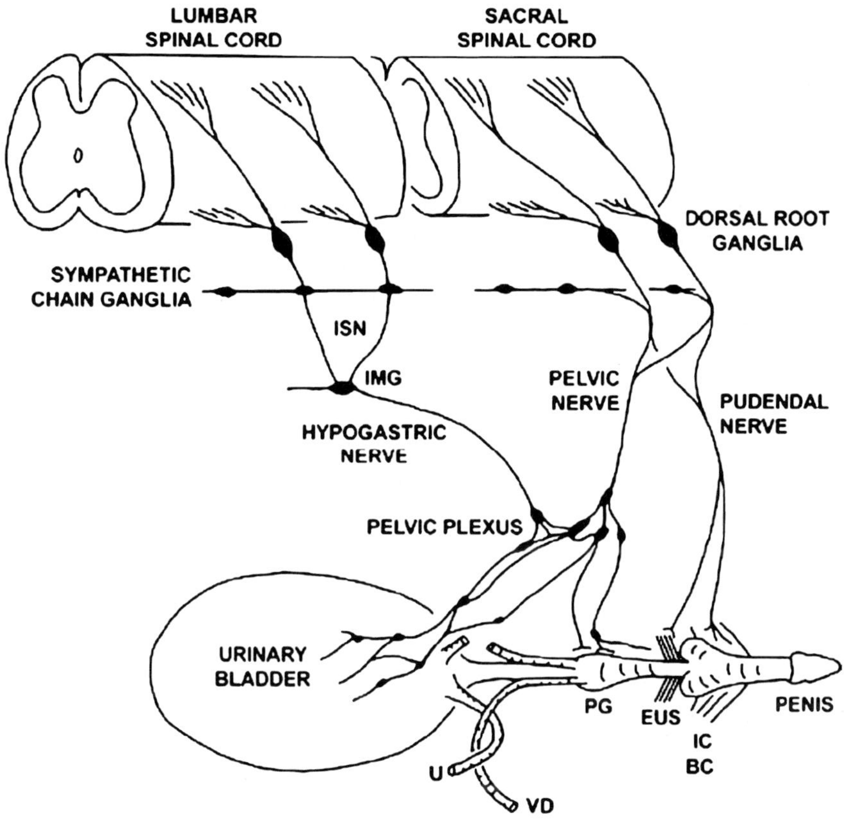

Fig. 1 Sympathetic, parasympathetic, and somatic innervation of the urogenital tract of the male cat. Sympathetic preganglionic pathways emerge from the lumbar spinal cord and pass to the sympathetic chain ganglia and then via the inferior splanchnic nerves (*ISN*) to the inferior mesenteric ganglia (*IMG*). Preganglionic and postganglionic sympathetic axons then travel in the hypogastric nerve to the pelvic plexus and the urogenital organs. Parasympathetic preganglionic axons which originate in the sacral spinal cord pass in the pelvic nerve to ganglion cells in the pelvic plexus and to distal ganglia in the organs. Sacral somatic pathways are contained in the pudendal nerve, which provides an innervation to the penis, the ischiocavernosus (*IC*), bulbocavernosus (*BC*), and external urethral sphincter (*EUS*) muscles. The pudendal and pelvic nerves also receive postganglionic axons from the caudal sympathetic chain ganglia. These three sets of nerves contain afferent axons from the lumbosacral dorsal root ganglia. *U* ureter, *PG* prostate gland, *VD* vas deferens

1.1 Afferent Nerves

The afferent innervation of the human lower urinary tract arises from neurons located in the dorsal root ganglia (DRG) at S2–S4 and T11–L2 spinal segmental levels. Axons in the pelvic and pudendal nerves originate in sacral DRG, whereas those in the hypogastric nerves originate in the rostral lumbar and caudal thoracic DRG. A similar segmental organization occurs in nonhuman primates, cats (Fig. 1), and dogs. In rats, pelvic and pudendal afferent neurons are located in the sacral and most caudal lumbar DRG.

The urinary bladder, which is divided into two parts, the fundus (body) and the trigone (base or neck), consists of several layers: serosal, muscularis, lamina propria, and urothelium. Afferent axons, identified primarily by neuropeptide immunoreactivity for calcitonin-gene-related peptide (CGRP), pituitary adenylate cyclase activating polypeptide (PACAP), or substance P (SP), are distributed throughout the bladder wall (Gabella and Davis 1998; Smet et al. 1997; Uemura et al. 1973) from the serosal layer to the lamina propria, including a dense suburothelial plexus that gives rise to axons extending into the urothelium (Birder et al. 2008; Fowler et al. 2008). In the cat bladder, sacral afferents are more abundant in the muscularis than in the suburothelium and have a more uniform distribution throughout the fundus and trigone regions, whereas the lumbar afferents are localized to the trigone and are more abundant in the suburothelium than in the muscularis (Uemura et al. 1975). In human and animal bladders, peptidergic afferent axons are also located around blood vessels and in close proximity to intramural ganglion cells where they may make synaptic connections and participate in local reflex networks within the bladder wall (Gillespie et al. 2006; Smet et al. 1997).

In the urethra, the afferent nerves are also distributed between the muscle fibers, around blood vessels, in the urothelium, and in a dense suburothelial plexus (Crowe et al. 1986; Fahrenkrug and Hannibal 1998; Tainio 1993). In some species afferent nerves extend to the luminal surface of the urothelium. The striated sphincter muscle that surrounds the urethra receives a very sparse afferent innervation that is localized primarily to nerve bundles passing between the muscle bundles. Specialized tension receptors (muscle spindles) which are innervated by large-diameter myelinated group IA afferents and which are prominent in most striated muscles are absent (Gosling et al. 1981) or are present in low density (Lassmann 1984) in striated sphincter muscles.

Retrograde axonal tracing methods have identified DRG cells innervating the bladder, urethra, and EUS (Fig. 2a). Afferent nerves arising in DRG on one side of the spinal cord appear to be distributed bilaterally in the bladder wall (Chai et al. 1996). Relatively small numbers, less than 3% of the total population of neurons in an individual DRG, innervate the lower urinary tract, e.g., fewer than 3,000 sacral afferent neurons innervate the bladder of the cat (de Groat 1986; Morgan et al. 1981). The neurons are small to medium-sized (mean, 32 μm × 23 μm in the cat) and are distributed randomly throughout the DRG.

When different axonal tracers are injected into multiple pelvic organs, e.g., bladder and colon, a small percentage (5–15%) of DRG neurons are doubled-labeled (Christianson et al. 2007; Keast and de Groat 1992; Malykhina et al. 2006), indicating that individual sensory neurons can innervate multiple target organs. As discussed in Sect. 12, this pattern of innervation may contribute to the phenomenon of cross-sensitization of afferent pathways and provide a mechanism by which disease in one organ can influence sensations in an adjacent organ (Christianson et al. 2007; Pezzone et al. 2005).

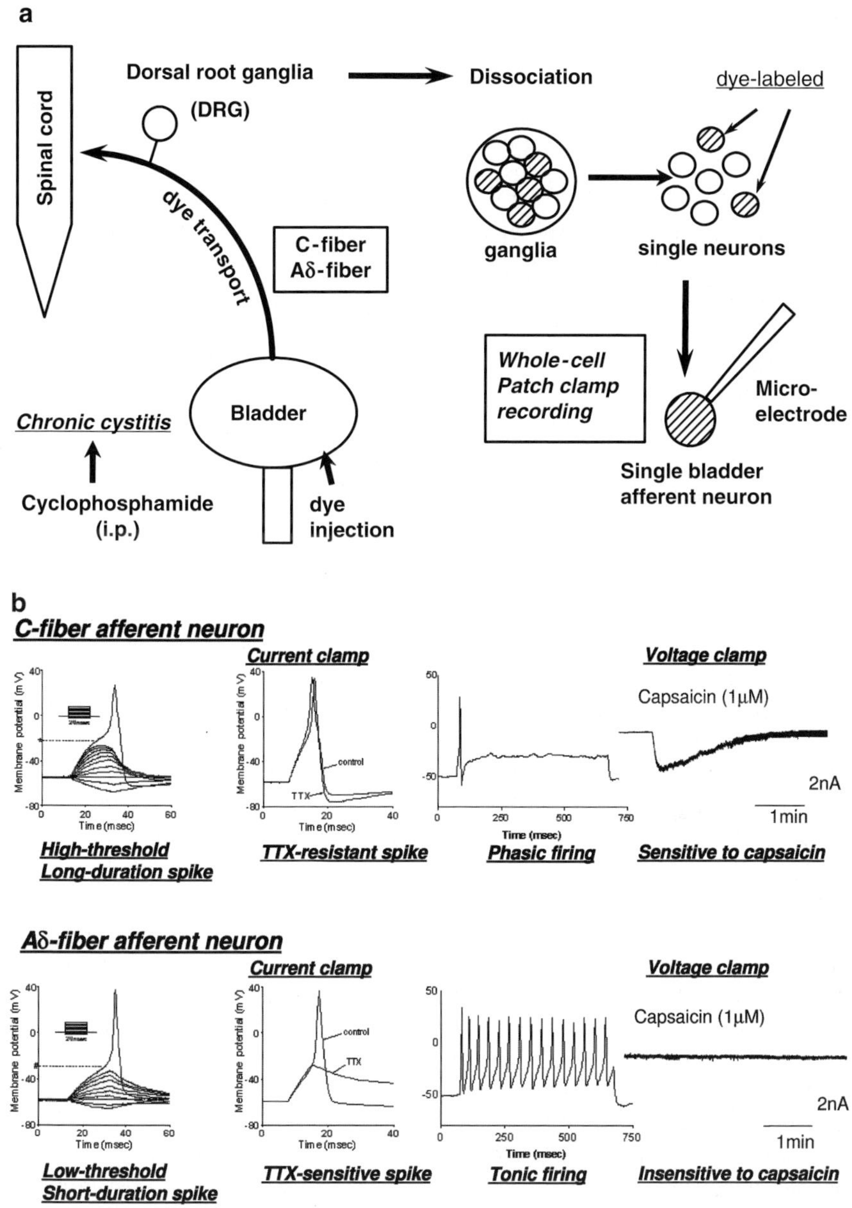

Fig. 2 **(a)** Experimental methods for performing patch-clamp recordings on bladder afferent neurons obtained from rats with chronic cystitis. Chronic cystitis was induced by intraperitoneal injection of cyclophosphamide. Fluorescent dye (fast blue) injected into the bladder wall was transported via Aδ- and C-fiber bladder afferent axons to neurons in the dorsal root ganglia (*DRG*). L6 and S1 DRG were dissected and dissociated into single neurons by enzymatic methods. Whole-cell patch-clamp recordings were then performed on fast blue-labeled bladder afferent neurons that were identified with a fluorescence microscope. **(b)** Characteristics of a bladder afferent neuron

1.2 Central Afferent Pathways

Central projections of afferent neurons innervating the lower urinary tract and the relationship between these projections and the spinal interneurons and efferent neurons have been studied by anterograde and retrograde axonal tracing methods. Parasympathetic preganglionic neurons are located in the intermediolateral gray matter (laminae V–VII) in the sacral segments of the spinal cord (de Groat et al. 1981; Morgan et al. 1993), whereas sympathetic preganglionic neurons are located in medial (lamina X) and lateral (laminae V–VII) sites in the rostral lumbar spinal cord. EUS motoneurons are located in lamina IX in Onuf's nucleus (Thor et al. 1989b; de Groat et al. 2001; Morrison et al. 2005). Parasympathetic preganglionic neurons and EUS motoneurons send dendrites to similar regions of the spinal cord (laminae I, V–VII, and X), indicating that these sites contain important pathways for coordinating bladder and sphincter function (Morgan et al. 1993).

Afferent pathways from the lower urinary tract labeled by transganglionic transport of tracers project to discrete regions of the dorsal horn that contain the soma and/or dendrites of efferent neurons innervating the lower urinary tract (Fig. 3b). Afferent pathways from the urinary bladder of the cat (Morgan et al. 1981; de Groat 1986) and rat (Jancso and Maggi 1987; Steers et al. 1991a) project into Lissauer's tract in the lumbosacral spinal cord and then pass rostrocaudally giving off collaterals that extend through lamina I laterally and medially around the dorsal horn into deeper laminae (laminae V–VII and X) at the base of the dorsal horn. The lateral pathway, which is the most prominent projection (Fig. 3b), terminates in the region of the sacral parasympathetic nucleus (SPN) and also sends some axons medially to the dorsal commissure. Bladder afferents have not been detected in the center of the dorsal horn (laminae III–IV) or in the ventral horn. Afferent axons from the pelvic viscera of the cat passing through sympathetic nerves to the rostral lumbar segments have similar sites of termination in laminae I, V–VII, and X (Morgan et al. 1986). Although afferents are distributed primarily to the ipsilateral side of the spinal cord, an estimated 10–20% also project to the opposite side of the cord (Applebaum et al. 1980; Jänig and Morrison 1986).

Fig. 2 (Continued) (24-μm diameter, C-fiber afferent neuron, *top record*) exhibiting tetrodotoxin (TTX)-resistant action potentials and a bladder afferent neuron (33-μm diameter, Aδ-fiber afferent neuron, *bottom record*) exhibiting TTX-sensitive action potentials. The *left panels* are voltage responses and action potentials evoked by 30-ms depolarizing current pulses injected through the patch pipette in current-clamp conditions. *Asterisks with dashed lines* indicate the thresholds for spike activation. The *second panels on the left side* show the effects of TTX application (1 μM) on action potentials. The *third panels from the left* show firing patterns during membrane depolarization (700-ms duration). The *panels on the right* show the responses to extracellular application of capsaicin (1 μM) in voltage-clamp conditions. Note that the TTX-resistant bladder afferent neuron (**a**) exhibited phasic firing (i.e., one to two spikes during prolonged membrane depolarization) and an inward current in response to capsaicin, while the TTX-sensitive afferent neuron exhibited tonic firing (i.e., repetitive firing during membrane depolarization) and no response to capsaicin

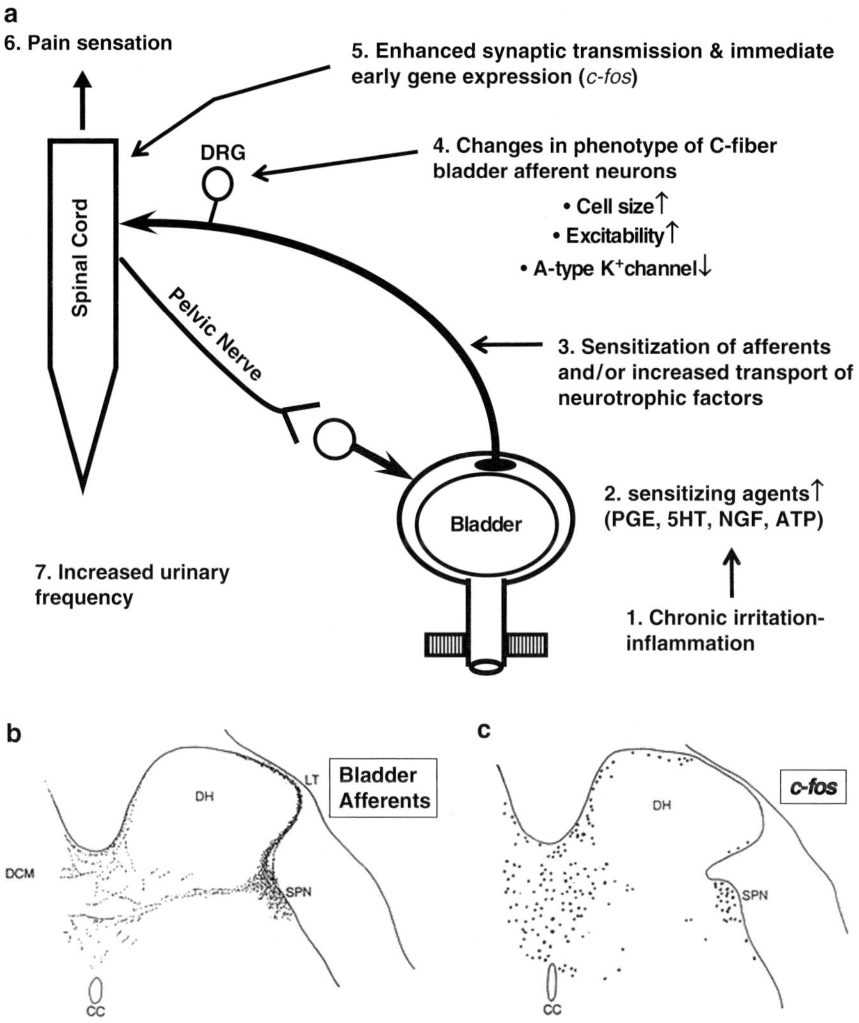

Fig. 3 (**a**) Summary of the events involved in chronic inflammation of the bladder and hyperexcitability of C-fiber bladder afferent neurons. The events that occur following chronic bladder inflammation (*1*) are indicated by sequential numbers (*2–7*). *DRG* dorsal root ganglia, *5-HT* serotonin, *PGE* prostaglandin E, *NGF* nerve growth factor. (**b**) Primary afferent pathways to the L6 spinal cord of the rat project to the dorsal commissure (*DCM*), the superficial dorsal horn (*DH*), and the sacral parasympathetic nucleus (*SPN*), which contains parasympathetic preganglionic neurons. The afferent nerves consist of myelinated Aδ axons, which respond to bladder distension and contraction, and unmyelinated C-fiber axons, which respond to noxious stimuli. (**c**) Spinal neurons that express *c-fos* following the activation of bladder afferents by a noxious stimulus (acetic acid) to the bladder are located in the same regions of the L6 spinal segment that receive afferent input

Pudendal nerve afferent pathways from the EUS of the cat have central terminations that overlap in part with those of bladder afferents in lateral laminae I and V–VII and in lamina X (de Groat 1986; Thor et al. 1989b). These afferents differ markedly from other populations of pudendal nerve afferents that terminate in the deeper layers of the dorsal horn (laminae II–IV). The latter innervate sex organs as well as cutaneous and subcutaneous tissues of the perineum (Ueyama et al. 1984; Thor et al. 1989b).

The spinal neurons involved in processing afferent input from the lower urinary tract have been identified by the expression of the immediate early gene *c-fos* (Fig. 3c). In the rat, noxious or nonnoxious stimulation of the bladder and urethra increases the levels of Fos protein primarily in the dorsal commissure, the superficial dorsal horn, and in the area of the SPN (Birder and de Groat 1993; Birder et al. 1999; Vizzard 2000a). Noxious stimulation induces *c-fos* expression in a greater number of spinal neurons and in a larger number of neurons in the dorsal commissure (Fig. 3c). Some of these interneurons send long projections to the brain, whereas others make local connections in the spinal cord and participate in segmental spinal reflexes (Birder et al. 1999).

2 Histological and Chemical Properties of Afferent Nerves

Light and electron microscopy has revealed that the visceral nerves innervating the lower urinary tract are composed primarily of small myelinated (Aδ) and unmyelinated (C-fiber) axons (Hulsebosch and Coggeshall 1982; Gabella and Davis 1998; Uvelius and Gabella 1998). The cat pelvic and hypogastric nerves contain axons less than 2–3 μm in diameter, with a few larger axons 5–10 μm in diameter. The rat pelvic and hypogastric nerves contain approximately 25,000 and 21,000 axons, respectively, of which 94% are unmyelinated (Hulsebosch and Coggeshall 1982). On the other hand, the pudendal nerve in the rat contains larger-diameter myelinated as well as unmyelinated axons (Hulsebosch and Coggeshall 1982). The total number of axons in these nerves is considerably larger than the number of afferent neurons in the DRG and efferent neurons in the spinal cord sending axons into the nerves. For example, the pelvic nerve of the cat has approximately 18,000 axons (Morgan et al. 1981), compared with approximately 5,000 afferent and efferent neurons projecting into the nerve (Morgan et al. 1981). This suggests that there is considerable branching of afferent axons as they pass from the DRG into the periphery (Langford and Coggeshall 1981).

DRG neurons giving rise to myelinated Aδ-fiber and unmyelinated C-fiber axons can also be distinguished by immunohistochemical staining for neurofilament protein. Neurofilament is a cytoskeletal protein that is synthesized in cell bodies and delivered to axons by axoplasmic transport. The level of neurofilament expression is known to correlate with axonal caliber and myelination. The 200-kDa neurofilament subunit is exclusively expressed in myelinated A-fiber DRG neurons, but not in unmyelinated C-fiber neurons (Lawson et al. 1993). Approximately two thirds of bladder afferent neurons in rats are neurofilament-poor (i.e., C-fiber neurons), while the remaining one third of cells exhibit intense neurofilament immunoreactivity (Aδ-fiber neurons) (Yoshimura et al. 1998). Neurofilament immunoreactivity in bladder afferent neurons negatively correlates with the sensitivity to capsaicin (Fig. 2b). Approximately 80% of neurofilament-poor C-fiber bladder afferent neurons are sensitive to capsaicin (Yoshimura et al. 1998). The predominance of neurofilament-poor, C-fiber afferent cells in the bladder afferent population is also in line with studies using conduction velocity measurement or histological analysis of the pelvic nerve which revealed that unmyelinated C-fiber bladder afferents are more numerous than myelinated Aδ-fiber afferents in bladder afferent pathways (Hulsebosch and Coggeshall 1982; Vera and Nadelhaft 1990).

In the rhesus monkey, pelvic and pudendal nerves have axons conducting at 2–31 and 34–119 ms^{-1}, respectively, reflecting the larger fiber diameter in the pudendal nerve (Rockswold et al. 1980a, b). Bladder afferent axons in the pelvic and hypogastric nerves in the cat have conduction velocities of 1–22 and 1–16 ms^{-1}, respectively (Winter 1971).

Afferent neurons innervating the lower urinary tract exhibit immunoreactivity for various neuropeptides, such as SP, CGRP, PACAP, leucine enkephalin, corticotropin releasing factor, and vasoactive intestinal polypeptide (VIP) (de Groat 1986, 1989; Maggi 1993; Keast and de Groat 1992; Vizzard 2001, 2006) as well as growth-associated protein 43 and, nitric oxide synthase (NOS) (Vizzard et al. 1996), glutamic acid, and aspartic acid (Keast and Stephensen 2000). These substances have been identified in many species and at one or more locations in the afferent pathways, including (1) afferent neurons in lumbosacral DRG, (2) afferent nerves in the peripheral organs, and (3) afferent axons and terminals in the lumbosacral spinal cord (Kawatani et al. 1985, 1986, 1996; Morrison et al. 2005). The majority (more than 70%) of bladder DRG neurons in rats appear to contain multiple neuropeptides, CGRP, SP, and PACAP being the most common. In cats, VIP is also contained in a large percentage of bladder DRG neurons (de Groat 1989).

Peptide-containing axons are distributed throughout all layers of the bladder but are particularly dense in the lamina propria just beneath the urothelium. In the spinal cord of rats and cats, peptidergic afferents are present in Lissauer's tract, in lamina I, where they are very prominent on the lateral edge of the dorsal horn and in the region of the parasympathetic nucleus (Kawatani et al. 1985, 1996; Vizzard 2001). This distribution is similar to that of the central projections of bladder afferent neurons labeled by axonal tracers (de Groat 1986; Steers et al. 1991a). Acute treatment with C-fiber afferent neurotoxins, capsaicin or resiniferatoxin, releases CGRP, SP, and PACAP in the bladder wall and can trigger inflammatory responses, including plasma extravasation or vasodilation (i.e., neurogenic inflammation) (Maggi 1993). Chronic treatment with these toxins reduces peptidergic afferent staining in the bladder wall of animals and humans, indicating that the majority of peptidergic bladder afferent nerves are capsaicin-sensitive C-fibers (Fowler et al. 2008).

Bladder afferent neurons and axons, especially C-fiber afferents, also express various receptors, including transient receptor potential vanilloid 1 (TRPV1, the capsaicin receptor), transient receptor potential ankyrin 1 (TRPA1), transient receptor potential cation channel subfamily M member 8 (TRPM8), a cold receptor, tropomyosin-related kinase A (TrkA), which responds to nerve growth factor (NGF), α and β estrogen receptors (Bennett et al. 2003), tropomyosin-related kinase B (TrkB), which responds to brain-derived neurotrophic factor (BDNF), glial cell line derived neurotrophic factor (GDNF) receptors, which respond to GDNF (GRFα1) and artemin (GRFα3) (Forrest and Keast 2008), isolectin B4 (IB4) binding sites, muscarinic receptors, endothelin receptors, and purinergic receptors ($P2X_2$, $P2X_3$ P2Y), receptors that can be activated by adenosine 5′-triphosphate (ATP) (Bennett et al. 1996; Everaerts et al. 2008; Streng et al. 2008;Vizzard and Boyle 1999; Zhong et al. 2003). Many of these receptors have been detected not only in axons in the bladder but also in the lumbosacral spinal cord in the same locations as the projections of bladder afferent axons.

C-fiber afferents innervating the lower urinary tract of the rat have been subdivided into two populations on the basis of lectin binding; i.e., IB4-negative, peptidergic and IB4-positive, nonpeptidergic subpopulations (Bennett et al. 1996; Yoshimura et al. 2003). The IB4-negative, peptidergic subgroup represents the largest population (70–80%) of C-fiber afferents. IB4 binding has also been used to identify different types of somatic C-fiber afferents (Averill et al. 1995; Bennett et al. 1996). One type that does not exhibit IB4 binding is NGF-dependent, expresses TrkA receptors and contains neuropeptides (Averill et al. 1995), whereas a second type that binds IB4 is dependent on and expresses the GDNF family of growth factor receptors (GFRα) and is thought to be largely nonpeptidergic (Bennett et al. 1996). The IB4-binding somatic afferent neurons reportedly express a specific type of ATP receptor, $P2X_3$ (Vulchanova et al. 1998; Guo et al. 1999), as well as TRPV1 receptors (Guo et al. 1999).

Bladder afferent neurons have a lower percentage of IB4-positive cells (30%) than somatic afferent neurons innervating the skin (50%) (Bennett et al. 1996). In addition, afferent neurons innervating the bladder or proximal urethra contain a smaller population of IB4-positive, nonpeptidergic C-fiber cells than somatic afferent neurons innervating the distal urethra (20% vs. 49% of C-fiber neurons) (Yoshimura et al. 2003). The smaller numbers of the IB4-positive bladder afferents is also reflected in the smaller numbers of GFRα receptor positive neurons. GRFα1 is present in 15.4%, GFRα3 in 8.4%, and GRFα2 in only 1% of lumbosacral bladder DRG neurons (Forrest and Keast 2008). The total percentage of GFRα-positive bladder neurons is similar to the percentage of IB4-positive bladder neurons.

The expression in bladder afferent nerves of multiple receptors indicates that sensory mechanisms in the bladder are likely to be complex and involve the summation of a variety of chemical and mechanical signaling mechanisms, many of which may interact to produce excitation, while others may produce the opposite effect and suppress afferent firing. It is clear that transient receptor potential channels such as TRPV1, TRPA1, and TRPM8, as well as TrkA receptors, P2X purinergic receptors, nicotinic and muscarinic receptors, and endothelin receptors when activated by intravesical administration of receptor agonists in in vivo experiments or by direct application to nerves in in vitro preparations can enhance afferent nerve activity (Fig. 3a), release afferent transmitters, or stimulate reflex bladder activity (Andrade et al. 2006; Avelino et al. 2002; Birder et al. 2001, 2002a; Chuang et al. 2001; Du et al. 2007; Lee et al. 2000; Nishiguchi et al. 2005; Ogawa et al. 2004; Pandita and Andersson 2002; Pandita et al. 2000; Rong et al. 2002; Streng et al. 2008; Studeny et al. 2005; Zhong et al. 2003). On the other hand, some putative transmitters/neuromodulators such as nitric oxide, nicotinic and muscarinic agonists also appear to have inhibitory effects (Beckel et al. 2006; Kullmann et al. 2008b; Masuda et al. 2007; Ozawa et al. 1999; Pandita et al. 2000). The complex chemical modulation of bladder afferent activity may be related not only to the expression of multiple receptors on afferent nerves, but may also be due to effects on nonneural cells (urothelial cells and myofibroblasts) that can interact with afferent nerves via chemical messengers (Birder et al. 2008; Birder and de Groat 2007).

3 Anatomy and Putative Sensory Functions of the Urothelium

The specialized epithelial lining of the urinary tract (termed "urothelium") which extends from the renal pelvis to the urethra is composed of at least three layers: a basal cell layer attached to a basement membrane, an intermediate layer, and a superficial apical layer with large hexagonal umbrella cells (diameters of 25–250 μm) (Birder et al. 2008). Cells in all cell layers may have direct connections to the basement membrane. Basal cells, which are thought to be precursors for other cell types, normally exhibit a low (3–6 month) turnover rate, but have an accelerated proliferation after injury (Lavelle et al. 2002).

The major function of the urothelium is to act as a barrier to block the passage of potentially noxious substances from the urine into the bladder wall. When this function is compromised during injury or inflammation, it can result in damage to the underlying tissue (neural/muscle layers), resulting in urgency, frequency, and pain during bladder distention. The superficial umbrella cells, which exhibit a number of unusual characteristics, including specialized membrane lipids, asymmetric unit membrane particles, and a plasmalemma with stiff plaques, play a prominent role in maintaining this barrier (Hu et al. 2002). The "watertight" function of the apical membrane is due in part to these specialized lipid molecules and uroplakin proteins which reduce the permeability of the urothelium to small molecules (water, urea, protons), while the tight-junction complexes reduce the movement of ions and solutes between cells.

While the urothelium has been historically viewed as primarily a "barrier," it is becoming increasingly appreciated as a responsive structure capable of detecting physiological and chemical stimuli, and releasing a number of signaling molecules (Birder and de Groat 2007; Birder et al. 2008; de Groat 2004) (Fig. 4). Thus, urothelial cells display a number of properties similar to those of nociceptive and

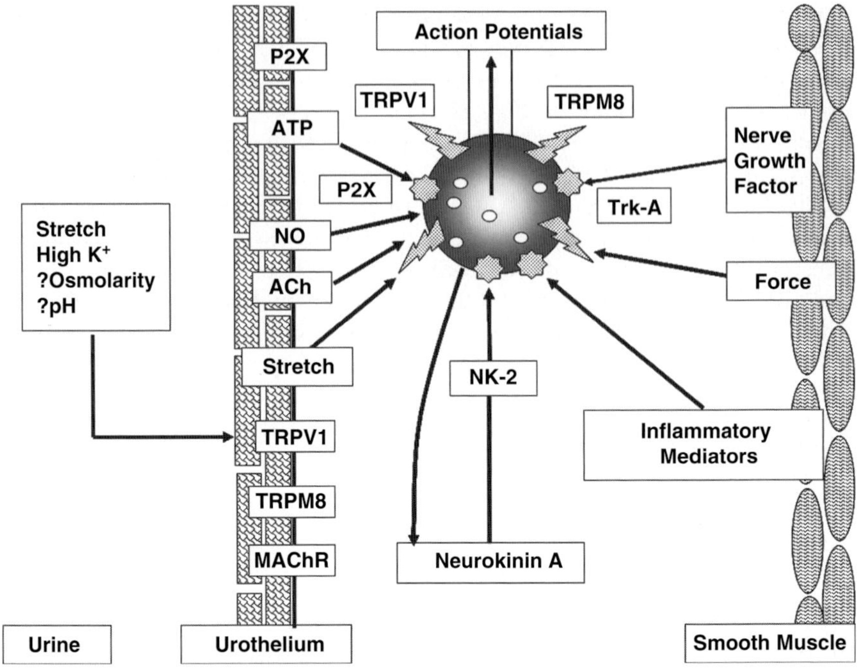

Fig. 4 Receptors present in the urothelium (*left side*) and in sensory nerve endings in the bladder mucosa (*center*) and putative chemical mediators that are released by the urothelium, nerves, or smooth muscle (*right side*) that can modulate the excitability of sensory nerves. Urothelial cells and sensory nerves express common receptors (P2X, TRPV1, and TRPM8). Distension of the bladder activates stretch receptors and triggers the release of urothelial transmitters such as ATP, acetylcholine, and nitric oxide that may interact with adjacent nerves. Receptors in afferent nerves or the urothelium can respond to changes in pH, osmolality, high K^+ concentration, chemicals in the urine, or inflammatory mediators released in the bladder wall. Neuropeptides (neurokinin A) released from sensory nerves in response to distension or chemical stimulation can act on neurokinin-2 autoreceptors to sensitize the mechanosensitive nerve endings. The smooth muscle can generate force which may influence some mucosal endings. Nerve growth factor released from muscle or urothelium can exert an acute and chronic influence on the excitability of sensory nerves via an action on TrkA receptors. *ACh* acetylcholine, *MAChR* muscarinic acetylcholine receptor, *TRPV1* transient receptor potential vanilloid receptor 1 that are sensitive to capsaicin, *TRPM8* menthol/cold receptor, *NO* nitric oxide, *Trk-A* tropomyosin-related kinase A receptor

mechanosensitive sensory neurons and can use diverse signal-transduction mechanisms to detect physiological stimuli. The urothelium expresses "sensor molecules" (i.e., receptors/ion channels) that have been identified in afferent neurons, including receptors for bradykinin (Chopra et al. 2005), neurotrophins (TrkA and p75) (Murray et al. 2004), purines (P2X and P2Y) (Birder et al. 2004; Hu et al. 2002; Lee et al. 2000; Tempest et al. 2004), norepinephrine (α and β) (Birder et al. 1998, 2002b), acetylcholine (nicotinic and muscarinic) (Beckel et al. 2006; Chess-Williams 2002; Kullmann et al. 2008a, b), protease-activated receptors, amiloride/mechanosensitive Na^+ channels (Wang et al. 2003), and a number of transient receptor potential channels (TRPV1, TRPV2, TRPV4, TRPM8) (Birder et al. 1998,

2001, 2002a, b, 2008; Stein et al. 2004; Gevaert et al. 2007). In addition, urothelial cells can release neurotransmitters and signaling molecules such as nitric oxide, ATP, acetylcholine, prostaglandins, SP, and NGF (Birder et al. 1998, 2002a, b; Ferguson et al. 1997; Yoshida et al. 2004) that influence the excitability of afferent nerves (Fig. 4). Chemicals released from urothelial cells may act directly on afferent nerves or indirectly via an action on suburothelial myofibroblasts (also referred to as "interstitial cells") that lie in close proximity to afferent nerves. Myofibroblasts are extensively linked by gap junctions and can release chemicals that in turn act on afferent nerves (Fowler et al. 2008). Thus, it is believed that urothelial cells and myofibroblasts can participate in sensory mechanisms in the urinary tract by chemical coupling to the adjacent sensory nerves.

4 Properties of Afferent Receptors in the Lower Urinary Tract

4.1 Sacral Afferents

The properties of small myelinated Aδ and unmyelinated C-fiber afferent axons that innervate the bladder and urethra have been studied with single-unit and multiunit recording in in vitro and in vivo preparations of various mammalian species. Aδ mechanoreceptor afferents in the pelvic nerve (Bahns et al. 1987; Downie and Armour 1992; Winter 1971; Satchell and Vaughan 1994) and sacral dorsal roots (Jänig and Morrison 1986; Häbler et al. 1993) of the cat respond to both passive distension as well as active contraction of the bladder, indicating that that they are in series tension receptors (Fig. 5). These afferents, which have conduction velocities ranging between 2.5 and 15 ms^{-1} (Häbler et al. 1993), are silent when the bladder is empty, but during slow filling of the bladder they display a graded increase in discharge frequency at bladder pressures above threshold, which generally is below 25 mmHg. Multiunit recordings exhibit a successive recruitment of mechanoreceptors with different thresholds during bladder filling. The maximal firing rates range from 15 to 30 Hz. All afferents behave like slowly adapting mechanoreceptors with both a dynamic and a static component of their discharge. Pressure thresholds for mechanosensitive afferents in the cat fall on the flat, compliant part of the bladder pressure-volume curve at about 25–75% of the pressure at which the curve becomes steep. These thresholds are consistent with the conditions in which humans report the first sensation of bladder filling. However, one study in cats (Downie and Armour 1992) which simultaneously measured intravesical pressure and orthogonal receptive field dimensions with a piezoelectric crystal revealed that afferent activity did not correlate with maximal bladder volume or pressure. Furthermore, activity was not linearly related to intravesical pressure, receptor field dimensions, or calculated wall tension. Thus, it was concluded that afferent receptors are also influenced by the viscoelastic properties of the bladder wall. Urethral afferents do not respond to bladder distension, but are

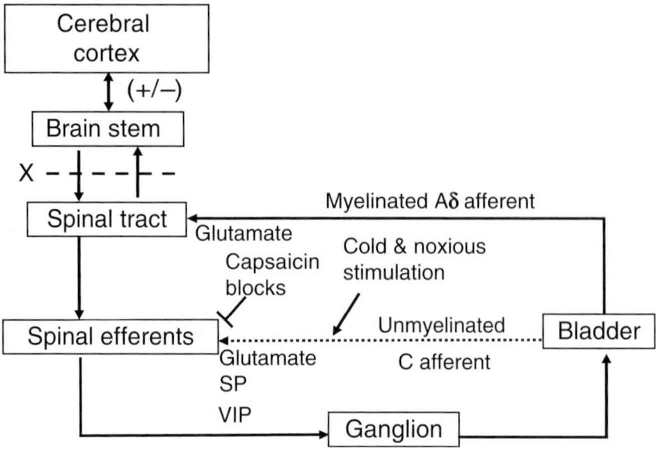

Fig. 5 Organization of the parasympathetic excitatory reflex pathway to the detrusor muscle. The scheme is based on electrophysiological studies in cats. In animals with an intact spinal cord, micturition is initiated by a supraspinal reflex pathway passing through a center in the brainstem. The pathway is triggered by myelinated afferents (Aδ-fibers), which are connected to the tension receptors in the bladder wall. Injury to the spinal cord above the sacral segments interrupts the connections between the brain and spinal autonomic centers and initially blocks micturition. However, over a period of several weeks following cord injury, a spinal reflex mechanism emerges, which is triggered by unmyelinated vesical afferents (C-fibers); the A-fiber afferent inputs are ineffective. The C-fiber reflex pathway is usually weak or undetectable in animals with an intact nervous system. Stimulation of the C-fiber bladder afferents by instillation of ice-water into the bladder (cold stimulation) activates voiding responses in patients with spinal cord injury. Capsaicin (20–30 mg, subcutaneously) blocks the C-fiber reflex in chronic spinal cats, but does not block micturition reflexes in intact cats. Intravesical capsaicin also suppresses detrusor hyperreflexia and cold-evoked reflexes in patients with neurogenic bladder dysfunction. Glutamate is the main neurotransmitter released by Aδ and C afferent fibers at synapses in the spinal cord; C-fiber afferents additionally release neuropeptides such as substance P (*SP*) or vasoactive intestinal polypeptide (*VIP*) as neurotransmitters. In animals with an intact spinal cord, noxious stimulation can activate C-fiber afferents, which leads to a facilitation of the micturition reflex pathway

excited by low-threshold mechanical stimulation induced by movements of a urethral catheter.

The firing of pelvic nerve Aδ afferents in the cat also reflects the size and timing of bladder contractions, and the afferent responses are larger under isovolumetric than under isotonic conditions (Jänig and Morrison 1986). When the thresholds for afferent firing were studied using small neurally evoked bladder contractions or irregular contractions that occurred spontaneously, the thresholds ranged from 5 to 15 mmHg. These pressures are within the physiological range for contractions during micturition in people with normal bladders or the pressures during involuntary detrusor contractions in people with detrusor overactivity (DO). Thus, the pelvic nerve afferents provide the central nervous system with accurate information about the size and timing of bladder contractions.

Activity of unmyelinated C-fiber bladder afferent axons recorded in the sacral dorsal roots of the cat revealed only a small population (seven of 297 units) of mechanosensitive afferents that have high intravesical pressure thresholds ranging from 30 to 50 mmHg (Häbler et al. 1990). These pressures are within the range of intravesical pressures at which humans report discomfort and pain. The afferents are silent with the bladder empty, but exhibit a graded increase in firing at pressures between 30 and 100 mmHg. Among the mechanoinsensitive "silent" C-fiber units which have a mean conduction velocity of 1.4 ms^{-1} approximately 10% could be activated by intravesical injection of the irritant substance mustard oil (Fig. 5). After irritation of the bladder with mustard oil or turpentine oil, some mechanoinsensitive units became mechanosensitive. Some C-fiber bladder afferents also respond to cold temperatures and intravesical administration of menthol, an agent that sensitizes TRPM8 receptors (Fall et al. 1990; Jiang et al. 2002; Lindstrom et al. 2004). C-fiber bladder afferents have also been identified in the sacral ventral roots (Clifton et al. 1976) as well as in the dorsal roots.

Bladder afferent nerves have also been studied in the rat (Dmitrieva and McMahon 1996; Mitsui et al. 2001; Moss et al. 1997; Namasivayam et al. 1999; Sengupta and Gebhart 1994; Shea et al. 2000; Su et al. 1997; Vera and Nadelhaft 1990; Yu and de Groat 2008), mouse (Rong et al. 2002; Daly et al. 2007; Xu and Gebhart 2008), guinea pig (Zagorodnyuk et al. 2006, 2007), and dog. In the rat, 70% of bladder afferents in the pelvic nerve have conduction velocities in the C-fiber range and 30% in the Aδ-fiber range. The mechanoreceptive afferents are subdivided into a large population (80%) of low-threshold (6 mmHg) fibers and a smaller population (20%) of high-threshold (34 mmHg) fibers. Conduction velocity does not correlate with response threshold, each population consisting of Aδ as well as C-fiber axons. The majority of axons exhibit resting activity with the bladder empty (Dmitrieva and McMahon 1996; Sengupta and Gebhart 1994; Shea et al. 2000), show a monotonic increase in firing with graded bladder distension, and slow adaptation in response to a maintained distension. Receptive fields are located in the body, base, and at the ureterovesical junction and are punctuate or oval in shape. The majority of afferents respond to distension or contraction of the bladder and therefore have been defined as tension receptors. However, some afferents with C-fiber axons respond to distension but not to contraction and have been defined as volume receptors (Morrison 1997). Some bladder afferents that do not respond to bladder distension can be excited by intravesical application of potassium or capsaicin.

In the mouse pelvic nerve, four classes of bladder afferents (serosal, muscular, muscular/urothelial, and urothelial) have been identified on the basis of responses to receptive field stimulation with different mechanical stimuli, including probing, stretch, and stroking the urothelium. Both low-threshold, representing 65–80% of the total population, and high-threshold stretch-sensitive muscular afferents are present (Daly et al. 2007; Xu and Gebhart 2008). The muscular afferents can be sensitized by application of a combination of inflammatory mediators (bradykinin, serotonin, prostaglandin, and histamine at pH 6.0) (Xu and Gebhart 2008).

In the guinea pig bladder, four classes of afferents have also been detected (Zagorodnyuk et al. 2006, 2007). These include (1) stretch-sensitive afferents in muscle which behave as in-series tension receptors, (2) tension-mucosal mechanoreceptors which can be activated by stretch, mucosal stroking with light von

Frey hairs, or hypertonic solutions applied locally to the receptive fields in the mucosa, (3) stretch-insensitive afferents consisting of mucosal mechanoreceptors and chemoreceptors, and (4) muscle mechanoreceptors activated by stretch but not by mucosal stroking or by hypertonic solution or capsaicin. Removal of the urothelium does not affect the stretch-induced firing.

Muscle-mucosal mechanoreceptors are activated by both stretch and mucosal stroking, by hypertonic solution, by α,β-methylene-ATP but not by capsaicin. Stroking- and stretch-induced firing is significantly reduced by removal of the urothelium. The third class of afferents, mucosal high-responding mechanoreceptors, are stretch-insensitive but can be activated by mucosal stroking, hypertonic solution, α,β-methylene-ATP, and capsaicin. Stroking-induced activity is reduced by removal of the urothelium. The fourth class of afferents, mucosal low-responding mechanoreceptors, are stretch-insensitive but can be weakly activated by mucosal stroking but not by hypertonic solution, α,β-methylene-ATP, or capsaicin. Removal of the urothelium reduces stroking-induced firing. All four populations of afferents conducted in the C-fiber range and showed class-dependent differences in spike amplitude and duration.

4.2 *Lumbar Afferents*

Activity of Aδ and C-fiber bladder and urethral afferent axons with conduction velocities of 3–15 ms^{-1} and below 2 ms^{-1}, respectively, has been identified in the hypogastric nerves (Winter 1971; Floyd et al. 1976), lumbar splanchnic nerves (LSN), and the lumbar white rami (Bahns et al. 1986). The receptive fields of the units are either single or multiple punctuate sites on the bladder or urethral surface or associated with blood vessels in the peritoneal attachments to the bladder base. Afferents with receptive fields on or in the bladder wall respond in a graded manner to passive distension or isovolumetric contraction at intravesical pressures ranging from 10 to 70 mmHg, with threshold pressures generally below 20 mmHg. Urethral afferents exhibit either no responses to bladder stimulation or low discharge rates at higher intravesical pressures. No functional differences between the Aδ and C-fiber afferent populations in the hypogastric nerve have been reported, except that firing rates are lower in the latter group. In contrast to pelvic nerve afferents, the hypogastric afferents are often active with the bladder empty (Winter 1971; Bahns et al. 1986).

Bladder afferents in the LSN in the mouse consist of low-threshold and high-threshold subtypes with receptive fields in the serosal and mucosal layers of the bladder (Xu and Gebhart 2008). The serosal afferents are the most abundant. Virtually all of these afferents possess small (0.5-mm), punctuate receptive fields that tend to be clustered at the base of the bladder. Some of the afferents exhibit low rates of spontaneous activity. LSN afferents do not exhibit a dynamic response to probing or adaptation during a maintained force, whereas pelvic afferents in the mouse give dynamic responses at the onset of stimulation and adaptation to a maintained stimulus.

5 Electrophysiological Properties of Afferent Neurons

Functional properties of bladder afferent neurons have been extensively investigated using patch-clamp techniques combined with retrograde axonal transport of fluorescent dyes injected into the wall of the bladder or urethra to label the neurons (Dang et al. 2005, 2008; Sculptoreanu et al. 2005a, b; Yoshimura 1999; Yoshimura and de Groat 1997, 1999; Yoshimura et al. 1996, 2001a, b, 2003; Zhong et al. 2003) (Fig. 2a).

5.1 Passive Membrane Properties and Action Potentials

On the basis of current clamp recordings, bladder afferent neurons are divided into two populations according to the electrical characteristics of their action potentials (Yoshimura et al. 1996) (Fig. 2b). The most common population of bladder afferent neurons (greater than 70%) exhibit high-threshold, long-duration action potentials with an inflection on the repolarization phase. These neurons are small in size and have action potentials that are resistant to application of tetrodotoxin (TTX), a Na^+ channel blocker (Fig. 2b). The other population of bladder afferent neurons, which is larger in size, exhibits low-threshold, short-duration action potentials that are reversibly blocked by TTX (Fig. 2b). The population of neurons with TTX-resistant spikes usually exhibits a phasic firing pattern (i.e., one to two spike generation), while the neurons with TTX-sensitive spikes have a tonic firing pattern (i.e., multiple spikes) when stimulated with long-duration depolarizing current pulses (Fig. 2b). Since the majority of bladder afferent neurons with TTX-resistant spikes are sensitive to capsaicin (Fig. 2b), TTX-resistant neurons are likely to be the origin of C-fiber afferent axons (Yoshimura and de Groat 1999). The correlation of spike characteristics with other electrical and morphological properties of the neuron such as somal size, capsaicin sensitivity, action potential threshold, and duration has also been reported by other investigators in unspecified DRG neurons (Waddell and Lawson 1990).

Another distinctive characteristic of bladder afferent neurons with TTX-resistant action potentials is the prominent effect of 4-aminopyridine (4-AP), an A-type K^+ (I_A) channel blocker, on the spike threshold and firing pattern (Yoshimura et al. 1996; Yoshimura and de Groat 1999). When depolarizing currents were injected into these cells, they usually exhibited a relaxation in the membrane potential at voltages (−45 to −40 mV) below the threshold for spike activation (Fig. 2b). Since application of 4-AP suppresses this membrane potential relaxation, lowers the threshold for spike activation, and switches the phasic firing pattern to tonic firing (Yoshimura et al. 1996; Yoshimura and de Groat 1999), I_A currents activated by small depolarizations from resting membrane potential are likely to contribute to high thresholds for spike activation and the phasic firing pattern in these TTX-resistant neurons. This is discussed further in Sect. 5.3.

5.2 Sodium Channels

Voltage-clamp recordings of Na^+ currents in bladder afferent neurons have revealed a similar correlation between cell size and sensitivity to TTX (Yoshimura et al. 1996, 2001a). Although both TTX-resistant and TTX-sensitive Na^+ currents can occur in single neurons, usually one type of current predominates. TTX-resistant currents are prominent, representing more than 85% of the total Na^+ current in small bladder neurons, whereas TTX-sensitive currents represent 60–100% of the total Na^+ current in large bladder afferent neurons. These two types of Na^+ currents exhibit different voltage-dependence. The threshold for activation of the TTX-resistant Na^+ current is shifted in the depolarizing direction by approximately 15 mV relative to the threshold of the TTX-sensitive Na^+ current. Steady-state activation and inactivation of TTX-resistant Na^+ currents are also displaced to more depolarized levels by 10 and 30 mV, respectively, in comparison with the value for the TTX-sensitive Na^+ current. Thus, these different properties of the Na^+ currents likely contribute to the higher spike thresholds in C-fiber bladder afferent neurons with TTX-resistant action potentials.

Two different Na^+ channel subunits ($Na_v1.8$ and $Na_v1.9$) are responsible for TTX-resistant Na^+ currents in DRG neurons (Novakovic et al. 1998). $Na_v1.8$ channels, which are expressed at higher levels than $Na_v1.9$ channels in bladder DRG neurons (Black et al. 2003), are thought to have an important role in bladder nociceptive mechanisms because intrathecal administration of an $Na_v1.8$ antisense oligodeoxynucleotide suppresses reflex bladder hyperactivity induced by bladder irritation in addition to reducing $Na_v1.8$ expression in lumbosacral DRG neurons and TTX-resistant Na^+ currents in bladder afferent neurons (Yoshimura et al. 2001a). The relatively greater contribution of the $Na_v1.8$ channel to bladder sensory mechanisms is in line with previous findings that the two types of TTX-resistant channels are expressed in different types of C-fiber afferent neurons: (1) $Na_v1.8$ in peptidergic, IB4-negative neurons and (2) $Na_v1.9$ in nonpeptidergic, IB4-positive neurons.

5.3 Potassium Channels

Several types of transient I_A K^+ currents are expressed in sensory neurons (Gold et al. 1996). One of these I_A currents exhibits slowly inactivating decay kinetics (time constant between 150 and 300 ms) that is considerably shorter than that of other fast inactivating I_A currents. This slowly inactivating I_A current has a half-maximal inactivation voltage that is displaced to a more positive membrane potential when compared with that of the fast inactivating I_A current. The slowly inactivating I_A current is selectively expressed in small capsaicin-sensitive DRG neurons that have action potentials with inflections on the repolarization phase, whereas the fast inactivating I_A current is present in large-diameter DRG neurons without action potential inflections. Bladder afferent neurons exhibit a similar distribution of two types of I_A current; i.e., small neurons with TTX-resistant humped spikes exhibiting slow-inactivating I_A currents and large neurons with TTX-sensitive spikes exhibiting fast inactivating I_A currents (Yoshimura et al. 1996; Yoshimura and de Groat 1999). In bladder afferent neurons, the steady-state inactivation of slowly inactivating I_A currents is displaced by approximately 20 mV in a more depolarizing direction than fast inactivating I_A currents. Thus, 20% of the slow I_A current is available at the resting membrane potential between −50 and −60 mV, while the fast I_A current is almost completely inactivated at this membrane potential (Yoshimura et al. 1996; Yoshimura and de Groat 1999). This is inconsistent with the current clamp recordings showing that small bladder afferent neurons exhibit a 4-AP-sensitive membrane potential relaxation during depolarization. Thus, in small C-fiber bladder afferent neurons, TTX-resistant high-threshold Na^+ currents and slow I_A currents contribute to the high thresholds for spike activation.

SP, which is known to act on afferent terminals in the bladder to enhance afferent firing (Morrison et al. 2005), mimics the effect of 4-AP on small-diameter DRG neurons, reducing I_A currents and converting phasic firing to tonic firing (Sculptoreanu and de Groat 2007). The effects of SP are blocked by neurokinin-2 anatgonists. Similar effects are elicited by neurokinin A analogs that act selectively on neurokinin-2 receptors. However, other agonists that activate neurokinin-1 or neurokinin-3 receptors do not elicit these effects. These observations raise the possibility that neurokinins which are released from afferent nerves terminals in the bladder might participate in a positive autofeedback mechanism to increase the excitability at C-fiber afferent terminals.

5.4 *Calcium Channels*

Voltage-sensitive Ca^{2+} channels are divided into high-voltage-activated (HVA) and low-voltage-activated types according to their voltage thresholds for activation. HVA channels, which are known to be involved in neurotransmitter release from nerve terminals, are further classified into L, N, P/Q, and R subtypes on the basis of electrophysiological and pharmacological properties. N and L channels are major subtypes of HVA Ca^{2+} channels in both types of bladder afferent neurons. However, expression of L-type Ca^{2+} channels is greater in C-fiber than in Aδ bladder afferent neurons, while the proportion of N-type channels is similar in the two types of neurons (Yoshimura et al. 2001b).

HVA Ca^{2+} channels can be modulated by neurotransmitters. Nitric coxide donors inhibit N-type Ca^{2+} currents in bladder afferent neurons (Yoshimura et al. 2001b), raising the possibility that nitric oxide released from the urothelium might exert an inhibitory effect on the excitability or neurotransmitter release from afferent terminals in the bladder. Neurokinin-2 receptor activation enhances L- and N-type Ca^{2+} channels via protein kinase C (PKC)-induced phosphorylation in rat DRG neurons (Sculptoreanu and de Groat 2003). This effect could occur in combination with the blockade of I_A channels to enhance the excitability of afferent terminals in the bladder.

Low-voltage-activated T-type Ca^{2+} currents, which are important in controlling cell excitability, are expressed in somatic afferent neurons innervating the urethra and pelvic floor muscles, but not in visceral afferent neurons innervating the bladder or urethra (Yoshimura et al. 2003).

5.5 *Purinergic Channels*

ATP or α,β-methylene-ATP activates purinergic receptors and evokes persistent inward currents in a large percentage (88%) of cultured L6–S1 (LS) bladder DRG neurons of the rat (Zhong et al. 2003; Dang et al. 2008). The remaining neurons exhibit biphasic, transient, or no responses. In contrast, the majority (66%) of cutaneous afferent neurons in L3–L4 DRG exhibit transient or biphasic responses to a purinergic agonist (Zhong et al. 2003). The subtype-selective purinergic antagonist trinitrophenyl ATP (TNP-ATP), which is a 1,000-fold more potent in inhibiting $P2X_{2/3}$ receptors than $P2X_2$ receptors, inhibits the persistent currents evoked by purinergic agonists. TNP-ATP is also effective in inhibiting ATP or α,β-methylene-ATP induced facilitation of bladder afferent nerve activity in the rat (Yu and de Groat 2008) and mouse (Rong et al. 2002). Thus, it likely that heteromeric $P2X_{2/3}$ receptors are primarily involved in mediating the persistent purinergic evoked currents in bladder sensory neurons. This conclusion is supported by patch-clamp studies in unidentified DRG neurons from $P2X_3$ and $P2X_{2/3}$ knockout mice showing that homomeric $P2X_3$ receptors mediate transient currents and heteromeric $P2X_{2/3}$ receptors mediate sustained currents (Cockayne et al. 2000).

Bladder afferent neurons in the thoracic and rostral lumbar (TL) DRG in rats exhibit different responses to purinergic agonists (Dang et al. 2005, 2008). Only 50% of these neurons respond to ATP or α,β-methylene-ATP. In addition, the predominant responses are transient or biphasic currents, in contrast to the persistent currents in LS bladder DRG neurons, suggesting that in TL bladder neurons homomeric $P2X_3$ receptors rather than heteromeric $P2X_{2/3}$ receptors mediate the ATP-evoked responses. ATP also produces a low-magnitude depolarization and fewer action potentials in TL than in LS bladder neurons.

5.6 *Transient Receptor Potential Channels*

Capsaicin stimulates TRPV1 receptors and evokes an inward current (Fig. 2b) and cobalt uptake in rat LS and TL bladder afferent neurons (Yoshimura et al. 2003;

Dang et al. 2005) and in sacral bladder afferent neurons in the cat (Sculptoreanu et al. 2005a). In one study (Yoshimura et al. 2003) 70% of LS neurons responded to capsaicin, but in another study (Dang et al. 2005) more than 90% of the LS and TL neurons responded to capsaicin. The capsaicin-evoked inward currents are significantly smaller in TL than in LS neurons. More than 90% of capsaicin-sensitive LS neurons have TTX-resistant Na^+ currents and action potentials. Nearly all capsaicin-responsive LS and TL neurons respond to α,β-methylene-ATP or acid solution (pH 5) (Dang et al. 2005); and 75% of LS neurons respond to all three stimuli, whereas only 48% of TL neurons respond to the three stimuli. Among the α,β-methylene-ATP sensitive neurons, 60% of LS neurons and 85% of TL neurons exhibit IB4 binding, indicating that not all P2X receptor expressing bladder afferents are IB4-positive.

5.7 *Acid-Sensing Ion Channels*

The response of bladder afferent neurons to acid solutions was analyzed to determine if it was related to activation of TRPV1 channels or acid-sensing ion channels (ASICs) (Dang et al. 2005). The large majority of LS (78%) and TL (86%) neurons respond to application of pH 5 solutions. The neurons exhibit (1) transient currents that can be separated into rapidly and slowly desensitizing components and (2) sustained currents. Transient currents occur in 20% of LS neurons and 11% of TL neurons. Sustained currents occur in 31% of LS neurons and 44% of TL neurons. The remaining neurons exhibit mixed currents. Capsazepine, a TRPV1 antagonist, significantly reduces the sustained currents without affecting the transient currents, indicating that the sustained currents are mediated in part by activation of TRPV1 channels. On the other hand, amiloride, a nonselective ASIC blocker, almost completely blocks the transient currents while reducing the sustained currents, indicating that ASIC channels are expressed in LS and TL bladder afferent neurons.

6 Role of Afferent Neurons in the Normal Control of the Lower Urinary Tract

Afferent nerves innervating the bladder, urethra, and EUS have different roles in the regulation of urine storage and elimination. Mechanosensitive afferents in the bladder are activated during bladder filling and transmit information to the brain about the degree of bladder distension and, in turn, the amount of urine stored in the bladder. Studies in healthy volunteers have shown that the first sensation of filling occurs when about 40% of bladder capacity is reached, but this sensation is indistinct and easily disregarded. The first desire to void is reported at approximately 60% of capacity and has been defined by the International Continence Society (ICS) standardization committee as "the feeling, during filling cystometry that would lead to the patient to pass urine at the next convenient moment, but voiding can be delayed if necessary." At more than 90% of capacity, people report a strong desire to void, which is defined by ICS as a "persistent desire to void without fear of leakage." On the basis of studies in animals which examined the effects of C-fiber afferent neurotoxins on voiding and studies in humans after transection of sympathetic or parasympathetic nerves, it appears that the normal sensations of bladder filling are dependent on Aδ afferents carried in the pelvic nerves to the sacral spinal cord (Fowler et al. 2008). These afferents are also essential for the generation of storage and voiding reflexes.

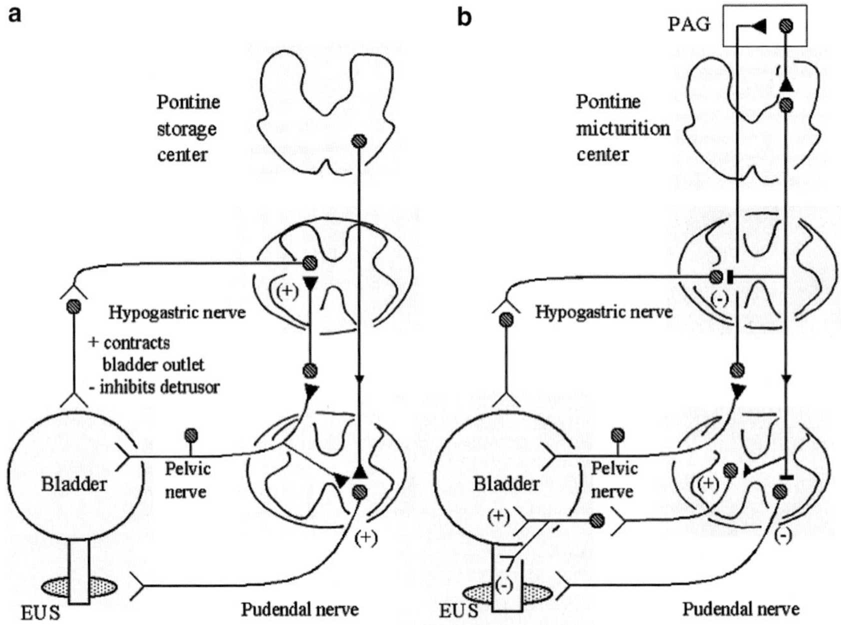

Fig. 6 Neural circuits controlling continence and micturition. (**a**) Urine storage reflexes. During the storage of urine, distension of the bladder produces low-level afferent firing in the pelvic nerve, which in turn stimulates (1) the sympathetic outflow to the bladder outlet (base and urethra) and (2) pudendal outflow to the external urethral sphincter. These responses occur by spinal reflex pathways and represent guarding reflexes, which promote continence. Sympathetic firing also inhibits detrusor muscle and modulates transmission in bladder ganglia. A region in the rostral pons (the pontine storage center) increases external urethral sphincter activity. (**b**) Voiding reflexes. During elimination of urine, intense bladder afferent firing activates spinobulbospinal reflex pathways passing through the pontine micturition center, which stimulate the parasympathetic outflow to the bladder and internal sphincter smooth muscle and inhibit the sympathetic and pudendal outflow to the urethral outlet. Ascending afferent input from the spinal cord may pass through relay neurons in the periaqueductal gray (*PAG*) before reaching the pontine micturition center

6.1 Sympathetic Storage Reflexes

Although the integrity of the sympathetic input to the lower urinary tract is not essential for the performance of micturition, it does contribute to the storage function of the bladder. Surgical interruption or pharmacological blockade of the sympathetic innervation can reduce urethral outflow resistance, reduce bladder capacity, and increase the frequency and amplitude of bladder contractions recorded under constant-volume conditions (Morrison et al. 2005). Sympathetic reflex activity is elicited by a sacrolumbar intersegmental spinal reflex pathway that is triggered by Aδ vesical afferent activity in the pelvic nerves (Fig. 6a). The reflex pathway is inhibited when bladder pressure is raised to the threshold for producing micturition (Fig. 6b). This inhibitory response is abolished by transection of the spinal cord at the lower thoracic level, indicating that it originates at a supraspinal site, possibly the pontine micturition center. Thus, the vesicosympathetic reflex represents a negative-feedback mechanism that allows the bladder to accommodate larger volumes.

6.2 Urethral Sphincter Storage Reflexes

Motoneurons innervating the striated muscles of the EUS exhibit a tonic discharge which increases during bladder filling. This activity, which is termed the "guarding reflex" because it closes the urethral outlet and prevents urine leakage, is mediated by a reflex pathway in the lumbosacral spinal cord that is activated by low-level afferent input from the bladder traveling in the pelvic nerve (Fig. 6a). Electrical stimulation of Aδ afferents in the pelvic nerve of the cat and rat evokes reflex discharges in pudendal nerve motor axons innervating the EUS and increases in EUS EMG activity, indicating that Aδ bladder afferents initiate the guarding reflex (Chang et al. 2007; Thor et al. 1989a). Cold stimulation of the rat urinary bladder also induces tonic activity of the EUS EMG. This reflex response is abolished by pretreatment with capsaicin, indicating that it is dependent on bladder C-fiber afferent nerves.

Sphincter-to-bladder reflexes may also contribute to urine storage because afferent activity arising in the striated EUS muscles during contractions can suppress reflex bladder activity and, in turn, increase bladder capacity. Studies in cats and monkeys revealed that direct electrical stimulation of the EUS muscles or electrical stimulation of motor pathways to induce a contraction of the sphincters suppresses reflex bladder activity (McGuire et al. 1983; de Groat et al. 2001). Similar inhibitory responses are elicited by electrical stimulation of afferent axons in the pudendal nerve, some of which must arise in the sphincter muscles.

6.3 Voiding Reflexes

Micturition is mediated by activation of the sacral parasympathetic efferent pathway to the bladder and the urethra as well as reciprocal inhibition of the somatic pathway to the EUS (Fig. 6b). Studies in anesthetized and decerebrate cats and rats revealed that reflex activation of the bladder is mediated by a spinobulbospinal pathway passing through the pontine micturition center (PMC; Barrington's nucleus) at the level of the inferior colliculus (de Groat et al. 1981, 1993). The reflex pathway is activated by Aδ bladder afferents traveling in the pelvic nerve to the sacral spinal cord (Fig. 5). Activation of the PMC also induces reflex inhibition of the spinal EUS and sympathetic storage reflexes. Micturition is accompanied by relaxation of the urethral smooth muscle mediated by activation of a sacral parasympathetic pathway and release of an inhibitory transmitter, nitric oxide, in the urethra. This reflex is activated by Aδ bladder afferents in the pelvic nerve. During micturition the flow of urine through the urethra also activates urethral afferents which travel in the pudendal nerve to the sacral spinal cord and facilitate the excitatory bladder reflex pathways.

In some species (rat, mouse, dog), micturition is accompanied by rhythmic contractions of the EUS (EUS bursting) rather than complete EUS relaxation (Chang et al. 2007). The pulsatile urethral contractile activity is thought to enhance urine flow. The EUS bursting is activated by bladder distension and by Aδ bladder afferents in the pelvic nerve. The EUS bursting is dependent on input from the PMC in rats with an intact spinal cord, but is mediated by lumbosacral spinal pathways in chronic spinal cord transected rats (Chang et al. 2007).

7 Plasticity of Afferent Neurons Induced by Spinal Cord Injury

7.1 Emergence of a C-Fiber Afferent Micturition Reflex

Spinal-cord injury (SCI) rostral to the lumbosacral level eliminates voluntary and supraspinal control of voiding, leading initially to an areflexic bladder and complete urinary retention, followed by a slow development of automatic micturition and bladder hyperactivity mediated by spinal reflex pathways (de Groat and Yoshimura 2006). However, voiding is commonly inefficient owing to simultaneous contractions of the bladder and urethral sphincter (detrusor-sphincter dyssynergia, DSD).

Electrophysiological studies in cats have shown that the recovery of bladder function after SCI is mediated by a change in the afferent limb of the micturition reflex pathway and remodeling of synaptic connections in the spinal cord. In chronic spinal cats, unmyelinated C-fiber afferents rather than Aδ afferents initiate voiding; and the spinal micturition reflex occurs with a short central delay (15 ms), in contrast to the long central delay (60 ms) of the reflex in cats with an intact spinal cord (de Groat et al. 1981) (Fig. 5). These findings are supported by pharmacological studies showing that subcutaneous administration of capsaicin, a C-fiber neurotoxin, completely blocks reflex bladder contractions induced by bladder distension in chronic spinal cats, whereas capsaicin has no inhibitory effect on reflex bladder contractions in cats with an intact spinal cord (de Groat et al. 1990; Cheng et al. 1999). Thus, it is plausible that C-fiber bladder afferents which usually do not respond to bladder distension (i.e., silent C-fibers) (Häbler et al. 1990) become mechanosensitive and initiate automatic micturition after SCI.

Studies in humans have revealed an increased density of TRPV1 and $P2X_3$ immunoreactivity as well as immunoreactivity to a pan-neuronal marker (protein gene product 9.5) in suburothelial nerves and increased TRPV1 immunoreactivity in the basal layer of the urothelium in patients with neurogenic detrusor overactivity (NDO) resulting from multiple sclerosis or various types of SCI (Brady et al. 2004a, b; Apostolidis et al. 2005a). Treatment of NDO patients with intravesical capsaicin or another C-fiber neurotoxin, resiniferatoxin, produces symptomatic improvement in a subpopulation of these patients and reduces the density of TRPV1, P2X3, and protein gene product 9.5 immunoreactive nerve fibers and urothelial TRPV1 immunoreactivity (Brady et al. 2004a, b). Injections into the bladder wall of botulinum neurotoxin type A, an agent that blocks the release of neurotransmitters from urothelial cells and from afferent and efferent nerves, also reduces NDO (Apostolidis and Fowler 2008; Popat et al. 2005; Schurch et al., 2005; Cruz and Dinis 2007) and reduces the density of TRPV1- and $P2X_3$-immunoreactive nerves but does not alter TRPV1 and P2X3 staining in the urothelium (Apostolidis et al. 2005a, b, 2008). These results suggest that an abnormality of the C-fiber afferent innervation contributes to NDO.

The effect in cat spinal cord of VIP, a putative bladder C-fiber afferent transmitter (Morgan et al. 1999), is also changed after SCI. Intrathecal administration of VIP, which suppresses reflex bladder activity in cats with an intact spinal cord, enhances or unmasks reflex bladder activity in chronic SCI cats. In addition, VIP-immunoreactive C-fiber afferent projections to the sacral spinal cord expand and reorganize after SCI (Thor et al. 1986). This is evident as (1) a wider distribution of VIP-immunoreactive axons in lateral lamina I of the dorsal horn forming an almost continuous band of axons in the rostrocaudal direction in comparison with a discontinuous distribution in normal cats, (2) appearance of rostrocaudal axons in this region where they are not normally present, (3) more extensive contralateral projections to lamina I, and (4) a more extensive ipsilateral projection to lateral lamina VII which contains bladder preganglionic neurons. These observations raise the possibility that C-fiber bladder afferents sprout and contribute to the synaptic remodeling in the spinal micturition reflex pathway that occurs after SCI.

Changes in morphology and neuropeptide expression in C-fiber afferents have also been detected in the rat after SCI. The changes include (1) somal hypertrophy of bladder afferent neurons (45–50% increase in cross-sectional area) in the LS DRG (Kruse et al. 1995; Yoshimura and de Groat 1997; Yoshimura et al. 1998), (2) increase in expression of PACAP immunoreactivity in bladder DRG neurons and expansion of PACAP-immunoreactive afferent axons in the lumbosacral spinal cord (Zvarova et al. 2005), (3) expansion of CGRP-containing primary afferent fibers in the spinal cord (Weaver et al. 2006), and (4) increase in Fos protein expression in the spinal cord in response to bladder distension (Vizzard 2000a).

Six weeks after SCI in the rat, PACAP immunoreactivity markedly increases in spinal segments and DRG (L1, L2, L6, S1) involved in micturition reflexes, but no changes occur in adjacent spinal segments (L4–L5) (Zvarova et al. 2005). PACAP immunoreactivity increases in the superficial laminae (I–II) of the relevant spinal segments and in a fiber bundle extending ventrally from Lissauer's tract in lamina I along the lateral edge of the dorsal horn to the SPN in the LS spinal segments. This is the same region in which VIP immunoreactivity increases in the cat after SCI (Thor et al. 1986). After SCI, PACAP immunoreactivity increases in cells in the L1, L2, L6, and S1 DRG and the percentage of bladder afferent cells expressing PACAP immunoreactiviy also significantly increases. These studies raise the possibility that upregulation of PACAP expression in C-fiber bladder afferent neurons may contribute to urinary bladder dysfunction or reemergence of primitive voiding reflexes after SCI.

The possible role of PACAP as a transmitter in bladder afferent pathways prompted an investigation of the physiological effects of PACAP on micturition reflex pathways in the spinal cord. Intrathecal administration of PACAP-27 (Ishizuka et al. 1995) or PACAP-38 (Yoshiyama and de Groat 2008a, b) in spinal cord intact unanesthetized rats decreases bladder capacity, decreases micturition volume, and increases micturition pressure, whereas PACAP-38 (Yoshiyama and de Groat 2008a, b) reduces EUS EMG activity. Thus, in spinal cord intact rats, PACAP-38 seems to facilitate micturition by enhancing the parasympathetic excitatory pathway to the bladder and inhibiting the somatic excitatory pathway to the EUS.

The effects of PACAP-38 in chronic SCI rats are somewhat different. During continuous-infusion cystometrograms in SCI rats, intrathecal injections of PACAP-38 decrease the amplitude of bladder contractions and suppress EUS EMG activity (Yoshiyama and de Groat 2008a). This unexpected result is most reasonably attributed to the combined effect of PACAP-38 on bladder and sphincter, where the excitatory effect of PACAP-38 on bladder activity is masked by a simultaneous inhibitory effect on the EUS that in turn blocks DSD and reduces urethral outlet resistance. This would indirectly lower intravesical pressure during voiding.

The physiological role of PACAP in the control of bladder function in chronic SCI rats was examined by administering PACAP6-38, a PAC1 receptor antagonist, during continuous-infusion cystometrograms in awake rats (Zvara et al. 2006). Intrathecal administration of the antagonist reduces premicturition contractions during bladder filling and reduces maximal voiding pressure, suggesting that activation of PAC1 receptors by endogenous PACAP contributes to the micturition reflex and bladder hyperreflexia. Capsaicin also suppresses premicturition contractions in SCI rats, indicating that they are induced by C-fiber bladder afferent pathways (Cheng et al. 1999). However, voiding contractions in SCI rats still occur, presumably triggered by capsaicin-resistant Aδ-fiber afferents.

The site and mechanism of action of PACAP on spinal micturition reflex pathways has been explored using patch-clamp recording in lumbosacral parasympathetic preganglionic neurons in spinal-slice preparations (Miura et al. 2001). The experiments revealed that PACAP-38 has direct excitatory effects on the preganglionic neurons and enhances excitatory input to the neurons, suggesting that it might act at several sites in the spinal micturition reflex pathway. In parasympathetic preganglionic neurons PACAP-38 decreases the electrical threshold for triggering action potentials, increases the number of action potentials induced by depolarizing current pulses, increases input resistance, and suppresses a 4-AP-sensitive outward current. PACAP-38 also induces spontaneous firing and increases the frequency of spontaneous excitatory postsynaptic potentials in the presence of TTX. Because excitatory synaptic inputs are mediated primarily by α-amino-3-hydroxy-5-methyl-4-isoxazolepropionate and *N*-methyl D-aspartate glutamatergic synapses, it was proposed that PACAP-38 facilitates glutamatergic excitatory synaptic input to the parasympathetic neurons in addition to directly enhancing the excitability of the neurons by blocking K^+ channels. PACAP-38 could act presynaptically to enhance the firing of excitatory interneurons and enhance glutamate release from interneuronal terminals or act postsynaptically directly on parasympathetic neurons to enhance glutamatergic currents.

Chronic spinal injury in humans also causes the emergence of an unusual bladder reflex that is elicited by infusion of cold water into the bladder (the Bors Ice Water Test) (Geirsson et al. 1993, 1994). The response to cold water does not occur in normal adults but does occur in (1) infants, (2) patients with suprasacral cord lesions, (3) patients with multiple sclerosis and Parkinson's disease, and (4) elderly patients with hyperactive bladders. Studies in animals indicate that cold temperature activates TRPM8 and possibly other temperature-sensitive receptors in bladder C-fiber afferents (Fig. 5) and/or urothelial cells (Fig. 4) (Fall et al. 1990; Stein et al. 2004). Intravesical administration of capsaicin to paraplegic patients blocks the cold-induced bladder reflexes, indicating that they are mediated by C-fiber afferents in humans as well (Geirsson et al. 1995, Jiang et al. 2002; Mazieres et al. 1998). Cold stimulation of the rat bladder also induces DSD and capsaicin pretreatment prevents this response (Cheng et al. 1997). The presence of the cold reflex in infants, its disappearance with maturation of the nervous system, and its reemergence under conditions in which higher brain functions are disrupted suggests that it may reflect a primitive spinal involuntary voiding reflex activated by C-fiber afferents.

Patients with SCI at the level of T6 or higher often exhibit autonomic dysreflexia, which is characterized by arterial pressor responses induced by visceral stimuli such as bladder distension, fecal impaction, or bladder inflammation below the level of spinal cord lesion (Fam and Yalla 1988; Weaver et al. 2006). These stimuli cause excitation of sympathetic reflex pathways and induce arteriolar vasoconstriction and high blood pressure, as well as piloerection and sweating below the level of injury. Studies in rats revealed that autonomic dysreflexia is associated with sprouting of CGRP-containing afferent nerves in the spinal cord (Weaver et al. 2006).

7.2 Role of Neurotrophic Factors

NGF has been implicated as a chemical mediator of injury or disease-induced changes in C-fiber afferent nerve excitability and reflex bladder activity (Vizzard 2000b; Yoshimura 1999). The levels of neurotrophic factors, including NGF, increase in the bladder after SCI (Vizzard 2000b, 2006) and increased levels of NGF have been detected in the lumbosacral spinal cord and DRG of rats after SCI (Seki et al. 2003). It is known that NGF upregulates PACAP expression in DRG neurons and it has been demonstrated that chronic administration of NGF into the spinal cord or chronic administration of NGF into the bladder of rats induces bladder hyperactivity and increases the firing frequency of dissociated bladder afferent neurons (Lamb et al. 2004; Seki et al. 2003; Yoshimura 1999; Yoshimura et al. 2006; Zvara and Vizzard 2007). Endogenous NGF seems to contribute to the lower urinary tract dysfunction after SCI because intrathecal application of NGF antibodies, which neutralize NGF in the spinal cord, suppresses detrusor hyperreflexia and DSD in SCI rats (Seki et al. 2002, 2004). This treatment with NGF antibodies produced effects similar to the effect of desensitizing C-fiber afferents with capsaicin or resiniferatoxin (Cheng et al. 1999). Intrathecal administration of NGF antibodies also blocks autonomic dysreflexia induced by bladder or distal bowel distension in SCI rats (Weaver et al. 2006). Thus, NGF and its receptors in the bladder and/or the spinal cord are potential targets for new therapies to reduce voiding dysfunction after SCI.

7.3 Changes in Firing Properties of Bladder Afferent Neurons After Spinal Cord Injury

The ionic mechanisms underlying the hyperexcitability of C-fiber bladder afferents were investigated using whole-cell patch-clamp recording in bladder DRG neurons (Yoshimura and de Groat 1997). Chronic SCI in rats produced hypertrophy of dissociated bladder DRG neurons as reflected by an increase in cell diameter and cell input capacitance. This is consistent with results from histological sections of LS DRG showing that bladder afferent neurons undergo somal hypertrophy (45–50% increase in cross-sectional area) in SCI rats (Kruse et al. 1995). In addition to neuronal hypertrophy, bladder afferent neurons from chronic SCI rats increased their excitability. In contrast to neurons from spinal cord intact rats where the majority (approximately 70%) of bladder afferent neurons exhibit high-threshold TTX-resistant action potentials (Yoshimura et al. 1996) (Fig. 2b), in chronic SCI rats, 60% of bladder afferent neurons exhibit low-threshold TTX-sensitive action potentials.

7.4 Plasticity in Sodium and Potassium Channels After Spinal Cord Injury

The alteration of electrophysiological properties in bladder afferent neurons after SCI was also reflected in changes in Na^+ current distribution (Yoshimura and de Groat 1997). Consistent with the increment in the proportion of neurons with TTX-sensitive spikes, the number of bladder afferent neurons which predominantly expressed TTX-sensitive Na^+ currents (60–100% of total Na^+ currents) also increased. The density of TTX-sensitive Na^+ currents in bladder afferent neurons significantly increased from 32.1 to 80.6 pA/pF, while TTX-resistant current density decreased from 60.5 to 17.9 pA/pF following SCI. In addition, an increase in TTX-sensitive Na^+ currents was detected in some bladder afferent neurons that still retained a predominance of TTX-resistant currents (more than 50% of total Na^+ currents) after SCI. These data indicate that SCI induces a switch in expression of Na^+ channels from TTX-resistant type to TTX-sensitive type. Since TTX-sensitive Na^+ currents have a lower threshold for activation than TTX-resistant currents, it is reasonable to assume that these changes in expression of Na^+ channels in bladder afferent neurons after SCI contribute to a low threshold for spike activation in these neurons.

Bladder afferent neurons with TTX-sensitive spikes in chronic SCI rats also do not exhibit membrane potential relaxation during low-intensity depolarizing current pulses. Furthermore, the voltage responses induced by current injections are not altered by application of 4-AP as noted in cells from control animals (Yoshimura et al. 1996). Therefore, it is likely that following SCI, A-type K^+ channels are suppressed in parallel with an increased expression of TTX-sensitive Na^+ currents, thereby increasing the excitability of C-fiber bladder afferent neurons. If the changes occurring in afferent cell bodies also occur at peripheral receptors in the bladder or in the spinal cord, these changes could contribute to the emergence of the C-fiber-mediated spinal micturition reflex following SCI.

8 Afferent Nerves and Idiopathic Detrusor Overactivity

Urgency incontinence with underlying idiopathic detrusor overactivity (IDO) is a common condition but its fundamental cause remains to be discovered. There is accumulating evidence that aberrant afferent activity plays an important role in IDO because women with IDO, like patients with NDO (see Sect. 7.1), have increased density of suburothelial afferent nerves that are immunoreactive for SP, CGRP, TRPV1, and P2X3 (Fowler et al. 2008). Moreover, intravesical administration of resiniferatoxin delays or suppresses involuntary detrusor contractions in patients with IDO (Apostolidis et al. 2005a; Fowler et al. 2008). In addition, biopsies from patients with IDO who exhibited decreased urgency symptoms after botulinum neurotoxin type A treatment also had a normalization of the density of suburothelial TRPV1- and P2X3-immunoreactive nerves (Apostolidis et al. 2005b, 2006).

Although IDO and NDO patients respond to neurotoxins that target afferent nerves, this does not necessarily mean that a common pathophysiological mechanism underlies both conditions.

9 Afferent Nerves and Urethral Outlet Obstruction

Plasticity of bladder afferent fibers in a setting of bladder outlet obstruction (BOO) resulting from benign prostatic hyperplasia likely plays a critical role in the subsequent manifestation of clinical symptoms. Evidence obtained from ice-water cystometry, which elicits a C-fiber-dependent spinal micturition reflex, suggests considerable C-fiber upregulation in symptomatic subjects with BOO (Chai et al. 1998; Hirayama et al. 2003). Among BOO patients with a positive ice-water test, the incidence of DO is significantly greater in those who report nocturia three times or more per night than in those who reported fewer episodes (Hirayama et al. 2003).

Histological and electrophysiological confirmation of neural plasticity in bladder afferent and bladder reflex pathways was obtained using a rat model of partial BOO. A significant increase in the size of bladder afferent and postganglionic efferent neurons innervating an enlarged bladder was documented in animals following 6 weeks of partial urethral obstruction (Steers et al. 1991a). Remodeling of the spinal cord components of the micturition reflex pathway was also evident following experimental BOO. With use of axonal labeling to identify afferent axonal projections to spinal cord, it was demonstrated that bladder afferent terminals expand to cover a larger area (60% increase) in the lateral dorsal horn and in the region of the SPN in BOO rats (Steers et al. 1991a). Electrophysiological experiments revealed that a spinal micturition reflex mechanism was unmasked in rats with BOO. An immunohistochemical analysis of the distribution and density of GAP-43 showed that this protein was increased in the spinal cord in the region of the SPN in BOO rats (Steers and Tuttle 2006). Because this protein is a marker for axonal sprouting, its upregulation provides further indirect support for morphological plasticity in afferent pathways after BOO.

Subsequent experiments using the same BOO rat model revealed that hypertrophied bladder tissue contained significantly greater amounts of NGF protein than normal bladders (Steers et al. 1991b). To determine if the changes induced by BOO were due to an action of NGF, BOO was carried out in NGF-immune animals in which endogenous NGF antibody prevents access of NGF to nerves. BOO in the NGF-immune animals does not elicit hypertrophy of bladder sensory neurons, increase in afferent projections in the spinal cord, or increase GAP-43 expression in afferent pathways (Steers et al. 1996). Removal of the urethral obstruction in BOO rats causes a partial reversal of both the elevated NGF levels in the bladder and the neuronal hypertrophy; however, bladder overactivity persists in the presence of the elevated NGF levels.

The stimulus for NGF production in the bladder is due in part to urinary retention and stretch of the bladder after BOO. Stretching bladder smooth muscle cells in vitro increases messenger RNA for NGF and stimulates the secretion of NGF (Steers and Tuttle 2006). Protein synthesis inhibitors suppress the stretch-evoked secretion. NGF levels also increase in the urothelium of BOO rats. These results indicate that mechanical stretch activates cellular machinery for the production and secretion of NGF, which in turn acts on sensory nerves in the bladder to enhance afferent input to the spinal cord and enhance reflex bladder activity.

Patch-clamp recordings from bladder sensory neurons in BOO rats have explored the mechanisms underlying the changes in afferent neuron excitability. The neurons exhibit increased amplitude and altered kinetics of TTX-sensitive Na^{+} currents that result in lowered firing thresholds (Steers and Tuttle 2006). An experimental drug (ICMI-136) that preferentially blocks TTX-sensitive currents reduces bladder overactivity in BOO rats.

Human bladder tissue obtained from subjects undergoing suprapubic prostatectomy for outlet obstruction had more than twice the level of NGF than tissue obtained by cystoscopy from patients who were being evaluated for conditions other than obstruction (Steers et al. 1991b). Increased levels of urinary NGF have also been detected in BOO patients exhibiting overactive bladder (OAB) symptoms. Total urinary NGF levels were low in controls (0.5 pg ml^{-1}) and in patients with BOO without OAB symptoms (1 pg ml^{-1}), but considerably higher in patients with BOO and OAB symptoms (41 pg ml^{-1}) or BOO and DO (50 pg ml^{-1}) (Liu and Kuo 2008). Following successful medical treatment with a combination of an α-adrenergic blocking agent and a 5α-reductase inhibitor that reduce symptoms, the urinary NGF levels were reduced to 3.2 pg ml^{-1}. It was concluded that urinary NGF levels can be used as a biomarker for OAB and DO and as a method for assessing successful therapies.

10 Afferent Nerves and Cystitis

Cystitis, which is an inflammatory condition of the urinary bladder that can occur as a result of infection, radiation-induced damage, irritant chemicals in the urine, or unknown causes (painful bladder syndrome, PBS/interstitial cystitis, IC), is accompanied by pain, unusual hypersensitivity to bladder distension, edema, and accumulation of large numbers of inflammatory cells in the bladder mucosa and musculature. Activation of sensory nerves (Aδ or C-fibers) by mechanical or chemical stimuli plays a key role in this condition by transmitting signals to the central nervous system to induce painful sensations and by releasing chemicals such as tachykinins that induce or enhance inflammatory mechanisms in the periphery. Because sensitization of the relatively inexcitable bladder C-fiber afferent nerves seems to play a key role in the symptoms of cystitis, considerable attention has been focused on disease-induced plasticity in these nerves.

Histological analysis of bladders from patients with PBS/IC revealed marked edema, vasodilation, proliferation of nerve fibers, and infiltration of mast cells (Johansson and Fall 1997). Chemically induced cystitis in animals using cyclophosphamide, mustard oil, turpentine oil, low-pH solutions, or acrolein, which increase urinary frequency, is initiated by sensitizing mechanosensitive afferents and/or recruitment of afferents normally unresponsive to mechanical stimulation (i.e., silent C-fibers) (Dmitrieva and McMahon 1996; Dmitrieva et al. 1997; Häbler et al. 1990; Sengupta and Gebhart 1994) (Fig. 3a). Proinflammatory agents such as prostaglandin E_2, serotonin, histamine, bradykinin, and adenosine, as well as neurotrophic factors such as NGF, which are released during chemical irritation can induce bladder hyperactivity as well as functional and chemical changes in C-fiber afferents that can lead to hyperexcitability (Dmitrieva and McMahon 1996; Gold et al. 1996) (Fig. 3a). For example, chronic chemical irritation of the bladder changes ion channel function in bladder afferent neurons and also increases the expression of various markers, including NOS (Vizzard et al. 1996), GAP-43 (Vizzard and Boyle 1999), PACAP, SP (Vizzard 2001), and protease-activated receptors (Dattilio and Vizzard 2005). The density of peptidergic afferent nerves also increases in the bladder mucosa and detrusor muscle (Dickson et al. 2006) and afferent peptidergic axons and parasympathetic efferent axons/varicosities are commonly observed in close contact, suggesting that sprouting of peripheral nerves occurs during chronic cystitis.

NGF has attracted considerable attention as a key player in the link between inflammation and altered pain signaling. NGF is expressed widely in various cells, including urothelial cells, smooth muscle cells, and mast cells, and can activate mast cells to degranulate and proliferate. In patients with PBS/IC, neurotrophins, including NGF, neurotrophin-3, and GDNF, have been detected in the urine (Okragly et al. 1999). Increased expression of NGF is also present in bladder biopsies from women with IC (Lowe et al. 1997). Thus, target organ-neural interactions mediated by an increase of neurotrophins in the bladder and increased transport of neurotrophins to the neuronal cell bodies in afferent pathways may contribute to the emergence of bladder pain in PBS/IC (Yoshimura 1999).

In the cyclophoshamide-induced chronic cystitis model in rats, increased expression of neurotrophic growth factors such as NGF, BDNF and CTNF in the bladder as well as phosphorylation of tyrosine kinase receptors (TrkA, TrkB) in bladder afferent neurons has been presented as direct evidence for increased neurotrophin-mediated signaling in chronic bladder inflammation (Qiao and Vizzard 2002; Vizzard 2000b). The enhanced neurotrophic factor mechanisms are also associated with increased phosphorylated cyclic AMP response element binding protein (CREB) in bladder afferent neurons. Phosphorylated CREB, which is a transcription factor in the neurotrophin intracellular signaling pathway, is coexpressed with phophorylated TrkA in a subpopulation of bladder afferent neurons (Qiao and Vizzard 2004). Resiniferatoxin, a C-fiber neurotoxin, reduced cyclophosphamide-induced upregulation of phosphorylated CREB in DRG cells, suggesting that cystitis is linked with an altered CREB phosphorylation in capsaicin-sensitive C-fiber bladder afferents (Qiao and Vizzard 2004). These results suggest that upregulation of phosphorylated CREB may be mediated by a neurotrophin/TrkA signaling pathway, and that CREB phosphorylation may play a role as a transcription factor in lower urinary tract plasticity induced by cystitis.

Exogenous NGF can induce bladder nociceptive responses and bladder overactivity in rats when applied acutely into the bladder lumen (Chuang et al. 2001; Dmitrieva et al. 1997) or chronically to the bladder wall or intrathecal space (Lamb et al. 2004; Seki et al. 2003; Zvara and Vizzard 2007). Conversely, application of NGF-sequestering molecules (TrkA-IgG or REN1820) can reduce referred thermal hyperalgesia elicited by bladder inflammation induced by intravesically applied turpentine oil (Jaggar et al. 1999) or bladder overactivity elicited by cyclophosphamide-induced cystitis (Hu et al. 2005), suggesting that increased NGF expression is directly involved in the emergence of bladder-related nociceptive responses in cystitis. Thus, NGF-activated mechanisms might be a potential target for the treatment of painful symptoms in PBS/IC.

Purinergic mechanisms may also contribute to the bladder dysfunction following chronic inflammation. ATP release from the urothelium is enhanced in patients and cats with PBS/IC (Birder et al. 2003, 2008; Sun et al. 2001). In conscious rats with cyclophosphamide-induced cystitis, purinergic receptor antagonists (PPADS and A-317491) reduce nonvoiding contractions and decrease voiding frequency (Ito et al. 2007). In in vitro whole bladder pelvic afferent nerve preparations from rats with cyclophosphamide-induced cystitis, afferent nerve firing induced by bladder distension or by direct electrical stimulation is markedly increased in comparison with firing in normal rats (Yu and de Groat 2008). Exogenous purinergic agonists mimic the facilitatory effects of cyclophosphamide treatment; and P2X purinergic receptor antagonists suppress the effects of purinergic agonists and cystitis. These results suggest that endogenous purinergic agonists released in the inflamed bladder can enhance the excitability of bladder afferent nerves by activating P2X receptors.

Patch-clamp studies on bladder afferent neurons from rats revealed that chronic cyclophosphamide treatment increases the currents induced by purinergic agonists in both TL and LS neurons (Dang et al. 2008). Analysis of the kinetics of the currents indicated that increased receptor expression and/or properties of homomeric $P2X_3$ in TL neurons and $P2X_{2/3}$ in LS neurons contribute to the enhanced responses during cystitis.

Cystitis also induces chemical changes in the spinal cord. Acute or chronic bladder irritation increases immediate early gene expression (*c-fos*) in spinal neurons (Birder and de Groat 1993) (Fig. 3) as well as an increase in GFRα1 immunoreactivity in the spinal dorsal horn and in areas associated with autonomic neurons (Forrest and Keast 2008). There was a much smaller increase in GFRα3 immunoreactivity and no change in GFRα2 immunoreactivity. Changes in spinal cord mitogen-activated-protein kinases [extracellular-signal-related kinase (ERK) 1 and ERK 2] may also play a role in the facilitation of reflex voiding after bladder inflammation. Immunohistochemical studies revealed that in noninflamed rat bladders noxious but not nonnoxious stimulation significantly increased phospho-ERK immunoreactivity (Cruz et al. 2007). However, after bladder inflammation innocuous and noxious bladder distension increased the number of spinal neurons exhibiting phospho-ERK immunoreactivity. The activation was rapid within a few minutes and transient. Desensitization of vanilloid-sensitive afferents by intravesical administration of resiniferatoxin does not decrease phospho-ERK immunoreactivity in normal or inflamed bladder preparations. ERK inhibition with intrathecal injection of PD98059 decreases reflex bladder activity and spinal *c-fos* expression in animals with inflamed bladders but not in normal animals (Cruz et al. 2007). The results suggest that activation of spinal cord ERK contributes to acute and chronic inflammatory pain perception and mediates reflex bladder overactivity accompanying chronic bladder inflammation.

Cystitis affects not only the bladder function but also alters somatic nociceptive mechanisms. Irritation of the bladder of mice by intravesical administration of NGF reduces the threshold for producing paw withdrawal in response to mechanical stimulation of the paw (mechanical hyperalgesia). The response occurs within 4 h after application of NGF and is blocked by administration of NGF antiserum. Systemic administration of cyclophosphamide or intravesical administration of its irritant metabolite, acrolein (Lanteri-Minet et al. 1995), produces a similar effect that occurs 24–48 h after administration of the irritants, at times when the bladder exhibits edema and areas of hemorrhage. These models of chemically induced cystitis do not influence the paw withdrawal responses induced by nociceptive thermal stimuli (thermal hyperalgesia) (Wang et al. 2008). On the other hand, bacterial cystitis or intravesical administration of turpentine oil increases thermal sensitivity. These selective sensitizing effects of different forms of cystitis on somatic sensory pathways, a phenomenon that may represent a type of visceral referred pain, raise the possibility that distinct populations of peripheral or central bladder sensory pathways can be activated by different nociceptive stimuli in the bladder. It is noteworthy that humans with bladder-associated pain also have a higher incidence of other painful disorders such as fibromyalgia. It would be interesting to determine if the location or type of somatic symptoms varies with the type of bladder disorder.

Direct evidence linking chronic bladder inflammation with functional changes in C-fiber afferents has been obtained from the rat cyclophosphamide chronic cystitis model. In this model, the electrical properties of bladder afferent neurons dissociated from L6 and S1 DRG as well as the activity of the inflamed bladder were measured. The majority of bladder afferent neurons from both control and cyclophosphamide-treated rats are capsaicin-sensitive and exhibit high-threshold TTX-resistant action potentials and Na^+ currents. However neurons from rats with cystitis exhibit significantly lower thresholds for spike activation (−25.4 vs. −21.4 mV) and show tonic rather than phasic firing characteristics (12.3 vs. 1.2 action potentials per 500-ms depolarization) (Yoshimura and de Groat 1999). Other significant changes in bladder afferent neurons from cyclophosphamide-treated rats include increase in somal diameter, increase in input capacitance, and decrease in density of slowly inactivating I_A currents (Yoshimura and de Groat 1999). Similar somal hyperexcitability due to reduced I_A current expression after chronic tissue inflammation has also been detected in afferent neurons innervating the rat stomach or the guinea pig ileum (Stewart et al. 2003). Thus, the reduction in I_A current size could be a key mechanism inducing afferent hyperexcitability and pain in pelvic visceral organs, including the bladder.

A recent study using cats with naturally occurring feline-type PBS/IC has also demonstrated that capsaicin-sensitive DRG neurons exhibit an increase in cell size and increase in firing rates to depolarizing current pulses owing to a reduction in low-threshold K^+ currents (Sculptoreanu et al. 2005a). Taken together, these data indicate that chronic inflammation in PBS/IC induces both cell hypertrophy and hyperexcitability of C-fiber bladder afferent neurons. If these changes in neuronal cell bodies also occur at C-fiber afferent terminals in the bladder wall, such hyperexcitability may represent an important mechanism for inducing pain in the inflamed bladder. Therefore, suppression of C-fiber activity represents a mechanism by which to treat bladder pain. This is supported by some clinical studies showing that C-fiber desensitization induced by intravesical application of capsaicin or resiniferatoxin is effective for treating painful symptoms in patients with PBS/IC (Lazzeri et al. 1996, 2000). However, a previous prospective, randomized clinical trial using intravesical resiniferatoxin application was not effective in patients with PBS/IC (Payne et al. 2005).

Although there is little information available about the neuroplasticity of Aδ-fiber bladder afferents in PBS/IC, a previous study (Roppolo et al. 2005) using single nerve fiber recordings has documented that Aδ-fiber bladder afferents in IC cats are more sensitive to bladder pressure changes than afferents in normal cats, suggesting that, in addition to neuroplasticity of C-fiber afferents, Aδ-fiber bladder afferents might also undergo functional changes in PBS/IC.

Chronic bladder inflammation can also induce changes in functional properties of chemosensitive receptors such as TRPV1 in sensory neurons. Sculptoreanu et al. (2005b) reported that DRG neurons obtained from IC cats exhibit capsaicin-induced responses that are larger in amplitude and desensitize more slowly compared with those obtained from normal cats, and that altered TRPV1 receptor activity in IC cats is reversed by an application of an inhibitor of PKC, suggesting that PBS/IC can alter TRPV1 activity owing to enhanced endogenous PKC activity. Since TRPV1 receptors are reportedly responsible at least in part for bladder overactivity elicited by cyclophosphamide-induced cystitis (Dinis et al. 2004), enhanced activity of TRPV1 receptors could contribute to bladder pain in PBS/IC.

Studies in mice have also demonstrated a role of TRPV1 in cystitis. Systemic treatment with cyclophosphamide or intravesical administration of acrolein, the irritant metabolite of cyclophosphamide, produces not only bladder hyperactivity but also a sensitization of the paw withdrawal responses to mechanical stimulation of the paw (mechanical hyperalgesia). These responses do not occur in TRPV1 knockout mice (Charrua et al. 2007; Wang et al. 2008). However, the lack of functional TRPV1 does not inhibit the development of the histological changes associated with bladder inflammation, including submucosal edema and areas of hemorrhage, and does not alter the increased expression of various markers of cystitis (messenger RNA for NGF, endothelial NOS, cyclooxygenase-2, and bradykinin receptors) in the urothelium.

The neurotoxin saporin, which is contained in the seeds of the soapwort plant, has been used to examine the roles of two types of afferent pathways in the transmission of nociceptive sensory information from the bladder to the spinal cord of the rat. After intrathecal administration of saporin conjugated with IB4 to selectively eliminate the IB4-positive C-fiber population, the bladder overactivity induced by bladder irritation is suppressed (Nishiguchi et al. 2004). Similarly when saporin conjugated to SP is administered to eliminate neurokinin-1 receptor expressing, pain-related spinal cord neurons, the bladder overactivity induced by bladder irritation is also suppressed (Seki et al. 2005). Thus, both IB4-binding, nonpeptidergic and IB4-negative, peptidergic C-fiber afferents seem to play an important role in bladder nociceptive mechanisms even though the former represents a smaller component of the total population of bladder afferent neurons.

11 Afferent Nerves and Diabetes Mellitus

Diabetes mellitus is often accompanied by urological complications characterized by impaired sensation of bladder fullness, increased bladder capacity, reduced bladder contractility, and elevated residual urine (Kebapci et al. 2007; Yoshimura et al. 2005). These changes are attributable in part to afferent neuropathy that is evident as a reduced afferent nerve conduction velocity (Nadelhaft and Vera 1992) and reduced axonal transport of neurotrophic factors, such as NGF (Steers et al. 1994; Tong and Cheng 2007; Yoshimura et al. 2005). In streptozotocin-induced diabetic rats, an increase in bladder capacity, an increase in postvoid residual volumes, and a decrease in bladder activation by intravesical administration of an irritant chemical occurs 12 weeks after injection of streptozotocin (Sasaki et al. 2002). In the same animals, NGF levels decrease in the bladder and in the lumbosacral DRG. NGF gene therapy using a replication-defective herpes simplex virus vector injected into the bladder wall reverses these changes (Sasaki et al. 2004). These data suggest that diabetic cystopathy is related to a reduced production or axonal transport of NGF in bladder nerves leading to a defect in the functions of Aδ or C-fiber bladder afferent pathways.

12 Afferent Nerves and Interorgan Cross-Sensitization

Axonal tracing studies revealed that a subpopulation (6–21%) of afferent neurons in the lumbosacral DRG of the rat and mouse can innervate multiple pelvic organs (Christianson et al. 2007; Keast and de Groat 1992). In the rat, the larger percentage of these neurons is present in the TL DRG, whereas in the mouse the larger percentage is in the LS DRG. Subsequent studies provided evidence that chemical irritation of one organ (either the urinary bladder or the colon) can facilitate/sensitize the activity of the other organ (Pezzone et al. 2005). Electrophysiological experiments showed that acute colonic irritation can sensitize bladder C-fiber afferents to mechanical and chemical stimuli (Ustinova et al. 2006) and enhance the firing of lumbosacral spinal interneurons receiving afferent input from the bladder (Qin et al. 2005). Lumbosacral afferent neurons in the L6–S2 DRG innervating both the colon and bladder ("convergent neurons") exhibited decreased voltage and current thresholds for action potential firing 3 days after colonic irritation with trinitrobenzene sulfonic acid (Malykhina et al. 2006). The effect persisted for 30 days in the absence of overt colonic inflammation. Colitis also enhanced the responses to capsaicin and increased the peak amplitude of TTX-resistant Na^+ currents in bladder afferent neurons isolated from the L6–S2 DRG (Malykhina et al. 2004).

Changes in bladder function after colonic inflammation also appear to be mediated by a change in the cholinergic efferent pathway to the bladder (Noronha et al. 2007). During the active colonic inflammation 3 days after instillation of trinitrobenzene sulfonic acid into the colon, the bladder was not inflamed, but the contractions of bladder strips induced by electrical field stimulation or carbachol, a muscarinic receptor agonist, were reduced, while the contractions induced by KCl were not changed. During and after recovery of the colonic inflammation (15–30 days) the contractile responses of the bladder returned to normal. It was suggested that the bladder dysfunction was mediated by visceral organ cross talk induced by sensitization of a subpopulation of afferents innervating both the bladder and the colon.

13 Perspectives

The afferent innervation of the lower urinary tract plays an important role in both reflex and voluntary control of voiding. Myelinated Aδ afferent nerves which are mechanosensitive and respond to bladder distension are essential for the initiation of urine storage reflexes and for signaling the brain about the level of bladder filling and the need to void. On the other hand, unmyelinated C-fiber afferent nerves seem to function primarily as nociceptors that respond to noxious chemical and mechanical stimuli. Activation of these afferents triggers painful sensations as well as body defense mechanisms such as inflammation and bladder hyperactivity that eliminate infectious or irritating, potentially injurious agents from the urinary tract. C-fiber bladder afferent neurons are sensitized by a variety of endogenous substances (neurotransmitters, neurotrophic factors and inflammatory mediators) released by neural and nonneural cells within the bladder wall and exhibit a remarkable degree of morphological, chemical, and electrophysiological plasticity. Thus C-fiber bladder afferents are involved in many pathophysiological processes and are important targets for drugs and neurotoxins used to treat lower urinary tract dysfunction.

References

Andrade EL, Ferreira J, Andre E, Calixto JB (2006) Contractile mechanisms coupled to TRPA1 receptor activation in rat urinary bladder. Biochem Pharmacol 72:104–114

Apostolidis A, Fowler CJ (2008) The use of botulinum neurotoxin type A (BoNTA) in urology. J Neural Transm 115:593–605

Apostolidis A, Brady CM, Yiangou Y, Davis J, Fowler CJ, Anand P (2005a) Capsaicin receptor TRPV1 in urothelium of neurogenic human bladders and effect of intravesical resiniferatoxin. Urology 65:400–405

Apostolidis A, Popat R, Yiangou Y, Cockayne D, Ford AP, Davis JB, Dasgupta P, Fowler CJ, Anand P (2005b) Decreased sensory receptors P2X3 and TRPV1 in suburothelial nerve fibers following intradetrusor injections of botulinum toxin for human detrusor overactivity. J Urol 174:977–982

Apostolidis A, Dasgupta P, Fowler CJ (2006) Proposed mechanism for the efficacy of injected botulinum toxin in the treatment of human detrusor overactivity. Eur Urol 49:644–650

Apostolidis A, Jacques TS, Freeman A, Kalsi V, Popat R, Gonzales G, Datta SN, Ghazi-Noori S, Elneil S, Dasgupta P, Fowler CJ (2008) Histological changes in the urothelium and suburothelium of human overactive bladder following intradetrusor injections of botulinum neurotoxin type A for the treatment of neurogenic or idiopathic detrusor overactivity. Eur Urol 53:1245–1253

Applebaum AE, Vance WH, Coggeshall RE (1980) Segmental localization of sensory cells that innervate the bladder. J Comp Neurol 192:203–209

Avelino A, Cruz C, Nagy I, Cruz F (2002) Vanilloid receptor 1 expression in the rat urinary tract. Neuroscience 109:787–798

Averill S, McMahon SB, Clary DO, Reichardt LF, Priestley JV (1995) Immunocytochemical localization of trkA receptors in chemically identified subgroups of adult rat sensory neurons. Eur J Neurosci 7:1484–1494

Bahns E, Ernsberger U, Janig W, Nelke A (1986) Functional characteristics of lumbar visceral afferent fibres from the urinary bladder and the urethra in the cat. Pflugers Arch 407:510–518

Bahns E, Halsband U, Janig W (1987) Responses of sacral visceral afferents from the lower urinary tract, colon and anus to mechanical stimulation. Pflugers Arch 410:296–303

Beckel JM, Kanai A, Lee SJ, de Groat WC, Birder LA (2006) Expression of functional nicotinic acetylcholine receptors in rat urinary bladder epithelial cells. Am J Physiol Renal Physiol 290: F103–F110

Bennett DL, Dmietrieva N, Priestley JV, Clary D, McMahon SB (1996) trkA, CGRP and IB4 expression in retrogradely labelled cutaneous and visceral primary sensory neurones in the rat. Neurosci Lett 206:33–36

Bennett HL, Gustafsson JA, Keast JR (2003) Estrogen receptor expression in lumbosacral dorsal root ganglion cells innervating the female rat urinary bladder. Auton Neurosci 105:90–100

Birder LA, de Groat WC (1993) Induction of *c-fos* expression in spinal neurons by nociceptive and nonnociceptive stimulation of LUT. Am J Physiol 265:R326–R333

Birder LA, de Groat WC (2007) Mechanisms of disease: involvement of the urothelium in bladder dysfunction. Nat Clin Pract Urol 4:46–54

Birder LA, Apodaca G, de Groat WC, Kanai AJ (1998) Adrenergic- and capsaicin-evoked nitric oxide release from urothelium and afferent nerves in urinary bladder. Am J Physiol 275:F226–F229

Birder LA, Barrick S, Roppolo JR, Kanai A, de Groat WC, Kiss S, Buffington CA (2003) Feline interstitial cystitis results in mechanical hypersensitivity and altered ATP release from bladder urothelium Am J Physiol 285:F423–F429

Birder LA, Roppolo JR, Erickson VL, de Groat WC (1999) Increased *c-fos* expression in spinal lumbosacral projection neurons and preganglionic neurons after irritation of the lower urinary tract in the rat. Brain Res 834:55–65

Birder LA, Kanai AJ, de Groat WC, Kiss S, Nealen ML, Burke NE, Dineley KE, Watkins S, Reynolds IJ, Caterina MJ (2001) Vanilloid receptor expression suggests a sensory role for urinary bladder epithelial cells. Proc Natl Acad Sci USA 98:13396–13401

Birder LA, Nakamura Y, Kiss S, Nealen ML, Barrick S, Kanai AJ, Wang E, Ruiz G, De Groat WC, Apodaca G, Watkins S, Caterina MJ (2002a) Altered urinary bladder function in mice lacking the vanilloid receptor TRPV1. Nat Neurosci 5:856–860

Birder LA, Nealen ML, Kiss S, de Groat WC, Caterina MJ, Wang E, Apodaca G, Kanai AJ (2002b) Beta-adrenoceptor agonists stimulate endothelial nitric oxide synthase in rat urinary bladder urothelial cells. J Neurosci 22:8063–8070

Birder LA, Ruan HZ, Chopra B, Xiang Z, Barrick S, Buffington CA, Roppolo JR, Ford AP, de Groat WC, Burnstock G (2004) Alterations in P2X and P2Y purinergic receptor expression in urinary bladder from normal cats and cats with interstitial cystitis. Am J Physiol Renal Physiol 287:F1084–F1091

Birder LA, de Groat WC, Apodaca G (2008) Physiology of the urothelium. In: Schick E, Corcos J (eds) Textbook of the neurogenic bladder, 2nd edn. Taylor and Francis, London, chap 3

Black JA, Cummins TR, Yoshimura N, de Groat WC, Waxman SG (2003) Tetrodotoxin-resistant sodium channels Na(v)1.8/SNS and Na(v)1.9/NaN in afferent neurons innervating urinary bladder in control and spinal cord injured rats. Brain Res 963:132–138

Brady CM, Apostolidis A, Yiangou Y, Baecker PA, Ford AP, Freeman A, Jacques TS, Fowler CJ, Anand P (2004a) P2X3-immunoreactive nerve fibres in neurogenic detrusor overactivity and the effect of intravesical resiniferatoxin. Eur Urol 46:247–253

Brady CM, Apostolidis AN, Harper M, Yiangou Y, Beckett A, Jacques TS, Freeman A, Scaravilli F, Fowler CJ, Anand P (2004b) Parallel changes in bladder suburothelial vanilloid receptor TRPV1 and pan-neuronal marker PGP9.5 immunoreactivity in patients with neurogenic detrusor overactivity after intravesical resiniferatoxin treatment. BJU Int 93:770–776

Chai TC, Steers WD, Broder SR, Rauchenwald M, Tuttle JB (1996) Characterization of laterality of innervation of the rat bladder. Scand J Urol Nephrol Suppl 179:87–92

Chai TC, Gray ML, Steers WD (1998) The incidence of a positive ice water test in bladder outlet obstructed patients: evidence for bladder neural plasticity. J Urol 160:34–38

Chang HY, Cheng CL, Chen JJ, de Groat WC (2007) Serotonergic drugs and spinal cord transections indicate that different spinal circuits are involved in external urethral sphincter activity in rats. Am J Physiol Renal Physiol 292:F1044–F1053

Charrua A, Cruz CD, Cruz F, Avelino A (2007) Transient receptor potential vanilloid subfamily 1 is essential for the generation of noxious bladder input and bladder overactivity in cystitis. J Urol 177:1537–1541

Cheng CL, Chai CY, de Groat WC (1997) Detrusor-sphincter dyssynergia induced by cold stimulation of the urinary bladder of rats. Am J Physiol 272:R1271–R1282

Cheng CL, Liu JC, Chang SY, Ma CP, de Groat WC (1999) Effect of capsaicin on the micturition reflex in normal and chronic spinal cord-injured cats. Am J Physiol 277:R786–R794

Chess-Williams R (2002) Muscarinic receptors of the urinary bladder: detrusor, urothelial and prejunctional. Auton Autacoid Pharmacol 22:133–145

Chopra B, Barrick SR, Meyers S, Beckel JM, Zeidel ML, Ford AP, de Groat WC, Birder LA (2005) Expression and function of bradykinin B1 and B2 receptors in normal and inflamed rat urinary bladder urothelium. J Physiol 562:859–871

Christianson JA, Liang R, Ustinova EE, Davis BM, Fraser MO, Pezzone MA (2007) Convergence of bladder and colon sensory innervation occurs at the primary afferent level. Pain 128: 235–243

Chuang YC, Fraser MO, Yu Y, Chancellor MB, de Groat WC, Yoshimura N (2001) The role of bladder afferent pathways in bladder hyperactivity induced by the intravesical administration of nerve growth factor. J Urol 165:975–979

Clifton GL, Coggeshall RE, Vance WH, Willis WD (1976) Receptive fields of unmyelinated ventral root afferent fibres in the cat. J Physiol 256:573–600

Cockayne DA, Hamilton SG, Zhu QM, Dunn PM, Zhong Y, Novakovic S, Malmberg AB, Cain G, Berson A, Kassotakis L, Hedley L, Lachnit WG, Burnstock G, McMahon SB, Ford AP (2000) Urinary bladder hyporeflexia and reduced pain-related behaviour in P2X3-deficient mice. Nature 407:1011–1015

Crowe R, Light K, Chilton CP, Burnstock G (1986) Vasoactive intestinal polypeptide-, somatostatin- and substance P-immunoreactive nerves in the smooth and striated muscle of the intrinsic external urethral sphincter of patients with spinal cord injury. J Urol 136:487–491

Cruz F, Dinis P (2007) Resiniferatoxin and botulinum toxin type A for treatment of lower urinary tract symptoms. Neurourol Urodyn 26:920–927

Cruz CD, Ferreira D, McMahon SB, Cruz F (2007) The activation of the ERK pathway contributes to the spinal *c-fos* expression observed after noxious bladder stimulation. Somatosens Mot Res 24:15–20

Daly D, Rong W, Chess-Williams R, Chapple C, Grundy D (2007) Bladder afferent sensitivity in wild-type and TRPV1 knockout mice. J Physiol 583:663–674

Dang K, Bielefeldt K, Gebhart GF (2005) Differential responses of bladder lumbosacral and thoracolumbar dorsal root ganglion neurons to purinergic agonists, protons, and capsaicin. J Neurosci 25:3973–3984

Dang K, Lamb K, Cohen M, Bielefeldt K, Gebhart GF (2008) Cyclophosphamide-induced bladder inflammation sensitizes and enhances P2X receptor function in rat bladder sensory neurons. J Neurophysiol 99:49–59

Dattilio A, Vizzard MA (2005) Up-regulation of protease activated receptors in bladder after cyclophosphamide induced cystitis and colocalization with capsaicin receptor (VR1) in bladder nerve fibers. J Urol 173:635–639

de Groat WC (1986) Spinal cord projections and neuropeptides in visceral afferent neurons. Prog Brain Res 67:165–187

de Groat WC (1989) Neuropeptides in pelvic afferent pathways. In: Polak JM (ed) Regulatory peptides. Birkhauser, Basel, pp 334–336

de Groat WC (2004) The urothelium in overactive bladder: passive bystander or active participant? Urology 64:7–11

de Groat WC, Yoshimura N (2006) Mechanisms underlying the recovery of lower urinary tract function following spinal cord injury. Eds.: Weaver LC, Polosa C. Progress in Brain Research 152:59–84

de Groat WC, Nadelhaft I, Milne RJ, Booth AM, Morgan C, Thor K (1981) Organization of the sacral parasympathetic reflex pathways to the urinary bladder and large intestine. J Auton Nerv Sys 3:135–160

de Groat WC, Kawatani M, Hisamitsu T, Cheng C-L, Ma C-P, Thor K, Steers W, Roppolo JR (1990) Mechanisms underlying the recovery of urinary bladder function following spinal cord injury. J Auto Nerv Sys 30(Suppl):S71–S77

de Groat WC, Booth AM and Yoshimura N (1993) Neurophysiology of micturition and its modification in animal models of human disease. In: Maggi CA (ed) The autonomic nervous system, vol 3. Nervous control of the urogenital system. Harwood, London, pp 227–289

de Groat WC, Fraser MO, Yoshiyama M, Smerin S, Tai C, Chancellor MB, Yoshimura N, Roppolo JR (2001) Neural control of the urethra. Scand J Urol Nephrol Suppl 207:35–43; discussion 106–125

Dickson A, Avelino A, Cruz F, Ribeiro-da-Silva A (2006) Peptidergic sensory and parasympathetic fiber sprouting in the mucosa of the rat urinary bladder in a chronic model of cyclophosphamide-induced cystitis. Neuroscience 139:671–685

Dinis P, Charrua A, Avelino A, Yaqoob M, Bevan S, Nagy I, Cruz F (2004) Anandamide-evoked activation of vanilloid receptor 1 contributes to the development of bladder hyperreflexia and nociceptive transmission to spinal dorsal horn neurons in cystitis. J Neurosci 24:11253–11263

Dmitrieva N, McMahon SB (1996) Sensitisation of visceral afferents by nerve growth factor in the adult rat. Pain 66:87–97

Dmitrieva N, Shelton D, Rice AS, McMahon SB (1997) The role of nerve growth factor in a model of visceral inflammation. Neuroscience 78:449–459

Downie JW, Armour JA (1992) Mechanoreceptor afferent activity compared with receptor field dimensions and pressure changes in feline urinary bladder. Can J Physiol Pharmacol 70:1457–1467

Du S, Araki I, Yoshiyama M, Nomura T, Takeda M (2007) Transient receptor potential channel A1 involved in sensory transduction of rat urinary bladder through C-fiber pathway. Urology 70:826–831

Everaerts W, Gevaert T, Nilius B, De Ridder D (2008) On the origin of bladder sensing: Tr(i)ps in urology. Neurourol Urodyn 27:264–273

Fahrenkrug J, Hannibal J (1998) Pituitary adenylate cyclase activating polypeptide immunoreactivity in capsaicin-sensitive nerve fibres supplying the rat urinary tract. Neuroscience 83:1261–1272

Fall M, Lindström S, Mazieres L (1990) A bladder-to-bladder cooling reflex in the cat. J Physiol (Lond) 427:281–300

Fam B, Yalla SV (1988) Vesicourethral dysfunction in spinal cord injury and its management. Semin Neurol 8:150–155

Ferguson DR, Kennedy I, Burton TJ (1997) ATP is released from rabbit urinary bladder epithelial cells by hydrostatic pressure changes – a possible sensory mechanism? J Physiol 505:503–511

Floyd K, Hick VE, Morrison JF (1976) Mechanosensitive afferent units in the hypogastric nerve of the cat. J Physiol (Lond) 259:457–471

Forrest SL, Keast JR (2008) Expression of receptors for glial cell line-derived neurotrophic factor family ligands in sacral spinal cord reveals separate targets of pelvic afferent fibers. J Comp Neurol 506:989–1002

Fowler CJ, Griffiths D, de Groat WC (2008) The neural control of micturition. Nat Rev Neurosci 9:453–466

Gabella G, Davis C (1998) Distribution of afferent axons in the bladder of rats. J Neurocytol 27:141–155

Geirsson G, Fall M, Lindstrom S (1993) The ice-water test – a simple and valuable supplement to routine cystometry. Br J Urol 71:681–685

Geirsson G, Fall M, Sullivan L (1995) Clinical and urodynamic effects of intravesical capsaicin treatment in patients with chronic traumatic spinal detrusor hyperreflexia. J. Urol 154:1825–1829

Geirsson G, Lindstrom S, Fall M, Gladh G, Hermansson G, Hjalmas K (1994) Positive bladder cooling test in neurologically normal young children. J Urol 151:446–448

Gevaert T, Vriens J, Segal A, Everaerts W, Roskams T, Talavera K, Owsianik G, Liedtke W, Daelemans D, Dewachter I, Van Leuven F, Voets T, De Ridder D, Nilius B (2007) Deletion of the transient receptor potential cation channel TRPV4 impairs murine bladder voiding. J Clin Invest 117:3453–3462

Gillespie JI, Markerink-van Ittersum M, de Vente J (2006) Sensory collaterals, intramural ganglia and motor nerves in the guinea-pig bladder: evidence for intramural neural circuits. Cell Tissue Res 325:33–45

Gold MS, Shuster MJ, Levine JD (1996) Characterization of six voltage-gated K+ currents in adult rat sensory neurons. J Neurophysiol 75:2629–2646

Gosling JA, Dixon JS, Critchley HO, Thompson SA (1981) A comparative study of the human external sphincter and periurethral levator ani muscles. Br J Urol 53:35–41

Guo A, Vulchanova L, Wang J, Li X, Elde R (1999) Immunocytochemical localization of the vanilloid receptor 1 (VR1): relationship to neuropeptides, the P2X3 purinoceptor and IB4 binding sites. Eur J Neurosci 11:946–958

Häbler HJ, Jänig W, Koltzenburg M (1990) Activation of unmyelinated afferent fibres by mechanical stimuli and inflammation of the urinary bladder in the cat. J Physiol (Lond) 425: 545–562

Häbler HJ, Jänig W, Koltzenburg M (1993) Myelinated primary afferents of the sacral spinal cord responding to slow filling and distension of the cat urinary bladder. J Physiol 463:449–460

Hirayama A, Fujimoto K, Matsumoto Y, Ozono S, Hirao Y (2003) Positive response to ice water test associated with high-grade bladder outlet obstruction in patients with benign prostatic hyperplasia. Urology 62:909–913

Hu P, Meyers S, Liang FX, Deng FM, Kachar B, Zeidel ML, Sun TT (2002) Role of membrane proteins in permeability barrier function: uroplakin ablation elevates urothelial permeability. Am J Physiol Renal Physiol 283:F1200–F1207

Hu VY, Zvara P, Dattilio A, Redman TL, Allen SJ, Dawbarn D, Stroemer RP, Vizzard MA (2005) Decrease in bladder overactivity with REN1820 in rats with cyclophosphamide induced cystitis. J Urol 173:1016–1021

Hulsebosch CE, Coggeshall RE (1982) An analysis of the axon populations in the nerves to the pelvic viscera in the rat. J Comp Neurol 211:1–10

Ishizuka O, Alm P, Larsson B, Mattiasson A, Andersson KE (1995) Facilitatory effect of pituitary adenylate cyclase activating polypeptide on micturition in normal, conscious rats. Neuroscience 66:1009–1014

Ito K, Iwami A, Katsura H, Ikeda M (2007) Therapeutic effects of the putative P2X(3)/P2X (2/3) antagonist A-317491 on cyclophosphamide-induced cystitis in rats. Naunyn Schmiedebergs Arch Pharmacol 377(4–6):483–490

Jaggar SI, Scott HC, Rice AS (1999) Inflammation of the rat urinary bladder is associated with a referred thermal hyperalgesia which is nerve growth factor dependent. Br J Anaesth 83: 442–448

Jancso G, Maggi CA (1987) Distribution of capsaicin-sensitive urinary bladder afferents in the rat spinal cord. Brain Res 418:371–376

Jänig W, Morrison JFB (1986) Functional properties of spinal visceral afferents supplying abdominal and pelvic organs, with special emphasis on visceral nociception. Prog Brain Res 67:87–114

Jiang CH, Mazieres L, Lindstrom S (2002) Cold- and menthol-sensitive C afferents of cat urinary bladder. J Physiol 543:211–220

Johansson S, Fall M (1997) The pathology of interstitial cystitis. In: Sant GR (ed) Interstitial cystitis. Lippincott-Raven, Philadelphia, pp 143–151

Kawatani M, Erdman SL, de Groat WC (1985) Vasoactive intestinal polypeptide and substance P in primary afferent pathways to the sacral spinal cord of the cat. J Comp Neurol 241:327–347

Kawatani M, Nagel J, de Groat WC (1986) Identification of neuropeptides in pelvic and pudendal nerve afferent pathways to the sacral spinal cord of the cat. J Comp Neurol 249:117–132

Kawatani M, Suzuki T, de Groat WC (1996) Corticotropin releasing factor-like immunoreactivity in afferent projections to the sacral spinal cord of the cat. J Auton Nerv Syst 61:218–226

Keast JR, de Groat WC (1992) Segmental distribution and peptide content of primary afferent neurons innervating the urogenital organs and colon of male rats. J Comp Neurol 319:615–623

Keast JR, Stephensen TM (2000) Glutamate and aspartate immunoreactivity in dorsal root ganglion cells supplying visceral and somatic targets and evidence for peripheral axonal transport. J Comp Neurol 424:577–587

Kebapci N, Yenilmez A, Efe B, Entok E, Demirustu C (2007) Bladder dysfunction in type 2 diabetic patients. Neurourol Urodyn 26:814–819

Kruse MN, Bray LA, de Groat WC (1995) Influence of spinal cord injury on the morphology of bladder afferent and efferent neurons. J Auto Nerv Sys 54:215–224

Kullmann FA, Artim D, Beckel J, Barrick S, de Groat WC, Birder LA (2008a) Heterogeneity of muscarinic receptor-mediated Ca^{2+} responses in cultured urothelial cells from rat. Am J Physiol Renal Physiol 294:F971–F981

Kullmann FA, Artim DE, Birder LA, de Groat WC (2008b) Activation of muscarinic receptors in rat bladder sensory pathways alters reflex bladder activity. J Neurosci 28:1977–1987

Lamb K, Gebhart GF, Bielefeldt K (2004) Increased nerve growth factor expression triggers bladder overactivity. J Pain 5:150–156

Langford LA, Coggeshall RE (1981) Branching of sensory axons in the peripheral nerve of the rat. J Comp Neurol 203:745–750

Lanteri-Minet M, Bon K, de Pommery J, Michiels JF, Menetrey D (1995) Cyclophosphamide cystitis as a model of visceral pain in rats: model elaboration and spinal structures involved as revealed by the expression of *c-fos* and *Krox-24* proteins. Exp Brain Res 105:220–232

Lassmann G (1984) Muscle spindles and sensory nerve endings in the urethral sphincter. Acta Neuropathol 63:344–346

Lavelle J, Meyers S, Ramage R, Bastacky S, Doty D, Apodaca G, Zeidel ML (2002) Bladder permeability barrier: recovery from selective injury of surface epithelial cells. Am J Physiol Renal Physiol 283:F242–F253

Lawson SN, Perry MJ, Prabhakar E, McCarthy PW (1993) Primary sensory neurones: neurofilament, neuropeptides, and conduction velocity. Brain Res Bull 30:239–243

Lazzeri M, Beneforti P, Benaim G, Maggi CA, Lecci A, Turini D (1996) Intravesical capsaicin for treatment of severe bladder pain: a randomized placebo controlled study. J Urol 156:947–952

Lazzeri M, Beneforti P, Spinelli M, Zanollo A, Barbagli G, Turini D (2000) Intravesical resiniferatoxin for the treatment of hypersensitive disorder: a randomized placebo controlled study. J Urol 164:676–679

Lee HY, Bardini M, Burnstock G (2000) Distribution of P2X receptors in the urinary bladder and the ureter of the rat. J Urol 163:2002–2007

Lindstrom S, Mazieres L, Jiang CH (2004) Inhibition of the bladder cooling reflex in the awake state: an experimental study in the cat. J Urol 172:2051–2053

Liu HT, Kuo HC (2008) Urinary nerve growth factor levels are increased in patients with bladder outlet obstruction with overactive bladder symptoms and reduced after successful medical treatment. Urology 72(1):104–108

Lowe EM, Anand P, Terenghi G, Williams-Chestnut RE, Sinicropi DV, Osborne JL (1997) Increased nerve growth factor levels in the urinary bladder of women with idiopathic sensory urgency and interstitial cystitis. Br J Urol 79:572–577

Maggi CA (1993) The dual, sensory and efferent function of the capsaicin-sensitive primary sensory nerves in the bladder and urethra. In: Maggi CA (ed) Nervous control of the urogenital system, vol 1. Harwood, London, pp 383–422

Malykhina AP, Qin C, Foreman RD, Akbarali HI (2004) Colonic inflammation increases Na^+ currents in bladder sensory neurons. Neuroreport 15:2601–2605

Malykhina AP, Qin C, Greenwood-van Meerveld B, Foreman RD, Lupu F, Akbarali HI (2006) Hyperexcitability of convergent colon and bladder dorsal root ganglion neurons after colonic inflammation: mechanism for pelvic organ cross-talk. Neurogastroenterol Motil 18:936–948

Masuda H, Kim JH, Kihara K, Chancellor MB, de Groat WC, Yoshimura N (2007) Inhibitory roles of peripheral nitrergic mechanisms in capsaicin-induced detrusor overactivity in the rat. BJU Int 100:912–918

Mazieres L, Jiang C, Lindstrom S (1998) The C fibre reflex of the cat urinary bladder. J Physiol 513(2):531–541

McGuire EJ, Morrissey SG, Schichun Z, Horwinsk E (1983) Control of reflex detrusor activity in normal and spinal injured non-human primates. J Urol 129:197–199

Mitsui T, Kakizaki H, Matsuura S, Ameda K, Yoshioka M, Koyanagi T (2001) Afferent fibers of the hypogastric nerves are involved in the facilitating effects of chemical bladder irritation in rats. J Neurophysiol 86:2276–2284

Miura A, Kawatani M, de Groat WC (2001) Effects of pituitary adenylate cyclase activating polypeptide on lumbosacral preganglionic neurons in the neonatal rat spinal cord. Brain Res 895:223–232

Morgan C, Nadelhaft I, de Groat WC (1981) The distribution of visceral primary afferents from the pelvic nerve to Lissauer's tract and the spinal gray matter and its relationship to the sacral parasympathetic nucleus. J Comp Neurol 201:415–440

Morgan C, de Groat WC, Nadelhaft I (1986) The spinal distribution of sympathetic preganglionic and visceral primary afferent neurons that send axons into the hypogastric nerves of the cat. J Comp Neurol 243:23–40

Morgan CW, de Groat WC, Felkins LA, Zhang SJ (1993) Intracellular injection of neurobiotin or horseradish peroxidase reveals separate types of preganglionic neurons in the sacral parasympathetic nucleus of the cat. J Comp Neurol 331:161–182

Morgan CW, Ohara PT, Scott DE (1999) Vasoactive intestinal polypeptide in sacral primary sensory pathways in the cat. J Comp Neurol 407:381–394

Morrison JF (1997) The physiological mechanisms involved in bladder emptying. Scand J Urol Nephrol Suppl 184:15–18

Morrison JF, Birder L, Craggs M, de Groat WC, Downie JW, Drake M, Fowler CJ, Thor KB (2005) Neural control. In: Abrams P, Cardozo L, Khoury S, Wein A (eds) Incontinence. Health, Plymouth, pp 363–422

Moss NG, Harrington WW, Tucker MS (1997) Pressure, volume, and chemosensitivity in afferent innervation of urinary bladder in rats. Am J Physiol 272:R695–R703

Murray E, Malley SE, Qiao LY, Hu VY, Vizzard MA (2004) Cyclophosphamide induced cystitis alters neurotrophin and receptor tyrosine kinase expression in pelvic ganglia and bladder. J Urol 172:2434–2439

Nadelhaft I, Vera PL (1992) Reduced urinary bladder afferent conduction velocities in streptozocin diabetic rats. Neurosci Lett 135:276–8

Namasivayam S, Eardley I, Morrison JF (1999) Purinergic sensory neurotransmission in the urinary bladder: an in vitro study in the rat. BJU Int 84:854–860

Nishiguchi J, Sasaki K, Seki S, Chancellor MB, Erickson KA, de Groat WC, Kumon H, Yoshimura N (2004) Effects of isolectin B4-conjugated saporin, a targeting cytotoxin, on bladder overactivity induced by bladder irritation. Eur J Neurosci 20:474–482

Nishiguchi J, Hayashi Y, Chancellor MB, de Miguel F, de Groat WC, Kumon H, Yoshimura N (2005) Detrusor overactivity induced by intravesical application of adenosine 5′-triphosphate under different delivery conditions in rats. Urology 66:1332–1337

Noronha R, Akbarali H, Malykhina A, Foreman RD, Greenwood-Van Meerveld B (2007) Changes in urinary bladder smooth muscle function in response to colonic inflammation. Am J Physiol Renal Physiol 293:F1461–F1467

Novakovic SD, Tzoumaka E, McGivern JG, Haraguchi M, Sangameswaran L, Gogas KR, Eglen RM, Hunter JC (1998) Distribution of the tetrodotoxin-resistant sodium channel PN3 in rat sensory neurons in normal and neuropathic conditions. J Neurosci 18:2174–2187

Ogawa T, Kamo I, Pflug BR, Nelson JB, Seki S, Igawa Y, Nishizawa O, de Groat WC, Chancellor MB, Yoshimura N (2004) Differential roles of peripheral and spinal endothelin receptors in the micturition reflex in rats. J Urol 172:1533–1537

Okragly AJ, Niles AL, Saban R, Schmidt D, Hoffman RL, Warner TF, Moon TD, Uehling DT, Haak-Frendscho M (1999) Elevated tryptase, nerve growth factor, neurotrophin-3 and glial cell line-derived neurotrophic factor levels in the urine of interstitial cystitis and bladder cancer patients. J Urol 161:438–442

Ozawa H, Chancellor MB, Jung SY, Yokoyama T, Fraser MO, Yu Y, de Groat WC, Yoshimura N (1999) Effect of intravesical nitric oxide therapy on cyclophosphamide-induced cystitis. J Urol 162:2211–2216

Pandita RK, Andersson KE (2002) Intravesical adenosine triphosphate stimulates the micturition reflex in awake, freely moving rats. J Urol 168:1230–1234

Pandita RK, Mizusawa H, Andersson KE (2000) Intravesical oxyhemoglobin initiates bladder overactivity in conscious, normal rats. J Urol 164:545–550

Payne CK, Mosbaugh PG, Forrest JB, Evans RJ, Whitmore KE, Antoci JP, Perez-Marrero R, Jacoby K, Diokno AC, O'Reilly KJ, Griebling TL, Vasavada SP, Yu AS, Frumkin LR (2005) Intravesical resiniferatoxin for the treatment of interstitial cystitis: a randomized, double-blind, placebo controlled trial. J Urol 173:1590–1594

Pezzone MA, Liang R, Fraser MO (2005) A model of neural cross-talk and irritation in the pelvis: implications for the overlap of chronic pelvic pain disorders. Gastroenterology 128:1953–1964

Popat R, Apostolidis A, Kalsi V, Gonzales G, Fowler CJ, Dasgupta P (2005) A comparison between the response of patients with idiopathic detrusor overactivity and neurogenic detrusor overactivity to the first intradetrusor injection of botulinum-A toxin. J Urol 174:984–989

Qiao LY, Vizzard MA (2002) Cystitis-induced upregulation of tyrosine kinase (TrkA, TrkB) receptor expression and phosphorylation in rat micturition pathways. J Comp Neurol 454: 200–211

Qiao LY, Vizzard MA (2004) Up-regulation of phosphorylated CREB but not c-Jun in bladder afferent neurons in dorsal root ganglia after cystitis. J Comp Neurol 469:262–274

Qin C, Malykhina AP, Akbarali HI, Foreman RD (2005) Cross-organ sensitization of lumbosacral spinal neurons receiving urinary bladder input in rats with inflamed colon. Gastroenterology 129:1967–1978

Rockswold GL, Bradley WE, Chou SN (1980a) Innervation of the external urethral and external anal sphincters in higher primates. J Comp Neurol 193:521–528

Rockswold GL, Bradley WE, Chou SN (1980b) Innervation of the urinary bladder in higher primates. J Comp Neurol 193:509–520

Rong W, Spyer KM, Burnstock G (2002) Activation and sensitisation of low and high threshold afferent fibres mediated by P2X receptors in the mouse urinary bladder. J Physiol 541:591–600

Roppolo JR, Tai C, Booth AM, Buffington CA, de Groat WC, Birder LA (2005) Bladder Aδ afferent nerve activity in normal cats and cats with feline interstitial cystitis. J Urol 173:1011–1015

Sasaki K, Chancellor MB, Phelan MW, Yokoyama T, Fraser MO, Seki S, Kubo K, Kumon H, de Groat WC, Yoshimura N (2002) Diabetic cystopathy correlates with long-term decrease in nerve growth factor (NGF) levels in the bladder and lumbosacral dorsal root ganglia. J Urol 168:1259–1264

Sasaki K, Chancellor MB, Goins WF, Phelan MW, Glorioso JC, de Groat WC, Yoshimura N (2004) Gene therapy using replication-defective herpes simplex virus vectors expressing nerve growth factor in a rat model of diabetic cystopathy. Diabetes 53:2723–2730

Satchell P, Vaughan C (1994) Bladder wall tension and mechanoreceptor discharge. Pflugers Arch 426:304–309

Schurch B, de Seze M, Denys P, Chartier-Kastler E, Haab F, Everaert K, Plante P, Perrouin-Verbe B, Kumar C, Fraczek S, Brin MF (2005) Botulinum toxin type a is a safe and effective treatment for neurogenic urinary incontinence: results of a single treatment, randomized, placebo controlled 6-month study. J Urol 174:196–200

Schurch B, Denys P, Kozma CM, Reese PR, Slaton T, Barron RL (2007) Botulinum toxin A improves the quality of life of patients with neurogenic urinary incontinence. Eur Urol 52:850–858

Sculptoreanu A, de Groat WC (2003) Protein kinase C is involved in neurokinin receptor modulation of N- and L-type Ca2+ channels in DRG neurons of the adult rat. J Neurophysiol 90:21–31

Sculptoreanu A, de Groat WC (2007) Neurokinins enhance excitability in capsaicin-responsive DRG neurons. Exp Neurol 205:92–100

Sculptoreanu A, de Groat WC, Buffington CA, Birder LA (2005a) Abnormal excitability in capsaicin-responsive DRG neurons from cats with feline interstitial cystitis. Exp Neurol 193:437–443

Sculptoreanu A, de Groat WC, Buffington CA, Birder LA (2005b) Protein kinase C contributes to abnormal capsaicin responses in DRG neurons from cats with feline interstitial cystitis. Neurosci Lett 381:42–46

Seki S, Sasaki K, Fraser MO, Igawa Y, Nishizawa O, Chancellor MB, de Groat WC, Yoshimura N (2002) Immunoneutralization of nerve growth factor in lumbosacral spinal cord reduces bladder hyperreflexia in spinal cord injured rats. J Urol 168:2269–2274

Seki S, Sasaki K, Igawa Y, Nishizawa O, Chancellor M, de Groat W, Yoshimura N (2003) Detrusor overactivity induced by increased levels of nerve growth factor in bladder afferent pathways in rats. Neurourol Urodyn 22:375–377

Seki S, Sasaki K, Igawa Y, Nishizawa O, Chancellor MB, de Groat WC, Yoshimura N (2004) Suppression of detrusor-sphincter dyssynergia by immunoneutralization of nerve growth factor in lumbosacral spinal cord in spinal cord injured rats. J Urol 171:478–482

Seki S, Erickson KA, Seki M, Nishizawa O, Igawa Y, Ogawa T, de Groat WC, Chancellor MB, Yoshimura N (2005) Elimination of rat spinal neurons expressing neurokinin 1 receptors reduces bladder overactivity and spinal *c-fos* expression induced by bladder irritation. Am J Physiol Renal Physiol 288:F466–F473

Sengupta JN, Gebhart GF (1994) Mechanosensitive properties of pelvic nerve afferent fibers innervating the urinary bladder of the rat. J Neurophysiol 72:2420–2430

Shea VK, Cai R, Crepps B, Mason JL, Perl ER (2000) Sensory fibers of the pelvic nerve innervating the rat's urinary bladder. J Neurophysiol 84:1924–1933

Smet PJ, Moore KH, Jonavicius J (1997) Distribution and colocalization of calcitonin gene-related peptide, tachykinins, and vasoactive intestinal peptide in normal and idiopathic unstable human urinary bladder. Lab Invest 77:37–49

Steers WD, Tuttle JB (2006) Mechanisms of disease: the role of nerve growth factor in the pathophysiology of bladder disorders. Nat Clin Pract Urol 3:101–110

Steers WD, Ciambotti J, Etzel B, Erdman S, de Groat WC (1991a) Alterations in afferent pathways from the urinary bladder of the rat in response to partial urethral obstruction. J Comp Neurol 310:401–410

Steers WD, Kolbeck S, Creedon D, Tuttle JB (1991b) Nerve growth factor in the urinary bladder of the adult regulates neuronal form and function. J Clin Invest 88:1709–1715

Steers WD, Mackway-Gerardi AM, Ciambotti J, de Groat WC (1994) Alterations in neural pathways to the urinary bladder of the rat in response to streptozotocin-induced diabetes. J Auton Nerv Syst 47:83–94

Steers WD, Creedon DJ, Tuttle JB (1996) Immunity to nerve growth factor prevents afferent plasticity following urinary bladder hypertrophy. J Urol 155:379–385

Stein RJ, Santos S, Nagatomi J, Hayashi Y, Minnery BS, Xavier M, Patel AS, Nelson JB, Futrell WJ, Yoshimura N, Chancellor MB, De Miguel F (2004) Cool (TRPM8) and hot (TRPV1) receptors in the bladder and male genital tract. J Urol 172:1175–1178

Stewart T, Beyak MJ, Vanner S (2003) Ileitis modulates potassium and sodium currents in guinea pig dorsal root ganglia sensory neurons. J Physiol 552:797–807

Streng T, Axelsson HE, Hedlund P, Andersson DA, Jordt SE, Bevan S, Andersson KE, Hogestatt ED, Zygmunt PM (2008) Distribution and function of the hydrogen sulfide-sensitive TRPA1 ion channel in rat urinary bladder. Eur Urol 53:391–400

Studeny S, Torabi A, Vizzard MA (2005) P2X2 and P2X3 receptor expression in postnatal and adult rat urinary bladder and lumbosacral spinal cord. Am J Physiol Regul Integr Comp Physiol 289:R1155–R1168

Su X, Sengupta JN, Gebhart GF (1997) Effects of opioids on mechanosensitive pelvic nerve afferent fibers innervating the urinary bladder of the rat. J Neurophysiol 77:1566–1580

Sun Y, Keay S, De Deyne PG, Chai TC (2001) Augmented stretch activated adenosine triphosphate release from bladder uroepithelial cells in patients with interstitial cystitis. J Urol 166:1951–1956

Tainio H (1993) Neuropeptidergic innervation of the human male distal urethra and intrinsic external urethral sphincter. Acta Histochem 94:197–201

Tempest HV, Dixon AK, Turner WH, Elneil S, Sellers LA, Ferguson DR (2004) P2X and P2X receptor expression in human bladder urothelium and changes in interstitial cystitis. BJU Int 93:1344–1348

Thor K, Kawatani M, de Groat WC (1986) Plasticity in the reflex pathways to the lower urinary tract of the cat during postnatal development and following spinal cord injury. In: Goldberger M, Gorio A, Murray M (eds) Development and plasticity of the mammalian spinal cord. Fidia research series, vol III. Fidia, Padua, pp 65–81

Thor KB, Hisamitsu T, Roppolo JR, Tuttle P, Nagel J, de Groat WC (1989a) Selective inhibitory effects of ethylketocyclazocine on reflex pathways to the external urethral sphincter of the cat. J Pharmacol Exp Ther 248:1018–1025

Thor KB, Morgan C, Nadelhaft I, Houston M, de Groat WC (1989b) Organization of afferent and efferent pathways in the pudendal nerve of the female cat. J Comp Neurol 288:263–279

Tong YC, Cheng JT (2007) Aldose reductase inhibitor ONO-2235 restores the alterations of bladder nerve growth factor and neurotrophin receptor p75 genetic expression in streptozotocin induced diabetic rats. J Urol 178:2203–7

Uemura E, Fletcher TF, Dirks VA, Bradley WE (1973) Distribution of sacral afferent axons in cat urinary bladder. Am J Anat 136:305–313

Uemura E, Fletcher TF, Bradley WE (1975) Distribution of lumbar and sacral afferent axons in submucosa of cat urinary bladder. Anat Rec 183:579–587

Ueyama T, Mizuno N, Nomura S, Konishi A, Itoh K, Arakawa H (1984) Central distribution of afferent and efferent components of the pudendal nerve in cat. J Comp Neurol 222:38–46

Ustinova EE, Fraser MO, Pezzone MA (2006) Colonic irritation in the rat sensitizes urinary bladder afferents to mechanical and chemical stimuli: an afferent origin of pelvic organ cross-sensitization. Am J Physiol Renal Physiol 290:F1478–F1487

Uvelius B, Gabella G (1998) The distribution of intramural nerves in urinary bladder after partial denervation in the female rat. Urol Res 26:291–297

Vera PL, Nadelhaft I (1990) Conduction velocity distribution of afferent fibers innervating the rat urinary bladder. Brain Res 520:83–89

Vizzard MA (2000a) Increased expression of spinal cord Fos protein induced by bladder stimulation after spinal cord injury. Am J Physiol Regul Integr Comp Physiol 279:R295–R305

Vizzard MA (2000b) Changes in urinary bladder neurotrophic factor mRNA and NGF protein following urinary bladder dysfunction. Exp Neurol 161:273–284

Vizzard MA (2001) Alterations in neuropeptide expression in lumbosacral bladder pathways following chronic cystitis. J Chem Neuroanat 21:125–138

Vizzard MA (2006) Neurochemical plasticity and the role of neurotrophic factors in bladder reflex pathways after spinal cord injury. Prog Brain Res 152:97–115

Vizzard MA, Boyle MM (1999) Increased expression of growth-associated protein (GAP-43) in lower urinary tract pathways following cyclophosphamide (CYP)-induced cystitis. Brain Res 844:174–187

Vizzard MA, Erdman SL, de Groat WC (1996) Increased expression of neuronal nitric oxide synthase in bladder afferent pathways following chronic bladder irritation. J Comp Neurol 370:191–202

Vulchanova L, Riedl MS, Shuster SJ, Stone LS, Hargreaves KM, Buell G, Surprenant A, North RA, Elde R (1998) P2X3 is expressed by DRG neurons that terminate in inner lamina II. Eur J Neurosci 10:3470–3478

Waddell PJ, Lawson SN (1990) Electrophysiological properties of subpopulations of rat dorsal root ganglion neurons in vitro. Neuroscience 36:811–822

Wang EC, Lee JM, Johnson JP, Kleyman TR, Bridges R, Apodaca G (2003) Hydrostatic pressure-regulated ion transport in bladder uroepithelium. Am J Physiol Renal Physiol 285: F651–F663

Wang ZY, Wang P, Merriam FV, Bjorling DE (2008) Lack of TRPV1 inhibits cystitis-induced increased mechanical sensitivity in mice. Pain 139(1):158–167

Weaver LC, Marsh DR, Gris D, Brown A, Dekaban GA (2006) Autonomic dysreflexia after spinal cord injury: central mechanisms and strategies for prevention. Prog Brain Res 152:245–263

Winter DL (1971) Receptor characteristics and conduction velocites in bladder afferents. J Psych Res 8:225–235

Xu L, Gebhart GF (2008) Characterization of mouse lumbar splanchnic and pelvic nerve urinary bladder mechanosensory afferents. J Neurophysiol 99:244–253

Yoshida M, Miyamae K, Iwashita H, Otani M, Inadome A (2004) Management of detrusor dysfunction in the elderly: changes in acetylcholine and adenosine triphosphate release during aging. Urology 63:17–23

Yoshimura N (1999) Bladder afferent pathway and spinal cord injury: possible mechanisms inducing hyperreflexia of the urinary bladder. Prog Neurobiol 57:583–606

Yoshimura N, de Groat WC (1997) Plasticity of Na^+ channels in afferent neurones innervating rat urinary bladder following spinal cord injury. J Physiol 503:269–276

Yoshimura N, de Groat WC (1999) Increased excitability of afferent neurons innervating rat urinary bladder after chronic bladder inflammation. J Neurosci 19:4644–4653

Yoshimura N, White G, Weight FF, de Groat WC (1996) Different types of Na^+ and A-type K^+ currents in dorsal root ganglion neurons innervating the rat urinary bladder. J Physiol 494:1–16

Yoshimura N, Erdman SL, Snider MW, de Groat WC (1998) Effects of spinal cord injury on neurofilament immunoreactivity and capsaicin sensitivity in rat dorsal root ganglion neurons innervating the urinary bladder. Neuroscience 83:633–643

Yoshimura N, Seki S, de Groat WC (2001a) Nitric oxide modulates Ca^{2+} channels in dorsal root ganglion neurons rat urinary bladder. J Neurophysiol 86:304–311

Yoshimura N, Seki S, Novakovic SD, Tzoumaka E, Erickson VL, Erickson KA, Chancellor MB, de Groat WC (2001b) The involvement of the tetrodotoxin-resistant sodium channel Na(v)1.8 (PN3/SNS) in a rat model of visceral pain. J Neurosci 21:8690–8696

Yoshimura N, Seki S, Erickson KA, Erickson VL, Chancellor MB, de Groat WC (2003) Histological and electrical properties of rat dorsal root ganglion neurons innervating the lower urinary tract. J Neurosci 23:4355–4361

Yoshimura N, Chancellor MB, Andersson KE, Christ GJ (2005) Recent advances in understanding the biology of diabetes-associated bladder complications and novel therapy. BJU Int 95: 733–738

Yoshimura N, Bennett NE, Hayashi Y, Ogawa T, Nishizawa O, Chancellor MB, de Groat WC, Seki S (2006) Bladder overactivity and hyperexcitability of bladder afferent neurons after intrathecal delivery of nerve growth factor in rats. J Neurosci 26:10847–10855

Yoshiyama M, de Groat WC (2008a) Effects of intrathecal administration of pituitary adenylate cyclase activating polypeptide on lower urinary tract functions in rats with intact or transected spinal cords. Exp Neurol 211:449–455

Yoshiyama M, de Groat WC (2008b) The role of vasoactive intestinal polypeptide and pituitary adenylate cyclase activating polypeptide in the neural pathways controlling the lower urinary tract. J Mol Neurosci 36(1–3):227–240

Yu Y, de Groat WC (2008) Sensitization of pelvic afferent nerves in the in vitro rat urinary bladder-pelvic nerve preparation by purinergic agonists and cyclophosphamide pretreatment. Am J Physiol Renal Physiol 294:F1146–F1156

Zagorodnyuk VP, Costa M, Brookes SJ (2006) Major classes of sensory neurons to the urinary bladder. Auton Neurosci 126–127:390–397

Zagorodnyuk VP, Gibbins IL, Costa M, Brookes SJ, Gregory SJ (2007) Properties of the major classes of mechanoreceptors in the guinea pig bladder. J Physiol 585:147–163

Zhong Y, Banning AS, Cockayne DA, Ford AP, Burnstock G, McMahon SB (2003) Bladder and cutaneous sensory neurons of the rat express different functional P2X receptors. Neuroscience 120:667–675

Zvara P, Braas KM, May V, Vizzard MA (2006) A role for pituitary adenylate cyclase activating polypeptide (PACAP) in detrusor hyperreflexia after spinal cord injury (SCI). Ann N Y Acad Sci 1070:622–628

Zvara P, Vizzard MA (2007) Exogenous overexpression of nerve growth factor in the urinary bladder produces bladder overactivity and altered micturition circuitry in the lumbosacral spinal cord. BMC Physiol 7:1–11

Sensory Nerves and Airway Irritability

B.J. Canning and D. Spina

Contents

B.J. Canning (✉) and D. Spina (✉)
Johns Hopkins Asthma and Allergy Center, 5501 Hopkins Bayview Circle, Baltimore, MD, 21224, USA
bjc@jhmi.edu
The Sackler Institute of Pulmonary Pharmacology, Division of Pharmaceutical Science, 5th Floor Hodgkin Building, King's College London, London SE1 1UL, UK
domenico.spina@kcl.ac.uk

B.J. Canning and D. Spina (eds.), *Sensory Nerves*,
Handbook of Experimental Pharmacology 194, DOI: 10.1007/978-3-540-79090-7_5,

Abstract The lung, like many other organs, is innervated by a variety of sensory nerves and by nerves of the parasympathetic and sympathetic nervous systems that regulate the function of cells within the respiratory tract. Activation of sensory nerves by both mechanical and chemical stimuli elicits a number of defensive reflexes, including cough, altered breathing pattern, and altered autonomic drive, which are important for normal lung homeostasis. However, diseases that afflict the lung are associated with altered reflexes, resulting in a variety of symptoms, including increased cough, dyspnea, airways obstruction, and bronchial hyperresponsiveness. This review summarizes the current knowledge concerning the physiological role of different sensory nerve subtypes that innervate the lung, the factors which lead to their activation, and pharmacological approaches that have been used to interrogate the function of these nerves. This information may potentially facilitate the identification of novel drug targets for the treatment of respiratory disorders such as cough, asthma, and chronic obstructive pulmonary disease.

Keywords Rapidly adapting receptors, C-fibers, Cough receptor, Cough, Parasympathetic nervous system, Sympathetic nervous system, Cough, Bronchoconstriction, Mucus secretion, Bronchial hyperresponsiveness

1 Introduction

The primary function of the lung is gas exchange. The airways serve as a conduit for moving inspired air to the gas-exchanging regions of the lungs, and for expiration of CO_2. Airway and lung reflexes optimize lung capacity for gas exchange in response to a continually changing demand. Airway reflexes also serve to preserve airway patency. These reflexes can become aberrant, however, and may worsen the symptoms of diseases such as asthma and chronic obstructive pulmonary disease (COPD). Multiple afferent nerve subtypes regulate these homeostatic and defensive reflexes, each subtype with unique physiological, anatomical, and pharmacological attributes. The properties of airway afferent nerve subtypes will be reviewed, as will their role in regulating bronchopulmonary reflexes and bronchial responsiveness.

2 Airway and Lung Afferent Nerve Subtypes

Airway afferent nerve subtypes have been defined by their chemical and physical sensitivity, adaptation to mechanical stimulation, origin, myelination, conduction velocity, neurochemistry, basal activity, reflexes associated with their activation, and sites of termination in the airways, lungs, and brain stem. These various approaches to characterizing airway afferent nerves are hampered by their lack of specificity. But when used in combination, patterns of physiological and pharmacological attributes have emerged to help define at least four distinct subtypes of airway afferent nerves (Canning et al. 2006b).

2.1 Slowly Adapting Receptors

Slowly adapting receptors (SARs) are the prototypical airway mechanoreceptors. The mechanical forces produced during breathing are the primary stimulus for SAR activation, with SAR activity increasing during inspiration and peaking prior to expiration (Miserocchi and Sant'Ambrogio 1974; Ho et al. 2001; Schelegle and Green 2001). SARs regulate the Hering-Breuer reflex, which terminates inspiration and initiates expiration when the lungs are adequately inflated (Schelegle and Green 2001). SARs thus play a primary role in regulating respiratory rate.

SARs can be differentiated from rapidly adapting receptors (RARs) in some species on the basis of action potential conduction velocity, and in most species by their modest adaptation to sustained lung inflation (Fig. 1). SARs may be differentially distributed in the airways of commonly studied mammalian species (Schelegle and Green 2001). In cats, guinea pigs, and rats, few SARs but many RAR-like receptors and C-fibers can be found in the extrapulmonary airways. In dogs, SARs may also be localized to the extrapulmonary airways (Miserocchi and Sant'Ambrogio 1974; Sant'Ambrogio et al. 1988). SARs also differ from RARs with respect to the reflexes they precipitate (see later). Subtypes of SARs have been described (Miserocchi and Sant'Ambrogio 1974; Schelegle and Green 2001).

SARs are generally unresponsive to chemical stimuli. With the exception of the small population of SARs terminating in airway smooth muscle, this also includes an insensitivity to stimuli that initiate bronchospasm, pulmonary edema, pulmonary vascular congestion, or any stimulus that decreases lung compliance. The ion channels regulating the mechanical sensitivity of SARs are also poorly defined. Gadolinium (20 mM applied repeatedly for 30 min to SAR receptive fields) slightly (10–40%) reduced rabbit bronchial SAR discharge to different levels of inflation pressures (Ma et al. 2004). Other drugs reported to modify SAR discharge include the voltage-sensitive K^+-channel blocker 4-aminopyridine, the voltage-sensitive Na^+-channel opener veratradine, the Na^+–K^+–$2Cl^-$ transporter inhibitor furosemide, sulfur dioxide, and the Na^+–K^+–ATPase inhibitor ouabain (Davies et al. 1978; Matsumoto et al. 1998, 1999, 2000, 2005, 2006; Sudo et al. 2000; Guardiola et al. 2007).

An additional and unique physiological and pharmacological property of SARs is their sensitivity to alveolar CO_2 concentrations (Coleridge et al. 1978; Fisher and Sant'Ambrogio 1982; Green et al. 1986). As alveolar CO_2 increases, SAR activity decreases. This contrasts sharply with bronchopulmonary C-fibers, which may be activated or at least sensitized by elevated alveolar CO_2 and/or decreases in extracellular pH (Delpierre et al. 1981; Lin et al. 2005). The inhibitory effect of CO_2 on SARs contributes in part to the hyperpnea associated with hypercapnea. The actions of CO_2 on SAR excitability may occur secondary to effects on nerve

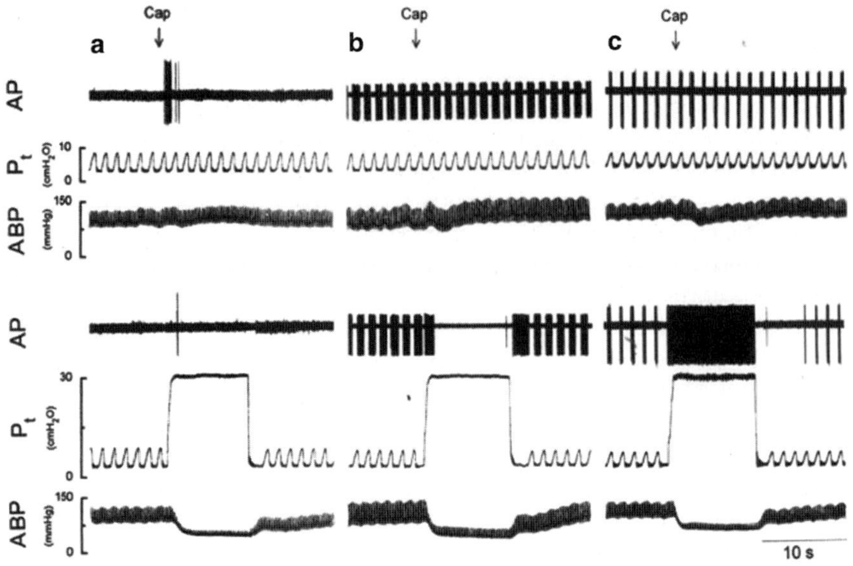

Fig. 1 The characteristic features of airway and lung vagal afferent nerve subtypes are shown in these single-fiber recordings in the rat. C-fibers are generally unresponsive to mechanical stimulation, including the mechanical consequences of lung inflation and deflation, but are vigorously activated by capsaicin. The rapidly adapting stretch receptors (RARs) and the slowly adapting stretch receptors (SARs) are largely insensitive to capsaicin. Both lung stretch receptor subtypes are responsive to lung inflation, with RAR activity more prominent in species with higher respiratory rates. RARs and SARs are differentiated in part by their responses to sustained lung inflation. These vagal afferent nerve subtypes differentially regulate airway autonomic outflow, respiratory pattern, respiratory sensations, and cough. Subtypes of each afferent class have been described and are found in all species thus far studied. (Reproduced with permission from Ho et al. 2001)

terminal pH as evidenced by the preventive effect of the carbonic anhydrase inhibitor acetazolamide during CO_2 challenges (Ravi 1985; Matsumoto 1996; Hempleman et al. 2000). The expression of a carbonic anhydrase isozyme in SARs has not been systematically evaluated.

2.2 *Rapidly Adapting Receptors*

The term "rapidly adapting receptor" (RAR) describes a subtype of airway and lung stretch receptor that are activated during the dynamic phase of lung inflation, but unlike SARs become quiescent during static lung inflation (Knowlton and Larrabee 1946; Widdicombe 1954a). Often inappropriately, airway afferents that rapidly adapt to any stimulus are grouped into a broad and heterogeneous class, all of which are called "RARs." This has proven misleading (Canning and Chou

2009). In this review, the term "RAR" refers to those intrapulmonary stretch receptors that rapidly adapt to sustained lung inflation (Fig. 1).

RARs are considerably less active than SARs during eupnea but more active than C-fibers. RARs are also activated (either directly or indirectly) by a variety of mechanical stimuli in the lung, including airway smooth muscle contraction, pulmonary edema, decreased lung compliance, lung collapse, and negative airway luminal pressures (Mills et al. 1970; Armstrong and Luck 1974; Bergren 1997; Ho et al. 2001; Canning et al. 2004; Canning and Chou 2009).

RARs are generally more responsive to chemical stimuli than SARs, prompting use of the term "irritant receptor" to describe this airway afferent nerve subtype. What has been less clear, however, is whether the ability of these chemical stimuli to activate RARs is through a direct action or secondary to a mechanical effect evoked in the lung. As mentioned above, RARs are exquisitely sensitive to decreases in lung compliance (Jonzon et al. 1986; Yu et al. 1987, 1989). Accordingly, bronchoconstrictors such as serotonin, methacholine, histamine, and substance P and many other stimuli that initiate bronchospasm likely activate RARs at least partly through their effects on lung mechanics (Mills et al. 1970; Mohammed et al. 1993; Bergren 1997; Canning et al. 2004; Chou et al. 2008). Similar mechanisms may underlie the ability of pulmonary embolism and pulmonary vascular congestion to activate RARs (Mills et al. 1969; Sellick and Widdicombe 1969; Ravi and Kappagoda 1992; Bonham et al. 1996) (Fig. 2). But there are several reports suggesting a direct effect of autacoids such as ATP, histamine, and serotonin

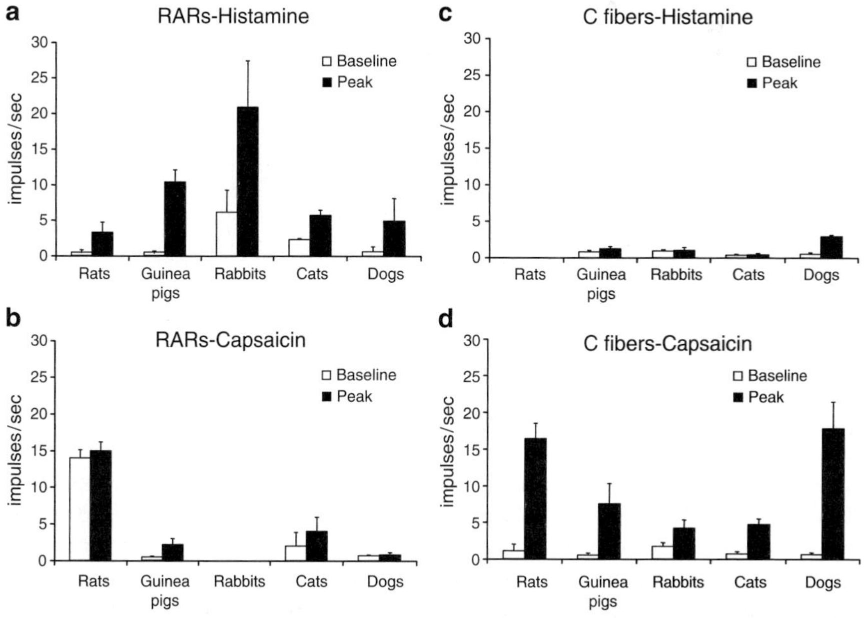

Fig. 2 Responsiveness to histamine and capsaicin differentiates RARs from C-fibers. (Reproduced from Canning and Chou 2009 and summarizes results published elsewhere)

on RARs (Vidruk et al. 1977; Dixon et al. 1979; Matsumoto and Shimizu 1989; Canning et al. 2004). Unlike SARs and C-fibers, however, RARs are largely unaffected by changes in alveolar CO_2 concentrations (Sampson and Vidruk 1975; Ravi 1985).

As with SARs, the ion channels regulating RAR activation secondary to mechanical stimulation are poorly defined. Gadolinium (20 mM applied repeatedly for 30 min to RAR receptive fields) is reported to have a profound effect on RAR excitation by lung inflation and pulmonary vascular congestion (Ma et al. 2004). Given the distinctive accommodative responses of RARs to sustained lung inflation, it seems possible that they express a unique set of ion channels that may be amenable to selective pharmacological modulation. This may prove useful in developing more selective drugs for treating respiratory disorders.

2.3 C-Fibers

With their defining physiological attribute of an axonal conduction velocity of 1 ms^{-1} or less, bronchopulmonary C-fibers are the most readily identifiable vagal afferent nerve subtype innervating the airways. C-fibers can be activated by several chemical and mechanical stimuli, with responses depending upon the stimulus and the C-fiber subtype studied (Coleridge and Coleridge 1984; Ricco et al. 1996; Lee and Pisarri 2001; Undem et al. 2004). The majority of C-fibers innervating the airways and lungs of all species are activated by the TRPV1 receptor agonist capsaicin (Figs. 1, 2), a predictable observation, given the known expression patterns of TRPV1 in afferent C-fibers throughout the body of most species (Caterina et al. 1997). But it is inappropriate to conclude from these data that responsiveness to capsaicin is the defining characteristic of airway C-fibers. C-fibers in dogs, rats, and mice that are not activated by lung capsaicin challenge have been described (Coleridge and Coleridge 1984; Ho et al. 2001; Kollarik et al. 2003). Moreover, perhaps secondary to the end organ effects associated with C-fiber activation (mucus secretion, vascular engorgement, airway smooth muscle contraction, altered respiratory pattern, and cough), other afferent nerve subtypes, especially intrapulmonary RARs, can be activated by capsaicin challenge (Mohammed et al. 1993; Bergren 1997; Morikawa et al. 1997). A lack of responsiveness to mechanical stimulation and basal activity may also fail to differentiate C-fibers from other subtypes of bronchopulmonary afferent nerves. While C-fibers are generally less responsive to mechanical stimulation, they can be activated by punctate mechanical stimulation or lung inflation, and can have basal activity comparable to that of some RARs (Coleridge and Coleridge 1984; Fox et al. 1993; Ricco et al. 1996; Lee and Pisarri 2001).

Subtypes of bronchopulmonary C-fibers have been described. The Coleridges defined C-fiber subtypes in dogs by their responsiveness to stimulants administered via the pulmonary or bronchial circulation (Coleridge and Coleridge 1984). More recently, Undem (Kollarik et al. 2003; Undem et al. 2004) described bronchopulmonary C-fiber subtypes in both guinea pigs and mice. In guinea pigs, C-fiber subtypes are differentiated on the basis of their ganglionic origin (nodose vs. jugular ganglia) and, by extension, their embryological origin, their sites of peripheral termination (extrapulmonary and intrapulmonary vs. exclusively intrapulmonary), expression of neurokinins, and responsiveness to adenosine, serotonin 5-HT$_3$, and ATP receptor agonists (Undem et al. 2004; Chuaychoo et al. 2005, 2006). These subtypes are known to have opposing effects on both cough and respiration, but both subtypes may initiate reflex bronchospasm upon activation (Canning et al. 2006a, b; Chou et al. 2008; Reynolds et al. 2008) (Fig. 3). C-fibers arising from dorsal root ganglia also innervate the airways (Martling 1987; Kummer et al. 1992; Dinh et al. 2004; Oh et al. 2006; Kwong et al. 2008b). Their physiological properties and reflex actions have been only partially described.

C-fibers are found throughout the airways and lungs of all species. In guinea pigs, the jugular-type C-fibers have been localized to both intrapulmonary and extrapulmonary airways, while the nodose-type C-fibers are found predominantly in the peripheral airways and lungs (Undem et al. 2004). The extensively branched terminals of C-fibers in guinea pig and rat tracheae can be immunohistochemically labeled for the neuropeptides calcitonin gene-related peptide (CGRP), substance P, and neurokinin A (McDonald et al. 1988; Baluk et al. 1992; Kummer et al. 1992; Hunter and Undem 1999; Yamamoto et al. 2007). Comparable structures can be

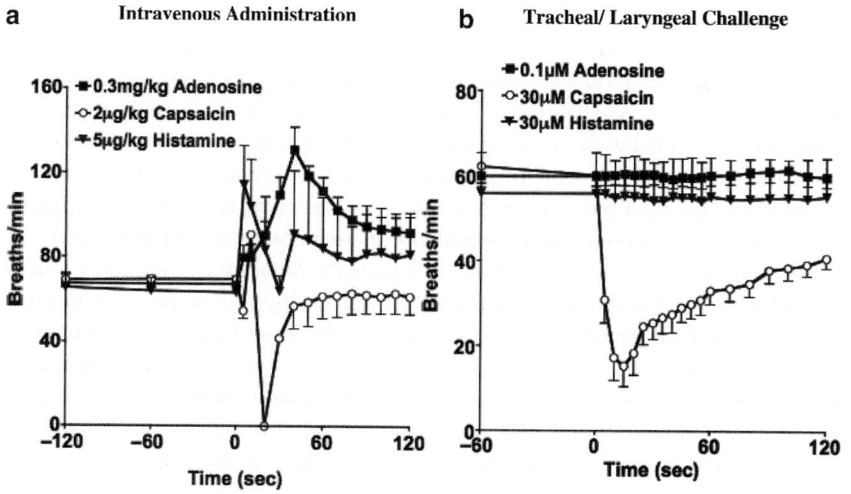

Fig. 3 Respiratory reflex effects evoked by histamine, adenosine, and capsaicin reveal the differential distribution of airway vagal afferent nerve subtypes and their distinct effects on respiratory pattern. Histamine selectively activates intrapulmonary RARs and initiates tachypnea. Adenosine selectively activates pulmonary C-fibers and also initiates tachypnea. Capsaicin activates both bronchial and pulmonary type C-fibers, initiating a profound slowing of respiration upon laryngeal challenge, tachypnea when capsaicin is inhaled (not shown), and both tachypnea and respiratory slowing following intravenous administration. (Data adapted from Chou et al. 2008)

found in the airways of other species and in the peripheral airways of guinea pigs (Dey et al. 1990; Yamamoto et al. 1998; Lamb and Sparrow 2002; Watanabe et al. 2006). C-fiber terminals can also be found in the airway microvasculature and airway smooth muscle layer, and comprise at least a portion of Paintal's J-receptors, suggesting peripheral/interstitial lung terminations (Paintal 1973; McDonald et al. 1988; Baluk et al. 1992).

A myelinated (based on an axonal conduction velocity of 5 ms^{-1}) afferent nerve subtype with many shared physiological and pharmacological attributes of jugular C-fibers has also been described in guinea pigs (Ricco et al. 1996). These afferents have their cell bodies in the jugular ganglia and are activated by acid, hypertonic saline, bradykinin, and capsaicin. Unlike jugular C-fibers, these capsaicin-sensitive Aδ-fibers terminate exclusively in the large airways (larynx, trachea, mainstem bronchi) and do not normally express the neuropeptide substance P (but can be labeled immunohistochemically for the structural protein neurofilament). TRPV1-positive, substance P-negative nerve terminals have been described in the airway epithelium of guinea pigs and may correspond to this afferent subtype (Watanabe et al. 2005, 2006). The existence of an Aδ afferent subpopulation expressing TRPV1 in other species and their reflex effects in any species upon activation are unknown.

In contrast to the indirect effects of autacoids and irritants thought to account for their activation of RARs, there is molecular, immunohistochemical, and electrophysiological evidence to suggest that many mediators associated with airway inflammation act directly on bronchopulmonary C-fibers. Stimuli known to activate airway and lung C-fibers include capsaicin and other TRPV1 receptor ligands, acid, cationic proteins, bradykinin, thrombin, and other protease-activated receptor 1 (PAR1) agonists, adenosine, 5-HT_3 receptor agonists, nicotine, ATP, prostanoids, and isoprostanes, and a variety of environmental irritants including acrolein, toluene diisocyanate, and ozone (Coleridge and Coleridge 1984; Lee and Pisarri 2001; Undem et al. 2004; Chuaychoo et al. 2005, 2006; Nassenstein et al. 2008; Taylor-Clark et al. 2008). Many of these stimuli work partly or entirely through gating of the ion channels TRPV1 and TRPA1. PCR analyses confirm the expression of TRPV1 and TRPA1, but also adenosine A_1, adenosine A_2, PAR1, and multiple subunits of nicotinic receptors in bronchopulmonary C-fibers (Chuaychoo et al. 2006; Gu et al. 2008; Kwong et al. 2008a, b; Nassenstein et al. 2008). The responsiveness to such a variety of inflammatory mediators and environmental toxins and the reflexes initiated upon the activation of C-fibers lends credence to the notion that bronchopulmonary C-fibers are analogous to the nociceptors innervating somatic tissues.

TRPV1-dependent signaling is not the same in all bronchopulmonary C-fibers and is at least suggestive of the differential expression of a ligand-transporting system in some C-fibers or perhaps unique gating mechanisms for TRPV1 in the various bronchopulmonary C-fiber subtypes. Olvanil and anandamide are reasonably effective and potent activators of intrapulmonary C-fibers in rats and in guinea pigs, but are minimally effective at evoking tracheal/bronchial C-fiber action potential discharge or tachykinin release from the peripheral terminals of bronchial and tracheal C-fibers (Tucker et al. 2001; Lin and Lee 2002; Kollarik and Undem 2004; Lee et al. 2005). This inability to activate bronchial C-fibers is overcome with sustained incubation times, suggesting an impaired access to the intracellular binding site of TRPV1. Conversely, cooling the terminals of pulmonary C-fibers rendered them considerably less responsive to olvanil and anandamide, but equally responsive to capsaicin. These data may predict the expression of an anandamide-transporting system in pulmonary C-fibers that is absent in bronchial and tracheal C-fibers (Ligresti et al. 2004). To date, however, no protein subserving this transporting function has been identified (Glaser et al. 2005). It is thus interesting that activation of TRPV1 has been shown to promote the movement of extraordinarily large molecules from the extracellular to the intracellular space through the open TRPV1 channel (Meyers et al. 2003; Binshtok et al. 2007). The Hill coefficient for TRPV1 activation is significantly different from unity, suggestive of cooperative binding properties (Szallasi 1994; Welch et al. 2000; Undem and Kollarik 2002). It seems possible that threshold TRPV1 activation resulting in transient channel opening promotes additional agonist influx and further receptor activation. Perhaps some subtle modification of TRPV1 channel gating in C-fiber subtypes determines the ability of anandamide and olvanil to move through the open TRPV1 channel.

In addition to the autacoids listed above that activate bronchopulmonary C-fibers, many other mediators can sensitize them to subsequent activation. These include histamine via H1 receptors, cysteinyl leukotrienes via cysLT1 receptors, epinephrine via β_3 receptors, and prostaglandin EP and TP receptor agonists (Karla et al. 1992; Lee and Morton 1993, 1995; McAlexander et al. 1998; Xiang et al. 2002; Gu et al. 2007). Prostaglandins also likely account for the sensitizing effects of protease-activated receptor 2 (PAR2) agonists on bronchopulmonary C-fibers (Gatti et al. 2006). Some mechanistic studies of these sensitizing effects have been carried out in patch-clamp analyses. Other unique characteristics regulating airway C-fiber activation include sensitivity to changes in extracellular Cl^- and Ca^{2+} concentrations, changes in airway surface liquid osmolarity, TRPV1-independent activation by acid (perhaps involving acid-sensing ion channels), and activation/sensitization by CO_2 (Delpierre et al. 1981; Pisarri et al. 1992; Fox et al. 1995; Pedersen et al. 1998; Kollarik and Undem 2002; Undem et al. 2003; Lin et al. 2005; Gu and Lee 2006).

2.4 *Cough Receptors*

C-fiber-selective stimulants that readily initiate coughing in awake human subjects and in awake guinea pigs have consistently failed to initiate cough in anesthetized cats, dogs, or guinea pigs. On the basis of the studies of Widdicombe (1954a, b) published in 1954 and the results of vagal cooling studies in cats and dogs by Tatar et al. (1988, 1994), it had become almost dogma that cough is initiated by activation of RARs. But many well-known and even selective stimuli for RARs, including a variety of bronchoconstrictors, negative airway luminal pressures, or inspiratory efforts against a closed glottis, have been consistently ineffective at evoking cough in either awake or anesthetized animals or humans. Recent studies carried out in guinea pigs and a reappraisal of Widdicombe's studies in cats suggest that a vagal afferent nerve subtype distinct from both C-fibers and RARs plays an essential role in regulating the cough reflex in anesthetized guinea pigs and cats and likely in any species that has a well-defined cough reflex. These afferents have thus been called "cough receptors" (Canning et al. 2004, 2006a, b; Canning and Chou 2009).

Cough receptors are differentiated from C-fibers and RARs in guinea pigs by conduction velocity. With a conduction velocity of approximately 5 ms^{-1}, these afferents conduct action potentials considerably faster than C-fibers (1 ms^{-1} or less) but considerably slower than either RARs or SARs (more than 20 ms^{-1}). Cough receptors are also differentiated from C-fibers and RARs by mechanical sensitivity, being exquisitely sensitive to punctate mechanical stimulation (5–10 times more sensitive than C-fibers) but utterly insensitive to changes in airway luminal pressure or airway smooth muscle contraction, both of which activate RARs. Also unlike C-fibers, the cough receptors are insensitive to capsaicin and bradykinin (Fig. 4). Cough receptors are activated by acid but entirely through TRPV1-independent mechanisms (Canning et al. 2004, 2006a, b).

By combination of electrophysiological studies with intravital labeling methods, retrograde neuronal tracing, organotypic cultures, and immunohistochemistry, the peripheral terminals of cough receptors in the guinea pig trachea and bronchus have been identified (Canning et al. 2006a, b). Terminating between the epithelium and smooth muscle layers of the airways mucosa, the cough receptors assume a

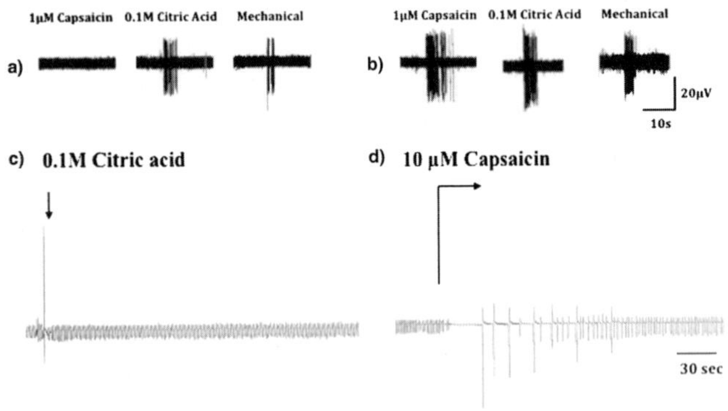

Fig. 4 Electrophysiological characteristics of the extrapulmonary vagal afferent nerves regulating cough of guinea pigs. Cough receptors and C-fibers are both activated by punctate mechanical stimulation and by acid, but the cough receptors are insensitive to capsaicin. Capsaicin and other C-fiber-selective stimulants initiate coughing in awake animals and in awake human subjects, but have consistently failed to initiate coughing in anesthetized animals. In anesthetized guinea pigs, topical acid challenge of the tracheal mucusa initiates coughing, while topical capsaicin challenge does not evoke coughing. Rather, capsaicin challenge in anesthetized guinea pigs evokes respiratory slowing and, occasionally, a profound apnea followed by gasping and a gradual recovery of a normal respiratory pattern. (Reproduced with permission from Canning et al. 2004)

circumferential position in the extracellular matrix. Branching is extensive at the terminals, with axons projecting from longitudinal nerve bundles through the smooth muscle layer. Similar structures have been described in the airway mucosa of other species but their identity as "cough receptors" is unclear (Larsell 1921, 1922; Gaylor 1934; Yamamoto et al. 1995; Yu 2005; De Proost et al. 2007). Immunohistochemistry confirms the selective expression of subtypes of Na^+–K^+–ATPase and Na^+–K^+–$2Cl^-$ transporter in guinea pig cough receptors (Canning et al. 2006a, b; Mazzone and McGovern 2006, 2008). More recently, tetrodotoxin-insensitive Na^+ channels have been localized to these cough receptors (Kwong et al. 2008a, b). Pharmacological analyses suggest that these regulators of ion flux and gradients, as well as Cl^- channels and voltage-sensitive K^+ channels, may be critical to the regulation of cough receptor responsiveness to chemical (acid) and punctate mechanical stimuli (Fox et al. 1995; McAlexander and Undem 2000; Canning et al. 2006a, b; Mazzone and McGovern 2006; Canning 2007). No other stimuli thus far studied, including a variety of autacoids and neurotransmitters and ion channel modulators, alter cough receptor excitability or the ability of acid or mechanical stimuli to initiate coughing in guinea pigs.

3 Autonomic Reflexes

3.1 Parasympathetic Nerve Regulation of Airway and Vascular Smooth Muscle and Mucus Secretion

Parasympathetic nerves play a primary role in regulating airway smooth muscle tone and glandular secretion in the airways and also regulate pulmonary and bronchial vascular tone (Canning 2006; Wine 2007). There are two anatomically, physiologically, and pharmacologically distinct parasympathetic pathways projecting to the airways with opposing effects on airway smooth muscle but synergistic effects on airway mucus secretion. Parasympathetic-cholinergic nerves initiate airway smooth muscle contraction, pulmonary vascular dilatation, and mucus secretion upon activation, with acetylcholine acting in each target tissue via muscarinic M3 receptors. Parasympathetic noncholinergic nerves also innervate the airways of most species, including humans. Noncholinergic parasympathetic nerves utilize the peptide transmitter vasoactive intestinal peptide and related peptides (pituitary adenylate cyclase activating peptide, peptide histidine isoleucine, peptide histidine methionine) as well as the gaseous transmitter nitric oxide (formed from arginine by the neuronal isoform of nitric oxide synthase). Upon activation, noncholinergic parasympathetic nerves evoke bronchodilatation, airway vascular dilatation, and mucus secretion. Coincident activation of cholinergic and noncholinergic parasympathetic nerves may have synergistic effects on airway glandular secretion (Choi et al. 2007; Wine 2007).

Airway and lung afferent nerve activation initiates myriad patterns of airway parasympathetic nerve responses (Canning 2006). At eupnea, basal parasympathetic tone appears to be necessarily dependent upon the ongoing activity of airway vagal afferent nerves, either RARs or C-fibers (Jammes and Mei 1979; Kesler and Canning 1999). With challenge, activation of bronchopulmonary C-fibers or RARs increases airway cholinergic and noncholinergic parasympathetic nerve activity (Fig. 5). Activation of intrapulmonary stretch receptors (SARs) by lung

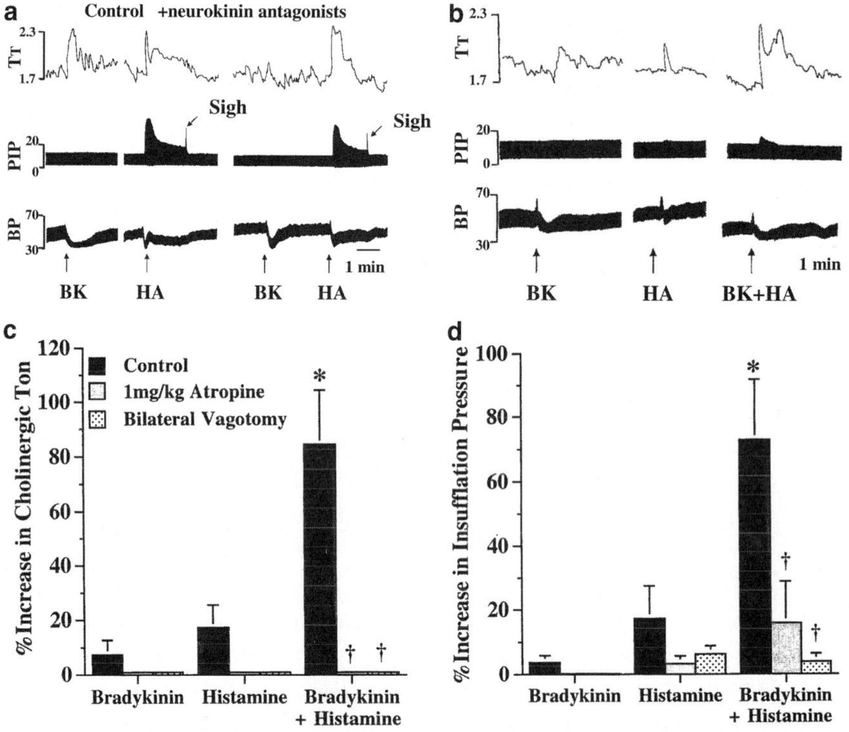

Fig. 5 Reflex-evoked, airway parasympathetic nerve-dependent regulation of airway smooth muscle tone in guinea pigs in situ. (**a**) The C-fiber-selective stimulant bradykinin evokes reflex bronchospasm largely independent of any direct effects on airway smooth muscle. Histamine-evoked reflex bronchospasm occurs secondary to its direct effects on airway smooth muscle, which in turn activates intrapulmonary RARs. Evidence for the selective effects of bradykinin and histamine on C-fibers and RARs, respectively, is apparent from the marked inhibition of bradykinin-evoked reflex bronchospasm by intravenous or intracerebroventricular administration of neurokinin receptor antagonists, which are without effect on histamine-evoked reflexes. Neurokinins are selectively expressed by C-fibers in guinea pigs. (**b**) When RARs and C-fibers are activated simultaneously, marked synergism is apparent. This synergistic effect of RAR and C-fiber activation on airway parasympathetic tone may result from central convergence in the nucleus of the solitary tract of these afferent nerve subtypes. (**c**, **d**) The mean data for reflex bronchospasm and whole-lung-inflation pressures evoked by histamine, bradykinin, or the combination of histamine and bradykinin. (Reproduced with permission from Canning et al. 2001 and Mazzone and Canning 2002a, b)

inflation or during the hyperpnea associated with exercise induces a withdrawal of parasympathetic cholinergic nerve activity and bronchodilatation, but has no effect on parasympathetic noncholinergic nerves.

Reflex regulation of airway parasympathetic nerves by vagal afferents may not be entirely unidirectional. Secondary to the end-organ effects precipitated by parasympathetic nerve stimulation (e.g., mucus secretion, bronchospasm), action potential patterning in airway mechanoreceptors may change dramatically (Coleridge et al. 1982; Richardson et al. 1984). This is especially true under conditions in which tidal volumes are held constant (e.g., mechanical ventilation). An increase in parasympathetic cholinergic tone will decrease airway volume and deadspace, resulting in an increase in end-inspiratory pressure with mechanical ventilation and an increase in alveolar stretch under any mode of static volume ventilation. The increase in alveolar distension will favor an increase in SAR activation and a resulting withdrawal of cholinergic tone. In this way, airway afferent and efferent nerves may work in concert to establish a set point for airway parasympathetic tone (Fisher and Sant'Ambrogio 1982; Richardson et al. 1984; Matsumoto 1996). Perhaps in COPD, with alveolar destruction and increases in lung compliance, SAR activation may be diminished, prompting the elevation in airway cholinergic tone observed in this disease (Gross et al. 1989; Canning 2006).

Reflexes regulating noncholinergic airway parasympathetic nerves have been studied in guinea pigs, cats, and human subjects (Szarek et al. 1986; Ichinose et al. 1987, 1988; Michoud et al. 1987; Inoue et al. 1989; Lammers et al. 1989; Canning et al. 2001; Kesler et al. 2002; Mazzone and Canning 2002a). Unlike cholinergic contractions of the airway smooth muscle, which reach a near maximum within 30 s and can reverse at the same rate, noncholinergic parasympathetic nerve mediated relaxations of airway smooth muscle are slow in both onset and reversal (Chesrown et al. 1980; Diamond and O'Donnell 1980; Irvin et al. 1982; Matsumoto et al. 1985; Lama et al. 1988; Canning and Undem 1993; Canning et al. 2001; Kesler et al. 2002; Mazzone and Canning 2002a, b). Perhaps noncholinergic parasympathetic nerves function to restore or maintain airway patency during or at the conclusion of defensive reflexes (Coburn and Tomita 1973; Canning et al. 2006a). Consistent with this hypothesis, noncholinergic parasympathetic nerve activation is only modestly effective at preventing bronchospasm mediated reflexively or by direct actions on smooth muscle, but can gradually reverse an evoked contraction and modulate sustained cholinergic tone at eupnea (Aizawa et al. 1982, 1997, 1999; Bai et al. 1986; Szarek et al. 1986; Clerici et al. 1989; Miura et al. 1990; Inoue et al. 1991; Matsumoto et al. 1999; Canning et al. 2001; Kesler et al. 2002).

3.2 *Reflex Regulation of Airway Sympathetic Nerves*

Sympathetic nerves innervate the airways and lungs of all species. In most species, including humans, sympathetic-adrenergic innervation of intrapulmonary airway smooth muscle is limited or nonexistent (Canning 2006). In all species, sympathetic aderenergic nerves have been found innervating the airway vascular smooth muscle. Until recently, however, no study has directly addressed the reflex mechanisms controlling airway sympathetic nerve activity. We recently studied reflex regulation of airway sympathetic nerves innervating the trachealis of guinea pigs (Oh et al. 2006). The vagus nerves were cut bilaterally to limit the influence of airway parasympathetic nerves on smooth muscle tone. With the trachealis precontracted with histamine, capsaicin inhalation evoked a marked relaxation of the trachealis that was prevented by sympathetic denervation of the trachealis, propranolol, or dorsal rhizotomy (T1-T4). Retrograde tracing and electrophysiological analyses identified a population of capsaicin-sensitive spinal afferent nerves innervating the intrapulmonary airways and lungs. The majority of these spinal afferent nerves expressed substance P. Not surprisingly, then, neurokinin receptor antagonists prevented the reflex-mediated relaxations evoked by capsaicin inhalation.

Interestingly, we found that the sympathetic reflexes evoked in the airways by capsaicin inhalation occurred without any coincident cardiovascular responses (Oh et al. 2006). This adds further evidence against historical notions regarding sympathetic nerve function in homeostatic and defensive settings (Morrison 2001; Janig and Habler 2003). We also observed that stimulating the central cut ends of the vagus nerves evoked propranolol-sensitive relaxations of the trachealis (Oh et al. 2006). Vagal afferents are known to regulate sympathetic outflow to multiple organs, including the airways (Barman and Gebber 1976; Bachoo and Polosa 1987; Habler et al. 1994; Huang et al. 2000).

3.3 The Axon Reflex

In rats and in guinea pigs, bronchopulmonary C-fiber activation can also initiate an axon reflex, characterized by the peripheral release of neuropeptides that produce a variety of end-organ effects within the airways and lungs, including bronchospasm, mucus secretion, vascular engorgement, inflammatory cell recruitment, and plasma extravasation (Barnes 1986, 2001; Canning et al. 2006a, b). The prominent role of the axon reflex in the response to a variety of experimental challenges in rats and guinea pigs prompted a nearly two decade effort to address the hypothesis that respiratory disorders such as asthma and COPD were due in part to an axon reflex. This notion did not live up to its promise in rats and guinea pigs when evaluated in the human airways, in large part owing to the relative paucity of neuropeptide-containing afferent nerve terminals in the airways and lungs of humans (Hislop et al. 1990; Howarth et al. 1995; Chanez et al. 1998; Lamb and Sparrow 2002). It is nevertheless possible that axonal reflexes regulate human airway function, but through the actions of transmitters (e.g., ATP, glutamate) other than substance P, neurokinin A, and CGRP.

The most effective stimulants of the axon reflex work through the gating of the ion channel TRPV1. Capsaicin, for example, evokes a profound C-fiber discharge and an axon reflex, all of which are abolished when TRPV1 gating is prevented. By contrast, bradykinin, which acts only partially through TRPV1 gating on bronchopulmonary C-fibers, evokes little if any axon reflex (Mizrahi et al. 1982; Bramley et al. 1990; Schlemper and Calixto 2002). Other stimuli evoking an axon reflex include hypertonic saline, cold, dry air, PAR2 agonists, nicotine, immunosuppressants (cyclosporin A, FK 506), and TRPA1 receptor activation (Lundberg et al. 1983; Umeno et al. 1990; Mapp et al. 1991; Harrison et al. 1998; Pedersen et al. 1998; Yoshihara et al. 1998; Carr et al. 2000; Ricciardolo et al. 2000; Andresen and Saugstad 2008; Taylor-Clark et al. 2008).

A variety of stimuli have also been reported to inhibit the axon reflex through effects on the airway C-fiber terminal, including α_2 adrenoceptor agonists, β_2 adrenoceptor agonists, μ-opioid receptor agonists, $GABA_B$ receptor agonists, nociceptin, neurotensin, galanin, serotonin (via $5\text{-}HT_1$ receptors), prostaglandin E_1, adenosine, phosphodiesterase type 4 inhibitors, neuropeptide Y, vasoactive intestinal peptide/pituitary adenylate cyclase activating peptide, dopamine D_2 receptor agonists, bradykinin channel openers, and histamine H_3 receptor agonists (Grundstrom et al. 1984; Belvisi et al. 1988, 1989; Giuliani et al. 1989; Kamikawa 1989; Matran et al. 1989; Aikawa et al. 1990; Stretton 1991; Verleden et al. 1993; Takahashi et al. 1994; Undem et al. 1994; Spina et al. 1995; Fox et al. 1997; Fischer et al. 1998; Shah et al. 1998; Birrell et al. 2002). It is tempting to speculate that the ability of these agents to inhibit the action-potential-independent axon reflex predicts a peripheral site of action of these drugs on bronchopulmonary C-fiber activation. This seems unlikely. Thus, prostaglandin E and adenosine both inhibit the axon reflex but activate and/or sensitize C-fibers to action potential formation (Kamikawa and Shimo 1989; Aikawa et al. 1990; Hong et al. 1998; Ho et al. 2000). The PAR2 agonist initiates an axon reflex but fails to initiate action potentials on airway C-fibers (Carr et al. 2000). Removal of extracellular Ca^{2+} reduces neuropeptide release from capsaicin-sensitive nerves, but enhances airway C-fiber excitability (Hua et al. 1992; Undem et al. 2003). Together, the data argue for an almost complete dissociation of the axon reflex from C-fiber action potential formation.

4 Respiratory Reflexes

4.1 Respiratory Pattern Changes and Respiratory Sensations

Changes in respiratory pattern attributable to airway afferent nerve activation have been studied extensively in animals (Fig. 3). Respiratory sensations such as dyspnea are less amenable to study in animals, but have been studied in human subjects. The classic triad of the pulmonary chemoreflex includes bradycardia and apnea followed by rapid shallow breathing (Green and Jackman 1984; Lee et al. 1995). Both the apnea and the rapid shallow breathing depend upon pulmonary C-fiber activation (Green and Jackman 1984). Apnea/respiratory slowing can also be evoked by

C-fiber activation in the extrapulmonary airways of anesthetized animals (Palecek et al. 1989; Chou et al. 2008). In both animals and humans, activation of intrapulmonary C-fibers and RARs can initiate tachypnea (Mills et al. 1969; Green and Jackman 1984; Chou et al. 2008). In humans, the increase in respiratory rate evoked by pulmonary C-fiber activation with adenosine is accompanied by a sensation of dyspnea (Burki et al. 2005). Dyspnea and "breathlessness" can be reduced by airway or vagus nerve anesthesia or transection (Winning et al. 1985; Davies et al. 1987b; Taguchi et al. 1991). Prostaglandin E_2 worsens the sensation of dyspnea (Taguchi et al. 1992). Bradykinin, a selective stimulant for airway C-fibers, reproduces the sensation of "sore throat" associated with upper respiratory tract infections (Proud and Kaplan 1988). Enhanced breaths (or sighs) become more frequent as airway lung compliance decreases. These have been attributed to the activation of RARs and may serve to open closed airways during tidal breathing at rest or during bronchospasm (Matsumoto et al. 1998; Dybas et al. 2006).

For good reason, much of the focus on respiratory sensations in disease has been directed to the activation of pulmonary C-fibers. But a role for SARs in respiratory sensations should not be discounted. The accumulation of CO_2 in the alveoli would limit SAR discharge, delaying inspiratory termination and thus prompting hyperpnea. In COPD, with alveolar destruction, the lung stretch associated with a normal tidal volume may have limited stretching effects in the peripheral airways and thus may limit SAR discharge, prompting a compensatory increase in end expiratory lung volume or an enhanced sensation of air hunger despite normal or near-normal blood gases. The Na–K^+–2Cl transport inhibitor furosemide is reported to diminish air hunger sensation during breath hold, perhaps owing to an inhibition of RAR discharge but an enhancement of SAR discharge (Nishino 2000; Sudo et al. 2000).

4.2 Cough

The cough reflex is initiated by activation of the cough receptors and by activation of a C-fiber subtype innervating the large airways (Canning and Chou 2009). The role of C-fibers in cough has been the subject of considerable debate. The chemical stimuli most effective at activating bronchopulmonary C-fibers, including capsaicin, bradykinin, and acid, are similarly very effective at initiating cough in conscious human subjects and in conscious animals (Forsberg et al. 1988; Laude et al. 1993; Karlsson and Fuller 1999; Jia et al. 2002; Trevisani et al. 2004; Dicpinigaitis 2007). These stimuli work entirely or partly through TRPV1, and immunohistochemical and single-cell PCR confirms expression of TRPV1 in airway C-fibers (Myers et al. 2002; Groneberg et al. 2004; Watanabe et al. 2006; Kwong et al. 2008a, b). Prior capsaicin desensitization prevents citric acid induced coughing in awake guinea pigs, as does pretreatment with TRPV1 receptor antagonists (Forsberg et al. 1988; Bolser et al. 1991; Lalloo et al. 1995; Trevisani et al. 2004; Gatti et al. 2006; Leung et al. 2007). Taken together, these and other observations argue strongly for a role of bronchopulmonary C-fibers in cough (Canning et al. 2006a, b). But C-fiber-selective stimuli have consistently failed to evoke coughing in anesthetized animals (Tatar et al. 1988; Karlsson et al. 1993; Tatar et al. 1994; Canning et al. 2004, 2006a, b). Anesthesia has no effect on coughing evoked by mechanical or acid stimulation of the airway mucosa and does not prevent C-fiber activation or other C-fiber-dependent reflexes, and yet capsaicin and bradykinin do not evoke cough in anesthetized animals (Coleridge and Coleridge 1984; Tatar et al. 1988; Canning et al. 2006a, b).

Perhaps it should be expected that C-fiber-selective stimulants would fail to evoke coughing in anesthetized animals. Airway and lung C-fibers share many characteristics with somatosensory nociceptors, and it is the objective of general anesthesia to prevent the sensations and reflexes associated with nociceptor activation. But while the effects of anesthesia on nociceptor signaling may explain the inability of C-fiber-selective stimulants to evoke coughing in anesthetized animals, anesthesia cannot account for the known acute inhibitory effects C-fiber activation may have on cough in anesthetized animals, or the inability of some C-fiber stimuli to evoke coughing in conscious animals and in conscious human subjects (Tatar et al. 1988, 1994). We have recently addressed the hypothesis that C-fiber subtypes might account for these opposing effects on cough. Subtypes have been described in several species (Coleridge and Coleridge 1984; Kollarik et al. 2003; Undem et al. 2004). In guinea pigs, airway vagal C-fiber subtypes can be differentiated by their ganglionic origin, distribution in the airways, and responsiveness to ATP, adenosine, and serotonin 5-HT_3 receptor agonists (Undem et al. 2004; Chuaychoo et al. 2005, 2006). The ability of C-fiber activation to evoke coughing in awake guinea pigs is reasonably well established, and we also reported a facilitating effect of C-fiber activation on cough (Mazzone et al. 2005; Canning et al. 2006a, b). In these latter studies, capsaicin or bradykinin applied topically to the tracheal mucosa greatly enhanced sensitivity to subsequent tussive stimuli. On the basis of the location of these bradykinin and capsaicin challenges, C-fibers arising from the jugular ganglia likely promote coughing. By inference, then, we further speculated that nodose C-fiber activation might acutely inhibit coughing. Consistent with this hypothesis, we found that selective activation of nodose C-fibers with adenosine or 2-methyl-5-hydroxytryptamine did not evoke coughing but greatly reduced the ability of citric acid to evoke coughing in anesthetized animals. Prior adenosine inhalation also inhibited capsaicin-induced coughing in conscious guinea pigs.

The results of studies carried out in other species are at least consistent with the notion that C-fiber subtypes may have opposing effects on cough. In anesthetized dogs and cats, C-fiber activation by bradykinin, capsaicin, or phenyldiguanide (a 5-HT_3 receptor agonist) does not induce cough but can inhibit cough (Tatar et al. 1988, 1994; Karlsson et al. 1993). In rabbits, a species in which cough can be evoked by citric acid aerosol inhalation (consistent with a TRPV1- and C-fiber-dependent mechanism; Tatar et al. 1997, Adcock et al. 2003), it has also been reported that sulfur dioxide inhalation is acutely inhibitory for cough (Hanacek et al. 1984). Sulfur dioxide is known to activate lung C-fibers (Ho et al. 2001).

Adcock et al. (2003) speculated that the inhibitory effects of the compound RSD931 in cough induced in rabbits might be due to its ability to activate pulmonary C-fibers. Humans readily cough to capsaicin and bradykinin challenge, but are refractory to serotonin and adenosine challenge (Stone et al. 1993; Burki et al. 2005) while intravenous capsaicin infusion is only minimally effective at evoking cough (Winning et al. 1986). There is also a report of serotonin-mediated inhibition of cough in human subjects (Stone et al. 1993). A comparable inability of intravenously capsaicin to evoke coughing has been reported in studies using conscious nonhuman primates (Deep et al. 2001).

5 CNS Pharmacology and Central Interactions Between Airway Afferent Nerve Subtypes

Studies of airway reflexes in response to stimuli known to be selective for the various airway afferent nerve subtypes largely substantiate the accepted classification schemes for afferent nerves. Implicit in the observation that afferent nerve subtypes subserve distinct reflex functions is that central termination sites of the various afferent nerve subpopulations must diverge to some extent, allowing for reflex specificity. From the little published evidence available, this notion would seem to be substantiated. Most of the work on central terminations of airway sensory nerves has been carried out in cats and rats. Bronchopulmonary C-fibers and RARs terminate extensively and often bilaterally in the nucleus of the solitary tract (nTS), particularly in the commissural and medial subnuclei (Davies and Kubin 1986; Kalia and Richter 1988; Bonham and Joad 1991; Ezure et al. 1991; Kubin et al. 1991; Lipski et al. 1991; Otake et al. 1992; Mazzone and Canning 2002a, b; Kubin et al. 2006). SARs terminate primarily ipsilateral to their vagal origin, rostral to obex in the lateral and interstitial subnuclei (Kalia and Richter 1985; Davies et al. 1987a,b; Bonham and McCrimmon 1990; Ezure et al. 2002; Kubin et al. 2006). No attempt at differentiating termination sites of RAR, SAR, or C-fiber subtypes has been described. In addition to the studies of SAR, RAR, and bronchopulmonary C-fiber termination sites, some work has been done to identify the nTS subnuclei regulating the cough reflex (Gestreau et al. 1997; Ohi et al. 2005; Jakus et al. 2008).

Electrophysiological and functional studies show evidence for bronchopulmonary afferent nerve convergence in the CNS (Takagi et al. 1995; Paton 1998; Silva-Carvalho et al. 1998). Coincident activation of airway afferent nerve subtypes can have synergistic effects on airway reflexes, including reflex bronchospasm and cough (Mazzone and Canning 2002a, b; Mazzone et al. 2005) (Fig. 5). Such synergistic interactions may explain the association between extrapulmonary disorders (e.g., gastroesophageal reflux disease, allergic rhinitis) and cough.

Several studies have characterized the pharmacology of the primary central synapses for airway vagal afferent nerves and have revealed a prominent role for glutamate acting via non-NMDA receptors (Bonham et al. 1993; Vardhan et al.

1993; Karius et al. 1994; Chianca and Machado 1996; Wilson et al. 1996; Aylwin et al. 1997; Ezure et al. 1999; Haxhiu et al. 2000; Mutolo et al. 2007, 2008). Notably, however, NMDA receptor activation plays an essential role in the initiation of cough, explaining in part the ability of the antitussive agent dextromethorphan to prevent coughing in animals and in human subjects (Canning et al. 2004, 2006a, b; Mutolo et al. 2007). Other agents shown to act centrally in nTS to regulate airway vagal reflexes include μ-opioid receptor agonists (codeine, DAMGO), $GABA_B$ receptor agonists, sigma agonists, and TRPV1 receptor agonists (Mazzone and Geraghty 1999; Mazzone et al. 2005; Ohi et al. 2005, 2007; Mutolo et al. 2007, 2008). Serotonin (5-HT) receptor antagonists have also been shown to act centrally to modulate airway reflexes, but their site of action has not been determined (Bootle et al. 1996).

The tachykinins substance P and neurokinin A have been localized to airway afferent neurons, and tachykinin receptor antagonists have been shown to reduce or abolish coughing evoked in guinea pigs, dogs, rabbits, cats, and pigs (Advenier and Emonds-Alt 1996; Bolser et al. 1997; Moreaux et al. 2000; House et al. 2004; Mutolo et al. 2008). Capsaicin microinjection in nTS evokes respiratory reflexes in rats that are abolished by neurokinin receptor antagonists, while coughing evoked in rabbits and sensitization of cough induced in guinea pigs is markedly inhibited or abolished by nTS microinjection of neurokinin receptor antagonists (Mazzone and Geraghty 1999; Mazzone et al. 2005; Mutolo et al. 2008). A central site of action for neuroknin receptor antagonists in cough in cats and in guinea pigs has also been suggested (Bolser et al. 1997). Reflex bronchospasm evoked by laryngeal capsaicin and by intravenous bradykinin in guinea pigs is also prevented by centrally acting neurokinin receptor antagonists (Canning et al. 2001; Mazzone and Canning 2002a, b) (Fig. 5). Neurokinin-1 receptor antagonists are also used clinically to treat emesis, a vagal reflex in humans that has many similarities to the cough reflex (Hornby 2001; Warr 2006). It seems likely then that neurokinins released from the central terminals of airway afferent nerves may also modulate airway reflexes in humans and in other species. It is thus interesting and confusing that in electrophysiological recordings of nTS neurons receiving synaptic input from airway afferent nerves, little evidence for an excitatory effect of neurokinins in otherwise healthy animals has been reported. Indeed, in one study, exogenously administered substance P was found to act presynaptically to depress synaptic transmission in nTS (Sekizawa et al. 2003). Many of these studies involved recording from unidentified synapses or the synapses of RARs or SARs, which are unlikely to express substance P under normal conditions. But even in recordings in C-fiber relay neurons, synaptic transmission has been explained entirely by the actions of glutamate (Wilson et al. 1996; Mutoh et al. 2000). This suggests that under the experimental conditions used for the electrophysiological recordings done to date, solitary tract stimulation is subthreshold in intensity, frequency, or duration for tachykinin release, the neurons selected for recording (i.e., neurons receiving monosynaptic input) are typically devoid of direct tachykinin input, or the process of tissue harvest and slice preparation effectively silences neurokinin-mediated effects in nTS.

6 Airway Sensory Nerves and Bronchial Hyperresponsiveness

6.1 *Defining Characteristics of Bronchial Hyperresponsiveness*

A number of clinical features distinguish asthmatic subjects from other respiratory diseases and may be considered characteristic of this phenotype (Avital et al. 1995). These include an exacerbation of disease following exposure to β-adrenoceptor antagonists (Bond et al. 2007), an impairment in the ability to bronchodilate following deep inspiration (Slats et al. 2007), and their bronchoconstrictor sensitivity to a wide range of innocuous stimuli (Cockcroft and Davis 2006; Van Schoor et al. 2002).

It is well established that asthmatic subjects are invariably more responsive to a range of stimuli, as expressed by an increase in provocative concentration that induces a 20% fall in forced expiratory volume in 1 s termed "bronchial hyperresponsiveness" (BHR). However, not only is there an increase in the sensitivity of the airways to a stimulus, but there is also an increase in the maximum degree of airway narrowing for a given dose of agonist (Fig. 6). The importance of understanding the underlying mechanism contributing toward BHR is confirmed by a study showing that treating the underlying hyperresponsiveness leads to a better improvement in asthma symptoms (Sont et al. 1999). A number of mechanisms have been proposed to account for why asthmatic subjects are invariably more responsive to the external environment. These include an alteration in airway geometry due to an increase in airway smooth muscle thickness that would lead to a greater degree of airway narrowing for a given dose of agonist and/or perturbations in myosin-actin function resulting in a loss in the ability of smooth muscle to dilate in response to deep inspiration, thereby leading to enhanced bronchoconstrictor responses (An et al. 2007; Gil and Lauzon 2007); the release of cytokines and growth factors from epithelial cells which stimulate mesenchymal cells and promote structural changes in the airways leading to airway remodeling, airway inflammation, and BHR (Holgate 2007); and recruitment and activation of dendritic cells, T lymphocytes, and eosinophils whose cell-derived products trigger a cascade of events within the lung leading to epithelial cell damage, increased smooth muscle contractility, and airway remodeling (Beier et al. 2007; Hammad and Lambrecht 2007; Jacobsen et al. 2007; Kallinich et al. 2007; Lloyd and Robinson 2007; Rosenberg et al. 2007). These mechanisms are all thought to contribute toward BHR in asthma, are likely to be interrelated, and contribute to the overall expression of BHR. However, there is also good evidence for the contribution of airway sensory nerves in this phenomenon (Spina and Page 2002) that might be likened to allodynia and/or hyperalgesia, which are characteristic of pain syndromes (Carr and Undem 2003; Undem et al. 2002).

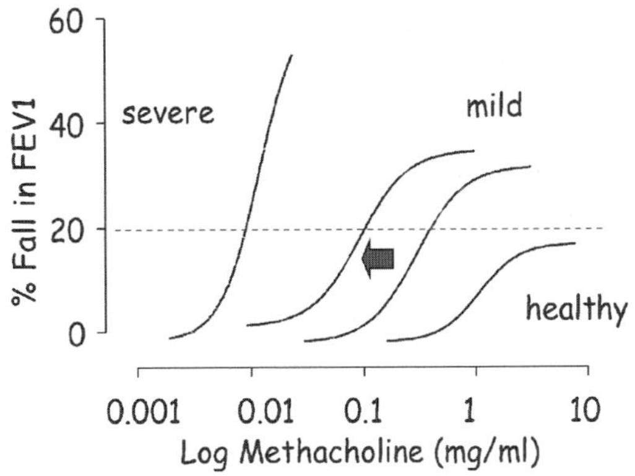

Fig. 6 Bronchial hyperresponsiveness (BHR) in asthma. It is convenient to measure changes in forced expiratory volume in 1 s (FEV_1) to increasing doses of methacholine. In asthma, there is an increase in sensitivity (leftward position of the dose–response curve) often measured in terms of PC20 (*dotted line*) and reactivity (increase in slope) and in severe cases of the disease an inability to define the maximum degree value for airway narrowing compared with healthy subjects. However, BHR as measured by changes in FEV_1 to increasing doses of methacholine may not be a sensitive indicator of the asthma phenotype (see the text). An increase in BHR can occur during exacerbation of disease as observed naturally during the pollen season, in the case of an allergic asthmatic, or following the deliberate exposure to a relevant antigen (*arrow*). However, asthmatic subjects are invariably responsive to a wide range of physiological stimuli that are otherwise refractory in healthy subjects. An understanding of the mechanisms by which these stimuli induce bronchoconstriction suggests that sensitization of afferent pathways may underlie this phenomenon

6.2 Bronchial Hyperresponsiveness and Sensory Nerves

It is common for clinicians to use stimuli such as methacholine and histamine to induce bronchoconstriction because these agents are relatively convenient to use. However, although there is a separation in airways responsiveness to these agents between asthmatic subjects and healthy individuals, there is a considerable degree of overlap and it has been suggested that these agents may not be sensitive indicators of the asthma phenotype (Avital et al. 1995; O'Connor et al. 1999). In contrast, asthmatic subjects invariably bronchoconstrict in response to the indirect-acting stimuli described earlier, which provoke little if any response in otherwise healthy individuals or in subjects with other respiratory diseases (Avital et al. 1995; Van Schoor et al. 2000).

Asthmatic subjects bronchoconstrict in response to a number of physiological stimuli such as exercise, distilled water, cold air, and hypertonic saline which are otherwise refractory in healthy subjects. Similarly, acidification, pollutants such as sulfur dioxide, and chemical substances, including adenosine, bradykinin, and neuropeptides, evoke bronchoconstriction in asthma but have little if any effect in nondiseased individuals. These agents are commonly referred to as "indirect-acting stimuli," since they do not appear to mediate bronchoconstriction by direct activation of airway smooth muscle. They are thought to elicit bronchospasm by activating a number of different cell types, including mast cells, vascular smooth muscle cells, and vascular endothelial cells, and/or airway nerves (Spina and Page 1996, 2002; Van Schoor et al. 2000). A number of studies which measured the generation of action potentials from individual afferent nerves using well-established electrophysiological techniques have shown that stimuli including sulfur dioxide, acidification, distilled water, bradykinin, neuropeptides, and adenosine can activate C-fiber and Aδ-fibers in vivo (Table 1). It is therefore of interest that asthmatic subjects are sensitive to such stimuli, whereas healthy subjects are invariably unresponsive to these agents (Van Schoor et al. 2000).

This suggests that the mechanisms by which these stimuli provoke bronchoconstriction are upregulated in asthma and characteristic of this phenotype. Furthermore, airways inflammation appears to be correlated better with BHR to indirect stimuli such as adenosine (van den Berge et al. 2001), bradykinin (Polosa et al. 1998; Roisman et al. 1996), and hypertonic saline (Sont et al. 1993) than it is to more direct acting stimuli such as methacholine. Similarly, during an exacerbation of BHR following the deliberate exposure of an asthmatic subject to an environmental allergen (e.g., house dust mite) there is a preferential increase in BHR to an indirect-acting stimulus such as bradykinin compared with methacholine (Berman et al. 1995). On the other hand, a number of pharmacological drugs used to treat asthma, including nedocromil sodium and ipratropium bromide, suppress airways responsiveness to these indirect-acting stimuli, suggesting the likely involvement of neural reflexes (Van Schoor et al. 2000). Furthermore, it is now recognized that glucocorticosteroids preferentially suppress BHR to adenosine (Ketchell et al. 2002; van den Berge et al. 2001) and bradykinin (Reynolds et al. 2002) compared with methacholine.

It is also noted that there is often a wide variability in airway sensitivity to spasmogens in subjects with mild asthma and there is little or very poor correlation between airway sensitivity to indirect-acting bronchoconstrictor agents such as adenosine and sensitivity to direct-acting stimuli such as methacholine. Also, BHR to an indirect-acting stimulus is greater during an exacerbation of asthma and lower following anti-inflammatory treatment compared with BHR to methacholine, which directly activates airway smooth muscle (O'Connor et al. 1999; Van Schoor et al. 2000). This apparent lack of correlation between bronchoconstrictor potency of these different types of stimuli suggest that alteration in the thickness of the airway wall (i.e., airway remodeling) alone cannot account for these discrepancies. If airway remodeling were responsible, then there would be a better correlation between bronchoconstrictor potency of indirect-acting and direct-acting stimuli. Furthermore, inflammatory insults to the airway wall would cause a similar change in BHR to these different agents and, finally, there would be no preferential effect of drug treatment on BHR to different stimuli.

Together, the findings of clinical studies support the notion that inflammatory insults to the lung might increase the activity of neuronal pathways, thereby

Table 1 Electrophysiological evidence for activation of afferent nerves in vivo by substances that elicit bronchoconstriction in asthmatic subjects

Stimulus	RARs	C-fibers	References
Sulfur dioxide	Cat, rabbit	Dog, rat	Widdicombe (1954a, b), Boushey et al. (1974), Ho et al. (2001), Matsumoto et al. (1997), Roberts et al. (1982)
Distilled water	Dog	Dog, guinea pig	Fox et al. (1995), Pisarri et al. (1992)
Bradykinin		Dog	Kaufman et al. (1980)
	Guinea pig	Guinea pig	Bergren (1997), Fox et al. (1993), Ricco et al. (1996)
		Mouse	Kollarik and Undem (2004)
Neuropeptides	Rabbit	Rabbit, guinea pig	Bergren (2006), Bonham et al. (1996), Prabhakar et al. (1987)
Capsaicin	Cat, guinea pig	Cat, dog, guinea pig, rat, mouse	Armstrong and Luck (1974), Bergren (1997)
			Mohammed et al. (1993), Morikawa et al. (1997)
			Coleridge and Coleridge (1977), Dixon et al. (1980), Fox et al. (1993), Ho et al. (2001), Jackson et al. (1989), Kollarik and Undem (2004), Ricco et al. (1996)
Adenosine		Rat, guinea pig	Chuaychoo et al. (2006), Hong et al. (1998), Kwong et al. (1998)
Endotoxin	Rat	Rat	Lai et al. (2005), Ruan et al. (2005)

RARs rapidly adapting receptors

resulting in heightened sensitivity of the lungs to these indirect-acting stimuli. Furthermore, one cannot view BHR as a nonspecific phenomenon, that is to say, that asthmatics are hyperresponsive to all stimuli, but rather it is increasingly apparent that BHR is more heterogeneous than is widely appreciated (O'Connor et al. 1999) and sensory nerves might be a common pathway through which BHR is manifested in respiratory diseases such as asthma.

6.3 TRPV1 and Bronchial Hyperresponsiveness

Transient receptor potential (TRP) channels are protein sensors for the perception of pain, taste, hearing, and smell and comprise at least six subfamilies (Nilius et al. 2007). One member of this superfamily (TRPV1) is predominantly localized to small-diameter afferent neurons in dorsal and vagal sensory ganglia (Szallasi and Blumberg 1999) and activation by capsaicin gives rise to feelings of warmth, heat, and pain. The cloning and expression of TRPV1 has increased our understanding of the role of this protein in neurogenic pain, but also with migraine, cough, irritable bladder disease, and gastrointestinal inflammation (Cortright et al. 2007; Geppetti and Trevisani 2004; Jia and Lee 2007; Kollarik et al. 2007; Liddle 2007; Ma and Quirion 2007; Okajima and Harada 2006; Storr 2007). The role of these proteins in contributing to BHR has been investigated in a number of experimental models. It has long been recognized that capsaicin selectively activates a subpopulation of afferent nerves, the neuropeptide containing C-fibers. However, it is now well established that capsaicin may also target a subset of airway Aδ-fibers whose cell nuclei reside within the jugular but not nodose ganglion (Myers et al. 2002). The activation of both of these nerve types can lead to a number of physiological changes within the airways, including reflex bronchoconstriction, release of sensory neuropeptides, edema, cough, and submucosal gland secretion (De Swert and Joos 2006).

Chronic treatment with capsaicin in various animal species leads to an impairment of somatosensory function as a consequence of depletion of sensory neuropeptide content, downregulation of TRPV1 receptor expression, and/or destruction and loss of sensory nerves (Watanabe et al. 2005, 2006). A consequence of chronic treatment with capsaicin upon neural function in the lung is an attenuation of BHR induced by a range of stimuli (Table 2). Thus, BHR induced by exposing nonallergic animals to lipid mediators, including platelet-activating factor and 15-hydroperoxyeicosatetraenoic acid, is attenuated. A similar observation was noted when BHR was elicited following exposure of nonallergic animals to lipopolysaccharide, ozone, citric acid, parainfluenza-3 virus, and poly(l-lysine) or exposure of allergic animals to inhaled antigens (Table 2). It has been concluded that the peripheral release of sensory neuropeptides per se was responsible for inducing BHR because depletion of sensory neuropeptides within the airways was a natural consequence of chronic treatment with capsaicin. Indeed a variety of animal experimental data have provided a wealth of information concerning the potential role of tachykinins

Table 2 Studies demonstrating a role for sensory nerves in bronchial hyperresponsiveness (*BHR*)

Stimulus[a]	Spasmogen	Species	Effect of chronic capsaicin treatment on BHR	Effect of chronic capsaicin treatment on inflammatory cell recruitment	References
Antigen	Acetylcholine	Guinea pig	Inhibited	No effect	Matsuse et al. (1991)
	Histamine	Rabbit	Inhibited	No effect	Herd et al. (1995)
	Histamine	Rabbit	Inhibited	No effect	Riccio et al. (1993)[f]
	Serotonin	Rat (BNxWi/Fu)	Increased[c]	Increased[e]	Ahlstedt et al. (1986)[f]
TDI	Acetylcholine	Guinea pig	Inhibited	Not measured	Thompson et al. (1987)
	Acetylcholine	Rabbit	Inhibited	Not measured	Marek et al. (1996)
SO_2	Methacholine	Rat (Sprague-Dawley)	Augmented[c]	Not measured	Long et al. (1997)[f]
			Not measured	Augmented	Long et al. (1999)[f]
LPS	Histamine	Guinea pig	Inhibited	Inhibited	Jarreau et al. (1994)
	Histamine	Guinea pig	Augmented[d]	Not measured	Loeffler et al. (1997)
Ozone	Histamine	Guinea pig	Inhibited	Not measured	Tepper et al. (1993)
	Histamine	Guinea pig	Inhibited	Inhibited	Koto et al. (1995)
	Methacholine	Rat (Sprague-Dawley)	Augmented[c]	Not measured	Jimba et al. (1995)[f]
		Rat (Wistar)	Not measured	Augmented	Vesely et al. (1999)[f]
	EFS[b]	Ferret	Inhibited	Not measured	Wu et al. (2003)
Citric acid	Acetylcholine	Guinea pig	Inhibited	Not measured	Girard et al. (1996)
Parainfluenza-3	Acetylcholine	Guinea pig	Inhibited	Not measured	Riedel et al. (1997)
Cigarette smoke	Acetylcholine	Guinea pig	Inhibited	Not measured	Daffonchio et al. (1990)
PAF	Histamine	Rabbit	Inhibited	Neutrophils inhibited; eosinophils not inhibited	Spina et al. (1991)
	Acetylcholine	Guinea pig		Not measured	Perretti and Manzini (1993)
15-HPETE	Histamine	Rabbit	Inhibited	No effect	Riccio et al. (1997)

(continued)

Table 2 (continued)

Stimulus[a]	Spasmogen	Species	Effect of chronic capsaicin treatment on BHR	Effect of chronic capsaicin treatment on inflammatory cell recruitment	References
Poly(l-lysine)	Methacholine	Rat (Sprague-Dawley)	Inhibited	Not determined	Coyle et al. (1994)[f]
		Nonallergic chronic rhinitis	Nasal resistance inhibited; symptom scores reduced		Lacroix et al. (1991)
		Allergic rhinitis	Hyperosmolar response inhibited; symptom scores reduced		Sanico et al. (1999)

15-HPETE 15-hydroperoxyeicosatetraenoic acid, *LPS* lipopolysaccharide, *PAF* platelet-activating factor, *TDI* toluene diioscyanate, *EFS* electrical field stimulation

[a]Stimulus denotes a substance used to induce bronchial hyperresponsiveness
[b]EFS and BHR was measured in vitro
[c]Unlike in guinea pigs, rabbits, ferrets and humans, neurokinins released from capsaicin-sensitive nerves are bronchodilators in rats (and mice), which may explain in part the augmentation of bronchial responsiveness seen with capsaicin pretreatment in rats (Manzini 1992; Szarek et al. 1995)
[d]BHR augmented at 2 h but not at 1 and 3 h after LPS challenge
[e]Data not analyzed statistically
[f]Treatment of neonates with capsaicin but measurement of bronchial hyperresponsiveness and inflammation performed in adult animals

such as substance P, neurokinin A, and CGRP in altering both resident lung and inflammatory cells, thereby perpetuating the inflammatory process in the lung and contributing to this process and inducing BHR (De Swert and Joos 2006).

It is therefore surprising that neurokinin antagonists have thus far proved disappointing in clinical trials in asthma (De Swert and Joos 2006). However, the rationale for the development of tachykinin antagonists was based on the assumption that local release of tachykinins from C-fibers was sufficient to perpetuate the inflammatory response. One can only conclude that other mediators released within the airways contribute to the inflammatory process, or the possibility that capsaicin is selective for C-fiber afferents in the airways needs to be revised since TRPV1 may also be localized to non-C-fiber afferents, or is not necessarily colocalized with sensory neuropeptides (Guo et al. 1999; Myers et al. 2002; Tominaga et al. 1998; Watanabe et al. 2005, 2006), and, therefore, sensory-neuropeptide-independent mechanisms may also operate in the lung. Furthermore, most studies showing an importance for tachykinins in mediating BHR stem from studies conducted in the guinea pig, an animal rich in sensory neuropeptide innervation in the lung. In contrast, the rabbit is relatively resistant to the neuropeptide-depleting effects of capsaicin despite the inhibition of BHR induced by nonimmunological and immunological methods (Herd et al. 1995; Riccio et al. 1997)and, therefore, mechanisms other than neuropeptide depletion must account for this phenomenon, and the peripheral release of sensory neuropeptides is not obligatory for the development of BHR. This may be one reason why, thus far, selective neurokinin antagonists have proved disappointing in the treatment of asthma (Spina and Page 2002).

Studies using capsaicin have shown that the functional effect of neuropeptides on airway smooth muscle is species-dependent. Rabbit, monkey, and human airways contract weakly on exposure to capsaicin in vitro (Ellis et al. 1997; Spina et al. 1998), whereas guinea-pig airways are very sensitive (Grundstrom et al. 1981). These variable functional effects are superficially consistent with the differential localization of substance P and CGRP in the airways across species, as the occurrence of these neuropeptide-containing nerves in human and rabbit tends to be sparse (Hislop et al. 1990; Howarth et al. 1995; Laitinen et al. 1983; Lundberg et al. 1984), whereas neuropeptides are found widely throughout the airways of guinea pigs (Hua et al. 1985; Nohr and Weihe 1991; Saria et al. 1985).

Hyperalgesia induced by chemical and thermal stimuli is suppressed in TRPV1 knockout mice, suggesting that this protein is an important transducer of pain (Gunthorpe et al. 2002; Julius and Basbaum 2001). It is therefore of interest that chronic treatment with capsaicin in humans can lead to a suppression of allodynia and hyperalgesia induced by intradermal injection of capsaicin (Davis et al. 1995) and when applied topically to the nose, capsaicin reduces nasal hyperresponsiveness in allergic rhinitis patients (Sanico et al. 1999). A loss in TRPV1 signaling might help explain the loss in BHR observed in various experimental animal models (Spina and Page 2002).

6.4 TRPV1 Antagonist and Knockout Studies

If the activation of TRPV1 is important for the sensitization of primary afferent nerves in the lung, then it would seem reasonable to suggest that pharmacological antagonism of this protein might reduce BHR. Unfortunately, very few studies have specifically addressed this question in the context of BHR. In one study, BHR was induced in the guinea pig by acute challenge with platelet-activating factor, which was inhibited following pretreatment with ruthenium red, a nonselective TRP channel blocker (Perretti and Manzini 1993). Studies using TRPV1 antagonists may require an additional control to rule out any possible bronchorelaxant capabilities that may confound any potential effect on BHR (Skogvall et al. 2007).

The effect of TRPV1 antagonists on cellular recruitment has been investigated in a number of inflammatory models. The TRPV1 antagonist *N*-(4-chlorobenzyl)-*N′*-(4-hydroxy-3-iodo-5-methoxybenzyl) thiourea had no effect on neutrophil recruitment induced by injection of complete Freund's adjuvant into the hindpaw of mice (Tang et al. 2007). In contrast, capsazepine inhibited neutrophil recruitment to the lung induced by systemic administration of hydrogen sulfide donor (Bhatia et al. 2006) and inhibited neutrophil recruitment in a model of colitis (Kihara et al. 2003) and pancreatitis (Hutter et al. 2005). Differences in the severity of the inflammatory models utilized in these studies may account for the lack of general consensus concerning the role of TRPV1 in inflammatory cell recruitment; however, as indicated earlier, the findings of most chemical ablation studies using chronic treatment with capsaicin are consistent with the peripheral involvement of sensory neuropeptides in neutrophil recruitment to sites of inflammation (Table 2).

There has also been a paucity of studies utilizing TRPV1 gene deficient mice to study the role of this protein in BHR and inflammation. In one study, BHR in response to lipopolysaccharide challenge was significantly augmented in TRPV1 knockout mice, and highlighted the existence of an anti-inflammatory substance (e.g., somatostatin) released from TRPV1-positive cells, which could act in a negative-feedback mechanism to limit the inflammatory response (Helyes et al. 2007). However, these data are not consistent with those form chemical ablation studies showing that BHR to lipopolysaccharide is inhibited in the guinea pig (Jarreau et al. 1994). This discrepancy may be due to the two different methods employed to "impair" TRPV1 signaling. It could be envisaged that sensory nerves would be bombarded by multiple signals by a plethora of mediators released following the initial insult, resulting in the activation of various receptor proteins (e.g., bradykinin and NGF receptor, other TRPs) on primary afferent terminals. These signals would be processed at the level of the nTS, but would also require the activation of TRPV1 for a facilitated response (i.e., gain in function). However, the interpretation of these signals by the nTS would be lost following chemical ablation with capsaicin, owing to destruction of the peripheral terminations of C-fibers in the airway, but these would be retained in TRPV1 knockout mice with an intact afferent nervous system and therefore would still able to signal to the nTS. Alternatively, compensatory mechanisms during the development of TRPV1 knockout mice might account for this anomaly. The implication is that impairment of sensory nerve function (e.g., via TRPV1 desensitization) may be required instead of TRPV1 antagonism to completely suppress BHR.

In terms of the inflammatory response, it appears that neutrophil recruitment in joint inflammation was either unaffected (Keeble et al. 2005) or augmented during inflammatory insults to the lung (Helyes et al. 2007) and gastrointestinal tract (Massa et al. 2006). Similarly, the amounts of TNF-α released within the extracellular space at sites of inflammation were either increased (Clark et al. 2007) or unaffected (Keeble et al. 2005) by gene deletion of TRPV1 in different inflammatory models. Hence, these murine models have been inconclusive concerning the role of TRPV1 in mediating BHR and/or inflammation. The observation that activation of TRPV1 may stimulate the release of an anti-inflammatory substance in the mouse also makes it difficult to elucidate the role of TRPV1 in BHR and inflammation in this species (Helyes et al. 2007).

7 Conclusions

Airway sensory nerves play an essential role in regulating airway and lung defensive and homeostatic reflexes. The afferent nerve subtypes regulating these reflexes have unique physiological and pharmacological attributes that are amenable to selective therapeutic interventions. There is extensive evidence to suggest that airway sensory nerves are dysregulated in disease. Therapeutic strategies that target the excitability of airway sensory nerves at their central and peripheral terminations may provide symptom relief in conditions such as cough, asthma, and COPD.

References

Adcock JJ, Douglas GJ, Garabette M, Gascoigne M, Beatch G, Walker M, Page CP (2003) RSD931, a novel anti-tussive agent acting on airway sensory nerves. Br J Pharmacol 138:407–416

Advenier C, Emonds-Alt X (1996) Tachykinin receptor antagonists and cough. Pulm Pharmacol 9:329–333

Ahlstedt S, Alving K, Hesselmar B, Olaisson E (1986) Enhancement of the bronchial reactivity in immunized rats by neonatal treatment with capsaicin. Int Arch Allergy Appl Immunol 80:262–266

Aikawa T, Sekizawa K, Itabashi S, Sasaki H, Takishima T (1990) Inhibitory actions of prostaglandin E1 on non-adrenergic non-cholinergic contraction in guinea-pig bronchi. Br J Pharmacol 101(1):13–14

Aizawa H, Matsuzaki Y, Ishibashi M, Domae M, Hirose T, Shigematsu N, Tanaka K (1982) A possible role of a nonadrenergic inhibitory nervous system in airway hyperreactivity. Respir Physiol 50:187–196

Aizawa H, Tanaka H, Sakai J, Takata S, Hara N, Ito Y (1997) L-NAME-sensitive and -insensitive nonadrenergic noncholinergic relaxation of cat airway in vivo and in vitro. Eur Respir J 10:314–321

Aizawa H, Takata S, Inoue H, Matsumoto K, Koto H, Hara N (1999) Role of nitric oxide released from iNANC neurons in airway responsiveness in cats. Eur Respir J 13(4):775–780

An SS, Bai TR, Bates JH, Black JL, Brown RH, Brusasco V, Chitano P, Deng L, Dowell M, Eidelman DH, Fabry B, Fairbank NJ, Ford LE, Fredberg JJ, Gerthoffer WT, Gilbert SH, Gosens R, Gunst SJ, Halayko AJ, Ingram RH, Irvin CG, James AL, Janssen LJ, King GG, Knight DA, Lauzon AM, Lakser OJ, Ludwig MS, Lutchen KR, Maksym GN, Martin JG, Mauad T, McParland BE, Mijailovich SM, Mitchell HW, Mitchell RW, Mitzner W, Murphy TM, Pare PD, Pellegrino R, Sanderson MJ, Schellenberg RR, Seow CY, Silveira PS, Smith PG, Solway J, Stephens NL, Sterk PJ, Stewart AG, Tang DD, Tepper RS, Tran T, Wang L (2007) Airway smooth muscle dynamics: a common pathway of airway obstruction in asthma. Eur Respir J 29:834–860

Andresen JH, Saugstad OD (2008) Effects of nicotine infusion on striatal glutamate and cortical non-protein-bound iron in hypoxic newborn piglets. Neonatology 94:284–292

Armstrong DJ, Luck JC (1974) A comparative study of irritant and type J receptors in the cat. Respir Physiol 21:47–60

Avital A, Springer C, Bar-Yishay E, Godfrey S (1995) Adenosine, methacholine, and exercise challenges in children with asthma or paediatric chronic obstructive pulmonary disease. Thorax 50:511–516

Aylwin ML, Horowitz JM, Bonham AC (1997) NMDA receptors contribute to primary visceral afferent transmission in the nucleus of the solitary tract. J Neurophysiol 77:2539–2548

Bachoo M, Polosa C (1987) Properties of the inspiration-related activity of sympathetic preganglionic neurones of the cervical trunk in the cat. J Physiol 385:545–564

Bai TR, Macklem PT, Martin JG (1986) The effects of parasympathectomy on serotonin-induced bronchoconstriction in the cat. Am Rev Respir Dis 133:110–115

Baluk P, Nadel JA, McDonald DM (1992) Substance P-immunoreactive sensory axons in the rat respiratory tract: a quantitative study of their distribution and role in neurogenic inflammation. J Comp Neurol 319:586–598

Barman SM, Gebber GL (1976) Basis for synchronization of sympathetic and phrenic nerve discharges. Am J Physiol 231:1601–1607

Barnes PJ (1986) Asthma as an axon reflex. Lancet 1(8475):242–245

Barnes PJ (2001) Neurogenic inflammation in the airways. Respir Physiol 125:145–154

Barnes PJ, Adcock IM (1997) NF-kappa B: a pivotal role in asthma and a new target for therapy. Trends Pharmacol Sci 18:46–50

Beier KC, Kallinich T, Hamelmann E (2007) T-cell co-stimulatory molecules: novel targets for the treatment of allergic airway disease. Eur Respir J 30:383–390

Belvisi MG, Chung KF, Jackson DM, Barnes PJ (1988) Opioid modulation of non-cholinergic neural bronchoconstriction in guinea-pig in vivo. Br J Pharmacol 95:413–418

Belvisi MG, Ichinose M, Barnes PJ (1989) Modulation of non-adrenergic, non-cholinergic neural bronchoconstriction in guinea-pig airways via GABAB-receptors. Br J Pharmacol 97: 1225–1231

Bergren DR (1997) Sensory receptor activation by mediators of defense reflexes in guinea-pig lungs. Respir Physiol 108:195–204

Bergren DR (2006) Prostaglandin involvement in lung C-fiber activation by substance P in guinea pigs. J Appl Physiol 100(6):1918–1927

Berman AR, Togias AG, Skloot G, Proud D (1995) Allergen-induced hyperresponsiveness to bradykinin is more pronounced than that to methacholine. J Appl Physiol 78:1844–1852

Bhatia M, Zhi L, Zhang H, Ng SW, Moore PK (2006) Role of substance P in hydrogen sulfide-induced pulmonary inflammation in mice. Am J Physiol Lung Cell Mol Physiol 291: L896–L904

Binshtok AM, Bean BP, Woolf CJ (2007) Inhibition of nociceptors by TRPV1-mediated entry of impermeant sodium channel blockers. Nature 449:607–610

Birrell MA, Crispino N, Hele DJ, Patel HJ, Yacoub MH, Barnes PJ, Belvisi MG (2002) Effect of dopamine receptor agonists on sensory nerve activity: possible therapeutic targets for the treatment of asthma and COPD. Br J Pharmacol 136:620–628

Bolser DC, Aziz SM, Chapman RW (1991) Ruthenium red decreases capsaicin and citric acid-induced cough in guinea pigs. Neurosci Lett 126:131–133
Bolser DC, DeGennaro FC, O'Reilly S, McLeod RL, Hey JA (1997) Central antitussive activity of the NK1 and NK2 tachykinin receptor antagonists, CP-99,994 and SR 48968, in the guinea-pig and cat. Br J Pharmacol 121:165–170
Bond RA, Spina D, Parra S, Page CP (2007) Getting to the heart of asthma: can "beta blockers" be useful to treat asthma? Pharmacol Ther 115:360–374
Bonham AC, Joad JP (1991) Neurones in commissural nucleus tractus solitarii required for full expression of the pulmonary C fibre reflex in rat. J Physiol 441:95–112
Bonham AC, McCrimmon DR (1990) Neurones in a discrete region of the nucleus tractus solitarius are required for the Breuer-Hering reflex in rat. J Physiol 427:261–280
Bonham AC, Coles SK, McCrimmon DR (1993) Pulmonary stretch receptor afferents activate excitatory amino acid receptors in the nucleus tractus solitarii in rats. J Physiol 464:725–745
Bonham AC, Kott KS, Ravi K, Kappagoda CT, Joad JP (1996) Substance P contributes to rapidly adapting receptor responses to pulmonary venous congestion in rabbits. J Physiol 493 (Pt 1):229–238
Bootle DJ, Adcock JJ, Ramage AG (1996) Involvement of central 5-HT1A receptors in the reflex activation of pulmonary vagal motoneurones by inhaled capsaicin in anaesthetized cats. Br J Pharmacol 117:724–728
Boushey HA, Richardson PS, Widdicombe JG, Wise JC (1974) The response of laryngeal afferent fibres to mechanical and chemical stimuli. J Physiol Lond 240:153–175
Bramley AM, Samhoun MN, Piper PJ (1990) The role of the epithelium in modulating the responses of guinea-pig trachea induced by bradykinin in vitro. Br J Pharmacol 99:762–766
Burki NK, Dale WJ, Lee LY (2005) Intravenous adenosine and dyspnea in humans. J Appl Physiol 98:180–185
Canning BJ (2006) Reflex regulation of airway smooth muscle tone. J Appl Physiol 101:971–985
Canning BJ (2007) Encoding of the cough reflex. Pulm Pharmacol Ther 20:396–401
Canning BJ, Chou YL (2009) Cough sensors. I. Physiological and pharmacological properties of the afferent nerves regulating cough. Handb Exp Pharmacol:23–47
Canning BJ, Undem BJ (1993) Relaxant innervation of the guinea-pig trachealis: demonstration of capsaicin-sensitive and -insensitive vagal pathways. J Physiol 460:719–739
Canning BJ, Reynolds SM, Mazzone SB (2001) Multiple mechanisms of reflex bronchospasm in guinea pigs. J Appl Physiol 91:2642–2653
Canning BJ, Mazzone SB, Meeker SN, Mori N, Reynolds SM, Undem BJ (2004) Identification of the tracheal and laryngeal afferent neurones mediating cough in anaesthetized guinea-pigs. J Physiol 557:543–558
Canning BJ, Farmer DG, Mori N (2006a) Mechanistic studies of acid-evoked coughing in anesthetized guinea pigs. Am J Physiol Regul Integr Comp Physiol 291:R454–R463
Canning BJ, Mori N, Mazzone SB (2006b) Vagal afferent nerves regulating the cough reflex. Respir Physiol Neurobiol 152:223–242
Carr MJ, Undem BJ (2003) Pharmacology of vagal afferent nerve activity in guinea pig airways. Pulm Pharmacol Ther 16:45–52
Carr MJ, Schechter NM, Undem BJ (2000) Trypsin-induced, neurokinin-mediated contraction of guinea pig bronchus. Am J Respir Crit Care Med 162(5):1662–1667
Caterina MJ, Schumacher MA, Tominaga M, Rosen TA, Levine JD, Julius D (1997) The capsaicin receptor: a heat-activated ion channel in the pain pathway. Nature 389:816–824
Chanez P, Springall D, Vignola AM, Moradoghi-Hattvani A, Polak JM, Godard P, Bousquet J (1998) Bronchial mucosal immunoreactivity of sensory neuropeptides in severe airway diseases. Am J Respir Crit Care Med 158:985–990
Chesrown SE, Venugopalan CS, Gold WM, Drazen JM (1980) In vivo demonstration of non-adrenergic inhibitory innervation of the guinea pig trachea. J Clin Invest 65:314–320
Chianca DA Jr, Machado BH (1996) Microinjection of NMDA antagonist into the NTS of conscious rats blocks the Bezold–Jarisch reflex. Brain Res 718:185–188

Choi JY, Joo NS, Krouse ME, Wu JV, Robbins RC, Ianowski JP, Hanrahan JW, Wine JJ (2007) Synergistic airway gland mucus secretion in response to vasoactive intestinal peptide and carbachol is lost in cystic fibrosis. J Clin Invest 117(10):3118–3127

Chou YL, Scarupa MD, Mori N, Canning BJ (2008) Differential effects of airway afferent nerve subtypes on cough and respiration in anesthetized guinea pigs. Am J Physiol Regul Integr Comp Physiol 295:R1572–R1584

Chuaychoo B, Lee MG, Kollarik M, Undem BJ (2005) Effect of 5-hydroxytryptamine on vagal C-fiber subtypes in guinea pig lungs. Pulm Pharmacol Ther 18:269–276

Chuaychoo B, Lee MG, Kollarik M, Pullmann R Jr, Undem BJ (2006) Evidence for both adenosine A1 and A2A receptors activating single vagal sensory C-fibres in guinea pig lungs. J Physiol 575:481–490

Clark N, Keeble J, Fernandes ES, Starr A, Liang L, Sugden D, de WP, Brain SD (2007) The transient receptor potential vanilloid 1 (TRPV1) receptor protects against the onset of sepsis after endotoxin. FASEB J 21:3747–3755

Clerici C, Macquin-Mavier I, Harf A (1989) Nonadrenergic bronchodilation in adult and young guinea pigs. J Appl Physiol 67(5):1764–1769

Coburn RF, Tomita T (1973) Evidence for nonadrenergic inhibitory nerves in the guinea pig trachealis muscle. Am J Physiol 224:1072–1080

Cockcroft DW, Davis BE (2006) Mechanisms of airway hyperresponsiveness. J Allergy Clin Immunol 118:551–559

Coleridge HM, Coleridge JC (1977) Impulse activity in afferent vagal C-fibres with endings in the intrapulmonary airways of dogs. Respir Physiol 29:125–142

Coleridge JC, Coleridge HM (1984) Afferent vagal C fibre innervation of the lungs and airways and its functional significance. Rev Physiol Biochem Pharmacol 99:1–110

Coleridge HM, Coleridge JC, Banzett RB (1978) II. Effect of CO2 on afferent vagal endings in the canine lung. Respir Physiol 34:135–151

Coleridge JC, Coleridge HM, Roberts AM, Kaufman MP, Baker DG (1982) Tracheal contraction and relaxation initiated by lung and somatic afferents in dogs. J Appl Physiol 52:984–990

Cortright DN, Krause JE, Broom DC (2007) TRP channels and pain. Biochim Biophys Acta 1772:978–988

Coyle AJ, Perretti F, Manzini S, Irvin CG (1994) Cationic protein-induced sensory nerve activation: role of substance P in airway hyperresponsiveness and plasma protein extravasation. J Clin Invest 94:2301–2306

Daffonchio L, Hernandez A, Gallico L, Omini C (1990) Airway hyperreactivity induced by active cigarette smoke exposure in guinea-pigs: possible role of sensory neuropeptides. Pulm Pharmacol 3:161–166

Davies RO, Kubin L (1986) Projection of pulmonary rapidly adapting receptors to the medulla of the cat: an antidromic mapping study. J Physiol 373:63–86

Davies A, Dixon M, Callanan D, Huszczuk A, Widdicombe JG, Wise JC (1978) Lung reflexes in rabbits during pulmonary stretch receptor block by sulphur dioxide. Respir Physiol 34:83–101

Davies RO, Kubin L, Pack AI (1987a) Pulmonary stretch receptor relay neurones of the cat: location and contralateral medullary projections. J Physiol 383:571–585

Davies SF, McQuaid KR, Iber C, McArthur CD, Path MJ, Beebe DS, Helseth HK (1987b) Extreme dyspnea from unilateral pulmonary venous obstruction. Demonstration of a vagal mechanism and relief by right vagotomy. Am Rev Respir Dis 136(1):184–188

Davis KD, Meyer RA, Turnquist JL, Filloon TG, Pappagallo M, Campbell JN (1995) Cutaneous pretreatment with the capsaicin analog NE-21610 prevents the pain to a burn and subsequent hyperalgesia. Pain 62:373–378

Deep V, Singh M, Ravi K (2001) Role of vagal afferents in the reflex effects of capsaicin and lobeline in monkeys. Respir Physiol 125:155–168

Delpierre S, Grimaud C, Jammes Y, Mei N (1981) Changes in activity of vagal bronchopulmonary C fibres by chemical and physical stimuli in the cat. J Physiol 316:61–74

De Proost I, Pintelon I, Brouns I, Timmermans JP, Adriaensen D (2007) Selective visualisation of sensory receptors in the smooth muscle layer of ex-vivo airway whole-mounts by styryl pyridinium dyes. Cell Tissue Res 329:421–431

De Swert KO, Joos GF (2006) Extending the understanding of sensory neuropeptides. Eur J Pharmacol 533:171–181

Dey RD, Altemus JB, Zervos I, Hoffpauir J (1990) Origin and colocalization of CGRP- and SP-reactive nerves in cat airway epithelium. J Appl Physiol 68:770–778

Diamond L, O'Donnell M (1980) A nonadrenergic vagal inhibitory pathway to feline airways. Science 208:185–188

Dicpinigaitis PV (2007) Experimentally induced cough. Pulm Pharmacol Ther 20:319–24

Dinh QT, Groneberg DA, Peiser C, Mingomataj E, Joachim RA, Witt C, Arck PC, Klapp BF, Fischer A (2004) Substance P expression in TRPV1 and trkA-positive dorsal root ganglion neurons innervating the mouse lung. Respir Physiol Neurobiol 144(1):15–24

Dixon M, Jackson DM, Richards IM (1979) The effects of histamine, acetylcholine and 5-hydroxytryptamine on lung mechanics and irritant receptors in the dog. J Physiol 287:393–403

Dixon M, Jackson DM, Richards IM (1980) The action of sodium cromoglycate on 'C' fibre endings in the dog lung. Br J Pharmacol 70:11–13

Dybas JM, Andresen CJ, Schelegle ES, McCue RW, Callender NN, Jackson AC (2006) Deep-breath frequency in bronchoconstricted monkeys (Macaca fascicularis). J Appl Physiol 100:786–791

Ellis JL, Sham JS, Undem BJ (1997) Tachykinin-independent effects of capsaicin on smooth muscle in human isolated bronchi. Am J Respir Crit Care Med 155:751–755

Ezure K, Otake K, Lipski J, She RB (1991) Efferent projections of pulmonary rapidly adapting receptor relay neurons in the cat. Brain Res 564:268–278

Ezure K, Tanaka I, Miyazaki M (1999) Electrophysiological and pharmacological analysis of synaptic inputs to pulmonary rapidly adapting receptor relay neurons in the rat. Exp Brain Res 128:471–480

Ezure K, Tanaka I, Saito Y, Otake K (2002) Axonal projections of pulmonary slowly adapting receptor relay neurons in the rat. J Comp Neurol 446:81–94

Fischer A, Forssmann WG, Undem BJ (1998) Nociceptin-induced inhibition of tachykinergic neurotransmission in guinea pig bronchus. J Pharmacol Exp Ther 285:902–907

Fisher JT, Sant'Ambrogio G (1982) Effects of inhaled CO2 on airway stretch receptors in the newborn dog. J Appl Physiol 53(6):1461–1465

Forsberg K, Karlsson JA, Theodorsson E, Lundberg JM, Persson CG (1988) Cough and bronchoconstriction mediated by capsaicin-sensitive sensory neurons in the guinea-pig. Pulm Pharmacol 1:33–39

Fox AJ, Barnes PJ, Urban L, Dray A (1993) An in vitro study of the properties of single vagal afferents innervating guinea-pig airways. J Physiol 469:21–35

Fox AJ, Barnes PJ, Dray A (1995) Stimulation of guinea-pig tracheal afferent fibres by non-isosmotic and low-chloride stimuli and the effect of frusemide. J Physiol 482(Pt 1):179–187

Fox AJ, Barnes PJ, Venkatesan P, Belvisi MG (1997) Activation of large conductance potassium channels inhibits the afferent and efferent function of airway sensory nerves in the guinea pig. J Clin Invest 99:513–519

Gatti R, Andre E, Amadesi S, Dinh TQ, Fischer A, Bunnett NW, Harrison S, Geppetti P, Trevisani M (2006) Protease-activated receptor-2 activation exaggerates TRPV1-mediated cough in guinea pigs. J Appl Physiol 101:506–511

Gaylor JB (1934) The intrinsic nervous mechanism of the human lung. Brain 57:143–160

Geppetti P, Trevisani M (2004) Activation and sensitisation of the vanilloid receptor: role in gastrointestinal inflammation and function. Br J Pharmacol 141:1313–1320

Gestreau C, Bianchi AL, Grelot L (1997) Differential brainstem fos-like immunoreactivity after laryngeal-induced coughing and its reduction by codeine. J Neurosci 17:9340–9352

Gil FR, Lauzon AM (2007) Smooth muscle molecular mechanics in airway hyperresponsiveness and asthma. Can J Physiol Pharmacol 85:133–140

Girard V, Yavo JC, Emonds-Alt X, Advenier C (1996) The tachykinin NK2 receptor antagonist SR 48968 inhibits citric acid-induced airway hyperresponsiveness in guinea-pigs. Am J Respir Crit Care Med 153:1496–1502

Giuliani S, Amann R, Papini AM, Maggi CA, Meli A (1989) Modulatory action of galanin on responses due to antidromic activation of peripheral terminals of capsaicin-sensitive sensory nerves. Eur J Pharmacol 163:91–96

Glaser ST, Kaczocha M, Deutsch DG (2005) Anandamide transport: a critical review. Life Sci 77:1584–1604

Green JF, Schmidt ND, Schultz HD, Roberts AM, Coleridge HM, Coleridge JC (1984) Pulmonary C-fibers evoke both apnea and tachypnea of pulmonary chemoreflex. J Appl Physiol 57(2): 562–567

Green JF, Schertel ER, Coleridge HM, Coleridge JC (1986) Effect of pulmonary arterial PCO2 on slowly adapting pulmonary stretch receptors. J Appl Physiol 60:2048–2055

Groneberg DA, Niimi A, Dinh QT, Cosio B, Hew M, Fischer A, Chung KF (2004) Increased expression of transient receptor potential vanilloid-1 in airway nerves of chronic cough. Am J Respir Crit Care Med 170:1276–1280

Gross NJ, Co E, Skorodin MS (1989) Cholinergic bronchomotor tone in COPD. Estimates of its amount in comparison with that in normal subjects. Chest 96:984–987

Grundstrom N, Andersson RG, Wikberg JE (1981) Prejunctional alpha 2 adrenoceptors inhibit contraction of tracheal smooth muscle by inhibiting cholinergic neurotransmission. Life Sci 28:2981–2986

Grundstrom N, Andersson RG, Wikberg JE (1984) Inhibition of the excitatory non-adrenergic, non-cholinergic neurotransmission in the guinea pig tracheo-bronchial tree mediated by alpha 2-adrenoceptors. Acta Pharmacol Toxicol (Copenh) 54:8–14

Gu Q, Lee LY (2006) Characterization of acid signaling in rat vagal pulmonary sensory neurons. Am J Physiol Lung Cell Mol Physiol 291:L58–L65

Gu Q, Lin YS, Lee LY (2007) Epinephrine enhances the sensitivity of rat vagal chemosensitive neurons: role of beta3-adrenoceptor. J Appl Physiol 102:1545–1555

Gu Q, Ni D, Lee LY (2008) Expression of neuronal nicotinic acetylcholine receptors in rat vagal pulmonary sensory neurons. Respir Physiol Neurobiol 161:87–91

Guardiola J, Proctor M, Li H, Punnakkattu R, Lin S, Yu J (2007) Airway mechanoreceptor deactivation. J Appl Physiol 103:600–607

Gunthorpe MJ, Benham CD, Randall A, Davis JB (2002) The diversity in the vanilloid (TRPV) receptor family of ion channels. Trends Pharmacol Sci 23:183–191

Guo A, Vulchanova L, Wang J, Li X, Elde R (1999) Immunocytochemical localization of the vanilloid receptor 1 (VR1): relationship to neuropeptides, the P2X3 purinoceptor and IB4 binding sites. Eur J Neurosci 11:946–958

Habler HJ, Janig W, Michaelis M (1994) Respiratory modulation in the activity of sympathetic neurones. Prog Neurobiol 43:567–606

Hammad H, Lambrecht BN (2007) Lung dendritic cell migration. Adv Immunol 93:265–278

Hanacek J, Davies A, Widdicombe JG (1984) Influence of lung stretch receptors on the cough reflex in rabbits. Respiration 45:161–168

Harrison S, Reddy S, Page CP, Spina D (1998) Stimulation of airway sensory nerves by cyclosporin A and FK506 in guinea-pig isolated bronchus. Br J Pharmacol 125:1405–1412

Haxhiu MA, Chavez JC, Pichiule P, Erokwu B, Dreshaj IA (2000) The excitatory amino acid glutamate mediates reflexly increased tracheal blood flow and airway submucosal gland secretion. Brain Res 883:77–86

Helyes Z, Elekes K, Nemeth J, Pozsgai G, Sandor K, Kereskai L, Borzsei R, Pinter E, Szabo A, Szolcsanyi J (2007) Role of transient receptor potential vanilloid 1 receptors in endotoxin-induced airway inflammation in the mouse. Am J Physiol Lung Cell Mol Physiol 292: L1173–L1181

Hempleman SC, Rodriguez TA, Bhagat YA, Begay RS (2000) Benzolamide, acetazolamide, and signal transduction in avian intrapulmonary chemoreceptors. Am J Physiol Regul Integr Comp Physiol 279:R1988–R1995

Herd CM, Gozzard N, Page CP (1995) Capsaicin pretreatment prevents the development of antigen induced airway hyperresponsiveness in neonatally immunized rabbits. Eur J Pharmacol 282:111–119

Hislop AA, Wharton J, Allen KM, Polak JM, Haworth SG (1990) Immunohistochemical localization of peptide-containing nerves in human airways: age-related changes. Am J Respir Cell Mol Biol 3:191–198

Ho CY, Gu Q, Hong JL, Lee LY (2000) Prostaglandin E(2) enhances chemical and mechanical sensitivities of pulmonary C fibers in the rat. Am J Respir Crit Care Med 162:528–533

Ho CY, Gu Q, Lin YS, Lee LY (2001) Sensitivity of vagal afferent endings to chemical irritants in the rat lung. Respir Physiol 127:113–124

Holgate ST (2007) The epithelium takes centre stage in asthma and atopic dermatitis. Trends Immunol 28:248–251

Hong JL, Ho CY, Kwong K, Lee LY (1998) Activation of pulmonary C fibres by adenosine in anaesthetized rats: role of adenosine A1 receptors. J Physiol 508 (Pt 1):109–118

Hornby PJ (2001) Central neurocircuitry associated with emesis. Am J Med 111(Suppl 8A): 106S–112S

House A, Celly C, Skeans S, Lamca J, Egan RW, Hey JA, Chapman RW (2004) Cough reflex in allergic dogs. Eur J Pharmacol 492:251–258

Howarth PH, Springall DR, Redington AE, Djukanovic R, Holgate ST, Polak JM (1995) Neuropeptide-containing nerves in endobronchial biopsies from asthmatic and nonasthmatic subjects. Am J Respir Cell Mol Biol 13:288–296

Hua XY, Yaksh TL (1992) Release of calcitonin gene-related peptide and tachykinins from the rat trachea. Peptides 13(1):113–120

Hua XY, Theodorsson-Norheim E, Brodin E, Lundberg JM, Hokfelt T (1985) Multiple tachykinins (neurokinin A, neuropeptide K and substance P) in capsaicin-sensitive sensory neurons in the guinea-pig. Regul Pept 13:1–19

Huang WX, Yu Q, Cohen MI (2000) Fast (3 Hz and 10 Hz) and slow (respiratory) rhythms in cervical sympathetic nerve and unit discharges of the cat. J Physiol 523(Pt 2):459–477

Hunter DD, Undem BJ (1999) Identification and substance P content of vagal afferent neurons innervating the epithelium of the guinea pig trachea. Am J Respir Crit Care Med 159:1943–1948

Hutter MM, Wick EC, Day AL, Maa J, Zerega EC, Richmond AC, Jordan TH, Grady EF, Mulvihill SJ, Bunnett NW, Kirkwood KS (2005) Transient receptor potential vanilloid (TRPV-1) promotes neurogenic inflammation in the pancreas via activation of the neurokinin-1 receptor (NK-1R). Pancreas 30:260–265

Ichinose M, Inoue H, Miura M, Yafuso N, Nogami H, Takishima T (1987) Possible sensory receptor of nonadrenergic inhibitory nervous system. J Appl Physiol 63:923–929

Ichinose M, Inoue H, Miura M, Takishima T (1988) Nonadrenergic bronchodilation in normal subjects. Am Rev Respir Dis 138:31–34

Inoue H, Ichinose M, Miura M, Katsumata U, Takishima T (1989) Sensory receptors and reflex pathways of nonadrenergic inhibitory nervous system in feline airways. Am Rev Respir Dis 139(5):1175–1178

Inoue H, Aizawa H, Miyazaki N, Ikeda T, Shigematsu N (1991) Possible roles of the peripheral vagal nerve in histamine-induced bronchoconstriction in guinea-pigs. Eur Respir J 4:860–866

Irvin CG, Martin RR, Macklem PT (1982) Nonpurinergic nature and efficacy of nonadrenergic bronchodilation. J Appl Physiol 52:562–569

Jackson DM, Norris AA, Eady RP (1989) Nedocromil sodium and sensory nerves in the dog lung. Pulm Pharmacol 2:179–184

Jacobsen EA, Ochkur SI, Lee NA, Lee JJ (2007) Eosinophils and asthma. Curr Allergy Asthma Rep 7:18–26

Jakus J, Poliacek I, Halasova E, Murin P, Knocikova J, Tomori Z, Bolser DC (2008) Brainstem circuitry of tracheal-bronchial cough: c-fos study in anesthetized cats. Respir Physiol Neurobiol 160:289–300

Jammes Y, Mei N (1979) Assessment of the pulmonary origin of bronchoconstrictor vagal tone. J Physiol 291:305–316

Janig W, Habler HJ (2003) Neurophysiological analysis of target-related sympathetic pathways–from animal to human: similarities and differences. Acta Physiol Scand 177:255–274

Jarreau PH, D'Ortho MP, Boyer V, Harf A, quin Mavier I (1994) Effects of capsaicin on the airway responses to inhaled endotoxin in the guinea pig. Am J Respir Crit Care Med 149:128–133

Jia Y, Lee LY (2007) Role of TRPV receptors in respiratory diseases. Biochim Biophys Acta 1772:915–927

Jia Y, McLeod RL, Wang X, Parra LE, Egan RW, Hey JA (2002) Anandamide induces cough in conscious guinea-pigs through VR1 receptors. Br J Pharmacol 137:831–836

Jimba M, Skornik WA, Killingsworth CR, Long NC, Brain JD, Shore SA (1995) Role of C fibers in physiological responses to ozone in rats. J Appl Physiol 78:1757–1763

Jonzon A, Pisarri TE, Coleridge JC, Coleridge HM (1986) Rapidly adapting receptor activity in dogs is inversely related to lung compliance. J Appl Physiol 61:1980–1987

Julius D, Basbaum AI (2001) Molecular mechanisms of nociception. Nature 413:203–210

Kalia M, Richter D (1985) Morphology of physiologically identified slowly adapting lung stretch receptor afferents stained with intra-axonal horseradish peroxidase in the nucleus of the tractus solitarius of the cat. I. A light microscopic analysis. J Comp Neurol 241:503–520

Kalia M, Richter D (1988) Rapidly adapting pulmonary receptor afferents: II. Fine structure and synaptic organization of central terminal processes in the nucleus of the tractus solitarius. J Comp Neurol 274:574–594

Kallinich T, Beier KC, Wahn U, Stock P, Hamelmann E (2007) T-cell co-stimulatory molecules: their role in allergic immune reactions. Eur Respir J 29:1246–1255

Kamikawa Y, Shimo Y (1989) Adenosine selectively inhibits noncholinergic transmission in guinea pig bronchi. J Appl Physiol 66:2084–2091

Karius DR, Ling L, Speck DF (1994) Nucleus tractus solitarius and excitatory amino acids in afferent-evoked inspiratory termination. J Appl Physiol 76:1293–1301

Karla W, Shams H, Orr JA, Scheid P (1992) Effects of the thromboxane A2 mimetic, U46,619, on pulmonary vagal afferents in the cat. Respir Physiol 87:383–396

Karlsson JA, Fuller RW (1999) Pharmacological regulation of the cough reflex–from experimental models to antitussive effects in Man. Pulm Pharmacol Ther 12:215–228

Karlsson JA, Sant'Ambrogio FB, Forsberg K, Palecek F, Mathew OP, Sant'Ambrogio G (1993) Respiratory and cardiovascular effects of inhaled and intravenous bradykinin, PGE2, and PGF2 alpha in dogs. J Appl Physiol 74:2380–2386

Kaufman MP, Coleridge HM, Coleridge JC, Baker DG (1980) Bradykinin stimulates afferent vagal C-fibers in intrapulmonary airways of dogs. J Appl Physiol 48:511–517

Keeble J, Russell F, Curtis B, Starr A, Pinter E, Brain SD (2005) Involvement of transient receptor potential vanilloid 1 in the vascular and hyperalgesic components of joint inflammation. Arthritis Rheum 52:3248–3256

Kesler BS, Canning BJ (1999) Regulation of baseline cholinergic tone in guinea-pig airway smooth muscle. J Physiol 518 (Pt 3):843–855

Kesler BS, Mazzone SB, Canning BJ (2002) Nitric oxide-dependent modulation of smooth-muscle tone by airway parasympathetic nerves. Am J Respir Crit Care Med 165:481–488

Ketchell RI, Jensen MW, Lumley P, Wright AM, Allenby MI, O'Connor BJ (2002) Rapid effect of inhaled fluticasone propionate on airway responsiveness to adenosine 5′-monophosphate in mild asthma. J Allergy Clin Immunol 110:603–606

Kihara N, de la Fuente SG, Fujino K, Takahashi T, Pappas TN, Mantyh CR (2003) Vanilloid receptor-1 containing primary sensory neurones mediate dextran sulphate sodium induced colitis in rats. Gut 52:713–719

Knowlton GC, Larrabee MG (1946) A unitary analysis of pulmonary volume receptors. Am J Physiol Lung Cell Mol Physiol 147:100–114

Kollarik M, Undem BJ (2002) Mechanisms of acid-induced activation of airway afferent nerve fibres in guinea-pig. J Physiol 543:591–600

Kollarik M, Undem BJ (2004) Activation of bronchopulmonary vagal afferent nerves with bradykinin, acid and vanilloid receptor agonists in wild-type and TRPV1−/− mice. J Physiol 555:115–123

Kollarik M, Dinh QT, Fischer A, Undem BJ (2003) Capsaicin-sensitive and -insensitive vagal bronchopulmonary C-fibres in the mouse. J Physiol 551:869–879

Kollarik M, Ru F, Undem BJ (2007) Acid-sensitive vagal sensory pathways and cough. Pulm Pharmacol Ther 20:402–411

Koto H, Aizawa H, Takata S, Inoue H, Hara N (1995) An important role of tachykinins in ozone-induced airway hyperresponsiveness. Am J Respir Crit Care Med 151:1763–1769

Kubin L, Kimura H, Davies RO (1991) The medullary projections of afferent bronchopulmonary C fibres in the cat as shown by antidromic mapping. J Physiol 435:207–228

Kubin L, Alheid GF, Zuperku EJ, McCrimmon DR (2006) Central pathways of pulmonary and lower airway vagal afferents. J Appl Physiol 101:618–627

Kummer W, Fischer A, Kurkowski R, Heym C (1992) The sensory and sympathetic innervation of guinea-pig lung and trachea as studied by retrograde neuronal tracing and double-labelling immunohistochemistry. Neuroscience 49:715–737

Kwong K, Hong JL, Morton RF, Lee LY (1998) Role of pulmonary C fibres in adenosine-induced respiratory inhibition in anesthetized rats. J Appl Physiol 84:417–424

Kwong K, Carr MJ, Gibbard A, Savage TJ, Singh K, Jing J, Meeker S, Undem BJ (2008a) Voltage-gated sodium channels in nociceptive versus non-nociceptive nodose vagal sensory neurons innervating guinea pig lungs. J Physiol 586:1321–1336

Kwong K, Kollarik M, Nassenstein C, Ru F, Undem BJ (2008b) P2X2 receptors differentiate placodal vs. neural crest C-fiber phenotypes innervating guinea pig lungs and esophagus. Am J Physiol Lung Cell Mol Physiol 295:L858–L865

Lacroix JS, Buvelot JM, Polla BS, Lundberg JM (1991) Improvement of symptoms of non-allergic chronic rhinitis by local treatment with capsaicin. Clin Exp Allergy 21:595–600

Lai CJ, Ruan T, Kou YR (2005) The involvement of hydroxyl radical and cyclooxygenase metabolites in the activation of lung vagal sensory receptors by circulatory endotoxin in rats. J Appl Physiol 98:620–628

Laitinen LA, Laitinen A, Panula PA, Partanen M, Tervo K, Tervo T (1983) Immunohistochemical demonstration of substance P in the lower respiratory tract of the rabbit and not of man. Thorax 38:531–536

Lalloo UG, Fox AJ, Belvisi MG, Chung KF, Barnes PJ (1995) Capsazepine inhibits cough induced by capsaicin and citric acid but not by hypertonic saline in guinea pigs. J Appl Physiol 79:1082–1087

Lama A, Delpierre S, Jammes Y (1988) The effects of electrical stimulation of myelinated and non-myelinated vagal motor fibres on airway tone in the rabbit and the cat. Respir Physiol 74:265–274

Lamb JP, Sparrow MP (2002) Three-dimensional mapping of sensory innervation with substance p in porcine bronchial mucosa: comparison with human airways. Am J Respir Crit Care Med 166:1269–1281

Lammers JW, Minette P, McCusker MT, Chung KF, Barnes PJ (1989) Capsaicin-induced bronchodilation in mild asthmatic subjects: possible role of nonadrenergic inhibitory system. J Appl Physiol 67(2):856–861

Larsell O (1921) Nerve termination in the lung of the rabbit. J Comp Neurol 33:105–131

Larsell O (1922) The ganglia, plexuses and nerve-termination of the mammalian lung and pleura pulmonis. J Comp Neurol 35:97–132

Laude EA, Higgins KS, Morice AH (1993) A comparative study of the effects of citric acid, capsaicin and resiniferatoxin on the cough challenge in guinea-pig and man. Pulm Pharmacol 6:171–175
Lee LY, Morton RF (1993) Histamine enhances vagal pulmonary C-fiber responses to capsaicin and lung inflation. Respir Physiol 93:83–96
Lee LY, Morton RF (1995) Pulmonary chemoreflex sensitivity is enhanced by prostaglandin E2 in anesthetized rats. J Appl Physiol 79:1679–1686
Lee LY, Pisarri TE (2001) Afferent properties and reflex functions of bronchopulmonary C-fibers. Respir Physiol 125:47–65
Lee MG, Weinreich D, Undem BJ (2005) Effect of olvanil and anandamide on vagal C-fiber subtypes in guinea pig lung. Br J Pharmacol 146:596–603
Leung SY, Niimi A, Williams AS, Nath P, Blanc FX, Dinh QT, Chung KF (2007) Inhibition of citric acid- and capsaicin-induced cough by novel TRPV-1 antagonist, V112220, in guinea-pig. Cough 3:10
Liddle RA (2007) The role of Transient Receptor Potential Vanilloid 1 (TRPV1) channels in pancreatitis. Biochim Biophys Acta 1772:869–878
Ligresti A, Morera E, Van Der Stelt M, Monory K, Lutz B, Ortar G, Di Marzo V (2004) Further evidence for the existence of a specific process for the membrane transport of anandamide. Biochem J 380:265–272
Lin YS, Lee LY (2002) Stimulation of pulmonary vagal C-fibres by anandamide in anaesthetized rats: role of vanilloid type 1 receptors. J Physiol 539:947–955
Lin RL, Gu Q, Lin YS, Lee LY (2005) Stimulatory effect of CO_2 on vagal bronchopulmonary C-fiber afferents during airway inflammation. J Appl Physiol 99:1704–1711
Lipski J, Ezure K, Wong She RB (1991) Identification of neurons receiving input from pulmonary rapidly adapting receptors in the cat. J Physiol 443:55–77
Lloyd CM, Robinson DS (2007) Allergen-induced airway remodelling. Eur Respir J 29:1020–1032
Loeffler BS, Arden WA, Fiscus RR, Lee LY (1997) Involvement of tachykinins in endotoxin-induced airway hyperresponsiveness. Lung 175:253–263
Long NC, Martin JG, Pantano R, Shore SA (1997) Airway hyperresponsiveness in a rat model of chronic bronchitis: role of C fibers. Am J Respir Crit Care Med 155:1222–1229
Long NC, Abraham J, Kobzik L, Weller EA, Krishna Murthy GG, Shore SA (1999) Respiratory tract inflammation during the induction of chronic bronchitis in rats: role of C-fibres. Eur Respir J 14:46–56
Lundberg JM, Martling CR, Saria A, Folkers K, Rosell S (1983) Cigarette smoke-induced airway oedema due to activation of capsaicin-sensitive vagal afferents and substance P release. Neuroscience 10:1361–1368
Lundberg JM, Hokfelt T, Martling CR, Saria A, Cuello C (1984) Substance P-immunoreactive sensory nerves in the lower respiratory tract of various mammals including man. Cell Tissue Res 235:251–261
Ma AA, Ravi K, Bravo EM, Kappagoda CT (2004) Effects of gadolinium chloride on slowly adapting and rapidly adapting receptors of the rabbit lung. Respir Physiol Neurobiol 141: 125–135
Ma W, Quirion R (2007) Inflammatory mediators modulating the transient receptor potential vanilloid 1 receptor: therapeutic targets to treat inflammatory and neuropathic pain. Expert Opin Ther Targets 11:307–320
Manzini S (1992) Bronchodilatation by tachykinins and capsaicin in the mouse main bronchus. Br J Pharmacol 105(4):968–972
Mapp CE, Boniotti A, Graf PD, Chitano P, Fabbri LM, Nadel JA (1991) Bronchial smooth muscle responses evoked by toluene diisocyanate are inhibited by ruthenium red and by indomethacin. Eur J Pharmacol 200:73–76
Marek W, Potthast JJW, Marczynski B, Baur X (1996) Role of substance P and neurokinin A in toluene diisocyanate- induced increased airway responsiveness in rabbits. Lung 174:83–97

Martling CR (1987) Sensory nerves containing tachykinins and CGRP in the lower airways. Functional implications for bronchoconstriction, vasodilatation and protein extravasation. Acta Physiol Scand Suppl 563:1–57

Massa F, Sibaev A, Marsicano G, Blaudzun H, Storr M, Lutz B (2006) Vanilloid receptor (TRPV1)-deficient mice show increased susceptibility to dinitrobenzene sulfonic acid induced colitis. J Mol Med 84:142–146

Matran R, Martling CR, Lundberg JM (1989) Inhibition of cholinergic and non-adrenergic, non-cholinergic bronchoconstriction in the guinea pig mediated by neuropeptide Y and alpha 2-adrenoceptors and opiate receptors. Eur J Pharmacol 163:15–23

Matsumoto S (1996) Effects of vagal stimulation on slowly adapting pulmonary stretch receptors and lung mechanics in anesthetized rabbits. Lung 174:333–344

Matsumoto S (1998) Effects of sustained constant artificial ventilation on rapidly adapting pulmonary stretch receptors and lung mechanics in rabbits. Life Sci 62(4):319–325

Matsumoto S, Shimizu T (1989) Effects of 5-hydroxytryptamine on rapidly adapting pulmonary stretch receptor activity in the rabbit. J Auton Nerv Syst 27:35–38

Matsumoto N, Inoue H, Ichinose M, Ishii M, Inoue C, Sasaki H, Takishima T (1985) Effective sites by sympathetic beta-adrenergic and vagal nonadrenergic inhibitory stimulation in constricted airways. Am Rev Respir Dis 132:1113–1117

Matsumoto S, Okamura H, Suzuki K, Sugai N, Shimizu T (1996) Inhibitory mechanism of CO_2 inhalation on slowly adapting pulmonary stretch receptors in the anesthetized rabbit. J Pharmacol Exp Ther 279(1):402–409

Matsumoto S, Takeda M, Saiki C, Takahashi T, Ojima K (1997) Effects of vagal and carotid chemoreceptor afferents on the frequency and pattern of spontaneous augmented breaths in rabbits. Lung 175:175–186.

Matsumoto S, Takahashi T, Tanimoto T, Saiki C, Takeda M, Ojima K (1998) Excitatory mechanism of veratridine on slowly adapting pulmonary stretch receptors in anesthetized rabbits. Life Sci 63:1431–1437

Matsumoto S, Takahashi T, Tanimoto T, Saiki C, Takeda M (1999) Effects of potassium channel blockers on CO_2-induced slowly adapting pulmonary stretch receptor inhibition. J Pharmacol Exp Ther 290:974–979

Matsumoto S, Ikeda M, Nishikawa T (2000) Effects of sodium and potassium channel blockers on hyperinflation-induced slowly adapting pulmonary stretch receptor stimulation in the rat. Life Sci 67:2167–2175

Matsumoto S, Ikeda M, Yoshida S, Nishikawa T, Itoh Y, Fujimi Y, Tanimoto T, Saiki C, Takeda M (2005) The inhibitory effect of ouabain on the response of slowly adapting pulmonary stretch receptors to hyperinflation in the rabbit. Life Sci 78:112–120

Matsumoto S, Saiki C, Yoshida S, Takeda M, Kumagai Y (2006) Effect of ouabain on the afterhyperpolarization of slowly adapting pulmonary stretch receptors in the rat lung. Brain Res 1107:131–139

Matsuse T, Thomson RJ, Chen XR, Salari H, Schellenberg RR (1991) Capsaicin inhibits airway hyperresponsiveness but not lipoxygenase activity or eosinophilia after repeated aerosolized antigen in guinea pigs. Am Rev Respir Dis 144:368–372

Mazzone SB, Canning BJ (2002a) Evidence for differential reflex regulation of cholinergic and noncholinergic parasympathetic nerves innervating the airways. Am J Respir Crit Care Med 165(8):1076–1083

Mazzone SB, Canning BJ (2002b) Synergistic interactions between airway afferent nerve subtypes mediating reflex bronchospasm in guinea pigs. Am J Physiol Regul Integr Comp Physiol 283: R86–R98

Mazzone SB, Geraghty DP (1999) Respiratory action of capsaicin microinjected into the nucleus of the solitary tract: involvement of vanilloid and tachykinin receptors. Br J Pharmacol 127:473–481

Mazzone SB, McGovern AE (2006) Na^+–K^+–$2Cl^-$ cotransporters and Cl^- channels regulate citric acid cough in guinea pigs. J Appl Physiol 101:635–643

Mazzone SB, McGovern AE (2008) Immunohistochemical characterization of nodose cough receptor neurons projecting to the trachea of guinea pigs. Cough 4:9

Mazzone SB, Mori N, Canning BJ (2005) Synergistic interactions between airway afferent nerve subtypes regulating the cough reflex in guinea-pigs. J Physiol 569:559–573

McAlexander MA, Undem BJ (2000) Potassium channel blockade induces action potential generation in guinea-pig airway vagal afferent neurones. J Auton Nerv Syst 78:158–164

McAlexander MA, Myers AC, Undem BJ (1998) Inhibition of 5-lipoxygenase diminishes neurally evoked tachykinergic contraction of guinea pig isolated airway. J Pharmacol Exp Ther 285:602–607

McDonald DM, Mitchell RA, Gabella G, Haskell A (1988) Neurogenic inflammation in the rat trachea. II. Identity and distribution of nerves mediating the increase in vascular permeability. J Neurocytol 17:605–628

Meyers JR, MacDonald RB, Duggan A, Lenzi D, Standaert DG, Corwin JT, Corey DP (2003) Lighting up the senses: FM1-43 loading of sensory cells through nonselective ion channels. J Neurosci 23:4054–4065

Michoud MC, Amyot R, Jeanneret-Grosjean A, Couture J (1987) Reflex decrease of histamine-induced bronchoconstriction after laryngeal stimulation in humans. Am Rev Respir Dis 136:618–622

Mills JE, Sellick H, Widdicombe JG (1969) Activity of lung irritant receptors in pulmonary microembolism, anaphylaxis and drug-induced bronchoconstrictions. J Physiol 203:337–357

Mills JE, Sellick H, Widdicombe JG (1970) Epithelial irritant receptors in the lungs. In: Ruth P (ed) Breathing: Hering–Breuer Centenary Symposium. J. & A. Churchill, London, pp 77–99

Miserocchi G, Sant'Ambrogio G (1974) Responses of pulmonary stretch receptors to static pressure inflations. Respir Physiol 21:77–85

Miura M, Inoue H, Ichinose M, Kimura K, Katsumata U, Takishima T (1990) Effect of nonadrenergic noncholinergic inhibitory nerve stimulation on the allergic reaction in cat airways. Am Rev Respir Dis 141:29–32

Mizrahi J, D'Orleans-Juste P, Caranikas S, Regoli D (1982) Effects of peptides and amines on isolated guinea pig tracheae as influenced by inhibitors of the metabolism of arachidonic acid. Pharmacology 25:320–326

Mohammed SP, Higenbottam TW, Adcock JJ (1993) Effects of aerosol-applied capsaicin, histamine and prostaglandin E2 on airway sensory receptors of anaesthetized cats. J Physiol Lond 469:51–66

Moreaux B, Nemmar A, Vincke G, Halloy D, Beerens D, Advenier C, Gustin P (2000) Role of substance P and tachykinin receptor antagonists in citric acid-induced cough in pigs. Eur J Pharmacol 408:305–312

Morikawa T, Gallico L, Widdicombe J (1997) Actions of moguisteine on cough and pulmonary rapidly adapting receptor activity in the guinea pig. Pharmacol Res 35:113–118

Morrison SF (2001) Differential control of sympathetic outflow. Am J Physiol Regul Integr Comp Physiol 281:R683–R698

Mutoh T, Joad JP, Bonham AC (2000) Chronic passive cigarette smoke exposure augments bronchopulmonary C-fibre inputs to nucleus tractus solitarii neurones and reflex output in young guinea-pigs. J Physiol 523(Pt 1):223–233

Mutolo D, Bongianni F, Fontana GA, Pantaleo T (2007) The role of excitatory amino acids and substance P in the mediation of the cough reflex within the nucleus tractus solitarii of the rabbit. Brain Res Bull 74:284–293

Mutolo D, Bongianni F, Cinelli E, Fontana GA, Pantaleo T (2008) Modulation of the cough reflex by antitussive agents within the caudal aspect of the nucleus tractus solitarii in the rabbit. Am J Physiol Regul Integr Comp Physiol 295:R243–R251

Myers AC, Kajekar R, Undem BJ (2002) Allergic inflammation-induced neuropeptide production in rapidly adapting afferent nerves in guinea pig airways. Am J Physiol Lung Cell Mol Physiol 282:L775–L781

Nassenstein C, Kwong K, Taylor-Clark T, Kollarik M, Macglashan DM, Braun A, Undem BJ (2008) Expression and function of the ion channel TRPA1 in vagal afferent nerves innervating mouse lungs. J Physiol 586:1595–1604

Nilius B, Owsianik G, Voets T, Peters JA (2007) Transient receptor potential cation channels in disease. Physiol Rev 87:165–217

Nishino T (2000) Physiological and pathophysiological implications of upper airway reflexes in humans. Jpn J Physiol 50:3–14

Nohr D, Weihe E (1991) Tachykinin-, calcitonin gene-related peptide-, and protein gene product 9.5-immunoreactive nerve fibers in alveolar walls of mammals. Neurosci Lett 134:17–20

O'Connor BJ, Crowther SD, Costello JF, Morley J (1999) Selective airway responsiveness in asthma. Trends Pharmacol Sci 20:9–11

Oh EJ, Mazzone SB, Canning BJ, Weinreich D (2006) Reflex regulation of airway sympathetic nerves in guinea-pigs. J Physiol 573:549–564

Ohi Y, Yamazaki H, Takeda R, Haji A (2005) Functional and morphological organization of the nucleus tractus solitarius in the fictive cough reflex of guinea pigs. Neurosci Res 53:201–209

Ohi Y, Kato F, Haji A (2007) Codeine presynaptically inhibits the glutamatergic synaptic transmission in the nucleus tractus solitarius of the guinea pig. Neuroscience 146(3):1425–1433

Okajima K, Harada N (2006) Regulation of inflammatory responses by sensory neurons: molecular mechanism(s) and possible therapeutic applications. Curr Med Chem 13:2241–2251

Otake K, Ezure K, Lipski J, Wong She RB (1992) Projections from the commissural subnucleus of the nucleus of the solitary tract: an anterograde tracing study in the cat. J Comp Neurol 324:365–378

Paintal AS (1973) Vagal sensory receptors and their reflex effects. Physiol Rev 53:159–227

Palecek F, Sant'Ambrogio G, Sant'Ambrogio FB, Mathew OP (1989) Reflex responses to capsaicin: intravenous, aerosol, and intratracheal administration. J Appl Physiol 67:1428–1437

Paton JF (1998) Pattern of cardiorespiratory afferent convergence to solitary tract neurons driven by pulmonary vagal C-fiber stimulation in the mouse. J Neurophysiol 79:2365–2373

Pedersen KE, Meeker SN, Riccio MM, Undem BJ (1998) Selective stimulation of jugular ganglion afferent neurons in guinea pig airways by hypertonic saline. J Appl Physiol 84:499–506

Perretti F, Manzini S (1993) Activation of capsaicin-sensitive sensory fibers modulates PAF-induced bronchial hyperresponsiveness in anesthetized guinea pigs. Am Rev Respir Dis 148:927–931

Pisarri TE, Jonzon A, Coleridge HM, Coleridge JC (1992) Vagal afferent and reflex responses to changes in surface osmolarity in lower airways of dogs. J Appl Physiol 73:2305–2313

Polosa R, Renaud L, Cacciola R, Prosperini G, Crimi N, Djukanovic R (1998) Sputum eosinophilia is more closely associated with airway responsiveness to bradykinin than methacholine in asthma. Eur Respir J 12:551–556

Prabhakar NR, Runold M, Yamamoto Y, Lagercrantz H, Cherniack NS, von Euler C (1987) Role of the vagal afferents in substance P-induced respiratory responses in anaesthetized rabbits. Acta Physiol Scand 131:63–71

Proud D, Reynolds CJ, Lacapra S, Kagey-Sobotka A, Lichtenstein LM, Naclerio RM (1988) Nasal provocation with bradykinin induces symptoms of rhinitis and a sore throat. Am Rev Respir Dis 137(3):613–616

Ravi K (1985) Effect of carbon dioxide on the activity of slowly and rapidly adapting pulmonary stretch receptors in cats. J Auton Nerv Syst 12:267–277

Ravi K, Kappagoda CT (1992) Responses of pulmonary C-fibre and rapidly adapting receptor afferents to pulmonary congestion and edema in dogs. Can J Physiol Pharmacol 70:68–76

Reynolds CJ, Togias A, Proud D (2002) Airways hyper-responsiveness to bradykinin and methacholine: effects of inhaled fluticasone. Clin Exp Allergy 32:1174–1179

Reynolds SM, Docherty R, Robbins J, Spina D, Page CP (2008) Adenosine induces a cholinergic tracheal reflex contraction in guinea pigs in vivo via an adenosine A1 receptor-dependent mechanism. J Appl Physiol 105:187–196

Ricciardolo FL, Steinhoff M, Amadesi S, Guerrini R, Tognetto M, Trevisani M, Creminon C, Bertrand C, Bunnett NW, Fabbri LM, Salvadori S, Geppetti P (2000) Presence and bronchomotor activity of protease-activated receptor-2 in guinea pig airways. Am J Respir Crit Care Med 161:1672–1680

Riccio MM, Manzini S, Page CP (1993) The effect of neonatal capsaicin on the development of bronchial hyperresponsiveness in allergic rabbits. Eur J Pharmacol 232:89–97

Riccio MM, Matsumoto T, Adcock JJ, Douglas GJ, Spina D, Page CP (1997) The effect of 15-HPETE on airway responsiveness and pulmonary cell recruitment in rabbits. Br J Pharmacol 122:249–256

Ricco MM, Kummer W, Biglari B, Myers AC, Undem BJ (1996) Interganglionic segregation of distinct vagal afferent fibre phenotypes in guinea-pig airways. J Physiol 496(Pt 2): 521–530

Richardson CA, Herbert DA, Mitchell RA (1984) Modulation of pulmonary stretch receptors and airway resistance by parasympathetic efferents. J Appl Physiol 57:1842–1849

Riedel F, Benden C, Philippou S, Streckert HJ, Marek W (1997) Role of sensory neuropeptides in PIV-3-infection-induced airway hyperresponsiveness in guinea pigs. Respiration 64:211–219

Roberts AM, Hahn HL, Schultz HD, Nadel JA, Coleridge HM, Coleridge J (1982) Afferent vagal C-fibres are responsible for the reflex airway constriction and secretion evoked by pulmonary administration of SO_2 in dogs. Physiologist 250:226

Roisman GL, Lacronique JG, Desmazes DN, Carre C, Le-Cae A, Dusser DJ (1996) Airway responsiveness to bradykinin is related to eosinophilic inflammation in asthma. Am J Respir Crit Care Med 153:381–390

Rosenberg HF, Phipps S, Foster PS (2007) Eosinophil trafficking in allergy and asthma. J Allergy Clin Immunol 119:1303–1310

Ruan T, Lin YS, Lin KS, Kou YR (2005) Sensory transduction of pulmonary reactive oxygen species by capsaicin-sensitive vagal lung afferent fibres in rats. J Physiol 565:563–578

Sampson SR, Vidruk EH (1975) Properties of ‘irritant’ receptors in canine lung. Respir Physiol 25:9–22

Sanico AM, Philip G, Lai GK, Togias A (1999) Hyperosmolar saline induces reflex nasal secretions, evincing neural hyperresponsiveness in allergic rhinitis. J Appl Physiol 86: 1202–1210

Sant’Ambrogio FB, Sant’Ambrogio G, Fisher JT (1988) Lung mechanics and activity of slowly adapting airway stretch receptors. Eur Respir J 1:685–690

Saria A, Martling CR, Dalsgaard CJ, Lundberg JM (1985) Evidence for substance P-immunoreactive spinal afferents that mediate bronchoconstriction. Acta Physiol Scand 125:407–414

Schelegle ES, Green JF (2001) An overview of the anatomy and physiology of slowly adapting pulmonary stretch receptors. Respir Physiol 125:17–31

Schlemper V, Calixto JB (2002) Mechanisms underlying the contraction induced by bradykinin in the guinea pig epithelium-denuded trachea. Can J Physiol Pharmacol 80:360–367

Sekizawa S, Joad JP, Bonham AC (2003) Substance P presynaptically depresses the transmission of sensory input to bronchopulmonary neurons in the guinea pig nucleus tractus solitarii. J Physiol 552:547–559

Sellick H, Widdicombe JG (1969) The activity of lung irritant receptors during pneumothorax, hyperpnoea and pulmonary vascular congestion. J Physiol 203:359–381

Shah S, Page CP, Spina D (1998) Nociceptin inhibits non-adrenergic non-cholinergic contraction in guinea-pig airway. Br J Pharmacol 125:510–516

Silva-Carvalho L, Paton JF, Rocha I, Goldsmith GE, Spyer KM (1998) Convergence properties of solitary tract neurons responsive to cardiac receptor stimulation in the anesthetized cat. J Neurophysiol 79:2374–2382

Skogvall S, Berglund M, ence-Guzman MF, Svensson K, Jonsson P, Persson CG, Sterner O (2007) Effects of capsazepine on human small airway responsiveness unravel a novel class of bronchorelaxants. Pulm Pharmacol Ther 20:273–280

Slats AM, Janssen K, van SA, van der Plas DT, Schot R, van den Aardweg JG, de Jongste JC, Hiemstra PS, Mauad T, Rabe KF, Sterk PJ (2007) Bronchial inflammation and airway responses to deep inspiration in asthma and chronic obstructive pulmonary disease. Am J Respir Crit Care Med 176:121–128

Sont JK, Booms P, Bel EH, Vandenbroucke JP, Sterk PJ (1993) The determinants of airway hyperresponsiveness to hypertonic saline in atopic asthma in vivo. Relationship with subpopulations of peripheral blood leucocytes. Clin Exp Allergy 23:678–688

Sont JK, Willems LN, Bel EH, van Krieken JH, Vandenbroucke JP, Sterk PJ (1999) Clinical control and histopathologic outcome of asthma when using airway hyperresponsiveness as an additional guide to long-term treatment. The AMPUL Study Group. Am J Respir Crit Care Med 159:1043–1051

Spina D, Page CP (1996) Airway sensory nerves in asthma – targets for therapy? Pulm Pharmacol 9:1–18

Spina D, Page CP (2002) Pharmacology of airway irritability. Curr Opin Pharmacol 2:264–272

Spina D, McKenniff MG, Coyle AJ, Seeds EA, Tramontana M, Perretti F, Manzini S, Page CP (1991) Effect of capsaicin on PAF-induced bronchial hyperresponsiveness and pulmonary cell accumulation in the rabbit. Br J Pharmacol 103:1268–1274

Spina D, Harrison S, Page CP (1995) Regulation by phosphodiesterase isoenzymes of non-adrenergic non-cholinergic contraction in guinea-pig isolated main bronchus. Br J Pharmacol 116:2334–2340

Spina D, Matera MG, Riccio MM, Page CP (1998) A comparison of sensory nerve function in human, guinea-pig, rabbit and marmoset airway. Life Sci 63:1629–1643

Stone RA, Worsdell YM, Fuller RW, Barnes PJ (1993) Effects of 5-hydroxytryptamine and 5-hydroxytryptophan infusion on the human cough reflex. J Appl Physiol 74:396–401

Storr M (2007) TRPV1 in colitis: is it a good or a bad receptor? – a viewpoint. Neurogastroenterol Motil 19:625–629

Stretton CD, Belvisi MG, Barnes PJ (1991) Modulation of neural bronchoconstrictor responses in the guinea pig respiratory tract by vasoactive intestinal peptide. Neuropeptides 18(3):149–157

Sudo T, Hayashi F, Nishino T (2000) Responses of tracheobronchial receptors to inhaled furosemide in anesthetized rats. Am J Respir Crit Care Med 162(3 Pt 1):971–975

Szallasi A (1994) The vanilloid (capsaicin) receptor: receptor types and species differences. Gen Pharmacol 25:223–243

Szallasi A, Blumberg PM (1999) Vanilloid (capsaicin) receptors and mechanisms. Pharmacol Rev 51:159–211

Szarek JL, Gillespie MN, Altiere RJ, Diamond L (1986) Reflex activation of the nonadrenergic noncholinergic inhibitory nervous system in feline airways. Am Rev Respir Dis 133:1159–1162

Szarek JL, Stewart NL, Spurlock B, Schneider C (1995) Sensory nerve- and neuropeptide-mediated relaxation responses in airways of Sprague-Dawley rats. J Appl Physiol 78(5): 1679–1687

Taguchi O, Kikuchi Y, Hida W, Iwase N, Satoh M, Chonan T, Takishima T (1991) Effects of bronchoconstriction and external resistive loading on the sensation of dyspnea. J Appl Physiol 71:2183–2190

Taguchi O, Kikuchi Y, Hida W, Iwase N, Okabe S, Chonan T, Takishima T (1992) Prostaglandin E2 inhalation increases the sensation of dyspnea during exercise. Am Rev Respir Dis 145:1346–1349

Takagi S, Umezaki T, Shin T (1995) Convergence of laryngeal afferents with different natures upon cat NTS neurons. Brain Res Bull 38:261–268

Takahashi T, Belvisi MG, Barnes PJ (1994) Modulation of neurotransmission in guinea-pig airways by galanin and the effect of a new antagonist galantide. Neuropeptides 26(4):245–251

Tang L, Chen Y, Chen Z, Blumberg PM, Kozikowski AP, Wang ZJ (2007) Antinociceptive pharmacology of *N*-(4-chlorobenzyl)-*N*′-(4-hydroxy-3-iodo-5-methoxybenzyl) thiourea, a high-affinity competitive antagonist of the transient receptor potential vanilloid 1 receptor. J Pharmacol Exp Ther 321:791–798

Tatar M, Sant'Ambrogio G, Sant'Ambrogio FB (1994) Laryngeal and tracheobronchial cough in anesthetized dogs. J Appl Physiol 76:2672–2679

Tatar M, Pecova R, Karcolova D (1997) Sensitivity of the cough reflex in awake guinea pigs, rats and rabbits. Bratisl Lek Listy 98:539–543

Tatar M, Webber SE, Widdicombe JG (1988) Lung C-fibre receptor activation and defensive reflexes in anaesthetized cats. J Physiol 402:411–420

Taylor-Clark TE, McAlexander MA, Nassenstein C, Sheardown SA, Wilson S, Thornton J, Carr MJ, Undem BJ (2008) Relative contributions of TRPA1 and TRPV1 channels in the activation of vagal bronchopulmonary C-fibres by the endogenous autacoid 4-oxononenal. J Physiol 586:3447–3459

Tepper JS, Costa DL, Fitzgerald S, Doerfler DL, Bromberg PA (1993) Role of tachykinins in ozone-induced acute lung injury in guinea pigs. J Appl Physiol 75:1404–1411

Thompson JE, Scypinski LA, Gordon T, Sheppard D (1987) Tachykinins mediate the acute increase in airway responsiveness caused by toluene diisocyanate in guinea pigs. Am Rev Respir Dis 136:43–49

Tominaga M, Caterina MJ, Malmberg AB, Rosen TA, Gilbert H, Skinner K, Raumann BE, Basbaum AI, Julius D (1998) The cloned capsaicin receptor integrates multiple pain-producing stimuli. Neuron 21:531–543

Trevisani M, Milan A, Gatti R, Zanasi A, Harrison S, Fontana G, Morice AH, Geppetti P (2004) Antitussive activity of iodo-resiniferatoxin in guinea pigs. Thorax 59:769–772

Tucker RC, Kagaya M, Page CP, Spina D (2001) The endogenous cannabinoid agonist, anandamide stimulates sensory nerves in guinea-pig airways. Br J Pharmacol 132:1127–1135

Umeno E, McDonald DM, Nadel JA (1990) Hypertonic saline increases vascular permeability in the rat trachea by producing neurogenic inflammation. J Clin Invest 85:1905–1908

Undem BJ, Kollarik M (2002) Characterization of the vanilloid receptor 1 antagonist iodo-resiniferatoxin on the afferent and efferent function of vagal sensory C-fibers. J Pharmacol Exp Ther 303(2):716–722

Undem BJ, Meeker SN, Chen J (1994) Inhibition of neurally mediated nonadrenergic, noncholinergic contractions of guinea pig bronchus by isozyme-selective phosphodiesterase inhibitors. J Pharmacol Exp Ther 271(2):811–817

Undem BJ, Carr MJ, Kollarik M (2002) Physiology and plasticity of putative cough fibres in the Guinea pig. Pulm Pharmacol Ther 15:193–198

Undem BJ, Oh EJ, Lancaster E, Weinreich D (2003) Effect of extracellular calcium on excitability of guinea pig airway vagal afferent nerves. J Neurophysiol 89:1196–1204

Undem BJ, Chuaychoo B, Lee MG, Weinreich D, Myers AC, Kollarik M (2004) Subtypes of vagal afferent C-fibres in guinea-pig lungs. J Physiol 556:905–917

van den Berge M, Kerstjens HA, Meijer RJ, de Reus DM, Koeter GH, Kauffman HF, Postma DS (2001) Corticosteroid-induced improvement in the PC20 of adenosine monophosphate is more closely associated with reduction in airway inflammation than improvement in the PC20 of methacholine. Am J Respir Crit Care Med 164:1127–1132

Van Schoor J, Joos GF, Pauwels RA (2000) Indirect bronchial hyperresponsiveness in asthma: mechanisms, pharmacology and implications for clinical research. Eur Respir J 16:514–533

Van Schoor J, Joos GF, Pauwels RA (2002) Effect of inhaled fluticasone on bronchial responsiveness to neurokinin A in asthma. Eur Respir J 19:997–1002

Vardhan A, Kachroo A, Sapru HN (1993) Excitatory amino acid receptors in the nucleus tractus solitarius mediate the responses to the stimulation of cardio-pulmonary vagal afferent C fiber endings. Brain Res 618:23–31

Verleden GM, Belvisi MG, Rabe KF, Miura M, Barnes PJ (1993) Beta 2-adrenoceptor agonists inhibit NANC neural bronchoconstrictor responses in vitro. J Appl Physiol 74:1195–1199

Vesely KR, Hyde DM, Stovall MY, Harkema JR, Green JF, Schelegle ES (1999) Capsaicin-sensitive C-fiber-mediated protective responses in ozone inhalation in rats. J Appl Physiol 86:951–962

Vidruk EH, Hahn HL, Nadel JA, Sampson SR (1977) Mechanisms by which histamine stimulates rapidly adapting receptors in dog lungs. J Appl Physiol 43:397–402

Warr D (2006) The neurokinin1 receptor antagonist aprepitant as an antiemetic for moderately emetogenic chemotherapy. Expert Opin Pharmacother 7:1653–1658

Watanabe N, Horie S, Michael GJ, Spina D, Page CP, Priestley JV (2005) Immunohistochemical localization of vanilloid receptor subtype 1 (TRPV1) in the guinea pig respiratory system. Pulm Pharmacol Ther 18:187–197

Watanabe N, Horie S, Michael GJ, Keir S, Spina D, Page CP, Priestley JV (2006) Immunohistochemical co-localization of transient receptor potential vanilloid (TRPV)1 and sensory neuropeptides in the guinea-pig respiratory system. Neuroscience 141:1533–1543

Welch JM, Simon SA, Reinhart PH (2000) The activation mechanism of rat vanilloid receptor 1 by capsaicin involves the pore domain and differs from the activation by either acid or heat. Proc Natl Acad Sci USA 97:13889–13894

Widdicombe JG (1954a) Receptors in the trachea and bronchi of the cat. J Physiol 123:71–104

Widdicombe JG (1954b) Respiratory reflexes from the trachea and bronchi of the cat. J Physiol 123:55–70

Wilson CG, Zhang Z, Bonham AC (1996) Non-NMDA receptors transmit cardiopulmonary C fibre input in nucleus tractus solitarii in rats. J Physiol 496 (Pt 3):773–785

Wine JJ (2007) Parasympathetic control of airway submucosal glands: central reflexes and the airway intrinsic nervous system. Auton Neurosci 133:35–54

Winning AJ, Hamilton RD, Shea SA, Knott C, Guz A (1985) The effect of airway anaesthesia on the control of breathing and the sensation of breathlessness in man. Clin Sci (Lond) 68(2):215–225

Winning AJ, Hamilton RD, Shea SA, Guz A (1986) Respiratory and cardiovascular effects of central and peripheral intravenous injections of capsaicin in man: evidence for pulmonary chemosensitivity. Clin Sci (Lond) 71(5):519–526

Wu ZX, Satterfield BE, Dey RD (2003) Substance P released from intrinsic airway neurons contributes to ozone-enhanced airway hyperresponsiveness in ferret trachea. J Appl Physiol 95:742–750

Xiang A, Uchida Y, Nomura A, Iijima H, Sakamoto T, Ishii Y, Morishima Y, Masuyama K, Zhang M, Hirano K, Sekizawa K (2002) Involvement of thromboxane A(2) in airway mucous cells in asthma-related cough. J Appl Physiol 92:763–770

Yamamoto Y, Atoji Y, Suzuki Y (1995) Nerve endings in bronchi of the dog that react with antibodies against neurofilament protein. J Anat 187(1):59–65

Yamamoto Y, Ootsuka T, Atoji Y, Suzuki Y (1998) Morphological and quantitative study of the intrinsic nerve plexuses of the canine trachea as revealed by immunohistochemical staining of protein gene product 9.5. Anat Rec 250:438–447

Yamamoto Y, Sato Y, Taniguchi K (2007) Distribution of TRPV1- and TRPV2-immunoreactive afferent nerve endings in rat trachea. J Anat 211:775–783

Yoshihara S, Nadel JA, Figini M, Emanueli C, Pradelles P, Geppetti P (1998) Endogenous nitric oxide inhibits bronchoconstriction induced by cold-air inhalation in guinea pigs: role of kinins. Am J Respir Crit Care Med 157:547–552

Yu J (2005) Airway mechanosensors. Respir Physiol Neurobiol 148:217–243

Yu J, Coleridge JC, Coleridge HM (1987) Influence of lung stiffness on rapidly adapting receptors in rabbits and cats. Respir Physiol 68:161–176

Yu J, Schultz HD, Goodman J, Coleridge JC, Coleridge HM, Davis B (1989) Pulmonary rapidly adapting receptors reflexly increase airway secretion in dogs. J Appl Physiol 67:682–687

Regulation of Cardiac Afferent Excitability in Ischemia

Liang-Wu Fu and John C. Longhurst

Contents

Abstract The heart at the time of Sir William Harvey originally was thought to be an insensate organ. Today, however, we know that this organ is innervated by sensory nerves that course centrally though mixed nerve pathways that also contain parasympathetic or sympathetic motor nerves. Angina or cardiac pain is now well recognized as a pressure-like pain that occurs during myocardial ischemia when coronary artery blood flow is interrupted. Sympathetic (or spinal) afferent fibers

J.C. Longhurst (✉)
Department of Medicine, C240 Medical Sciences I, University of California, Irvine, Irvine, CA 92697, USA
jcl@uci.edu

B.J. Canning and D. Spina (eds.), *Sensory Nerves*,
Handbook of Experimental Pharmacology 194, DOI: 10.1007/978-3-540-79090-7_6,

that are either finely myelinated or unmyelinated are responsible for the transmission of information to the brain that ultimately allows the perception of angina as well as activation of the sympathetic nervous system, resulting in tachycardia, hypertension, and sometimes arrhythmias. Although early studies defined the importance of the vagal and sympathetic cardiac afferent systems in reflex autonomic control, until recently there has been little appreciation of the mechanisms of activation of the sensory endings. This review examines the role of a number of chemical mediators and their sources that are activated by the ischemic process. In this regard, patients with ischemic syndromes, particularly myocardial infarction and unstable angina, are known to have platelet activation, which leads to release of a number of chemical mediators, including serotonin, histamine, and thromboxane A_2, all of which stimulate ischemically sensitive cardiac spinal afferent endings in the ventricles through specific receptor-mediated processes. Furthermore, protons from lactic acid, bradykinin, and reactive oxygen species, especially hydroxyl radicals, individually and frequently in combination, stimulate these endings during ischemia. Cyclooxygenase products appear to sensitize the endings to the action of bradykinin and histamine. These studies of the chemical mechanisms of activation of cardiac sympathetic afferent endings during ischemia have the potential to provide targeted therapies that can modify the angina and the deleterious reflex responses that have the potential to exacerbate ischemia and myocardial cell death.

Keywords Sympathetic nervous system, Cardiac spinal afferent, Myocardial ischemia, Ischemic mediator, Nociceptor

1 Introduction

Heart disease is rapidly becoming the single most important cause of death worldwide. Coronary artery disease is the major form of heart disease underlying the high morbidity and mortality. Coronary atherosclerosis, or what we now call "atherothrombosis," is now not only prevalent in developed countries but has eclipsed infections and injuries in developing nations. The rise in atherosclerotic heart disease is due mainly to the increase in risk factors that promote development of the atherosclerotic plaque, including hypertension, obesity, diabetes, hyperlipidemia, and physical inactivity. Plaques in the coronary vasculature can physically limit flow, particularly during times of increased myocardial oxygen demand, resulting in an imbalance between oxygen demand and supply and hence myocardial ischemia. This so-called demand-induced ischemia quickly reduces myocardial function and is perceived by the symptom we call "angina" or "cardiac chest pain." Acute myocardial infarction or heart attacks generally are associated with plaque rupture and local thrombus formation because the contents of the plaque activate platelets (Stormorken 1986; Flores and Sheridan 1994). Mortality during infarction is directly dependent on a number of factors, including the extent of myocardial necrosis, the resulting pump dysfunction, and both ventricular and supraventricular arrhythmias, all of which lower cardiac output and blood pressure. Infarction is associated with prolonged ischemia and hence angina as well as with both excitatory and inhibitory reflex responses that originate from activation of cardiac sensory neural pathways. We have been interested in mechanisms, particularly chemical events, associated with activation of cardiac sensory neural endings that ultimately produce angina and reflex responses associated with myocardial ischemia, since this knowledge may allow better treatment of this common and very serious condition. We have employed a combination of whole animal reflex, electrophysiological, and pharmacological methods in experimental preparations to investigate mechanisms of activation of cardiac ischemically sensitive afferents.

2 The Responses of Myocardial Reflex During Ischemia

Two distinctly separate sensory pathways innervate the myocardium, including those that travel side by side with vagal preganglionic motor nerves and those that travel with sympathetic or spinal efferents. Thus, the somewhat confusing terms "vagal afferents" and "sympathetic (spinal) afferents" have been applied to describe anatomically these two sets of pathways that provide information from the heart to the central nervous system. It is useful to distinguish between these two types of afferents since, when stimulated, they elicit quite separate physiological responses. On one hand, when stimulated, vagal afferents cause a large decrease in heart rate and blood pressure, while, on the other hand, sympathetic afferent stimulation increases heart rate and blood pressure and pretty much is the sole pathway responsible for the sensation of angina (Longhurst 1984; White 1957). Furthermore, cardiac vagal afferent stimulation causes bradyarrhythmias, while sympathetic afferent stimulation leads to tachyarrhythmias. A number of studies highlight the roles of both finely myelinated Aδ and unmyelinated C-fibers in transmission of inhibitory cardiovascular reflex responses during stimulation of cardiac atrial and ventricular vagal endings (Baker et al. 1980; Thoren 1973, 1976; Oberg and Thoren 1973; Kappagoda et al. 1977, 1979; Paintal 1973). However, there has been little study of cardiac sympathetic afferents (Malliani et al. 1981). Furthermore, there has been very little investigation of the mechanisms of activation of cardiac sympathetic afferent ending during myocardial ischemia. Since this system is so relevant to angina, the predominate warning sign for patients experiencing myocardial ischemia and infarction as well as the associated reflexes, including reflexes that can exacerbate the extent of ischemia and infarction and because of the attendant potentially lethal arrhythmias, we have been studying this area over the last decade. This review concentrates strictly on studies from our laboratory, not to minimize any of the prior elegant work in this area but because we wish to focus the discussion. Review of the original articles provides abundant evidence that much of the foundation for our work has been carried out in pioneering laboratories over the last 30 years. Our studies were conducted in a model of brief myocardial ischemia in which ischemia was induced by complete occlusion of an appropriate branch of the coronary artery supplying the regional receptive field of the cardiac afferent nerve fiber endings in cats (Fu and Longhurst 2002a; Huang et al.1995a).

3 Chemical Mediators in Activation of Cardiac Spinal Afferent

3.1 Protons

Protons, derived from lactic acid, CO_2, or abnormal fatty acid metabolism during local ischemia, have been shown to be capable of stimulating visceral afferents, including pulmonary vagal afferents and abdominal sympathetic afferent nerve endings (Hong et al. 1997; Stahl and Longhurst 1992). Protons also can evoke a somatic-cardiovascular reflex through activation of group III and IV afferent nerve endings in muscle (Rotto et al. 1989). In a rat-skin-saphenous nerve preparation, protons, derived from either lactic acid or CO_2, selectively stimulated polymodal cutaneous C-fiber rather than Aδ-fiber afferents (Steen et al. 1995). However, in studies of ischemically sensitive abdominal visceral sympathetic afferents in cats, we have observed that Aδ- and C-fiber afferents respond to administration of lactic acid but not to hypercapnia, despite the smaller changes in local tissue pH caused by lactic acid compared with hypercapnia (Stahl and Longhurst 1992). Likewise, it has been found that hypercapnia does not activate cardiac vagal chemoreceptors (Mark et al. 1974). Furthermore, a number of studies have documented that, during myocardial ischemia, protons are produced mainly from the acid products of glycolysis that are associated with the production of lactic acid and abnormal fatty acid metabolism (Opie et al. 1973; Poole-Wilson 1978). Finally, investigators previously have shown that exogenous lactic acid stimulates cardiac sympathetic afferents, including both myelinated and unmyelinated fibers (Uchida and Murao 1975; Pal et al. 1989). We therefore postulated that protons produced during myocardial ischemia might be important mediators in activation of ischemically sensitive cardiac sympathetic afferents.

We examined the effect of ischemia-induced alterations of epicardial pH on the activity of cardiac afferents in the absence and the presence of isotonic neutral phosphate buffer. We also evaluated the responses of these afferents to hypercapnia, acidic phosphate buffer, lactic acid, and sodium lactate since they are major sources of protons during myocardial ischemia (Poole-Wilson 1978; Stahl and Longhurst 1992). We continuously measured epicardial pH with a pH-sensitive needle electrode (0.9-mm outer diameter) because cardiac sympathetic afferent nerve endings generally are located near the epicardial surface (Baker et al. 1980). We found that epicardial pH decreased progressively during brief (5-min) ischemia, topical application of acidic phosphate buffer, lactic acid, or exposure to a hypercapnic gas mixture. Lactic acid, but not sodium lactate, stimulated cardiac sympathetic afferents to a greater extent than acidic phosphate buffer solution. Conversely, inhalation of a high CO_2 gas concentration failed to activate these afferents, despite similar or greater pH changes in the epicardial region. Compared with ischemically sensitive afferents, only 19% of ischemically insensitive afferents responded to epicardial application of lactic acid. Moreover, the neutral phosphate buffer, which reduced tissue acidosis in the epicardial layer of the ischemic region, attenuated the response of these afferents to brief myocardial ischemia (Fig. 1). These results suggest that endogenous protons, derived from lactic acid but not as a result of hypercapnia, contribute to activation or sensitization of cardiac sympathetic afferents during myocardial ischemia (Pan et al. 1999). Protons likely directly stimulate cardiac sympathetic afferent nerve endings by opening two different classes of cation channels, namely, the acid-sensing ion channels (ASIC) and transient receptor potential vanilloid receptors 1 (TRPV1), members of the vanilloid-receptor-like transient receptor potential channel family (Immke and McCleskey 2003; Jordt et al. 2000). Both ASIC and TRPV1 are enriched in cardiac spinal afferent nerves and have the capability of generating a sustained current that triggers sensory nerve action potential (Immke and McCleskey

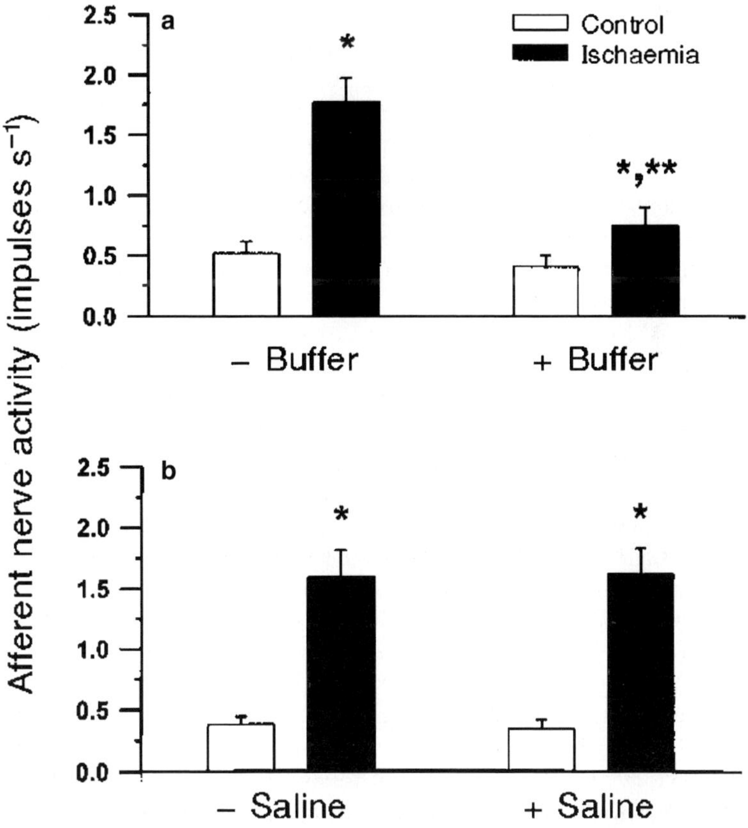

Fig. 1 Bar graphs displaying the responses of cardiac afferents to repeated 5 min of ischemia before and after treatment with isotonic neutral phosphate buffer (**a**, $n = 16$) or saline (**b**, $n = 14$). *Columns and brackets* are means ± the standard error of the mean (SEM). $*p < 0.05$ compared with the respective preischemia control. $**p < 0.05$ compared with the initial afferent response to ischemia (Pan et al. 1999)

2003; Jordt et al. 2000). Proton generation might also lead to the production of other mediators, such as bradykinin, since an acidic environment favors activation of kallikrein, the enzyme responsible for production of bradykinin (Stahl and Longhurst 1992). The role of bradykinin as a mediator of proton-induced cardiac afferent activation during ischemia requires further study.

3.2 Bradykinin and BK_2 Receptors

Bradykinin was first demonstrated to induce pain perception in humans when it was applied to an exposed blister base in volunteers (Armstrong et al. 1951). Since then, the role of bradykinin, as a mediator of pain and inflammation, has been extensively investigated (Rupniak et al. 2000; Couture et al. 2001). More recently, there has been interest in exploring the importance of bradykinin in excitation of cardiac afferents, particularly sympathetic afferents and the associated cardiac pain (Baker et al. 1980). In this respect, an increase in bradykinin concentration in coronary sinus blood was observed within 2 min of cardiac ischemia created by occlusion of the anterior descending left coronary artery (Hashimoto et al. 1977). Similarly, an increase in the concentration of bradykinin in the coronary sinus was detected within 2–5 min of occluding the left anterior descending coronary artery in dogs (Kimura et al. 1973). We have observed that bradykinin, in part, is responsible for stimulation of abdominal visceral afferents during ischemia (Lew and Longhurst 1986; Pan et al. 1994). Furthermore, exogenous bradykinin has been shown to stimulate cardiac afferent nerve endings (Nishi et al. 1977; Nerdrum et al. 1986; Kaufman et al. 1980; Baker et al. 1980) as well as sensory endings in skeletal muscle during muscle contraction (Kaufman et al. 1982; Stebbins and Longhurst 1985, 1986). Finally, in a study in humans undergoing cardiac catheterization (Schaefer et al. 1996), we demonstrated that administration of exogenous bradykinin into the coronary artery causes arterial hypotension and atypical (non-angina-like) chest pain in patients with or without coronary artery disease.

Bradykinin binds to two receptor subtypes: BK_1 and BK_2 receptors. Through activation of both receptors, this peptide stimulates a large number of cell types, including fibroblasts, endothelial cells, macrophages, kidney cells, and neurons (Bhoola et al. 1992). Moreover, activating cardiac sympathetic afferents evokes excitatory cardiovascular reflex responses such as tachycardia and hypertension (Uchida and Murao 1974; Baker et al. 1980; Staszewka-Barczak et al. 1976), which are either abolished or attenuated by a BK_2 receptor antagonist (Staszewska-Woolley and Woolley 1989). As such, we have investigated the possibility that endogenous bradykinin contributes to activation of cardiac sympathetic afferents during myocardial ischemia through a BK_2 receptor mechanism.

We first measured the responses of cardiac sympathetic afferents to exogenous bradykinin. Injection of bradykinin into the left atrium stimulated ischemically sensitive as well as ischemia-insensitive cardiac afferents, indicating that this peptide, in contrast to our observations with 5-hydroxytryptamine (5-HT; serotonin), is a less specific stimulus in cats (Fu and Longhurst 2002a). Because it lacks

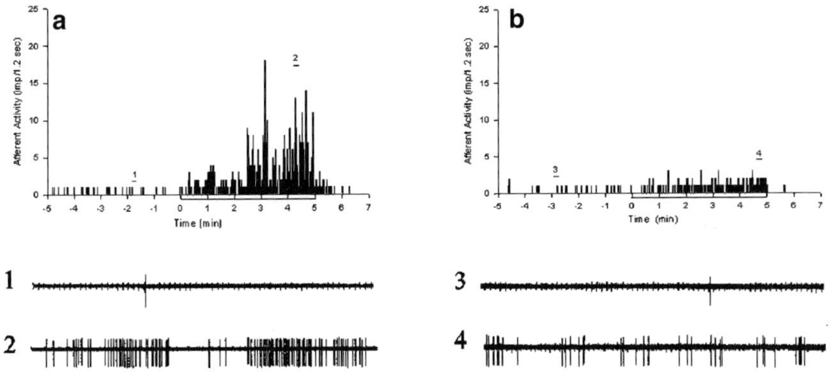

Fig. 2 Nerve activity of an ischemically sensitive cardiac C-fiber afferent during myocardial ischemia. (**a**, **b**) Afferent activity before and after treatment with HOE_{140}, a kinin B_2 receptor antagonist, respectively. Neurograms *1–4* display discharge activity of the afferent at the times indicated in the histograms. These data demonstrate that isotonic neutral phosphate buffer attenuates the response of cardiac afferents to ischemia (Tjen-A-Looi et al. 1998)

specificity for ischemically sensitive afferents and because it causes atypical chest pain in patients with coronary artery disease, it is unclear if bradykinin is responsible for cardiac pain (i.e., angina pectoris) during myocardial ischemia. However, it is clear that this peptide is capable of stimulating cardiac C-fibers in spinal pathways that could contribute to the overall afferent response as part of a group of chemicals released during ischemia.

To study the role of bradykinin during ischemia, we evaluated the responses of cardiac sympathetic afferents to endogenously produced bradykinin as well as the associated subtype receptor mechanism. Sufficient ischemia to induce a rise in bradykinin concentration that could potentially stimulate cardiac sympathetic afferents was achieved by occluding a branch of the coronary arterial system for 5 min. We observed a significant increase in discharge activity of single-unit afferents innervating this region during the initial period of ischemia. After blockade of BK_2 receptor with HOE_{140} and NPC-17731, two selective BK_2 receptor antagonists, the ischemia-induced increase in the activity of these afferents was significantly attenuated (Fig. 2) (Tjen-A-Looi et al. 1998). Conversely, we found that a kinin B_1 (or BK_1) receptor agonist, des-Arg^9-bradykinin, did not alter discharge activity of cardiac sympathetic afferents. These electrophysiological data suggest that endogenous bradykinin contributes to activation of cardiac afferents during myocardial ischemia through activation of BK_2 receptors.

3.3 Platelets and Glycoprotein IIb-IIIa Receptors

Thrombocytes (platelets) contain at least three distinct types of storage granules: dense granules, α-granules, and lysosomal vesicles. Dense granules contain mostly small molecules and ions, including adenosine 5′-triphosphate (ATP) and adenosine

5′-diphosphate (ADP), 5-HT, histamine, calcium, inorganic diphosphate, and inorganic phosphate (Stormorken 1986; Meyers et al. 1982). The αα-granules and lysosomal vesicles primarily contain macromolecular substances, including proteins, glycoproteins, proteoglycans, and a number of different acid hydrolytic enzymes (Rao 1993). Platelets normally circulate freely in the bloodstream as small, anucleate, disk-shaped cells, but are easily activated upon interaction with cell matrix components such as collagen, fibronectin, laminin, and von Willebrand factor, as well as with thrombin, ADP, and epinephrine. Pathophysiologically, this occurs with vascular injury during rupture of an atherosclerotic plaque that leads to myocardial ischemia and infarction as well as platelet activation (Stormorken 1986). Clinical studies have shown that platelet activation occurs in patients with spontaneous or unstable angina or during myocardial infarction (Flores et al. 1994; Fitzgerald 1991; Grande et al. 1990).

Upon activation, platelets release the contents of granules. 5-HT and histamine, two mediators released from activated platelets, stimulate ischemically sensitive abdominal visceral afferents (Fu et al. 1997; Fu and Longhurst 1998). Other platelet-derived mediators, including prostaglandins and other cyclooxygenase products, also can stimulate or sensitize cardiac sympathetic and vagal afferents (Ustinova and Schultz 1994; Nerdrum et al. 1986; Tjen-A-Looi et al. 1998). Intradermal injection of human platelets induces a distinct pain sensation in humans (Schmelz et al. 1997; Blunk et al. 1999). Furthermore, application of activated human platelet solutions to an ex vivo skin-nerve preparation of rats excites cutaneous nociceptors (Ringkamp et al. 1994). Thus, we hypothesized that activated platelets would be capable of exciting cardiac spinal afferents responsible for angina and sympathoexcitatory reflexes.

To test this hypothesis, we recorded the responses of ischemically sensitive cardiac sympathetic afferents to the presence of activated platelets. Ischemia-sensitive afferent nerve endings were identified on the anterior and posterior ventricles (Fig. 3). Platelets in enriched plasma were activated by either collagen or thrombin, since both function as strong platelet activators. Thrombin activates platelets without a measurable increase in cytoplasmic Ca^{2+} of platelets, whereas collagen activates platelets by increasing cytoplasmic Ca^{2+} (Holmsen 1985). Left atrial injection of platelets activated by collagen or thrombin increased discharge activity of ischemically sensitive afferents (Fu and Longhurst 2002b). Conversely, enriched plasma containing nonactivated platelets and platelet-poor plasma plus collagen or thrombin did not alter afferent activity (Fig. 4). These observations are reinforced by results of studies that have observed enhanced cutaneous C-fiber activity following application of platelets activated by ADP (Ringkamp et al. 1994). Similarly, intravenous injection of platelet-rich solutions induces burning pain and protracted hyperalgesia in humans (Schmelz et al. 1997). Finally, we have shown that depletion of circulating platelets with a polyclonal antibody attenuates the response of cardiac spinal afferents during myocardial ischemia (Fu and Longhurst 2002b). These findings are consistent with the demonstration that depletion of circulating platelets with anti-platelet antibody abolishes the reflex pulmonary pressor and systemic depressor responses following intravenous injection of autologous

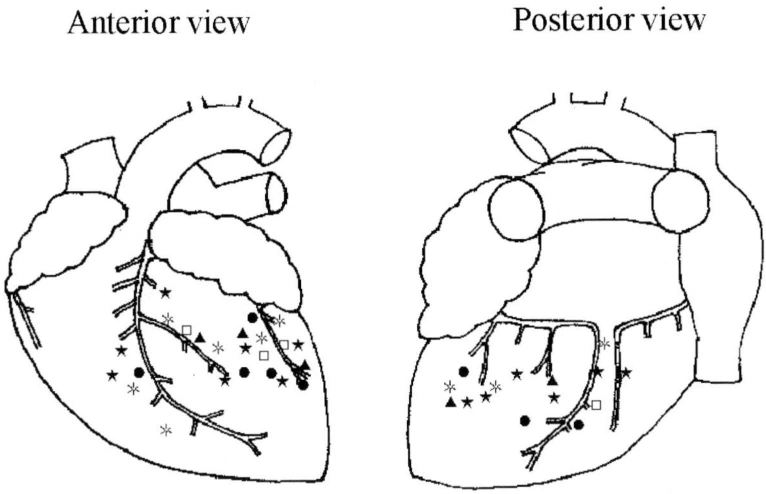

Fig. 3 Location of epicardial receptive fields of ischemically sensitive cardiac afferent nerve endings on the surface of left ventricle. *Symbols* indicate receptive fields of cardiac afferents ($n = 41$) (Fu and Longhurst 2002b)

bone marrow (Leanos et al. 1995). Taken together, these data suggest that activated platelets are capable of stimulating ischemically sensitive cardiac sympathetic afferents.

To further evaluate the role of activated platelets in stimulating cardiac spinal afferents during myocardial ischemia, we employed an inhibitor of platelet glycoprotein IIb-IIIa receptors. Platelet glycoprotein IIb-IIIa receptors located on plasma membranes of platelets are the final common pathway leading to platelet activation. The glycoprotein IIb-IIIa receptor, or αIIbβ3 (integrin nomenclature), is expressed only in megakaryocytes and platelets and thus is uniquely adapted to its role in platelet physiological function. The density of glycoprotein IIb-IIIa receptors on the surface of platelets is extraordinary (approximately 80,000 copies per platelet) and there is an additional internal pool of glycoprotein IIb-IIIa receptors in α-granules. Vessel damage, adhesion, and shear forces initiate signals that transform glycoprotein IIb-IIIa receptor into a high-affinity state that binds plasma-borne adhesive proteins such as fibrinogen and von Willebrand factor. This binding reaction leads to platelet aggregation irrespective of any of the agonists that stimulate platelets or of the stimulus-response-coupling pathway (Lefkovits et al. 1995; Coller 1997).

Highly specific competitive inhibitors of platelet glycoprotein IIb-IIIa receptors, including abciximab, eptifibatide, tirofiban, lamifibn, and fradafiban, are available. These inhibitors combine with the resting and active forms of platelet glycoprotein IIb-IIIa receptors and therefore bind to nonstimulated and stimulated platelets to completely inhibit platelet activation during stimulation by any of a number of platelet activators, including ADP, thrombin, collagen, and thromboxane A_2 (TxA_2), as shown in several animal models (Lefkovits et al. 1995; Coller 1997; Hiramatsu et al.

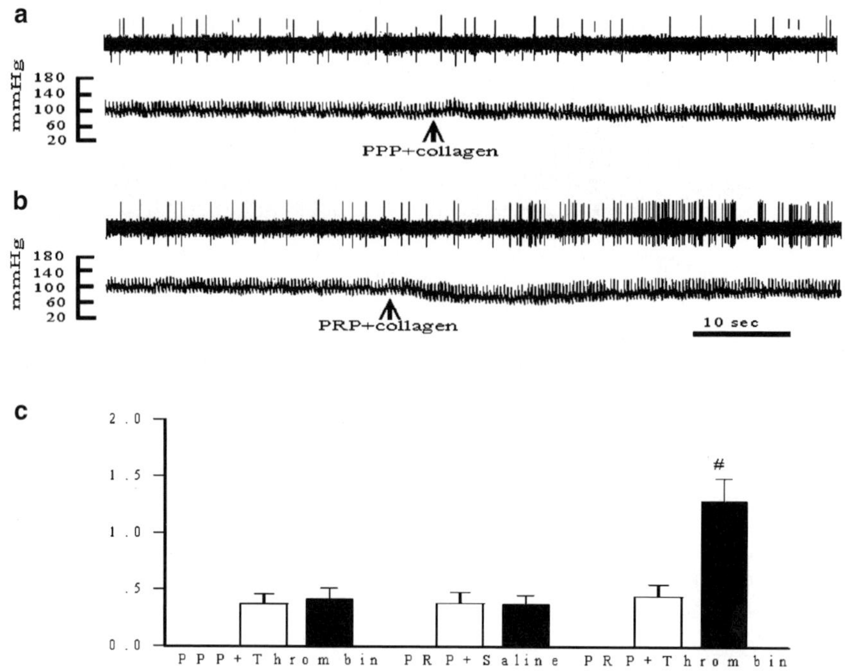

Fig. 4 Neurograms showing discharge frequencies of an ischemically sensitive cardiac spinal afferent during myocardial ischemia that increased the baseline activity of the afferent from 0.38 to 2.21 imp s^{-1}. (**a, b**) Responses of this afferent to application of platelet-poor plasma (PPP) plus collagen (**a**) or platelet-rich plasma (PRP) plus collagen (**b**) injected into the left atrium. (**c**) Peak impulse activity of cardiac spinal afferents before (*open bar*) and after (*closed bar*) application of PPP plus collagen, PRP plus saline, and PRP plus collagen ($n = 12$). *Bars* represent means ± SEM. $^{\#}p < 0.05$ versus the control (Fu and Longhurst 2002b)

1997). Clinical trials of glycoprotein IIb-IIIa antagonists have shown a high degree of inhibition of platelets leading to a significant reduction in the number of ischemic events in patients with myocardial infarction and unstable angina (Hiramatsu et al. 1997; Phillips and Scarborough 1997; Lincoff et al. 2000). We employed tirofiban to prevent ischemia-induced platelet activation while recording single-unit sensory nerve activity in the sympathetic chain or rami communicates of cats. Blockade of platelet glycoprotein IIb-IIIa receptors with tirofiban attenuated the response of cardiac afferents to brief myocardial ischemia, confirming that platelet glycoprotein IIb-IIIa receptors and activated platelets play an important role in ischemia-mediated excitation of cardiac sympathetic afferents during ischemia (Fig. 5).

3.4 5-Hydroxytryptamine and 5-HT$_3$ Receptors

5-HT is an important biogenic amine that functions as an excitatory neurotransmitter and as a neuromodulator. Its role in inflammation and nociception has been the

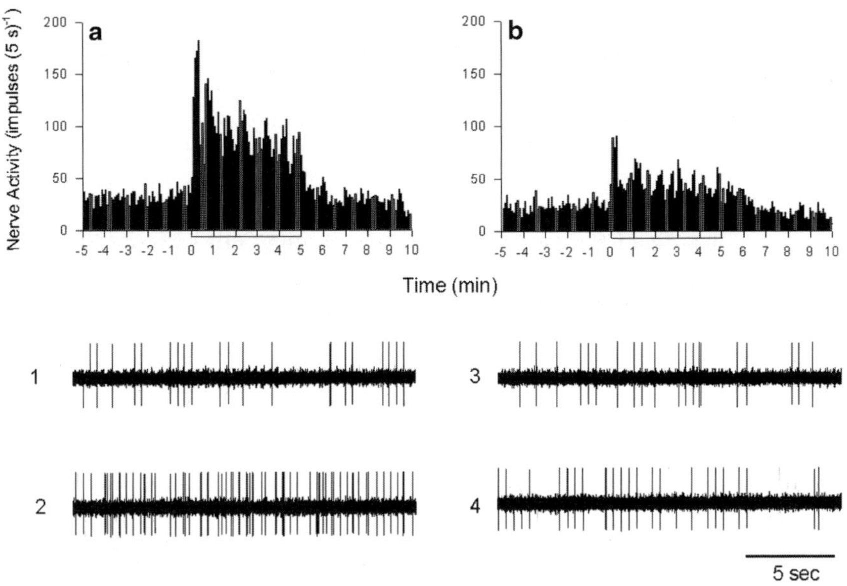

Fig. 5 Histograms displaying summed 5-s nerve activity of seven cardiac afferents during myocardial ischemia before (**a**) and after (**b**) administration of tirofiban. Neurograms *1–4* are representative tracings of a C-fiber cardiac afferent activity during preischemia (*1* and *3*) and ischemia (*2* and *4*) in the absence (*1* and *2*) and presence (*3* and *4*) of tirofiban, a platelet glycoprotein IIb-IIIa inhibitor. These data indicate that tirofiban attenuated the response of cardiac afferents to myocardial ischemia (Fu and Longhurst 2002a)

focus of much interest (Dray 1995; Richardson 1990). Numerous studies have demonstrated that 5-HT stimulates or sensitizes somatic sensory nerves and gastrointestinal afferents involved in hyperalgesia (Sommer 2004), visceral pain, as well as irritable bowel syndrome (Holzer 2001). Our group and others have shown that 5-HT stimulates visceral sympathetic afferents (Fu and Longhurst 1998; Nishi et al. 1977). The cellular sources of 5-HT with respect to peripheral nerve stimulation mainly include platelets and mast cells (Anden and Olsson 1967; Lehtosalo et al. 1984). As much as 0.9 μmol of 5-HT can be released from 100 million human platelets (Meyers et al. 1982). Platelet activators such as collagen induce the release of 5-HT from rabbit platelets in vitro (Packham et al. 1977; Fujimori et al. 1982; Packham et al. 1991), while thrombin stimulates the release of 5-HT from humans and rat platelets (Belville et al. 1979; Verhoeven et al. 1984). Both thrombin and collagen also activate feline platelets to release 5-HT (Fu and Longhurst 2002a, b). Because our previous investigations have documented that application of a suspension of activated platelets can stimulate cardiac spinal afferents (Fu and Longhurst 2002b), it is likely that 5-HT plays an important role in the stimulation of cardiac spinal sympathetic afferents by activated platelets. In this regard, we have evaluated the response of ischemically sensitive cardiac sympathetic afferents to platelets activated with collagen or thrombin before and after administration of tropisetron.

Blockade of 5-HT_3 receptors, in fact, abolishes the responses of these cardiac afferents to exogenously activated platelets (Fig. 6). Thus, through a 5-HT_3 mechanism, activated platelets stimulate cardiac sympathetic afferents that specifically respond to myocardial ischemia.

In addition to in vitro activation of platelets, myocardial ischemia likely stimulates the endogenous release of 5-HT, which then is available to stimulate cardiac sympathetic afferents. In support of this hypothesis is the observation that coronary sinus 5-HT in patients with coronary disease is significantly elevated compared with that in patients without coronary disease (Van den Berg et al. 1989). Furthermore, brief coronary occlusion during angioplasty increases 5-HT in coronary sinus blood of patients who have experienced angina (Golino et al. 1994). In addition, the

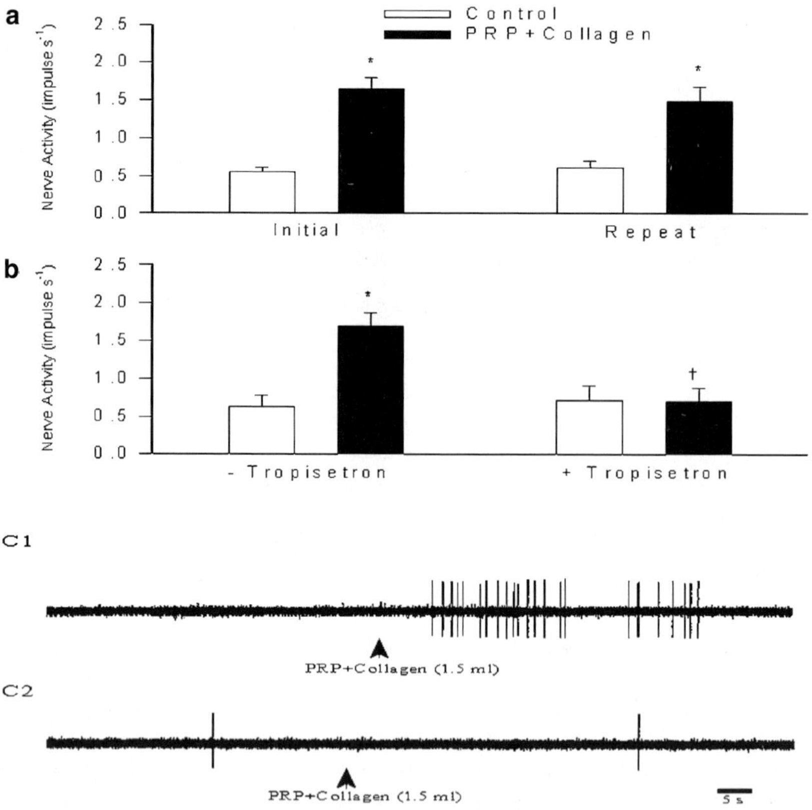

Fig. 6 (**a**) Discharge activity of nine cardiac afferents before (*open bar*) and after (*filled bar*) application of PRP plus collagen. (**b**) Effect of PRP plus collagen on the mean activity of eight separate cardiac afferents before and after 5-HT_3 blockade with tropisetron. (**c**) Neurograms showing responses of an ischemically sensitive cardiac C-fiber afferent to PRP plus collagen (1.5 ml, left atrium) before (*c1*) and after (*c2*) administration of tropisetron. This cardiac afferent innervated the posterior wall of the left ventricle. Data are presented as the mean ± SEM. $^{*}p < 0.05$ compared with the control. $^{\dagger}p < 0.05$ versus before tropisetron administration (Fu and Longhurst 2002a)

concentration of 5-HT is increased at the site of coronary arterial stenosis and in coronary sinus blood during thrombosis-induced coronary artery occlusion (Ashton et al. 1986; Benedict et al. 1986). We likewise have observed an increase in the concentration of 5-HT in cardiac venous plasma during brief myocardial ischemia and in the immediate reperfusion period in cats and that these increases can be reduced by blockade of the glycoprotein IIb-IIIa receptors with tirofiban.

Exogenous 5-HT excites cardiac sympathetic Aδ afferents (Nishi et al. 1977) and evokes hypertension in anesthetized dogs (Zucker and Cornish 1980). We have observed that 5-HT stimulates ischemically sensitive abdominal sympathetic afferents (Fu and Longhurst 1998). Although there are at least seven types of 5-HT receptors that have been described, pharmacological data indicate that at least five types, including 5-HT_1, 5-HT_2, 5-HT_3, 5-HT_4, and 5-HT_7 receptors, exist in the brain, spinal cord, and cells of the peripheral nervous system (Hoyer et al. 1994; Nandam et al. 2007; Jordan 2005). These receptors are coupled to a ligand-gated ion channel, intracellular adenyl cyclase, or phospholipase C (PLC) and inositol triphosphate (Hoyer et al. 1994). Four types of 5-HT receptors appear to be involved in activation of the sensory nervous system. Early studies demonstrated that 5-HT produces hyperalgesia through direct stimulation of 5-HT_{1A} receptors on the primary afferent nerves (Taiwo and Levine 1992). Likewise, activation of 5-HT_2 receptors potentiates pain produced by inflammatory mediators (Abbott et al. 1996) and increases transmission of nociception at the spinal level following stimulation of somatic C-fiber afferents (Peroutka 1994). Activation of 5-HT_4 receptors depolarizes the cervical vagus nerve (Rhodes et al. 1992). Furthermore, exogenous 5-HT stimulates vagal mucosal chemosensitive afferents through a 5-HT_3 receptor mechanism (Grundy et al. 1994). Activation of 5-HT_3 receptors in the heart and lungs also leads to a depressor reflex in conscious rabbits (Evans et al. 1990). Recordings of single-unit cardiac sympathetic afferents during ischemia, as well as during exogenous administration of 5-HT, specific 5-HT receptor agonists, and antagonists have demonstrated that 5-HT stimulates ischemically sensitive afferent endings but not those that are insensitive to ischemia (Fu and Longhurst 2002a). This relative specificity of 5-HT for a specific population of cardiac afferents is different from the activity of bradykinin, which, as noted earlier, has been found to broadly stimulate both ischemically sensitive and ischemically insensitive cardiac sympathetic afferents (Tjen-A-Looi et al. 1998; Baker et al. 1980). Similarly phenylbiguanide, a selective 5-HT_3 receptor agonist, activates most (83%) ischemically sensitive cardiac afferents, α-methyl-5-HT, a selective 5-HT_2 receptor agonist, stimulates a minority (33%) of the afferents tested, but selective 5-HT_1 and 5-HT_4 receptors agonists do not alter the activity of any afferents (Fig. 7). In concert with the agonist data, blockade of 5-HT_3 receptors with tropisetron completely abolishes the response of these afferents to exogenous 5-HT (data not shown in Fig. 8) and attenuates their responses to myocardial ischemia, providing further confirmation that endogenous 5-HT stimulates cardiac sympathetic afferents through a 5-HT_3 receptor mechanism (Fig. 8).

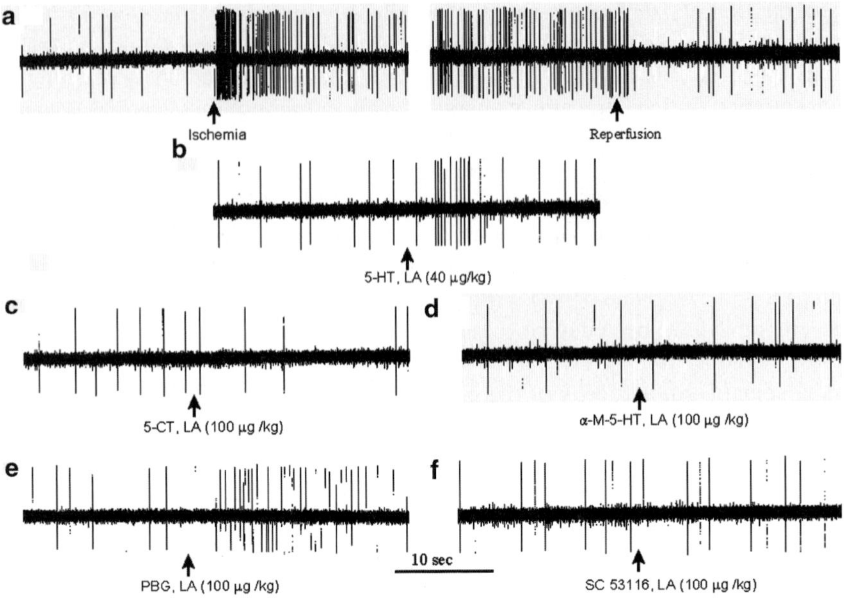

Fig. 7 Responses of cardiac sympathetic afferent to myocardial ischemia and to stimulation with 5-hydroxytryptamine (5-HT) and specific 5-HT receptor agonists. (**a**) Discharge activity of this afferent during myocardial ischemia, which increased nerve activity from 0.67 to 2.73 imp s^{-1}. (**b–f**) Responses of this afferent during injection of 5-HT (**b**), 5-CT (**c**), α-methyl-5-HT (**d**), phenylbiguanide (**e**) or SC 53116 (**f**) into the left atrium. This C-fiber afferent (CV = 0.53 ms^{-1}) innervated the posterior wall of the left ventricle (Fu and Longhurst 2002a)

3.5 Histamine and H_1 Receptors

Histamine has been considered to be a chemical stimulus of cardiac sympathetic afferent endings during ischemia for over a decade (Meller and Gebhart 1992). Myocardial ischemia activates platelets and degranulates mast cells, leading to an increase in histamine concentration in the coronary circulation and myocardial tissue. In this regard, clinical studies have documented increased histamine in patients with ischemic heart disease (Kounis and Zavras 1991). Coronary histamine is elevated shortly before spasm occurs in patients with variant angina (Sakata et al. 1996). Experimental studies likewise have documented that myocardial ischemia promotes the production and release of histamine in coronary sinus plasma (Flores and Sheridan 1994; Wolff and Levi 1988). As noted above, coronary histamine originates from cardiac mast cells (Frangogiannis et al. 1998) and activated platelets (Masini et al. 1998; Nakahodo et al. 1994). Most cardiac mast cells are located in the outer layer of the adventitia of coronary arteries (Stary 1990). Mast cell degranulation occurs following plaque rupture and in spastic atherosclerotic coronary segments (Laine et al. 1999). Myocardial ischemia and reperfusion or hypoxia

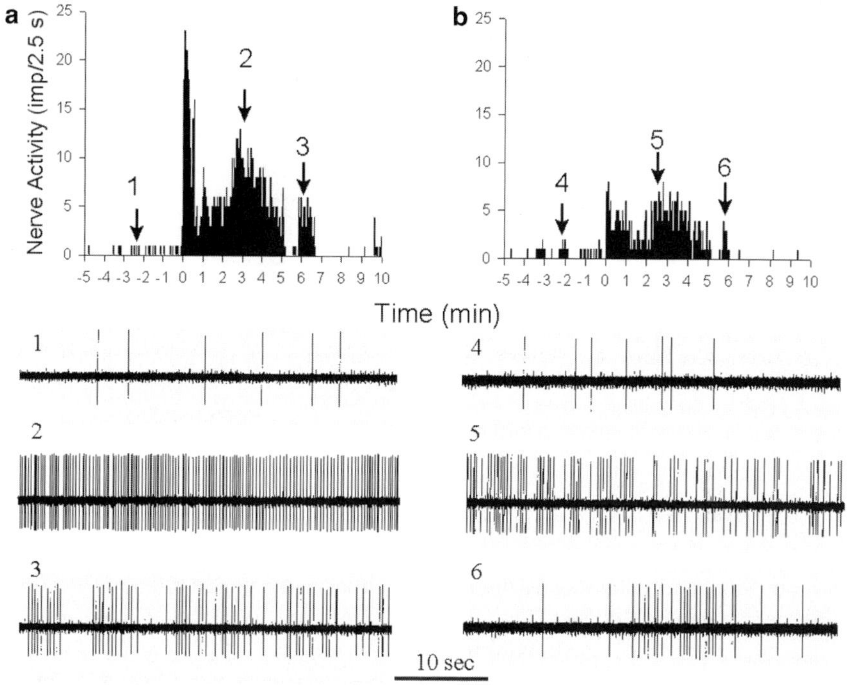

Fig. 8 Histograms displaying discharge frequency of a cardiac C-fiber afferent during myocardial ischemia before (**a**) and after (**b**) treatment with tropisetron. Neurograms *1–6* are representative tracings of the afferent at times indicated by *arrows* above the histogram. These data shows that 5 min of ischemia increased afferent activity from 0.09 to 2.90 imp s^{-1}; while blockade of 5-HT_3 with tropisetron attenuated the increase in the discharge activity of this afferent (0.12–1.40 imp s^{-1}) during repeated ischemia. This cardiac afferent innervated the anterior wall of the left ventricle (Fu and Longhurst 2002a)

also degranulates cardiac mast cells, leading to the release of histamine (Frangogiannis et al. 1998; Laine et al. 1999; Masini et al. 1987). Adventitial mast cells are closely associated with sensory nerve fibers in atherosclerotic coronary arteries (Laine et al. 2000). Thrombin and collagen as well as myocardial ischemia and hypoxia activate platelets to release histamine (Fu and Longhurst 2002b; Flores and Sheridan 1994; Nakahodo et al. 1994; Masini et al. 1998; Saxena et al. 1989).

Histamine stimulates visceral and somatic afferent nerve endings (Fu et al. 1997; Herbert et al. 2001). In this regard, application of histamine to an isolated rat-skin-nerve preparation increases discharge activity of polymodal C-fibers (Koppert et al. 2001). Histamine also stimulates group III and group IV articular afferents innervating the knee joint of cats (Herbert et al. 2001) as well as ischemically sensitive abdominal sympathetic afferents (Fu et al. 1997). Also, chest pain in patients with variant angina is triggered by coronary spasm provoked by histamine (Kounis and Zavras 1991; Ginsburg et al. 1981). In a recent single-unit cardiac

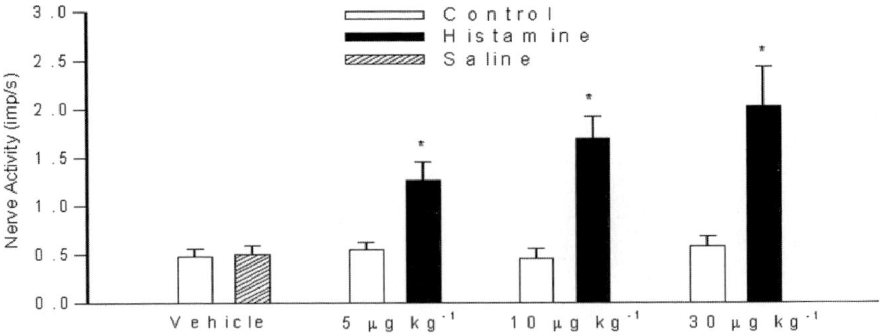

Fig. 9 Bar graphs displaying responses of seven ischemically sensitive cardiac afferents after injection of various doses of histamine, ranging from 5 to 30 μg kg^{-1}, or the vehicle control (saline) into the left atrium. *Columns* and *error bars* represent means ± SEM, respectively. $^*p < 0.05$ compared with the control (Fu et al. 2005)

spinal afferent recording study, we found that histamine stimulates both ischemically sensitive and ischemically insensitive cardiac sympathetic afferents in a dose-dependent manner (Fig. 9). Thus, like bradykinin, but unlike 5-HT and protons, histamine is a nonspecific stimulus of afferent endings.

The physiological action of histamine is mediated by several histamine receptors. Four distinct histamine receptor subtypes – H_1, H_2, H_3, and H_4 receptors – have been identified (Hill et al. 1997; Repka-Ramirez 2003). Three types have been implicated in the regulation of neural function. For example, stimulation of H_3 receptors inhibits the release of neuropeptides, including tachykinins and calcitonin gene-related peptide, from sensory C-fibers innervating the heart and airways (Imamura et al. 1996; Ichinose and Barnes 1990). Sympathetic nerve endings in the heart contain H_3 receptors that are capable of modulating adrenergic responses by inhibiting the release of norepinephrine (Imamura et al. 1995). H_2 receptors mediate histamine-induced postsynaptic excitation of submucosal plexus neurons in guinea pigs (Tokimasa and Akasu 1989). H_1 receptor messenger RNA is expressed in unmyelinated sensory neurons of guinea pigs (Kashiba et al. 1999) and H_1 receptors have been identified in sensory neurons located in the dorsal root ganglia (DRG) (Ninkovic and Hunt 1985). Furthermore, neurophysiological studies have shown that application of histamine depolarizes primary afferent fibers in mammals through an H_1 receptor mechanism (Koda et al. 1996).

Stimulation of H_1 receptors by histamine activates abdominal sympathetic afferents during ischemia (Fu et al. 1997) and evokes cardiovascular excitatory reflex responses (Stebbins et al. 1991). Recently, we observed that ischemically sensitive cardiac spinal afferents respond to 2-(3-chlorophenyl)histamine, a selective H_1 receptor agonist, but not to selective H_2 or H_3 receptor agonists. Blockade of H_1 receptors with pyrilamine, a selective H_1 receptor antagonist, eliminates cardiac afferent responses to histamine and significantly reduces the responses of afferents to myocardial ischemia, suggesting that histamine through an H_1 receptor mechanism, but not an H_2 or an H_3 receptor mechanism, participates in activation of cardiac spinal afferents during ischemia.

The PLC and protein kinase C (PKC) intracellular pathways play a pivotal role in signaling of sensory neurons in mammals (Bevan 1996). In fact, PKC underlies both activation and sensitization of sensory neurons in mammals (Bevan 1996; Guo et al. 1998). For example, we have shown that PKC contributes to ischemia-mediated activation of abdominal visceral afferents (Bevan 1996; Guo et al. 1998). Inhibition of PKC with the partial peptide antagonist PKC-(19-36) decreases C-fiber hyperexcitability and hyperalgesia in diabetic rats (Ahlgren and Levine 1994). More specifically, histamine may stimulate ischemically sensitive cardiac sympathetic afferents through a PLC–PKC mechanism. In this regard, histamine activates H_1 receptors through a PLC mechanism (Nicolson et al. 2002). We also have observed that single-unit cardiac sympathetic afferent responses to histamine are significantly (63%) attenuated by PKC-(19-36), indicating that the PLC–PKC pathway is involved in histamine-mediated activation of ischemically sensitive cardiac afferents (Fig. 10).

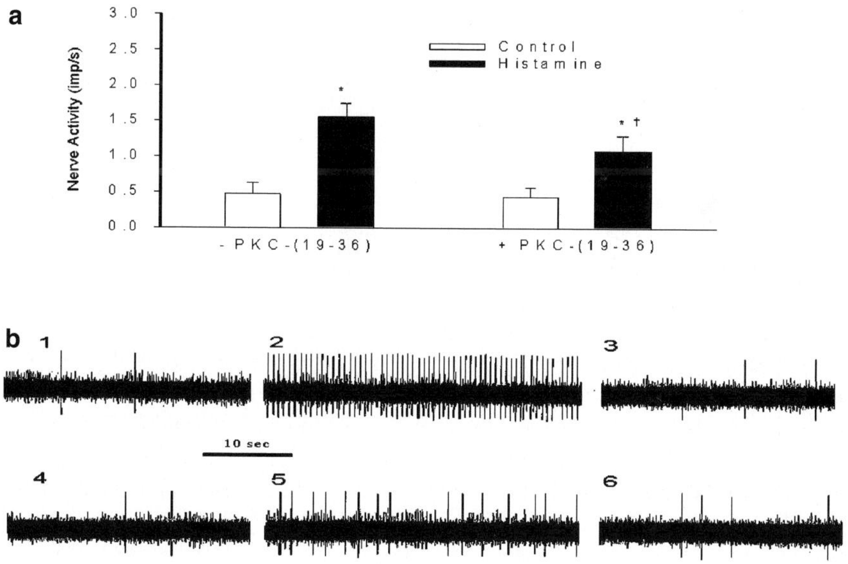

Fig. 10 (**a**) Bar graphs showing discharge activity of eight ischemically sensitive cardiac afferents before and after treatment with PKC-(19-36), a selective protein kinase C inhibitor. (**b**) Neurograms illustrating the response of an ischemically sensitive cardiac afferent to injection of histamine (10 μg kg^{-1}) into the left atrium before (*b1–b3*) and after (*b4–b6*) administration of 30 μg kg^{-1} of PKC-(19-36). Neurograms *b1–b6* display afferent activity before (*b1* and *b4*), during (*b2* and *b5*), and after (*b3* and *b6*) injection of histamine. This C-fiber afferent (CV = 2.32 ms^{-1}) innervated the posterior wall of the left ventricle. *Columns* and *error bars* represent means ± SEM, respectively. $*p < 0.05$ compared with the control, $^{\dagger}p < 0.05$ after PKC-(19-36) administration versus before PKC-(19-36) administration (Fu et al. 2005)

3.6 Thromboxane A_2 and Thromboxane A_2/Prostaglandin H_2 Receptors

TxA_2 is also released from activated platelets. This cyclooxygenase product is a potent vasoconstrictor (Furci et al. 1991) but also appears to have the potential to stimulate sensory endings during ischemic conditions. Previous studies have documented that TxA_2, which is formed from cyclic endoperoxides by the action of cyclooxygenase on arachidonic acid, is released from activated platelets during clinical conditions, including unstable angina and myocardial infarction as well as during provoked myocardial ischemia in experimental animals (Fitzgerald et al. 1986; Hirsh et al. 1981). For example, large increases in TxA_2 coincide with transient episodes of myocardial ischemia occurring in patients with unstable angina and during myocardial infarction (Fitzgerald et al. 1986). It has been demonstrated that TxA_2 is increased in coronary venous plasma during spontaneous and pacing-induced angina in patients with coronary artery disease (Mehta et al. 1984). Transcardiac TxA_2 is elevated during ischemia in animals with coronary artery stenosis (Lewy et al. 1980; Hirsh et al. 1981; Folts 1994; Folts et al. 1976). Furthermore, TxA_2 concentrations are increased in coronary venous plasma draining the ischemic region as early as 3 min after coronary artery branch occlusion (Parratt and Cokerm 1981).

Although previous studies have investigated extensively the role of TxA_2 in vascular smooth muscle constriction as well as platelet activation (Arita et al. 1989; Furci et al. 1991), the role of TxA_2 as a mediator of sensory neural activation has not been studied. Exogenous TxA_2 appears to be capable of stimulating hindlimb group III and group IV somatic afferent nerves (Kenagy et al. 1997). U46619, a stable TxA_2 receptor mimetic, inhibits the knee-jerk reflex through stimulation of vagal endings in the lung (Pickar 1998). U46619 additionally can evoke tachypnea and a depressor reflex response including bradycardia and hypotension through stimulation of the vagus nerve (Carrithers et al. 1994; Wacker et al. 2002) and can evoke vagally mediated rapid shallow breathing and airway hyperresponsiveness (Shams and Scheid 1990; Karla et al. 1992; Aizawa and Hirose 1988). Finally, epicardial application of exogenous TxA_2 is capable of stimulating cardiac vagal chemosensitive afferents in rats (Sun et al. 2001).

TxA_2 receptors or TxA_2/prostaglandin H_2 receptors (called “TP receptors”) are located on platelets and smooth muscle cells (Coleman et al. 1994). Recent investigations have suggested that TP receptors also exist on neurons and structural elements in the central and peripheral nervous systems. In this respect, immunohistochemical studies have revealed the presence of TP receptors on oligodendrocytes and astrocytes associated with myelinated fiber tracts, most notably in the striatum, spinal cord, and optic tract (Blackman et al. 1998; Borg et al. 1994). Stimulation of TxA_2 receptors in the brain stem of rats by intracerebroventricular injection of U46619 elevates arterial blood pressure (Gao et al. 1997), suggesting that TP receptors may be associated with neurons, although indirect effects stemming from activation of nearby cellular elements such as glia cannot be dismissed.

With respect to its peripheral neural elements, it was reported that TxA_2 receptors are located on Schwann cells in rat sciatic nerves (Muja et al. 2001). Furthermore, TP receptor messenger RNA has been detected in nodose ganglion neurons (Wacker et al. 2005) although the organ(s) innervated specifically by these neurons have not been identified. These studies led us to speculate that endogenous TxA_2 may stimulate cardiac spinal afferents during myocardial ischemia through a direct action on TP receptors located on cardiac sensory nerves.

To test this hypothesis, we recently recorded single-unit cardiac sympathetic afferent activity in cats during brief (5-min) myocardial ischemia and found that U46619 causes significant stimulation. In the same study, we administered BM13177, a selective TxA_2 receptor antagonist, which specifically blocks TxA_2 receptors but does not inhibit cyclooxygenase, prostacyclin, or thromboxane synthases (oude Egbrink et al. 1993; Stegmeier et al. 1984). BM13177 eliminated the excitatory response to U46619 and more importantly attenuated the responses of cardiac afferents to myocardial ischemia by 48% (Fig. 11) (Fu et al. 2008b). Theses data suggest that TxA_2 stimulates cardiac sympathetic afferents directly through activation of TP receptors located on afferent endings, an assumption

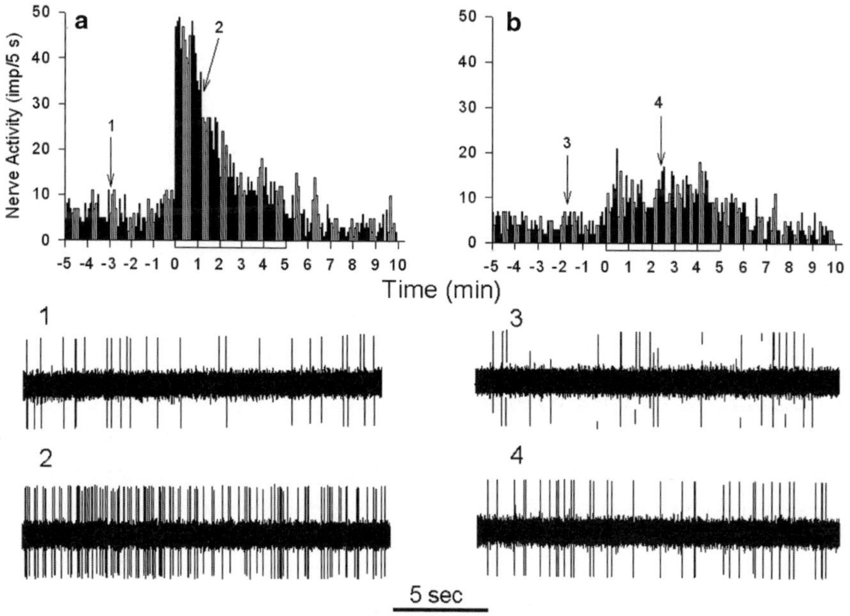

Fig. 11 Effect of thromboxane A_2 (TxA_2) receptor blockade with BM13177 (30 mg kg^{-1}, iv) on discharge activity of a C-fiber (CV = 0.33 ms^{-1}) cardiac sympathetic afferent during myocardial ischemia. (**a**) Initial brief (5 min) myocardial ischemia increased the baseline activity of this afferent from 1.23 to 4.47 imp s^{-1}. (**b**) Blockade of TxA_2 receptors with BM13177 attenuated the increase (0.99–2.31 imp s^{-1}) in activity of this afferent during repeated ischemia. Panels *1–4* are representative tracings showing the discharge activity of the afferent at times indicated by the *arrows* above the histograms (Fu et al. 2008b)

confirmed by immunohistochemical data showing that TP receptors are expressed in cardiac spinal afferent neurons in DRG. Data showing that vanilloid receptors are located on both DRG and cardiac spinal sensory nerve endings (Zahner et al. 2003) and on the nodose ganglia and vagal afferent nerve endings (Patterson et al. 2003) suggest that receptors found on neuronal cell bodies are also located on nerve endings. Thus, TxA_2, released from activated platelets, stimulates cardiac spinal sensory nerves and may contribute to reflex activation of the cardiovascular system during ischemia. The potential for TxA_2 to stimulate cardiac sympathoexcitatory reflexes has been demonstrated in preliminary studies of cats that develop a reflex pressor response during regional brief ischemia of the anterior cardiac wall (Fu et al. 2008a). Since BM13177 largely reverses this ischemic reflex, it seems very likely that TxA_2 participates in this cardiogenic response.

TxA_2 signals cellular events through a G protein coupled receptor, which, as noted above, is termed the "TP receptor." This receptor is coupled primarily to the Gq-dependent activation of PLC, which, in turn, produces phosphoinositide to mobilize intracellular Ca^{2+} and diacylglycerol, which activates PKC (Bevan 1996). Previous data have shown that PKC plays a pivotal role in processes underlying activation and sensitization of sensory neurons in mammals (Guo et al. 1998; Bevan 1996). For example, histamine and bradykinin activate sympathetic visceral afferents during ischemia, in part, through a PKC mechanism (Fu et al. 2005; Guo et al. 1998, 1999). TxA_2 also appears to alter neural transmission in the hippocampus through a PKC mechanism (Hsu and Han 1996). We therefore hypothesized that TxA_2 stimulates ischemically sensitive cardiac sympathetic afferents through an intracellular PKC signaling pathway. Treatment with PKC-(19-36) attenuated the responses of cardiac sympathetic afferents to U46619 by 38%. In sum, these data suggest strongly that endogenous TxA_2 directly stimulates cardiac spinal afferents through activation of TP receptors coupled to the PLC–PKC messaging system (Fu et al. 2008b).

3.7 *Reactive Oxygen Species*

Reactive oxygen species (ROS) are another source of chemical mediators that may activate cardiac sympathetic afferents during myocardial ischemia and reperfusion. Several of these species, including hydrogen peroxide, superoxide radicals, and hydroxyl radicals, increase in perfused rabbit hearts during myocardial ischemia and reperfusion (Grill et al. 1992). Furthermore, previous studies have demonstrated that ROS, produced during mesenteric ischemia, stimulate cardiac vagal afferents and abdominal visceral afferents to reflexly activate the cardiovascular system (Stahl et al. 1993; Ustinova and Schultz 1994); Application of H_2O_2 to the epicardial surface stimulates vagal afferents to produce reflex vasodepressor responses, while stimulation of sympathetic afferents causes sympathoexcitatory reflexes. A small dose-dependent increase in blood pressure occurs when both vagal and spinal pathways are intact (Fig. 12) (Huang et al. 1995b). Although hydroxyl

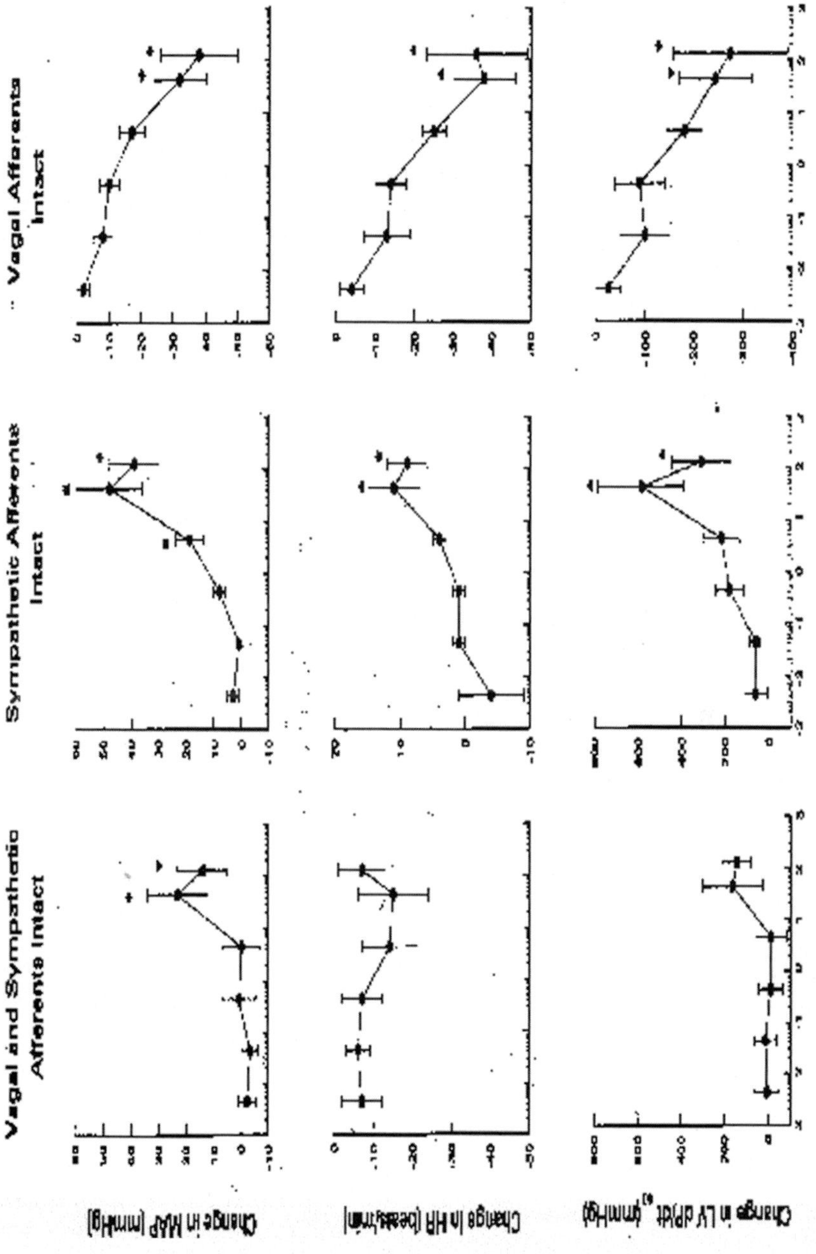
Vagal and Sympathetic Afferents Intact
Sympathetic Afferents Intact
Vagal Afferents Intact
Change in MAP (mmHg)
Change in HR (beats/min)
H_2O_2 (log µmol)
H_2O_2 (log µmol)
H_2O_2 (log µmol)

radicals are produced as early as 1 min during ischemia as well as during reperfusion (O'Neill et al. 1996), it is uncertain if ROS are produced in sufficient quantities to stimulate cardiac sympathetic afferent endings during ischemia and reperfusion.

Using single-unit recording techniques, we have found that epicardial application of H_2O_2 significantly stimulated cardiac sympathetic afferents. Dimethylthiourea, a nonspecific scavenger of ROS (Jackson et al. 1985), significantly attenuates the responses to H_2O_2 as well as the responses during ischemia and reperfusion (Fig. 13). In the presence of iron, $O_2^{\bullet-}$ and H_2O_2 form $^{\bullet}OH$ by the Haber–Weiss reaction (Grisham and Granger 1988). Deferoxamine, which chelates iron and thereby inhibits the Haber–Weiss reaction, inhibits $^{\bullet}OH$ generation (Halliwell 1989; Halliwell and Gutteridge 1990). Like dimethylthiourea, deferoxamine inhibits the

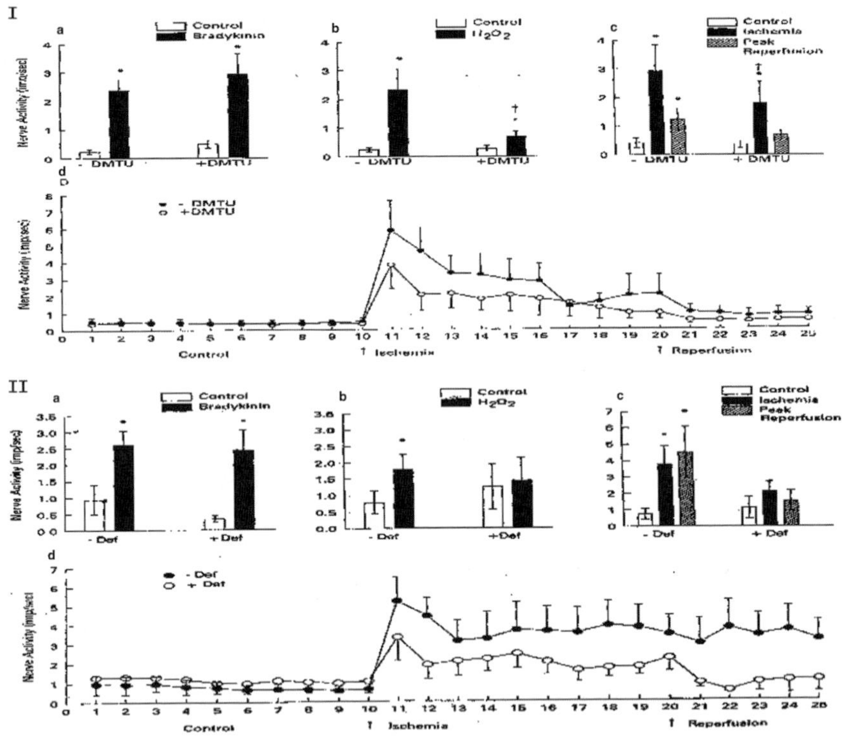

Fig. 13 *Top panels*: Bar graphs showing responses of ten cardiac afferents to topical application of bradykinin (**a**), H_2O_2 (**b**), and to myocardial ischemia/reperfusion (**c**) before (*–DMTU*) and after (*+DMTU*) treatment with dimethylthiourea. Discharge activity pattern of these cardiac afferents during control, ischemia, and reperfusion before and after dimethylthiourea treatment (*d*). *Bottom panels*: Bar graphs displaying nerve activity of seven cardiac afferents during topical application of bradykinin (**a**), H_2O_2 (**b**), and myocardial ischemia/reperfusion (**c**) before (*–Def*) and after (*+Def*) treatment with deferoxamine. Discharge pattern of these cardiac afferents during control, ischemia, and reperfusion before and after deferoxamine (**d**). *Circles* and *brackets* are means ± SEM. $*p < 0.05$ versus the control. $^{\dagger}p < 0.05$ versus before dimethylthiourea treatment (Huang et al. 1995a)

increased discharge activity of cardiac sympathetic afferents during ischemia and reperfusion (Fig. 13). In contrast, under an iron-loaded condition, deferoxamine does not alter the firing rate of these afferents during ischemia and reperfusion. These data thus suggest that $^{\bullet}OH$ contributes to activation of cardiac sympathetic afferents during ischemia and reperfusion (Huang et al. 1995a).

A second study has been conducted to identify the sources of ROS, including purine metabolites and polymorphonuclear leukocytes (PMNs) (Ferrari 1994). During ischemia, purine metabolites, hypoxanthine, and xanthine accumulate as a result of ATP breakdown (Jennings et al. 1981). In the presence of substrates such as hypoxanthine or xanthine, xanthine oxidase reduces molecular oxygen to $O_2^{\bullet-}$ and H_2O_2, which can react further to form the very reactive species •OH (Kuppusamy and Zweier 1989). Oxypurinol inhibits xanthine oxidase, decreases the synthesis of ROS such as $O_2^{\bullet-}$ and •OH during anoxia/reoxygenation (Zweier et al. 1994), and attenuates discharge activity of cardiac sympathetic afferents during ischemia and reperfusion by 44% (Fig. 14). Furthermore an anti-PMN polyclonal antibody decreased circulating PMNs by 94% and attenuated the firing rate of the cardiac afferents during myocardial ischemia and reperfusion by 66%. Thus, both purine metabolites and PMNs contribute to the production of ROS that stimulate cardiac sympathetic afferents during myocardial ischemia and reperfusion (Tjen-A-Looi et al. 2002).

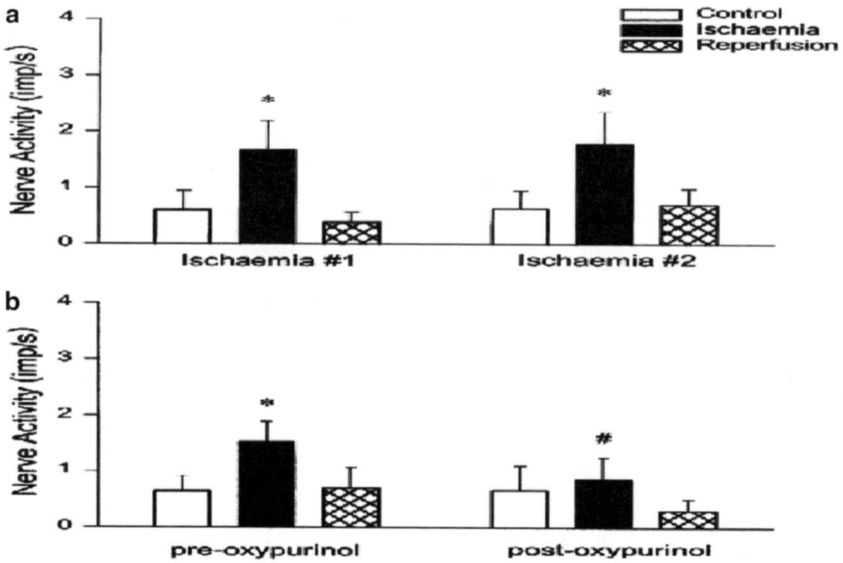

Fig. 14 **(a)** Histogram displaying group data of eight cardiac afferents yielding consistent responses during repeated ischemia. **(b)** Group data of nine cardiac afferents responsive to ischemia before and after administration of oxypurinol (10 mg kg^{-1}). *$p < 0.05$ versus the control. $^{\#}p < 0.05$ versus before oxypurinol administration (Tjen-A-Looi et al. 2002)

3.8 Adenosine

Adenosine is released from cells whenever there is decline in intracellular ATP. For instance, the concentration of adenosine increases in the ischemic region during brief myocardial ischemia (Delyani and Van Wylen 1994). Clinical studies have shown that intracoronary and intravenous adenosine cause angina-like pain in humans, likely through activation of adenosine A_1 receptors, whereas aminophylline, a nonselective adenosine receptor antagonist, attenuates the severity of chest pain induced by adenosine (Sylven et al. 1986; Crea et al. 1990, 1992). Some investigators therefore believe that adenosine is an important chemical mediator that activates cardiac sympathetic afferents during ischemia.

However, there is conflicting literature regarding the role of adenosine in stimulation of cardiac spinal afferents. On one hand, previous studies of cardiac-cardiovascular reflexes as well as direct recordings of cardiac afferents' activities suggested that adenosine might stimulate cardiac sympathetic afferents (Dibner-Dunlap et al. 1993; Cox et al. 1989). For example, intracoronary injection of adenosine or N^6-cyclopentyladenosine, an adenosine A_1 receptor agonist, reflexly increases renal sympathetic efferent activity (Dibner-Dunlap et al. 1993; Cox et al. 1989). Also, adenosine stimulates cardiac sympathetic afferents through activation of A_1 and A_2 receptors in dogs and cats (Gnecchi-Ruscone et al. 1995; Huang et al. 1995c). The issue with these studies is the failure to differentiate between the roles of endogenous and exogenous adenosine. In fact, a number of studies have demonstrated that endogenous adenosine does not play a role in activation of cardiac spinal afferents. For example, aminophylline, which blocks adenosine receptors, does not alter the response of cardiac sympathetic afferents to myocardial ischemia in cats, although exogenous adenosine is capable of stimulating these afferents (Gnecchi-Ruscone et al. 1995). Still, other investigators have observed that application of adenosine to epicardium does not evoke reflex responses, including changes in renal efferent nerve activity (Pagani et al. 1985). Likewise, we have found that even very high concentrations of adenosine and N^6-cyclopentyladenosine fail to stimulate ischemically sensitive cardiac afferent nerve endings in cats, the group of afferents that initiate excitatory cardiovascular reflexes from the heart during ischemia (Pan and Longhurst 1995). Moreover, blocking adenosine receptors with aminophylline does not attenuate the response of these C-fiber nerve endings to ischemia (Fig. 15). Similarly, others have observed that adenosine is unable to stimulate ischemically sensitive cardiac sympathetic afferents in cats (Abe et al. 1998). And, intracoronary adenosine fails to elicit cardiac pain in patients (Wilson et al. 1990). Taken together, studies evaluating the influence of adenosine on cardiac sympathetic afferent activity and symptomatic responses have led to mixed results. It is possible that differences in the dose of adenosine, exogenous application versus endogenous release, experimental species, and subgroups of afferent fibers have contributed to different results and conclusions. One firm conclusion, however, based on the data from our group as well as others (Abe et al. 1998) is that endogenous adenosine at least in some species does not appear to

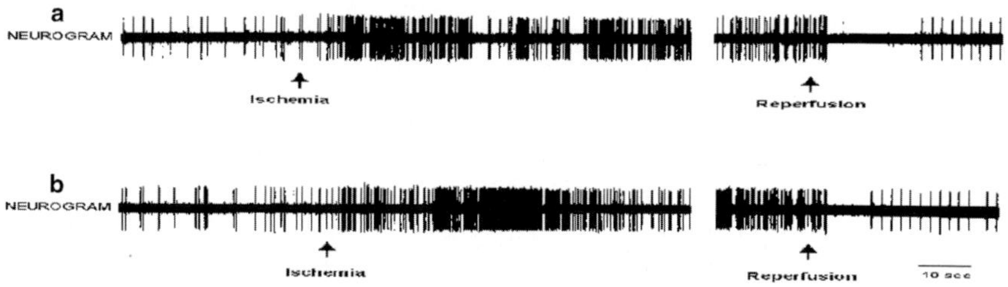

Fig. 15 Neurograms illustrating the response of a cardiac afferent to 5 min of myocardial ischemia and reperfusion before (**a**) and after (**b**) administration of aminophylline (5 mg kg^{-1} iv). This C-fiber (CV = 0.46 ms^{-1}) afferent innervated the posterior wall of the left ventricle (Pan and Longhurst 1995)

be an important contributor to the activation of cardiac sympathetic afferents during myocardial ischemia in cats.

4 Interactions Between Chemical Mediators

Myocardial ischemia leads to production and virtually simultaneous release of a number of chemical mediators that, as discussed earlier, stimulate and/or sensitize sensitive cardiac sympathetic afferents to ischemia. Inhibition of metabolite production or receptor blockade limits, but never fully prevents, activation of cardiac afferents during ischemia (Fu and Longhurst 2002a; Longhurst et al. 2001). We have concluded therefore that chemical stimulation of these endings during ischemia must be multifactorial, with individual mediators acting separately and in combination to contribute to afferent activation. Because many of the mediators are released virtually simultaneously within a relatively short period of time after the onset of ischemia and because our previous studies have shown that some, such as prostaglandins, sensitize abdominal visceral afferents to ischemia (Guo and Longhurst 2000), we have recently begun to explore interactions and their underlying mechanisms, particularly those associated with sensitization and desensitization, that might occur between various mediators that act individually on cardiac sympathetic afferent activity during ischemia.

4.1 *Prostaglandins and Bradykinin*

Prostaglandins are potent bioactive lipid messengers derived from the metabolism of arachidonic acid through the cyclooxygenase pathway. They were first extracted from semen, prostate, and seminal vesicles by Goldblatt and von Euler in the 1930s. It is well known that prostaglandins are hyperalgesic since they sensitize chemical receptors located on primary afferent nerve endings (Ferreira 1972). Sensitization refers to an increase in the magnitude of a response, sometimes accompanied by an increase in spontaneous activity and/or a decrease in response threshold (Gebhart 2000). Prostaglandin E_2 (PGE_2) and prostaglandin I_2 (PGI_2), for instance, produce hyperalgesia (Taiwo and Levine 1991). Prostaglandins also sensitize muscle mechanoreceptors to reflexly increase muscle sympathetic nerve activity in humans (Rotto et al. 1990; Middlekauff and Chiu 2004). Arachidonic acid metabolism is enhanced during myocardial ischemia and reperfusion (Hendrickson et al. 1997; Van der Vusse et al. 1997). Furthermore, the concentrations of plasma prostaglandins, including PGE_2, prostaglandin $F_{2\alpha}$, PGI_2, and TxA_2, are increased in patients with unstable angina as well as during acute myocardial infarction (Berger et al. 1977; Hirsh et al. 1981). Our data have shown that prostaglandins augment abdominal sympathetic afferent activity during ischemia and bradykinin stimulation (Longhurst and Dittman 1987; Longhurst et al. 1991; Pan et al. 1994; Guo and Longhurst 2000). Although exogenously administered cyclooxygenase products clearly sensitize cardiac afferents to the action of exogenous bradykinin, the role of endogenous prostaglandins in sensitizing or stimulating cardiac sympathetic afferents to chemical stimuli produced during myocardial ischemia has been unclear (Nerdrum et al. 1986). We therefore examined the interaction between prostaglandins and bradykinin in stimulation of cardiac sympathetic afferents during ischemia. Single-unit activity of cardiac sympathetic afferents was recorded during myocardial ischemia and bradykinin application before and after treatment with indomethacin. Cyclooxygenase blockade reduced cardiac sympathetic afferent responses to ischemia by almost 60%, while in a control group the afferents consistently responded to repeat ischemia after treatment with vehicle (8.4% $NaHCO_3$) (Fig. 16). Indomethacin also significantly attenuated the cardiac afferent responses to bradykinin stimulation. Thus, endogenous prostaglandins sensitize cardiac sympathetic afferents to the action of bradykinin and perhaps other metabolites produced during myocardial ischemia (Tjen-A-Looi et al. 1998).

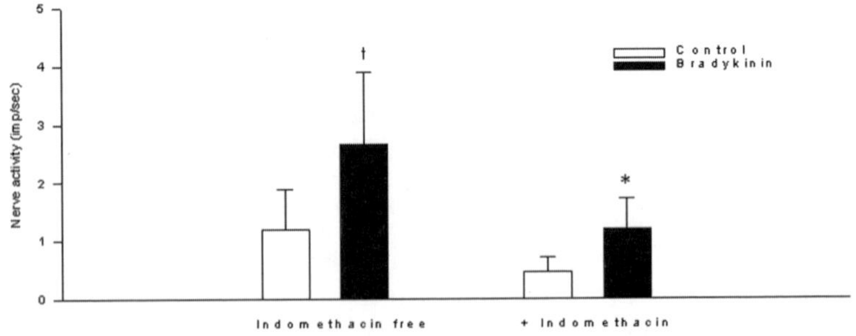

Fig. 16 Bar graphs showing that indomethacin reduces responses of six ischemically sensitive sympathetic cardiac afferents to bradykinin stimulation. Bradykinin (*closed bar*) increases afferent responses from the spontaneous baseline (control, *open bar*) level of afferent activity. *Columns* and *error bars* are means ± SEM. $^{\dagger}p < 0.05$ versus the control, $^{*}p < 0.05$ versus before indomethacin administration (Tjen-A-Looi et al. 1998)

4.2 Bradykinin and Histamine

As noted in earlier sections of this review, both bradykinin and histamine individually stimulate cardiac sympathetic afferents during myocardial ischemia (Fu et al. 2005; Tjen-A-Looi et al. 1998). Previous studies of sensory nerve activity have suggested that bradykinin may interact with histamine to stimulate these endings during vascular occlusion. In this regard, brief myocardial ischemia leads to the simultaneous release of both bradykinin and histamine (Frangogiannis et al. 1998; Kimura et al. 1973; Kounis and Zavras 1991). Furthermore, in vitro studies of somatic and testicular sensory nerve fibers have shown that bradykinin sensitizes these fibers to thermal and mechanical stimulation, while histamine sensitizes testicular polymodal afferents to thermal and mechanical stimulation (Koda et al. 1996; Koda and Mizumura 2002). Thus, these two mediators may interact during ischemia to enhance the degree of activation of cardiac sympathetic afferent endings.

To test this hypothesis, we examined the possibility that bradykinin potentiates the response of cardiac spinal afferents to histamine since earlier studies had suggested that bradykinin can potentiate histamine-evoked reflex bronchospasm as well as the response of polymodal cutaneous afferents in vitro (Koppert et al. 2001; Mazzone and Canning 2002). Bradykinin also sensitizes rat cutaneous nociceptive sensory fibers to mechanical stimulation, leading to hyperalgesia for more than 20 min (Taiwo et al. 1987). Thus, we recorded the responses of ischemically sensitive cardiac sympathetic afferents to histamine before and after application of bradykinin. We found that bradykinin augmented the response of these afferents to histamine by almost 60% and that the duration of this enhancement was 7 min (Fig. 17). These data indicate that bradykinin indeed sensitizes cardiac spinal afferents to stimulation by histamine (Fu and Longhurst 2005).

We next explored the mechanism underlying the interaction between bradykinin and histamine on cardiac spinal afferents. We thought that the cyclooxygenase products might be involved since bradykinin stimulates visceral spinal afferents originating from the cardiac and abdominal visceral organs, in part through a cyclooxygenase mechanism (Tjen-A-Looi et al. 1998). Also, bradykinin sensitizes polymodal somatic C-fiber afferents to thermal stimulation through a prostaglandin mechanism (Petho et al. 2001). We measured the influence of bradykinin on the responses of cardiac sympathetic afferents to histamine before and after administration of indomethacin, which fully eliminated the bradykinin-related facilitation of histamine's action on cardiac spinal afferents. Thus, bradykinin sensitizes ischemically sensitive afferent responses to histamine though a cyclooxygenase mechanism (Fig. 18).

Lastly, we explored the possibility that histamine potentiates the cardiac afferent response to bradykinin, since in vitro studies have shown that histamine sensitizes testicular polymodal afferents to thermal and mechanical stimulation (Koda et al. 1996; Koda and Mizumura 2002) and in high (pharmacological) concentrations (100 M) facilitates the response of visceral afferents to bradykinin stimulation

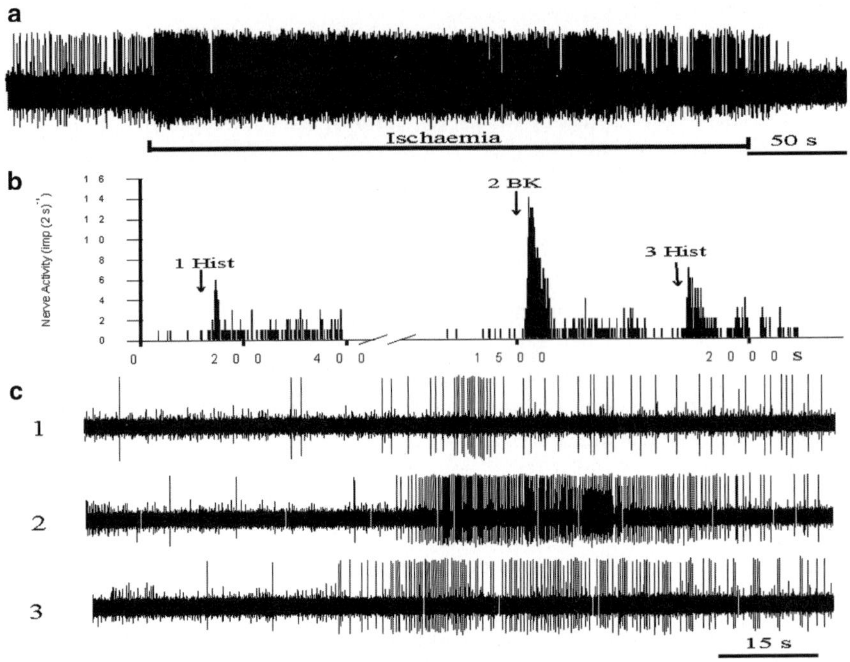

Fig. 17 **(a)** Discharge activity of cardiac C-fiber (CV = 0.66 ms^{-1}) spinal afferent during myocardial ischemia, application of histamine and bradykinin. Ischemia increased the afferent activity from 0.85 to 2.91 imp s^{-1} during brief (5-min) myocardial ischemia. **(b)** Neurohistogram showing responses of the afferent to histamine (*Hist*) before (*1*) and 4 min after (*3*) bradykinin (*BK*, *2*) application . Panels *c1–c3* contain representative tracings of the discharge activity of cardiac afferent at times indicated by the *arrows* above the histograms. This afferent innervated the posterior wall of the left ventricle (Fu and Longhurst 2005)

(Brunsden and Grundy 1999; Mizumura et al. 1995). We recorded the response of cardiac afferents to bradykinin stimulation before and after application of histamine. However, in contrast to our working hypothesis, we actually found that histamine reduced the responses of most cardiac spinal afferents to the action of bradykinin (Fig. 19). This finding is supported by other investigators who have observed that histamine is capable of suppressing responses of testicular polymodal afferents and abdominal visceral afferents to bradykinin stimulation (Mizumura et al. 1995; Stebbins et al. 1992).

Of particular interest was our finding that the result of bradykinin sensitization of the histamine response and the desensitization of the bradykinin response by histamine was a net additive response when afferent endings were simultaneously exposed to both mediators (Fig. 19). This situation is most relevant to the intact condition during myocardial ischemia, since bradykinin and histamine are released within the same time period during ischemia (Frangogiannis et al. 1998; Kimura

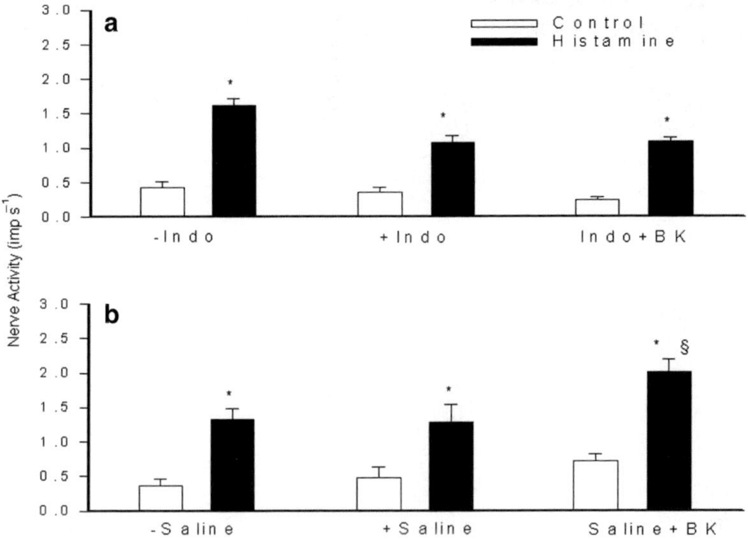

Fig. 18 **(a)** Bar graphs summarizing the effect of indomethacin (*Indo*) on histamine response in ten ischemically sensitive cardiac spinal afferents before and 4 min after administration of bradykinin. Indomethacin attenuated bradykinin-induced sensitization of this group of afferents to histamine. **(b)** Responses of five cardiac afferents to repeated application of histamine before and after application of bradykinin in the absence of indomethacin. *Columns* and *error bars* represent means ± S.E.M. $^{*}p < 0.05$ compared with the control, $^{\#}p < 0.05$ versus the first application of histamine. $^{\S}p < 0.05$ versus the second application of histamine (Fu and Longhurst 2005)

et al. 1973; Kounis and Zavras 1991). The combined action of the two mediators reflects the individual influences of histamine and bradykinin on each other (Fig. 20). Taken together, we believe that bradykinin sensitizes ischemically sensitive cardiac spinal afferents to histamine in a time-dependent fashion and that such sensitization requires an intact cyclooxygenase pathway. In contrast, histamine reduces the response of most cardiac afferents to bradykinin. However, when cardiac spinal afferents are exposed to bradykinin and histamine simultaneously, a condition that occurs normally during ischemia, the afferent response reflects summation of the individual responses to the two mediators (Fu and Longhurst 2005).

4.3 Thromboxane A_2 and Bradykinin

As noted in earlier sections of this review, TxA_2 and bradykinin contribute to activation of cardiac afferents during ischemia. Since both mediators are released virtually simultaneously during brief myocardial ischemia, there are several reasons why TxA_2 might interact reciprocally with bradykinin in stimulation of

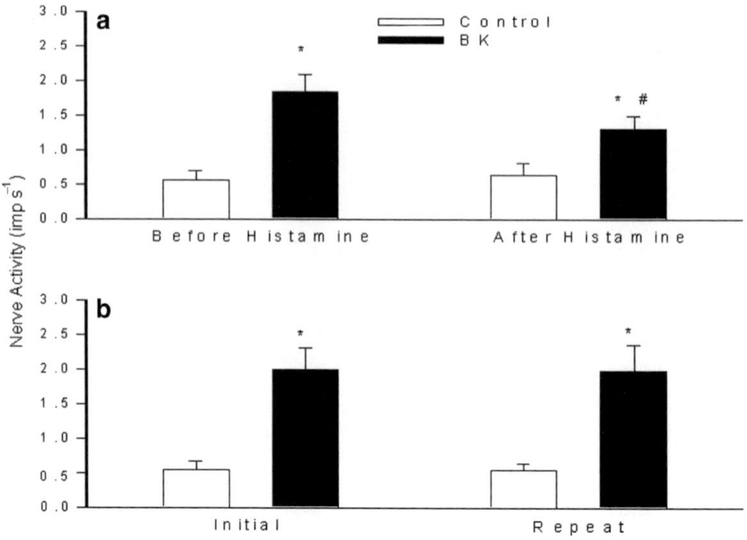

Fig. 19 **(a)** Histamine reduces the response of seven cardiac spinal afferents to bradykinin (1 μg, left atrium). **(b)** Bar graph showing responses of five other cardiac afferents to repeated application of bradykinin (1 μg, left atrium). *Columns* and *error bars* represents means ± SEM. $^*p < 0.05$ compared with the control. $^{\#}p < 0.05$ versus before histamine application (Fu and Longhurst 2005)

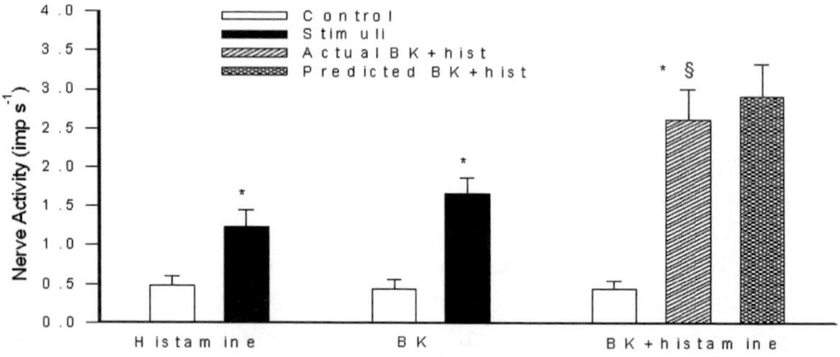

Fig. 20 Discharge activity of cardiac sympathetic afferents during injection of bradykinin (1 g, $n = 7$), histamine (10 g kg^{-1}, $n = 9$), and bradykinin (1 g) plus histamine (10 g kg^{-1}, $n = 16$) administered into the left atrium. *Columns* and *error bars* are means ± SEM. $^*p < 0.05$ compared with the control. $^{\S}p < 0.05$ compared with either bradykinin or histamine (Fu and Longhurst 2005)

ischemically sensitive cardiac afferents (Kimura et al. 1973; Parratt and Cokerm 1981). In this regard, bradykinin stimulates phospholipase A_2, which, in turn, generates arachidonic acid, the principal substrate for the cyclooxygenase pathway and TxA_2 formation (Rang et al. 1991). Once it has formed, TxA_2 diffuses out of the cell and through a TxA_2 receptor mechanism linked to the intracellular PKC pathway this cyclooxygenase product activates cardiac afferents (Fu et al. 2008b).

Thus, in addition to interactions with histamine and prostaglandins such as PGE_2 and PGE_1, bradykinin may initiate cyclooxygenase-mediated generation of TxA_2 (Nerdrum et al. 1986; Tjen-A-Looi et al. 1998; Fu and Longhurst 2005). The two chemical stimuli then would be available to activate cardiac sensory endings through subsequent activation of the individual receptors that both operate through the PKC messenger system.

In this regard, preliminary investigation has revealed that injection of TxA_2 into the left atrium 4 min after administration of bradykinin increases the cardiac afferent response to TxA_2 by 49% (Fu and Longhurst 2008). Additionally, administration of TxA_2 and bradykinin together causes a summated response that reflects simple addition of the individual responses. Lastly, blockade of TxA_2 receptors with BM13177 attenuates the cardiac afferent response to bradykinin by 47%. Thus, bradykinin and TxA_2 may reciprocally enhance the responses of ischemically sensitive cardiac afferent endings to the action of the other mediator.

5 Summary

Myocardial ischemia is a complex process. It is associated with a number of profound chemical and mechanical changes that have the potential to activate cardiac afferents. It is clear from our studies and those of others that there is not just one mechanism but that there are multiple mechanisms of activation of cardiac sensory nerve endings during and after myocardial ischemia. Typically, myocardial ischemia is associated with fissuring a rupture of an atherosclerotic plaque, discharge of the plaque into the vascular lumen, platelet activation, and formation of an occlusive thrombus with a rapid reduction of blood flow distal to the plaque. Sudden reduction in coronary blood flow causes a rapid shift to anaerobic glycolysis and the production of lactic acid, which releases protons and lowers the pH in the ischemic region. ATP breakdown leads to the production of adenosine. Phospholipids are released and arachidonic acid is produced, which through the cyclooxygenase pathway leads to the formation of a number of prostaglandin products such as PGE_2 and PGI_2. Platelet activation is associated with the release of histamine, 5-HT, and TxA_2 from platelet granules. Then, during the ischemia and, even more so, during reperfusion, ROS such as •OH are produced. Some chemical mediators such as bradykinin or TxA_2 are rapidly metabolized, while some such as protons are buffered and still others such as •OH are very reactive, and therefore are available to stimulate afferent endings for only a few minutes, seconds, or for even less than a second. Despite these relatively short half-lives, the sustained production of these mediators during ischemia can result in sufficiently high concentrations to allow interaction with specific receptors on afferent endings to depolarize the sensory axonal pathways. The receptors that underlie changes in the generator potential include BK_2 receptors for bradykinin, H_1 receptor for histamine, 5-HT_3 receptors for 5-HT, and the TP receptor for thromboxane. Some mediators, however, such as adenosine, do not seem to be produced in sufficient quantities to activate ischemically sensitive cardiac afferents. Current techniques for assessing concentrations do not have the resolution to accurately assess the time line of production. On the other hand, while it is clear that each of these chemical ligands exerts individual actions on the spinal afferent endings, it is also clear that many are produced early and nearly simultaneously. It comes as no surprise then that several of them interact to either increase or decrease the actions of other mediators. Prostaglandins, for example, sensitize endings to the action of kinins. Furthermore, bradykinin sensitizes afferent endings to the action of histamine through a mechanism involving the cyclooxygenase system. In contrast, however, histamine seems to reduce the action of bradykinin on cardiac sensory nerve endings. There is a net additive response when the ischemically sensitive endings are exposed simultaneously to both mediators, the most likely scenario to occur during myocardial ischemia. Recent preliminary findings suggest that bradykinin and TxA_2 also reciprocally interact and likely promote the action of the other mediator. It seems clear therefore that chemical stimulation of cardiac afferent nerve endings during myocardial ischemia is multifactorial and quite complex. Not only are a number of mediators produced during ischemia, each individually activating the endings, but they are produced very nearly simultaneously and interact to produce larger or smaller responses than would be expected from any single mediator. As we continue to examine these and still other mediators, such as endothelin, which work together to activate endings that ultimately subserve an important role in cardiac chest pain (angina) as well as with sympathoexcitatory reflex responses, we need to keep in mind that activation of the endings is simply the first step in the sensory reflex. Thus, the pattern of neural discharge and the central neural integration, likely involving a number of neurotransmitters, will be key components that we will need to study further to fully elucidate the mechanisms underlying cardiac reflex regulation of the cardiovascular system.

Acknowledgements This work was supported, in part, by National Heart, Lung, and Blood Institute grant HL-66217. J.C.L holds the Larry K. Dodge Chair in Integrative Biology and the Susan Samueli Chair in Integrative Medicine.

References

Abbott FV, Hong Y, Blier P (1996) Activation of 5-HT_{2A} receptors potentiates pain produced by inflammatory mediators. Neuropharmacology 35:99–110

Abe T, Morgan D, Sengupta JN, Gebhart GF, Gutterman DD (1998) Attenuation of ischemia-induced activation of cardiac sympathetic afferents following brief myocardial ischemia in cats. J Auton Nerv Syst 71:28–36

Ahlgren SC, Levine JD (1994) Protein kinase C inhibitors decrease hyperalgesia and C-fiber hyperexcitability in the streptozotocin-diabetic rat. J Neurophysiol 72:684–692

Aizawa H, Hirose T (1988) A possible mechanism of airway hyperresponsiveness induced by prostaglandin F_2 alpha and thromooxane A_2. Prosaglandins Leukot Essent Fatty Acids 33(3):185–189

Anden NE, Olsson Y (1967) 5-hydroxytryptamine in normal and sectioned rat sciatic nerve. Acta Pathol Microbiol Scand 70:537–540

Arita H, Nakano T, Hanasaki K (1989) Thromboxane A_2: its generation and role in platelet activation. Prog Lipid Res 28:273–301

Armstrong D, Dry RM, Keele CA, Markham JW (1951) Method for studying chemical excitants of cutaneous pain in man. J Physiol 115:59–60

Ashton JH, Benedict CR, Fitzgerald C, Raheja S, Taylor A, Campbell WB, Buja LM, Willerson JT (1986) Serotonin as a mediator of cyclic flow variation in stenosed canine coronoary arteries. Circulation 73:572–578

Baker D, Coleridge H, Coleridge J, Nerdrum T (1980) Search for a cardiac nociceptor: Stimulation by bradykinin of sympathetic afferent nerve endings in the heart of the cat. J Physiol 306:519–536

Belville JS, Bennett WF, Lynch G (1979) A method for investigating the role of calcium in the shape change, aggregation and secretion of rat platelets. J Physiol 297:289–297

Benedict CR, Mathew B, Rex KA, Cartwright J, Sordahl LA (1986) Correlation of plasma serotonin changes with platelet aggregation in an in vivo dog model of spontaneous occlusive coronary thrombus formation. Circ Res 58:58–67

Berger HJ, Zaret BL, Speroff L, Cohen LS, Wolfson S (1977) Cardiac prostaglandin release during myocardial ischemia induced by atrial pacing in patients with coronary artery disease. Am J Cardiol 39:481–486

Bevan S (1996) Intracellular messengers and signal transduction in nociceptors. In: Belmonte C, Cervero F (eds) Neurobiology of Nociceptors. Oxford University Press, Oxford, pp 298–324

Bhoola KD, Figueroa CD, Worthy K (1992) Bioregulation of kinins: kallikreins, kininogens, and kininases. Pharmacol Rev 44:1–80

Blackman SC, Dawson G, Antonakis K, Le Breton GC (1998) The identification and characterization of oligodendrocyte thromboxane A_2 receptors. J Biol Chem 273:475–483

Blunk J, Osiander G, Nischik M, Schmelz M (1999) Pain and inflammatory hyperalgesia induced by intradermal injections of human platelets and leukocytes. Eur J Pain 3:247–259

Borg C, Lim CT, Yeomans DC, Dieter JP, Komiotis D, Anderson EG, Le Breton GC (1994) Purification of rat brain, rabbit aorta, and human platelet thromboxane A_2/prostaglandin H_2 receptors by immunoaffinity chromatography employing anti-peptide and anti-receptor antibodies. J Biol Chem 269:6109–6116

Brunsden AM, Grundy D (1999) Sensitization of visceral afferents to bradykinin in rat jejunum in vitro. J Physiol 521 Pt 2:517–527

Carrithers JA, Liu F, Shirer HW, Orr JA (1994) Mechanisms for techypneic response to the thromboxane A_2 memetic U-46,619 in rabbits. Am J Physiol 266:R321–R327

Coleman RA, Smith WL, Narumiya S (1994) VIII. International union of pharmacology classification of prostanoid receptors: properties, distribution, and structure of the receptors and their subtypes. Pharmacol Rev 46:205–229

Coller BS (1997) Platelet GPIIb/IIIa antagonists: the first anti-integrin receptor therapeutics. J Clin Invest 100:S57–S60

Couture R, Harrisson M, Vianna RM, Cloutier F (2001) Kinin receptors in pain and inflammation. Eur J Pharmacol 429:167–176

Cox DA, Vita JA, Treasure CB, Fish RD, Seiwyn AP, Ganz P (1989) Reflex increase in blood pressure during intra-coronary administration of adenosine in man. J Clin Invest 84:592–596

Crea F, Pupita G, Galassi A, El-Tamimi H, Kaski JC, Davis G, Maseri A (1990) Role of adenosine in pathogenesis of angina pain. Circulation 81:164–182

Crea F, Gaspardone A, Kaski JC, Davis G, Maseri A (1992) Relation between stimulation site of cardiac afferent nerves by adenosine and distribution of cardiac pain: results of a study in patients with stable angina. JACC 20:1498–1502

Delyani JA, Van Wylen GL (1994) Endocardial and epicardial interstitial purines and lactate during graded ischemia. Am J Physiol 226:H1019–H1026

Dibner-Dunlap ME, Kinugawa T, Thames MD (1993) Activation of cardiac sympathetic afferents: effects of exogenous adenosine and adenosine analogues. Am J Physiol 265:H395–H400

Dray A (1995) Inflammatory mediators of pain. Br J Anaesth 75:125–131

Evans RG, Ludbrook J, Michalicek J (1990) Characteristis of cardiovascular reflexes originating from 5-HT_3 receptors in the heart and lungs of unanaethetized rabbits. Clin Exp Pharmacol Physiol 17:665–679

Ferrari R (1994) Oxygen-free radicals at myocardial level: effects of ischaemia and reperfusion. Adv Exp Med Biol 366:99–111

Ferreira SH (1972) Prostaglandins, aspirin-like drugs and analgesia. Nat New Biol 240:200–203

Fitzgerald DJ (1991) Platelet activation in the pathogenesis of unstable angina: importance in determining the response to plasminogen activators. Am J Cardiol 68:51B–57B

Fitzgerald DJ, Roy L, Catella F, Fitzgerald GA (1986) Platelet activation in unstable coronary disease. N Engl J Med 315:983–989

Flores NA, Sheridan DJ (1994) The pathophysiological role of platelets during myocardial ischemia. Cardiovasc Res 28:295–302

Flores NA, Goulielmos NV, Seghatchian MJ, Sheridan DJ (1994) Myocardial ischemia induces platelet activation with adverse electrophysiological and arrhythmogenic effects. Cardiovasc Res 28:1662–1671

Folts JD (1994) Platelet aggregation in partially obstructed vessels and its elimination with aspirin. Circulation 54:365–370

Folts JD, Crowell EB Jr, Rowe GG (1976) Platelet aggregation in partially obstructed vessels and its elimination with aspirin. Circulation 54:365–370

Frangogiannis N, ML Lindsey, LH Michael, KA Youker, RB Bressler, LH Mendoza, RN Spengler, CW Smith, ML Entman (1998) Resident cardiac mast cells degranulate and release preformed TNF-α, initiating the cytokine cascade in experimental canaine myocardial ischemia/reperfusion. Circulation 98:699–710

Fu L-W, Longhurst JC (1998) Role of 5-HT_3 receptors in activation of abdominal sympathetic C-fibre afferents during ischemia in cats. J Physiol (Lond) 509:729–740

Fu L-W, Longhurst JC (2002a) Activated platelets contribute to stimulation of cardiac afferents during ischaemia in cats: role of 5-HT_3 receptors. J Physiol (Lond) 544:897–912

Fu L-W, Longhurst JC (2002b) Role of activated platelets in excitation of cardiac afferents during myocardial ischemia in cats. Am J Physiol 282:H100–H109

Fu L-W, Longhurst JC (2005) Interactions between histamine and bradykinin in stimulation of ischaemically sensitive cardiac afferents in felines. J Physiol (Lond) 565:1007–1017

Fu L-W, Longhurst JC (2008) Reciprocal interactions between bradykinin and thromboxane A_2 during stimulation of ischemically sensitive cardiac spinal afferents. FASEB J 22:1230.4

Fu L-W, Pan H-L, Longhurst JC (1997) Endogenous histamine stimulates ischemically sensitive abdominal visceral afferents through H_1 receptors. Am J Physiol 273:H2726–H2737

Fu L-W, Phan A, Longhurst JC (2008a) Myocardial Ischemia-Mediated Excitatory Reflexes: A New Function for Thromboxane A_2? Am J Physiol 295:H2530–H2540

Fu L-W, Schunack W, Longhurst JC (2005) Histamine contributes to ischemia-related activation of cardiac spinal afferents: role of H_1 receptors and PKC. J Neurophysiol 93:713–722

Fu LW, Guo ZL, Longhurst JC (2008b) Undiscovered role of endogenous TxA_2 in activation of cardiac sympathetic afferents during ischemia. J Physiol 586(13):3287–3300

Fujimori T, Yamanishi Y, Yamatsu K, Tajima T (1982) High performance liquid chromatography (HPLC) determination of endogenous serotonin released from aggregating platelets. J Pharmacol Methods 7:105–113

Furci L, Fitzgerald DJ, Fitzgerald GA (1991) Heterogeneity of prostaglandin H_2/thromboxane A_2 receptors: distinct subtypes mediate vascular smooth muscle contraction and platelet aggregation. J Pharmacol Exp Ther 258:74–81

Gao H, Welch WJ, DiBona GF, Wilcox CS (1997) Sympathetic nervous system and hypertension during prolonged TxA_2/PGH_2 receptor activation in rats. Am J Physiol 273: H734–H739

Gebhart GF (2000) Pathobiology of visceral pain: molecular mechanisms and therapeutic implications IV. Visceral afferent contributions to the pathobiology of visceral pain. Am J Physiol Gastrointest Liver Physiol 278:G834–G838

Ginsburg R, Bristow M, Kantrowitz N, Baim D, Harrison D (1981) Histamine provocation of clinical coronary artery spasm: Implications concerning pathogenesis of variant angina pectoris. Am Heart J 102:819–822

Gnecchi-Ruscone T, Montano N, Contini M, Guazzi M, Lombardi F, Malliani A (1995) Adenosine activates cardiac sympathetic afferent fibers and potentiates the excitation induced by coronary occlusion. J Auton Nerv Syst 53:175–184

Golino P, Piscione F, Benedict C, Anderson H, Cappelli-Bigazzi M, Indolfi C, Condorelli M, Chiariello M, Willerson J (1994) Local effect of serotonin released during coronary angioplasty. N Engl J Med 330:523–528

Grande P, Grauholt A-M, Madsen JK (1990) Unstable angina pectoris: platelet behavior and prognosis in progressive angina and intermediate coronary syndrome. Circulation 81(suppl I): I16–I19

Grill HP, Zweier P, Kuppusamy ML, Weisfeldt ML, Flaherty JT (1992) Direct measurement of myocardial free radical generation in an in vivo model: effects of postischemic reperfusion and treatment with human recombinant superoxide dismutase. J Am Coll Cardiol 20:1604–1611

Grisham MB, Granger DN (1988) Neutrophil-mediated mucosal injury: role of reactive oxygen metabolites. Dig Dis Sci 33:6S–15S

Grundy D, Blackshae LA, Hillsley K (1994) Role of 5-hydroxytryptamine in gastrointestinal chemosensitivity. Dig Dis Sci 30(suppl):44S–47S

Guo Z-L, Longhurst J (2000) Role of cAMP in activation of ischemically sensitive abdominal visceral afferents. Am J Physiol 278:H843–H852

Guo Z-L, Fu L-W, Symons J, Longhurst J (1998) Signal transduction in activation of ischemically sensitive abdominal visceral afferents: role of PKC. Am J Physiol 275:H1024–H1031

Guo Z-L, JD Symons, JC Longhurst (1999) Activation of visceral afferents by bradykinin and ischemia: independent roles of PKC and prostaglandins. Am J Physiol 276:H1884–H1891

Halliwell B (1989) Protection against tissue damage in vivo by desferrioxamine: what is its mechanism of action? Free Radic Biol Med 7:645–651

Halliwell B, Gutteridge JMC (1990) Role of free radicals and catalytic metal ions in human disease. An overview. Meth Enzymol 186:1–85

Hashimoto K, Hirose M, Furukawa S, Hayakawa H, Kimura E (1977) Changes in hemodynamics and bradykinin concentration in coronary sinus blood in experimental coronary artery occlusion. Jpn Heart J 5:679–689

Hendrickson SC, St Louis JD, Lowe JE, bdel-Aleem S (1997) Free fatty acid metabolism during myocardial ischemia and reperfusion. Mol Cell Biochem 166:85–94

Herbert MK, Just H, Schmidt RF (2001) Histamine excites groups III and IV afferents from the cat knee joint depending on their resting activity. Neurosci Lett 305:95–98

Hill SJ, Ganellin CR, Timmerman H, Schwartz JC, Shankley NP, Young JM, Schunack W, Levi R, Haas HL (1997) International union of pharmacology. XIII. Classification of histamine receptors. Pharmacol Rev 49:253–278

Hiramatsu Y, Gikakis N, Anderson III HL, Gorman III JH, Marcinkiewicz C, Gould RJ, Niewiarowski S, Edmunds LH Jr (1997) Tirofiban provides "platelet anesthesia" during cardiopulmonary bypass in baboons. J Thorac Cardiovasc Surg 113:193

Hirsh P, Hillis L, Campbell W, Firth B, Willerson J (1981) Release of prostaglandins and thromboxane into the coronary circulation in patients with ischemic heart disease. N Engl J Med 304:685–691

Holmsen H (1985) Platelet metabolism and activation. Sem Hematol 22:219–240

Holzer P (2001) Gastroduodenal mucosal defense: coordination by a network of messengers and mediators. Curr Opin Gastroenterol 17:489–496

Hong JL, Kwong K, Lee LY (1997) Stimulation of pulmonary C fibers by lactic acid in rats: concentrations of H^+ and lactate ions. J Physiol 500:319–329

Hoyer D, Clarke DE, Fozard JR, Hartig PR, Martin GR, Mylecharane EJ (1994) International union of parmacology classification of receptors for 5-hydroxytryptamine (serotonin). Pharmacol Rev 46:157–203

Hsu KS, Han WM (1996) Thromboxane A_2 agonist modulation of excitatory synaptic transmission in hte rat hippocampal slice. Br J Pharmacol 118:2220–2227

Huang H-S, Pan H-L, Stahl G, Longhurst J (1995a) Ischemia- and reperfusion-sensitive cardiac sympathetic afferents: influence of H_2O_2 and hydroxyl radicals. Am J Physiol 269:H888–H901

Huang H-S, Stahl G, Longhurst J (1995b) Cardiac-cardiovascular reflexes induced by hydrogen peroxide in cats. Am J Physiol 268:H2114–H2124

Huang MH, Sylven C, Horackova M, Armour JA (1995c) Ventricular sensory neurons in canine dorsal root ganglia: effects of adenosine and substance P. Am J Physiol 269:R318–R324

Ichinose M, Barnes PJ (1990) Histamine H_3 receptors modulate antigen-induced bronchoconstriction in guinea pigs. J Allergy Clin Immunol 86:491–495

Imamura M, Seyedi N, Lander HM, Levi R (1995) Functional idendification of histamine H_3-receptors in the human heart. Circ Res 77:206–210

Imamura M, Smith NC, Garbarg M, Levi R (1996) Histamine H_3-receptor-mediated inhibition of calcitonin gene-related peptide release from cardiac C fibers. A regulatory negative-feedback loop. Circ Res 78:863–869

Immke DC, McCleskey EW (2003) Protons open acid-sensing ion channels by catalyzing relief of Ca^{2+} blockade. Neuron 37:75–84

Jackson JH, White CW, Parker NB, Ryan JW, Repine JE (1985) Dimethylthiourea consumption reflects H_2O_2 concentrations and severity of acute lung injury. J Appl Physiol 59:1995–1998

Jennings RB, Reimer KA, Hill ML, Mayer SE (1981) Total ischemia in dog heart in vitro. 1. Comparison of high energy phosphate production, utilization, an depletion, and of adenine nucleotide catabolism in total ischemia in vitro vs. severe ischemia in vivo. Circulation 49:892–900

Jordan D (2005) Vagal control of the heart: central serotonergic (5-HT) mechanisms. Exp Physiol 90:175–181

Jordt SE, Tominaga M, Julius D (2000) Acid potentiation of the capsaicin receptor determined by a key extracellular site. Proc Natl Acad Sci USA 97:8134–8139

Kappagoda CT, Linden RJ, Mary DASG (1977) Atrial receptors in the dog and rabbit. J Physiol 272:799–815

Kappagoda CT, Linden RJ, Sivananthan N (1979) The nature of the atrial receptors responsible for a reflex increase in heart rate in the dog. J Physiol 291:393–412

Karla W, Shams H, Orr JA, Scheid P (1992) Effects of the thromboxane A_2 mimetic, U46,619, on pulmonary vagal afferents in the cat. Respir Physiol 87:383–396

Kashiba H, Fukui H, Morikawa Y, Senba E (1999) Gene expression of histamine H_1 receptor in guinea pig primary sensory neurons: a relationship between H_1 receptor mRNA-expressing neurons and peptidergic neurons. Brain Res Mol Brain Res 66:24–34

Kaufman MP, Baker DG, Coleridge HM, Coleridge JCG (1980) Stimulation by bradykinin of afferent vagal C-fibers with chemosensitive endings in the heart and aorta of the dog. Circ Res 46:476–484

Kaufman MP, Iwamoto GA, Longhurst JC, Mitchell JH (1982) Effects of capsaicin and bradykinin on afferent fibers with endings in skeletal muscle. Circ Res 50:133–139

Kenagy J, VanCleave J, Pazdernik L, Orr JA (1997) Stimulation of group III and IV afferent nerves from the hindlimb by thromboxane A_2. Brain Res 744:175–178

Kimura E, Hashimoto K, Furukawa S, Hayakawa H (1973) Changes in bradykinin level in coronary sinus blood after the experimental occulsion of a coronary artery. Am Heart J 85:635–647

Koda H, Mizumura K (2002) Sensitization to mechanical stimulation by inflammatory mediators and by mild burn in canine visceral nociceptors in vitro. J Neurophysiol 87:2043–2051

Koda H, Minagawa M, Si-Hong L, Mizumura K, Kumazawa T (1996) H_1-receptor-mediated excitation and facilitation of the heat response by histamine in canine visceral polymodal receptors studied in vitro. J Neurophysiol 76:1396–1404
Koppert W, Martus P, Reeh PW (2001) Interactions of histamine and bradykinin on polymodal C-fibres in isolated rat skin. Eur J Pain 5:97–106
Kounis NG, Zavras GM (1991) Histamine-induced coronary artery spasm: the concept of allergic angina. Br J Clin Pract 45:121–127
Kuppusamy P, Zweier JL (1989) Characterization of free radical generation by xanthine oxidase. Evidence for hydroxyl radical generation. J Biol Chem 264:9880–9884
Laine P, Kaartinen M, Penttila A, Panula P, Paavonen T, Kovanen PT (1999) Association between myocardial infarction and the mast cells in the adventitia of the infarct-related coronary artery. Circulation 99:361–369
Laine P, Naukkarinen A, Heikkila L, Penttila A, Kovanen PT (2000) Adventitial mast cells connect with sensory nerve fibers in atherosclerotic coronary arteries. Circulation 101:1665–1669
Leanos OL, Hong E, Amezcua JL (1995) Reflex circulatory collapse following intrapulmonary entrapment of activated platelets: mediation via 5-HT_3 receptor stimulation. Br J Pharmacol 116:2048–2052
Lefkovits J, Plow EF, Topol EJ (1995) Platelet glycoprotein IIb/IIIa receptors in cardiovascular medicine. N Engl J Med 332:1553–1559
Lehtosalo JI, Uusitalo H, Laakso J, Palkama A, Harkonen M (1984) Biochemical and immunohistochemical determination of 5-hydroxytryptamine located in mast cells in the trigeminal ganglion of the rat and guinea pig. Histochemistry 80:219–223
Lew WYW, Longhurst JC (1986) Substance P, 5-hydroxytryptamine, and bradykinin stimulate abdominal visceral afferents. Am J Physiol 250:R465–R473
Lewy RI, Wiener L, Walinsky P, Lefer AM, Silver MJ, Smith JB (1980) Thromboxane release during pacing-induced angina pectoris: possible vasoconstrictor influence on the coronary vasculature. Circulation 61:1165–1171
Lincoff MA, Califf RM, Topol EJ (2000) Platelet glycoprotein IIb/IIia receptor blockade in coronary artery disease. J A Coll Cardiol 35:1103–1115
Longhurst JC (1984) Cardiac receptors: Their function in health and disease. Prog Cardiovasc Dis XXVII:201–222
Longhurst J, Dittman L (1987) Hypoxia, bradykinin, and prostaglandins stimulate ischemically sensitive visceral afferents. Am J Physiol 253:H556–H567
Longhurst J, Rotto D, Kaufman M, Stahl G (1991) Ischemically sensitive abdominal visceral afferents: response to cyclooxygenase blockade. Am J Physiol 261:H2075–H2081
Longhurst J, Tjen-A-Looi S, Fu L-W (2001) Cardiac sympathetic afferent activation provoked by myocardial ischemia and reperfusion: mechanisms and reflexes. Ann N Y Acad Sci 940:74–95
Malliani A, Lombardi F, Pagani M (1981) Functions of afferents in cardiovascular sympathetic nerves. J Auton Nerv Syst 3:231–236
Mark AL, Abboud FM, Heistad DD, Schmid PG, Johannsen UJ (1974) Evidence against the presence of ventricular chemoreceptors activated by hypoxia and hypercapnia. Am J Physiol 227:273–279
Masini E, Giannella E, Bianchi S, Mannaioni PF (1987) Histamine and lactate dehydrogenase (LDH) release in ischemic myocardium of the guinea-pig. Agents Actions 20:281–283
Masini E, Di Bello MG, Raspanti S, Fomusi Ndisang J, Baronti R, Cappugi P, Mannaioni PF (1998) The role of histamine in platelet aggregation by physiological and immunological stimuli. Inflamm Res 47:211–220
Mazzone SB, Canning BJ (2002) Synergistic interactions between airway afferent nerve subtypes mediating reflex bronchospasm in guinea pigs. Am J Physiol Regul Integr Comp Physiol 283: R86–R98
Mehta J, Mehta P, Feldman R, Horalek C (1984) Thromboxane release in coronary artery disease: spontaneous versus pacing-induced angina. Am Heart J 107:286–292

Meller ST, Gebhart GF (1992) A critical review of the afferent pathways and the potential chemical mediators involved in cardiac pain. Neuroscience 48:501–524

Meyers KM, Holsmen H, Seachord CL (1982) Comparative study of platelet dense granule constituents. Am J Physiol 243:R454–R461

Middlekauff HR, Chiu J (2004) Cyclooxygenase products sensitize muscle mechanoreceptors in healthy humans. Am J Physiol Heart Circ Physiol 5:H1944–H1949

Mizumura K, Minagawa M, Koda H, Kumazawa T (1995) Influence of histamine on the bradykinin response of canine testicular polymodal receptors in vitro. Inflamm Res 44:376–378

Muja N, Blackman SC, Le Breton GC, DeVries GH (2001) Identification and functional characterization of thromboxane A_2 receptors in Schwann cells. J Neurochem 78:446–456

Nakahodo K, Saitoh S, Nakamura M, Kosugi T (1994) Histamine release from rabbit platelets by platelet-activating factor (PAF). Arerugi 43:501–510

Nandam LS, Jhaveri D, Bartlett P (2007) 5-HT7, neurogenesis and antidepressants: a promising therapeutic axis for treating depression. Clin Exp Pharmacol Physiol 34:546–551

Nerdrum T, Baker D, Coleridge H, Coleridge J (1986) Interaction of bradykinin and prostaglandin E_1 on cardiac pressor reflex and sympathetic afferents. Am J Physiol 250:R815–R822

Nicolson TA, Bevan S, Richards CD (2002) Characterisation of the calcium responses to histamine in capsaicin-sensitive and capsaicin-insensitive sensory neurones. Neuroscience 110:329–338

Ninkovic M, Hunt SP (1985) Opiate and histamine H_1 receptors are present on some substance P-containing dorsal root ganglion cells. Neurosci Lett 53:133–137

Nishi K, Sakanashi M, Takenaka F (1977) Activation of afferent cardiac sympathetic nerve fibers of the cat by pain producing substances and by noxious heat. Pflugers Arch 372:53–61

O'Neill CA, Fu L-W, Halliwell B, Longhurst JC (1996) Hydroxyl radical production during myocardial ischemia and reperfusion in cats. Am J Physiol 271:H660–H667

Oberg B, Thoren PN (1973) Circulatory responses to stimulation of medullated and non-medullated afferents in the cardiac nerve in the cat. Acta Physiol Scand 87:121–132

Opie LH, Owen P, Thomas M, Samson R (1973) Coronary sinus lactic measurements in assessment of myocardial ischemia. Am J Cardiol 32:295–305

oude Egbrink MG, Tangelder GJ, Slaaf DW, Reneman RS (1993) Different roles of prostaglandins in thromboembolic processes in arterioles and venules in vivo. Thromb Haemost 70:826–833

Packham MA, Guccione MA, Greenberg JP, Kinlough-Rathbone RL, Mustard JF (1977) Release of 14C-serotonin during initial platelet changes induced by thrombin, collagen, or A23187. Blood 50:915–926

Packham MA, Rand ML, Ruben DH, Kinlough-Rathbone RL (1991) Effect of calcium concentration and inhibitors on the responses of platelets stimulated with collagen: contrast between human and rabbit platelets. Comp Biochem Physiol A 99:551–557

Pagani M, Pizzinelli R, furlan R, Guzzetti S, Rimoldi O, Sandrone G, Malliani A (1985) Analysis of the pressor sympathetic reflex produced by intracoronary injections of bradykinin in conscious dogs. Circ Res 56:175–183

Paintal AS (1973) Vagal sensory receptors and their reflex effects. Physiol Rev 53:159–227

Pal P, Koley J, Bhattacharyya S, Gupta JS, Koley B (1989) Cardiac nociceptors and ischemia: role of sympathetic afferents in cat. Jpn J Physiol 39:131–144

Pan H-L, Longhurst J (1995) Lack of a role of adenosine in activation of ischemically sensitive cardiac sympathetic afferents in cats. Am J Physiol 269:H106–H113

Pan H-L, Stahl GL, Rendig SV, Carretero OA, Longhurst JC (1994) Endogenous BK stimulates ischemically sensitive abdominal visceral C fiber afferents through kinin B_2 receptors. Am J Physiol 267:H2398–H2406

Pan H-L, Longhurst JC, Eisenach JC, Chen S-R (1999) Role of protons in activation of cardiac sympathetic C-fiber afferents during ischemia. J Physiol 518.3:857–866

Parratt JR, Cokerm S (1981) The significance of prostaglandin and thromboxane release in acute myocardial ischemia. In: Forster W (ed) Rostaglandins and Thromboxanes: Proceedings of the Third International Symposium on Prostaglandins and Thromboxanes in the Cardiovascular System. Pergamon, New York, pp 21–25

Patterson L, Patterson L, Patterso, Patterson LM, Zheng H, Ward SM, Berhoud H-R (2003) Vanilloid receptor (VR1) expression in vagal afferent neurons innervating the gastrointestinal tract. Cell Tissue Res 311:277–287

Peroutka SJ (1994) 5-Hydroxytryptamine receptors. J Neurochem 60:408–416

Petho G, Derow A, Reeh PW (2001) Bradykinin-induced nociceptor sensitization to heat is mediated by cyclooxygenase products in isolated rat skin. Eur J Neurosci 14:210–218

Phillips DR, Scarborough RM (1997) Clinical pharmacology of eptifibatide. Am J Cardiol 80:11B–20B

Pickar JG (1998) The thromboxane A_2 mimetic U-46619 inhibits somatomotor activity via a vagal reflex from the lung. Am J Physiol 275:R706–R712

Poole-Wilson PA (1978) Measurement of myocardial intracellular *p*H in pathological states. J Mol Cell Cardiol 10:511–526

Rang HP, Bevan SJ, Dray A (1991) Chemical activation of nociceptive peripheral neurons. Br Med Bull 47:534–548

Rao GHR (1993) Physiology of blood platelet activation. Indian J Physiol Pharmacol 37:263–275

Repka-Ramirez MS (2003) New concepts of histamine receptors and actions. Curr Allergy Asthma Rep 3:227–231

Rhodes KF, Coleman J, Lattimer N (1992) A component of 5-HT-evoked depolarization of the rat isolated vagus nerve is mediated by a putative 5-HT4 receptor. Naunyn Schemiedebergs Arch Pharmacol 346:496–503

Richardson BP (1990) Serotonin and nociception. Ann N Y Acad Sci 600:511–519

Ringkamp M, Schmelz M, Kress M, Allwang M, Ogilvie A, Reeh PW (1994) Activated human platelets in plasma excite nociceptors in rat skin, in vitro. Neurosci Lett 170:103–106

Rotto DM, Stebbins CL, Kaufman MP (1989) Reflex cardiovascular and ventilatory responses to increasing H^+ activity in cat hindlimb muscle. J Appl Physiol 67:256–263

Rotto D, Schultz H, Longhurst J, Kaufman M (1990) Sensitization of group III muscle afferents to static contraction by arachidonic acid metabolism. J Appl Physiol 68:861–867

Rupniak HT, Joy KA, Atkin C (2000) Oxidative neuropathology and putative chemical entities for Alzheimer's disease: neuroprotective effects of salen-manganese catalytic anti-oxidants. Neurotox Res 2:167–178

Sakata K, Yoshida H, Hoshino T, Kurata C (1996) Sympathetic nerve activity in the spasm-induced coronary artery region is associated with disease activity of vasospastic angina. J Am Coll Cardiol 28:460–464

Saxena SP, Brandes LJ, Becker AB, Simons KJ, LaBella FS, Gerrard JM (1989) Histamine is an intracellular messenger mediating platelet aggregation. Science 243:1596–1599

Schaefer S, RA Valente, LJ Laslett, JC Longhurst (1996) Cardiac reflex effects of intracoronary bradykinin in humans. J Investig Med 492:841–850

Schmelz M, Osiander G, Blunk J, Ringkamp M, Reeh PW, Handwerker HO (1997) Intracutaneous injections of platelets cause acute pain and protracted hyperalgesia. Neurosci Lett 226:171–174

Shams H, Scheid P (1990) Effects of thromboxane on respiration and pulmonary circulation in the cat: role of vagus nerve. J Appl Physiol 68:2042–2046

Sommer C (2004) Serotonin in pain and analgesia: actions in the periphery. Mol Neurobiol 30:117–125

Stahl G, Longhurst J (1992) Ischemically sensitive visceral afferents: importance of H^+ derived from lactic acid and hypercapnia. Am J Physiol 262:H748–H753

Stahl G, Pan H-L, Longhurst J (1993) Activation of ischemia and reperfusion-sensitive abdominal visceral C fiber afferents: role of hydrogen peroxide and hydroxyl radicals. Circ Res 72:1266–1275

Stary HC (1990) The sequence of cell and matrix changes in atherosclerotic lesions of coronary arteries in the first forty years of life. Eur Heart J 11(suppl E):3–19

Staszewka-Barczak J, Ferreira SH, Vane JR (1976) An excitatory nociceptive cardiac reflex elicited by bradykinin and potentiated by prostaglandins and myocardial ischaemia. Cardiovasc Res 10:314–327

Staszewska-Woolley J, Woolley G (1989) Participation of the kallikrein-kinin-receptor system in reflexes arising from neural afferents in the dog epicardium. J Physiol (Lond) 419:33–44
Stebbins CL, Longhurst JC (1985) Bradykinin-induced chemoreflexes from skeletal muscle: implications for the exercise reflex. J Appl Physiol 59:56–63
Stebbins CL, Longhurst JC (1986) Bradykinin in the reflex cardiovascular responses to static muscular contraction. J Appl Physiol 61:271–279
Stebbins CL, Theodossy SJ, Longhurst JC (1991) Cardiovascular reflexes evoked by histamine stimulation of the stomach. Am J Physiol 261:H1098–H1105
Stebbins C, Stahl G, Theodossy S, Longhurst J (1992) Modulation of bradykinin-induced gastric-cardiovascular reflexes by histamine. Am J Physiol 262:R112–R119
Steen KH, Steen AE, Reeh PW (1995) A dominant role of acid *p*H in inflammatory excitation and sensitization of nociceptors in rat skin, in vivo. J Neurosci 15:3982–3989
Stegmeier K, Pill J, Muller-Beckmann B, Schmidt FH, Witte EC, Wolff HP, Patscheke H (1984) The pharmacological profile of the thromboxane A_2 antagonist BM 13.177. A new anti-platelet and anti-thrombotic drug. Thromb Res 35:379–395
Stormorken H (1986) Platelets in hemostasis and thrombosis. In: Holmsen H (ed) Platelet responses and metabolism, vol 1. CRC, Boca Raton, pp 3–32
Sun SY, Wang W, Schultz HD (2001) Activation of cardiac afferents by arachidonic acid: relative contributions of metabolic pathways. Am J Physiol Heart Circ Physiol 281:H93–H104
Sylven C, Beemann B, Jonzon B, Brandt R (1986) Angina pectoris-like pain provoked by intravenous adenosine. Br Med J 293:227–230
Taiwo YO, Levine JD (1991) Further confirmation of the role of adenyl cyclase and of cAMP-dependent protein kinase in primary afferent hyperalgesia. Neuroscience 44:131–135
Taiwo YO, Levine JD (1992) Serotonin is a directly-acting hyperalgesic agent in the rat. Neuroscience 48:485–490
Taiwo Y, Goetzl EJ, Levine JD (1987) Hyperalgesia onset latency suggests a hierarchy of action. Brain Res 423:333–337
Thoren P (1973) Evidence for a depressor reflex elicited from left ventricular receptors during occlusion of one coronary artery in the cat. Acta Physiol Scand 88:23–34
Thoren PN (1976) Activation of left ventricular receptors with nonmedullated vagal afferent fibers during occlusion of a coronary artery in the cat. Am J Cardiol 37:1046–1051
Tjen-A-Looi S, H-L Pan, JC Longhurst (1998) Endogenous bradykinin activates ischaemically sensitive cardiac visceral afferents through kinin B2 receptors in cats. J Physiol (Lond) 510:633–641
Tjen-A-Looi S, Fu L-W, Longhurst JC (2002) Xanthine oxidase, but not neutrophils, contribute to activation of cardiac sympathetic afferents during myocardial ischaemia in cats. J Physiol (Lond) 543:327–336
Tokimasa T, Akasu T (1989) Histamine H_2 receptor mediates postsynaptic excitation and presynaptic inhibition in submucous plexus neurons of the guinea-pig. Neuroscience 28:735–744
Uchida Y, Murao S (1974) Bradykinin-induced excitation of afferent cardiac sympathetic nerve fibers. Jpn Heart J 15:84–91
Uchida Y, Murao S (1975) Acid-induced excitation of afferent cardiac sympathetic nerve fibers. Am J Physiol 228:27–33
Ustinova EE, Schultz HD (1994) Activation of cardiac vagal afferents in ischemia and reperfusion: prostaglandins vs. oxygen free radicals. Circ Res 74:904–911
Van den Berg EK, Schmitz JM, Benedict CR, Malloy CR, Willerson JT, Dehmer GJ (1989) Transcardiac serotonin concentration is increased in selected patients with limiting angina and complex coronary lesion morphology. Circulation 79:116–124
Van der Vusse GJ, Reneman RS, van Bilsen M (1997) Accumulation of arachidonic acid in ischemic/reperfused cardiac tissue: possible causes and consequences. Prostaglandins Leukot Essent Fatty Acids 57:85–93
Verhoeven AJM, Mommersteeg ME, Akkerman JWN (1984) Quantification of energy consumption in platelets during thrombin-induced aggregation and secretion. Biochem J 221:771–787

Wacker MJ, Tehrani RN, Smoot RL, Orr JA (2002) Thromboxane A_2 mimetic evokes a bradycardia mediated by stimulation of cardiac vagal afferent nerves. Am J Physiol Heart Circ Physiol 282:H482–H490

Wacker MJ, Tyburski JB, Ammar CP, Adams MC, Orr JA (2005) Detection of thromboxane A_2 receptor mRNA in rabbit nodose ganglion neurons. Neurosci Lett 386:121–126

White JC (1957) Cardiac pain: anatomic pathway and physiologic mechanisms. Circulation 16:644–655

Wilson RF, Wyche K, Christensen BV, Zimmer S, Laxson DD (1990) Effects of adenosine on human coronary arterial circulation. Circulation 82:1595–1606

Wolff AA, Levi R (1988) Ventricular arrhythmias parallel cardiac histamine efflux after coronary artery occlusion in the dog. Agents Actions 25:296–306

Zahner MR, Li D-P, Chen S-R, Pan H-L (2003) Cardiac vanilloid receptor 1-expressing afferent nerves and their role in the cardiogenic sympathetic reflex in rats. J Physiol (Lond) 551(2):515–523

Zucker IH, Cornish KG (1980) Reflex cardiovascular and respiratory effects of serotonin in conscious and anesthetized dogs. Circ Res 47:509–515

Zweier J, Broderick R, Kuppusamy P, Thompson-Gorman S, Lutty GA (1994) Determination of the mechanism of free radical generation in human aortic endothelial cells exposed to anoxia and reoxygenation. J Biol Chem 269:24156–24162

Roles of Gastro-oesophageal Afferents in the Mechanisms and Symptoms of Reflux Disease

Amanda J. Page and L. Ashley Blackshaw

Contents

Abstract Oesophageal pain is one of the most common reasons for physician consultation and/or seeking medication. It is most often caused by acid reflux from the stomach, but can also result from contractions of the oesophageal muscle. Different forms of pain are evoked by oesophageal acid, including heartburn and

---

L.A. Blackshaw (✉)
Nerve Gut Research Laboratory, Level 1 Hanson Institute, Frome Road, Adelaide, SA 5000, Australia
ashley.blackshaw@adelaide.edu.au

B.J. Canning and D. Spina (eds.), *Sensory Nerves*,
Handbook of Experimental Pharmacology 194, DOI: 10.1007/978-3-540-79090-7_7,

non-cardiac chest pain, but the basic mechanisms and pathways by which these are generated remain to be elucidated. Both vagal and spinal afferent pathways are implicated by basic research. The sensitivity of afferent fibres within these pathways may become altered after acid-induced inflammation and damage, but the severity of symptoms in humans does not necessarily correlate with the degree of inflammation. Gastro-oesophageal reflux disease (GORD) is caused by transient relaxations of the lower oesophageal sphincter, which are triggered by activation of gastric vagal mechanoreceptors. Vagal afferents are therefore an emerging therapeutic target for GORD. Pain in the absence of excess acid reflux remains a major challenge for treatment.

Keywords Visceral pain, Vagal afferents, Gastro-oesophageal reflux, Lower oesophageal sphincter

Abbreviations

AMPA	α-Amino-3-hydroxy-5-methylisoxazoleproprionate
(2R,4R)-APDC	(2R,4R)-4-Aminopyrrolidine-2,4-dicarboxylate
ATP	Adenosine triphosphate
CCK	Cholecystokinin
CGRP	Calcitonin gene-related peptide
CNQX	(6-cyano-7-nitroquinoxaline-2,3-dione)
DHPG	(RS)-3,5-Dihydroxyphenylglycine
GABA	γ-Aminobutyric acid
GORD	Gastro-oesophageal reflux disease
5-HT	5-Hydroxytryptamine
IGLE	Intraganglionic laminar endings
iGluR	Ionotropic glutamate receptor
IMA	Intramuscular array
L-AP4	L-(+)-2-Amino-4-phosphonobutyric acid
L-NAME	NG-nitro-L-arginine methyl ester
α,β-meATP	α,β-Methylene ATP
mGluR	Metabotropic glutamate receptor
MPEP	2-Methyl-6-(phenylethynyl)pyridine
MTEP	3-((2-Methyl-1,3-thiazol-4-yl)ethynyl)pyridine
NCCP	Non-cardiac chest pain
NMDA	*N*-Methyl D-aspartate
TLOSR	Transient lower oesophageal sphincter relaxation
TRPV1	Transient receptor potential vanilloid receptor 1

1 Pathways and Subtypes of Gastro-oesophageal Afferents

1.1 Anatomy of Gastro-oesophageal Afferents

1.1.1 Vagal Afferents

The axons of vagal afferents project directly to the nucleus of the solitary tract in the brain stem, whereupon connections with central pathways are made. The cell bodies of vagal afferents are located in the jugular and nodose ganglia. Viscerofugal neurones have cell bodies in the gastric and oesophageal myenteric plexus and project centrally in the vagal trunks, but their function is not understood. Vagal afferents innervate all layers of the gastro-oesophageal wall. They include various types of mucosal endings (Dutsch et al. 1998; Wank and Neuhuber 2001), intra-ganglionic laminar endings (IGLEs), and intramuscular arrays (IMAs) (Berthoud et al. 1997; Wang and Powley 2000). IGLEs have recently been identified as sites of mechanotransduction in response to gastro-oesophageal distension (Zagorodnyuk and Brookes 2000; Zagorodnyuk et al. 2001).

IGLEs are lamellar structures originating from the parent axon and covering enteric ganglia sandwiched between longitudinal and circular layers of the tunica muscularis (Rodrigo et al. 1975) (Fig. 1a). Some of the processes may penetrate within the ganglia. Anterograde tracing from the nodose ganglia identified them as vagal afferent endings in rat and guinea-pig oesophagus (Neuhuber 1987; Lindh et al. 1989) and rat and mouse stomach (Berthoud and Powley 1992; Fox et al. 2000). In the oesophagus, anterogradely traced IGLEs innervate virtually every myenteric ganglion (Neuhuber et al. 1998) and about 50% of gastric myenteric ganglia are innervated by IGLEs (Berthoud et al. 1997). IGLEs are more evenly scattered along the gastrointestinal tract than the IMAs, which appear to be confined to the gastric fundus and sphincter regions, particularly the lower oesophageal and pyloric sphincters (Berthoud and Powley 1992; Kressel et al. 1994; Neuhuber et al. 1998; Phillips and Powley 2000; Wang and Powley 2000). In in vitro preparations of the guinea-pig stomach, Zagorodnyuk et al. (Zagorodnyuk and Brookes 2000; Zagorodnyuk et al. 2001, 2003) identified IGLEs by anterograde tracing from branches of the vagus nerve attached to a wholemount of oesophagus and stomach and showed a convincing correlation with hot spots of mechanotransduction. Thus, the IGLEs can be considered as the mechanosensory endings of vagal afferents that respond to low-intensity stretch. Although the sensitivity of these afferents can be modulated (see Part 2), the sensory transduction process itself appears to be independent of chemical transmission and most likely involves mechanosensitive ion channels on the endings themselves (Zagorodnyuk et al. 2003). IMAs, which were also anterogradely labelled in vagus nerve stomach

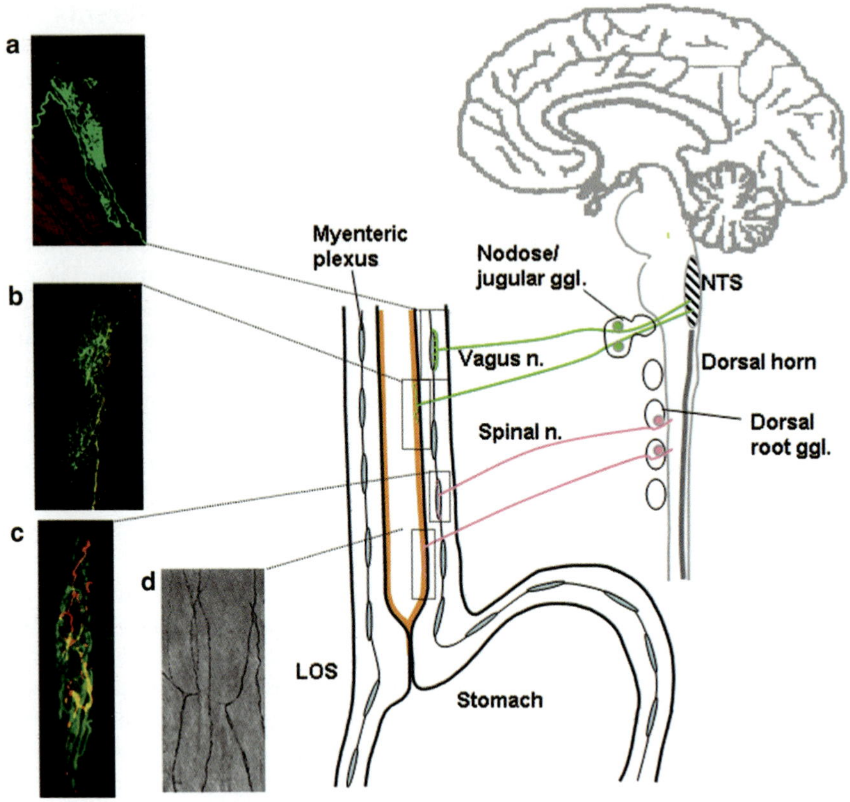

Fig. 1 Schematic and real examples of relative localization of spinal and vagal afferent endings within the oesophageal wall. Endings in the myenteric ganglia and mucosa are evident in both pathways (rostrocaudal localization is not representative). Only some of the documented types of ending are shown here for simplicity. (**a**) A typical oesophageal intraganglionic laminar ending (IGLE) in rat covering a myenteric ganglion and showing calbindin immunoreactivity (*green*). (**b**) Complex laminar type I vagal mucosal ending originating from a coarse parent axon coexpressing immunoreactivity for both calretinin and calbindin (*red* and *green*, respectively, resulting in *yellow*; wholemount). (**c**) Close contacts between calretinin-positive vagal IGLEs (*green*) and calcitonin gene related peptide (CGRP)-positive varicose spinal afferents (*red*) are indicated by *yellow* mixed colour in a section of rat oesophagus. No colocalization within the same nerve fibre is evident. (**d**) CGRP-positive spinal afferent endings (*black*) in a flat mount of rat cervical oesophagus. (Images taken from Dutsch et al. 1998 and Wank and Neuhuber 2001 with kind permission of the authors and the publisher Wiley-Liss Inc.)

preparations, could not be correlated with mechanosensory transduction sites (Zagorodnyuk et al. 2001). This is surprising considering the IMAs consist of long trails of branching varicose vagal afferent fibres embedded within the smooth muscle and arranged parallel to the muscle fibres (Berthoud and Powley 1992; Phillips and Powley 2000).

Vagal mucosal afferents are prominent in the upper cervical region of the oesophagus. The density of these afferents decreases in the lower cervical and thoracic oesophagus and then slightly increases again in the abdominal portion in rodents (Neuhuber 1987; Dutsch et al. 1998; Wank and Neuhuber 2001). In the upper cervical oesophagus, there are also thin varicose fibres that form a dense network in the submucosa. Many of these fibres have short fingerlike branches extending towards the epithelium, whereas other fibres are simple unbranched varicose fibres (Wank and Neuhuber 2001). In addition to these thin-calibre afferents, there are thick-calibre afferents exhibiting complex branching features, not dissimilar to IGLEs, in the upper segment of the oesophagus (Dutsch et al. 1998; Wank and Neuhuber 2001). Most of these fibres abut and even penetrate the epithelium with small branches (Fig. 1b).

1.1.2 Spinal Afferents

Spinal afferents have their cell bodies in the cervical and thoracic dorsal root ganglia, and central endings in the spinal dorsal horn, which may connect directly or indirectly with projection neurones that provide central input to sensory and reflex pathways. Specifically, the spinal afferent innervation of the gastro-oesophageal region spans from the cervical (C1) to the upper lumbar (L2) segment of the spinal cord (Clerc 1983; Brtva et al. 1989; Khurana and Petras 1991; Collman et al. 1992) via the thoracic spinal and greater splanchnic nerves. In the cat, labelled gastric cells were found in the dorsal root ganglia T4–L2 or T4–L1 (Brtva et al. 1989) and in the dog, labelling with horseradish peroxidase indicated two peak innervation fields for the cervical (C2–C6) and thoracic (T2–T4) parts of the oesophagus (Khurana and Petras 1991). Spinal afferents from the lower oesophageal sphincter extend from T1–L2 (Clerc 1983). Intestinofugal neurones with cell bodies in the myenteric plexus exist in the stomach and intestines (Furness et al. 2000) and project with spinal afferents from the gut to the coeliac ganglia and occasionally to the spinal cord. These neurones are responsible for reflex control of motility, but their contribution to sensory function would be indirect. It is not known if oesophagofugal neurones exist that project with thoracic sympathetic nerves. Up to 90% of oesophageal spinal afferent neurones in rodents contain calcitonin gene-related peptide (CGRP) (Green and Dockray 1987; Uddman et al. 1995; Dutsch et al. 1998), in marked contrast to vagal afferents, and so CGRP has been used as a fairly specific marker for spinal afferent endings in the oesophagus.

With use of CGRP as a marker, a delicate network of fine varicose fibres in wholemount specimens of mucosa has been observed (Dutsch et al. 1998) (Fig. 1d). In contrast to vagal mucosal afferents, spinal afferents are distributed evenly along the length of the oesophagus (Wank and Neuhuber 2001). Spinal afferents also innervate the myenteric plexus, either terminating there (Clerc and Mazzia 1994; Mazzia and Clerc 1997; Dutsch et al. 1998) or passing to other structures. In contrast to IGLEs, the spinal afferent ganglionic endings are less numerous and complex with fine varicosities rather than lamellar structures (Dutsch et al. 1998) (Fig. 1c).

1.2 *Functional Properties of Gastro-oesophageal Afferent Endings*

1.2.1 Vagal Afferents

Gastro-oesophageal vagal afferents may be divided into three classes on the basis of the layer of the gut containing the receptive field. The location of the afferent endings described earlier is important in determining sensitivity of the individual afferents, as anatomical and electrophysiological data concur. They have been studied by in vivo and in vitro techniques in a number of species, including mouse, rat, guinea pig, opossum, ferret, cat, dog and sheep, not all of which are described here.

Mucosal receptors are generally silent at rest, but will develop activity after acute inflammation or damage to the columnar epithelium presumably due to release of mediators (e.g. 5-hydroxytryptamine, 5-HT) (Blackshaw and Grundy 1993b). Vagal mucosal receptors are sensitive to light stroking of the mucosa, generating a brief burst of action potentials each time the stimulus passes over the receptive field (Page and Blackshaw 1998; Page et al. 2002). They are insensitive to distension and contraction of the gastro-oesophageal wall, except under circumstances when distortion of the mucosa occurs as a consequence. Mucosal receptors in the oesophagus may provide feedback to reflexes controlling peristaltic contraction, but they do not reach conscious perception. In the stomach and intestines, mucosal receptors are considered important in the initiation of satiety, nausea and vomiting.

Tension receptors often have a resting discharge of action potentials that is modulated in phase with any ongoing contractions. They are mechanosensitive to contractions and distension with a slowly adapting linear relationship to wall tension (Blackshaw et al. 1987; Sengupta et al. 1989; Page and Blackshaw 1998; Page et al. 2002) (Fig. 2). Tension receptors signal the amplitude, pattern and direction of luminal contractions to the central nervous system, which is important in triggering reflexes controlling gastrointestinal function. Their stimulus-response functions saturate within the physiological range (Sengupta et al. 1989), as distinct from those of spinal afferents, which signal well above this range (Sengupta et al. 1990). The responses to distension of gastric tension receptors are important in signalling of food intake and sensations such as satiety and fullness. In the oesophagus, the responses of vagal tension receptors were thought only to play a regulatory role in the generation of secondary peristalsis or perception of a bolus. However, recently oesophageal vagal afferents in the guinea pig have been further subdivided into "low-threshold mechanoreceptors" and "nociceptors" which are

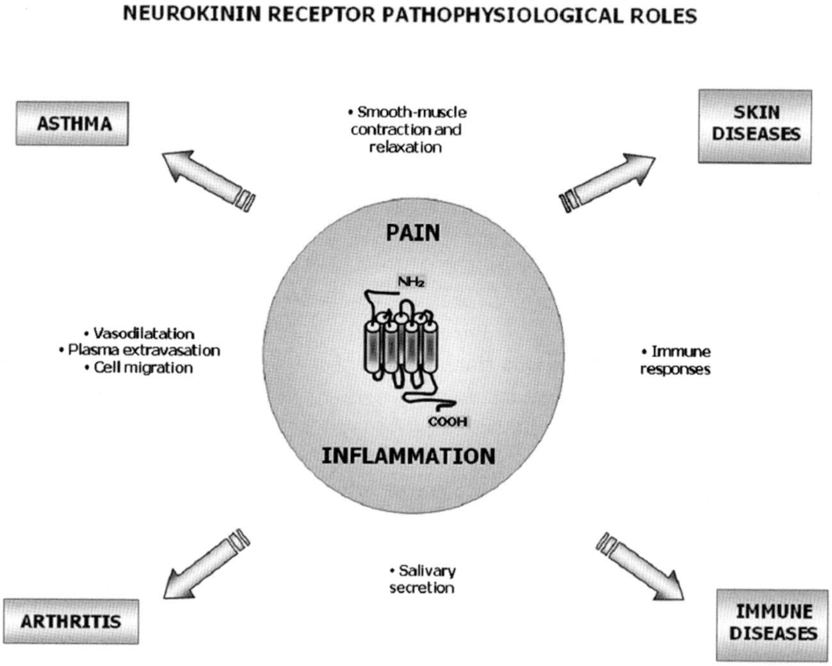

Fig. 2 Stimulus–response functions of vagal and spinal oesophageal afferents to distension in the opossum in vivo. Vagal responses saturate in the non-noxious range, but both classes of spinal afferents (wide dynamic range, and high threshold mechanonociceptor) respond well into the noxious range. The two populations of spinal afferents can be distinguished by their threshold. (Redrawn from Sengupta et al. 1989 and Sengupta et al. 1990)

activated by noxious mechanical force (Kollarik et al. 2007), and may play a role in signalling pain or the quality of pain.

Tension/mucosal receptors have so far been observed only in the striated oesophagus, not the stomach, of the ferret. They show mechanosensory responses of both tension receptors and mucosal receptors (Page and Blackshaw 1998). Tension/mucosal receptors would appear to have a spinal counterpart in the colonic muscular/mucosal pelvic nerve afferents observed in mice (Brierley et al. 2004). They may have a specialized role in the detection of a rapidly moving bolus of food and/or liquid along the oesophagus.

1.2.2 Spinal Afferents

Spinal afferents are generally considered to convey signals to the central nervous system that result in sensations such as discomfort and pain (Cervero 1994).

Low-threshold (tonic or wide dynamic range) mechanoreceptors respond to contractions and distension with a linear relationship to wall tension (Sengupta et al. 1990) (Fig. 2). In the oesophagus they are likely to contribute to a range of sensations, from the perception of bolus transit to mechanically induced pain. In the stomach they are likely to signal filling and give rise to sensations of fullness. Owing to the fact that they respond to gastric distension well into the noxious range, it is thought that it is these receptors that also contribute to sensations such as discomfort and pain, particularly in the presence of organ inflammation (Ozaki and Gebhart 2001).

High-threshold (phasic) mechanoreceptors have low resting activity and respond only to intensities of organ distension above approximately 40 mmHg, which would be painful in the stomach (Lee et al. 2004) but not necessarily in the oesophagus. Accordingly, they are considered mechanonociceptors (Sengupta et al. 1990; Cervero 1994; Ozaki and Gebhart 2001).

Other populations of spinal afferents have been described elsewhere in the gastrointestinal tract, including *mechanically insensitive afferents* (Coutinho et al. 2000; Brierley et al. 2005) and *mucosal receptors* (Lynn and Blackshaw 1999; Brierley et al. 2004), but their existence in the spinal innervation of the stomach and oesophagus is not yet established, despite compelling anatomical evidence for spinal mucosal endings (Clerc and Mazzia 1994; Dutsch et al. 1998).

2 Pharmacology of Gastro-oesophageal Afferents

The columnar epithelium of the small intestine is ideally suited to exocrine and endocrine secretion of endogenous mediators, as is the stomach. However, the squamous epithelium of the oesophagus has few secretory cells. Therefore, it needs to be remembered that their chemical environment, and therefore their pharmacological effects, may be quite different, although evidence to support this is mainly lacking. The pharmacological effects of the various receptors and channels on gastro-oesophageal afferents are described below and are summarized in Table 1, and we discuss evidence for how this may change in the diseased state. This is not intended to be an exhaustive list, but should provide the reader with the principles of excitatory and inhibitory modulation by receptors, and the ion channels involved in basic sensory function. For a review on ion channels involved in the regulation of excitability and axonal transmission, the reader is referred to Beyak and Vanner (2005).

2.1 Excitatory Receptors

In addition to *adenosine triphosphate* (ATP) release from viable cells, ATP is also released from damaged cells, making it a prime candidate for signalling of nociceptive events. It is also released from sympathetic and myenteric nerve terminals, and from mechanically deformed epithelia and endothelia. ATP activates ionotropic

Table 1 Summary of the published effects of receptor agonists/antagonists and receptor knockouts on the excitability of gastro-oesophageal afferents

Receptor/channel	Drug/intervention	Location	Effect	References	Comment
TRPV1	HCl	O	E/I	Kollarik et al. (2007)	Excites vagal "nociceptors"
	HCl	G-O	E	Page and Blackshaw (1998), Page et al. (2002)	Small proportion of afferents
	HCl	O	E	Sekizawa et al. (1999)	Small proportion of afferents
	Capsaicin	O	E	Sekizawa et al. (1999)	Small proportion of afferents
	Capsaicin	G-O	E	Page and Blackshaw (1998)	
	TRPV1−/−	G-O	I	Bielefeldt and Davis (2008)	
ASIC	Benzamil	G-O	I	Page et al. (2005a)	Greater effect on M than T
	Benzamil	O	I	Zagorodnyuk et al. (2003)	T and M
	ASIC1−/−	G-O	P	Page et al. (2004, 2005a)	Selective for T
	ASIC2−/−	G-O	I	Page et al. (2005a)	Selective for T
	ASIC3−/−	G-O	I	Page et al. (2005a)	
	ASIC3−/−	G-O	I	Bielefeldt and Davis (2008)	
Galanin	Galanin	G-O	I/P	Page et al. (2005b)	M, T and TM
Ghrelin	Ghrelin	G-O	I	Page et al. (2007d)	T in mouse, M in ferret
Bradykinin	Bradykinin	G-O	E	Page and Blackshaw (1998)	Only excites small proportion of afferents
	Bradykinin	O	E	Sengupta et al. (1992)	Vagal and splanchnic
5-HT	5-HT	G-O	E	Page and Blackshaw (1998)	Only excites small proportion of afferents
	5-HT	G	NE	Blackshaw and Grundy (1993a)	T afferents
	5-HT	G	E	Blackshaw and Grundy (1993b)	M afferents

(*continued*)

Table 1 (continued)

Receptor/channel	Drug/intervention	Location	Effect	References	Comment
Prosta-glandin	PGE_2	G-O	E	Page and Blackshaw (1998)	EP receptor agonist only excites a small proportion of afferents
iGluR	NMDA	G-O	P	Slattery et al. (2006)	NMDA receptor agonist
	AMPA	G-O	P	Slattery et al. (2006)	AMPA receptor agonist
	SYM-2081	G-O	P	Slattery et al. (2006)	Kainate receptor/M only
	Kynurenate	G-O	I	Slattery et al. (2006)	iGluR antagonist
	Various	G	I	Sengupta et al. (2004)	NMDA antagonists
	CNQX	G	I	Sengupta et al. (2004)	AMPA/kainate antagonist
mGluR	L-AP4	G-O	I	Page et al. (2005c)	Group III agonist
	(2*R*,4*R*)-APDC	G-O	I	Page et al. (2005c)	Group II agonist
	DHPG	G-O	NE	Page et al. (2005c)	Group I agonist
	MPEP/MTEP	G-O	I	Slattery et al. (2006), Young et al. (2007)	Group I antagonist
$GABA_B$	Baclofen	G-O	I	Page and Blackshaw (1999), Smid et al. (2001)	Baclofen inhibits M, T and a proportion of TM in vitro ferret
	Baclofen	G-O	NE	Zagorodnyuk et al. (2002)	Guinea pig
$GABA_A$	Muscimol	G	NE	Smid et al. (2001)	
Opioids	EMD61,753	G	I	Ozaki et al. (2000)	κ-Opioid agonist

(continued)

Table 1 (continued)

Receptor/channel	Drug/intervention	Location	Effect	References	Comment
	Morphine	G	NE	Ozaki et al. (2000)	μ-Opioid agonist
	SNC80	G	NE	Ozaki et al. (2000)	δ-Opioid agonist
Nitric oxide	L-NAME	G-O	P	Page et al. (2007b)	M receptors only
TRPV4	TRPV4−/−	G-O	NE	Brierley et al. (2008)	Colon-specific expression
P2X	α,β-meATP	G	E	Dang et al. (2005)	Gastric DRG and nodose
	ATP	G	E	Dang et al. (2005)	Gastric DRG and nodose
	α,β-meATP	G-O	E/P	Page and Blackshaw (1998), Page et al. (2000, 2002)	Potentiates M only in inflammation
	α,β-meATP	O	E	Zagorodnyuk et al. (2003)	Nodose, not jugular
	α,β-meATP	O	E	Yu et al. (2005)	

G gastric afferents, *O* oesophageal afferents, *G-O* gastro-oesophageal afferents, *E* excitation, *I* inhibition of response to mechanical stimuli, *P* potentiation of response to mechanical stimuli, *NE* no effect, *T* tension receptor, *M* mucosal receptor, *TM* tension/mucosal receptor, *TRPV1* transient receptor potential vanilloid receptor 1, *ASIC* acid-sensing ion channel, *5-HT* 5-hydroxytryptamine, *PGE*$_2$ prostaglandin E_2, *iGluR* ionotropic glutamate receptor, *NMDA* *N*-methyl D-aspartate, *AMPA* α-amino-3-hydroxy-5-methylisoxazoleproprionate, *mGluR* metabotropic glutamate receptor, *GABA* γ-aminobutyric acid, *DRG* dorsal root ganglion, *TRPV4* transient receptor potential vanilloid receptor 4, *α,β-meATP* α,β-methylene ATP, *CNQX* (6-cyano-7-nitroquinoxaline-2,3-dione, *L-AP4* L-(+)-2-Amino-4-phosphonobutyric acid, *L-NAME* NG-nitro-L-arginine methyl ester, *ATP* adenosine triphosphate, *(2R,4R)-APDC* (2R,4R)-4-Aminopyrrolidine-2,4-dicarboxylate, *MPEP* 2-Methyl-6-(phenylethynyl)pyridine, *MTEP* 3-((2-Methyl-1,3-thiazol-4-yl)ethynyl)pyridine, *DHPG* (RS)-3,5-Dihydroxyphenylglycine

(P2X) and metabotropic (P2Y) receptors, both of which are present in dorsal root and nodose ganglion neurones (Cook et al. 1997; Tominaga et al. 2001; Fong et al. 2002; Ruan and Burnstock 2003). ATP may have two types of effect on vagal and spinal gastrointestinal primary afferents: direct activation or sensitization to other stimuli (Kirkup et al. 1999; Page et al. 2000, 2002; Zagorodnyuk et al. 2003). Interestingly, the role of ATP in sensitization of gastro-oesophageal afferents may be more predominant after or during inflammation (Page et al. 2000; Dang et al. 2005). Vagal "nociceptive-like" fibres in the guinea-pig oesophagus have cell bodies in the nodose and jugular ganglia (Yu et al. 2005). Nodose "nociceptive-like" fibres are exclusively C-fibres sensitive to P2X receptor analogues, whereas jugular "nociceptive-like" fibres are both C- and Aδ-fibres which are insensitive to P2X receptor analogues (Yu et al. 2005), so purinergic pharmacology can in some circumstances distinguish afferent subtypes.

Adenosine is a breakdown product of ATP. Nothing is known about the effects of adenosine on gastro-oesophageal vagal or spinal afferents, but it has been shown that adenosine increases mesenteric nerve activity and intestinal motility in the rat through adenosine A_1 and A_{2B} receptors. Increased motor activity was responsible for part but not all of the adenosine-evoked excitation (Kirkup et al. 1998; Brunsden and Grundy 1999).

Bradykinin is a powerful algesic agent released during tissue damage which acts on bradykinin receptors (B_1–B_5). Bradykinin has been shown to have an excitatory effect on all subtypes of vagal and spinal afferents innervating the stomach and oesophagus (Sengupta et al. 1992; Page and Blackshaw 1998). These responses were shown in vitro to be resistant to blockade of smooth muscle contraction, indicating a direct action (Page and Blackshaw 1998), although many of the in vivo effects of bradykinin may be secondary to activation of afferents by potent contractile responses of smooth muscle (Sengupta et al. 1992)

Cholecystokinin (CCK) is released by nutrients from the small intestinal mucosa. CCK receptors have been reported in both the nodose ganglia and the dorsal root ganglia (Zhang et al. 1993; Moriarty et al. 1997; Broberger et al. 2000, 2001). It has been shown to have a direct excitatory effect on gastric vagal mucosal receptors (Blackshaw and Grundy 1990), but its effects on tension receptors are controversial, and may be indirect secondary to smooth muscle responses (Blackshaw and Grundy 1990). No reports exist on the action of CCK on spinal gastro-oesophageal afferents, but the action of CCK on a mixed population of afferents in the mesenteric nerves was abolished by chronic degeneration of vagal fibres, suggesting that these are the only targets for CCK (Richards et al. 1996).

5-Hydroxytryptamine (5-HT) is localized in enterochromaffin cells of the columnar epithelium, mast cells and enteric neurones. It is released from the gastrointestinal mucosa after a meal and may also be released in response to mechanical and chemical stimuli throughout the gastrointestinal tract. 5-HT receptors are classified into at least seven families of receptor subtypes (5-HT_{1-7}) (Hoyer and Martin 1997). Of these, so far only the 5-HT_3 receptor has been conclusively demonstrated to mediate actions on gastro-oesophageal afferents (Blackshaw and Grundy 1993b). However, there is some controversy as to the role of 5-HT_4

receptors (Hicks et al. 2001; Schikowski et al. 2002) in sensory function elsewhere in the gut, and the role of many other subtypes remains uninvestigated.

Ionotropic glutamate receptors (iGluRs) are ligand-gated cation channels that can be divided into three main groups: *N*-methyl D-aspartate (NMDA) receptors, α-amino-3-hydroxy-5-methylisoxazoleproprionate (AMPA) receptors and kainate receptors. There are several sources of glutamate, including the diet, intrinsic and extrinsic neurotransmission in the gut and also the epithelial cells. Slattery et al. (2006) have shown that AMPA and NMDA receptors are involved in the peripheral excitatory modulation of vagal afferent mechanosensitivity. These data in mouse complement findings of studies in ferret and rat, which suggest excitatory actions of glutamate on vagal afferents (Sengupta et al. 2004; Page et al. 2005c), although guinea-pig afferent endings in contrast lack functional receptors for glutamate (Zagorodnyuk et al. 2003). Expression of iGluRs in nodose ganglia has been demonstrated in several species with transport of the receptors towards the peripheral endings (Shigemoto et al. 1992; Chang et al. 2003; Slattery et al. 2006), suggesting a peripheral function. No reports exist on the effects of iGluR agonists and antagonists on gastro-oesophageal spinal afferents, but NMDA receptor antagonists have been shown to reduce responses to mechanical stimuli in pelvic and splanchnic afferents from the colon (McRoberts et al. 2001).

Prostaglandins are produced in a wide variety of cell types and blockade of prostaglandin synthesis is a common means to reduce pain and inflammation. Five classes of prostanoid receptors (DP, EP, FP, IP and TP receptors) have been identified and distinguished by rank order of agonist potency (e.g. PGE_2 acts at EP receptors). PGE_2 has been shown to directly excite a proportion of ferret gastro-oesophageal vagal afferents in vitro (Page and Blackshaw 1998), and sensory neurones in the nodose ganglia express receptors for PGE_2 (Ek et al. 1998). The effect of prostaglandins on spinal afferents in the gastro-oesophageal region is unknown; however, it has been shown that dorsal root ganglion neurones may be sensitized upon application of PGE_2 (Baccaglini and Hogan 1983; Nicol and Cui 1994; Gold et al. 1996).

Vanilloids, such as the hot chilli extract capsaicin, are well-established excitants of somatic nociceptors, giving rise to a burning sensation mediated through transient receptor potential vanilloid receptor 1 (TRPV1), which is also a natural receptor for heat and low pH (Caterina and Julius 2001). Capsaicin activates a proportion of all classes of vagal and spinal afferents throughout the gastrointestinal tract. An early report found that the majority of gastrointestinal afferents were activated by capsaicin (Longhurst et al. 1984), but recent reports have found that only 30% of vagal afferents (Blackshaw et al. 2000a) and 42% of nodose ganglion cells (Bielefeldt 2000) were activated. Gastric dorsal root ganglion neurones and nodose ganglion neurones both contain TRPV1 (Guo et al. 1999; Patterson et al. 2003) and expression of TRPV1 in gastric dorsal root ganglion neurones is increased upon acid insult of the gastric mucosa (Schicho et al. 2004). It has also been shown that mice lacking TRPV1 channels develop significantly less oesophagitis to acid exposure compared with wild-type mice (Fujino et al. 2006). In humans, it has been documented that oesophagitis leads to overexpression of

TRPV1 (Matthews et al. 2004). In the guinea pig, "non-nociceptive-like" oesophageal tension sensitive vagal afferents are distinguishable from "nociceptive-like" afferents not only by their saturable response to tension but also by the lack of response to capsaicin (Yu et al. 2005). In addition, "nociceptive-like" tension receptors in the oesophagus are stimulated by acid (Kollarik et al. 2007). In contrast, the responses of "non-nociceptive" tension receptors to acid are less well defined.

It is clear from studies of activation of central vagal neurones, and on reflex relaxation of the lower oesophageal sphincter, that intraoesophageal acid activates vagal reflexes (and therefore vagal afferents) (Blackshaw and Dent 1997; Partosoedarso and Blackshaw 1997; Medda et al. 2005). This reflex becomes sensitized with repeated exposure, possibly due to increased permeability of the squamous epithelium. This effect is mimicked by capsaicin, suggesting that the response to acid is mediated via TRPV1 (Blackshaw and Dent 1997; Partosoedarso and Blackshaw 1997). It is also clear that there is a component of the reflex mediated by splanchnic afferents that is resistant to vagotomy, and results in release of substance P from axon collaterals of these afferents either in the myenteric plexus or in the prevertebral ganglion (Smid et al. 1998). Thus, chronic splanchnic denervation in vivo abolishes the response of the isolated lower oesophageal sphincter to capsaicin subsequently in vitro (Staunton et al. 2000). In vitro studies of vagal afferents indicate that only a minority of fibres are sensitive to acid (Page and Blackshaw 1998; Page et al. 2002; Kollarik et al. 2007), indicating this reflex is initiated by only a few afferents.

2.2 Inhibitory Receptors

γ-Aminobutyric acid (GABA) exerts its effect through two ligand-gated channels, $GABA_A$ and $GABA_C$ receptors, and a metabotropic receptor, $GABA_B$, which acts through G proteins to regulate potassium and calcium channels. In vivo and in vitro recordings of ferret gastro-oesophageal vagal afferents showed that activation of $GABA_B$ receptors potently inhibited their mechanosensory stimulus-response relationships (Page and Blackshaw 1999; Partosoedarso et al. 2001; Smid et al. 2001). However, in the guinea pig although $GABA_B$ receptors are functionally expressed in the nodose ganglia they are not functionally expressed at the vagal afferent endings (Zagorodnyuk et al. 2002). These studies have stimulated clinical interest in the use of $GABA_B$ agonists as possible targets for the treatment of gastro-oesophageal reflux disease (GORD; see later). The ability of $GABA_B$ receptor agonists to reduce signalling of spinal afferents has so far only been demonstrated in the colon (Sengupta et al. 2002).

Galanin receptors fall into three types, each encoded by a different gene. GALR1 and GALR3 are inhibitory via actions on ion channels and adenylate cyclase, whereas GALR2 is excitatory, acting via phospholipase C. GALR1 and GALR2 have corresponding opposing actions on the mechanosensitivity of gastro-oesophageal vagal afferents, and there appears to be a role for endogenous galanin release in inhibitory modulation via GALR1 (Page et al. 2005b, 2007c)

Ghrelin is known for its inhibitory action on satiety signalling, which is mediated at least partly by actions on the inhibitory growth hormone secretagogue receptor GHS-1 on gastric afferents (Date et al. 2002). Its effects on different subtypes of afferents differ with species, such that in ferret, mucosal afferents are its major target for inhibition, whilst in the mouse, it prefers tension receptors (Page et al. 2007d). Either of these actions on gastric afferents could explain the inhibitory effect of ghrelin on satiety signalling from the stomach. The consequences of the inhibitory action of ghrelin on oesophageal afferents are not yet clear. An action of endogenous ghrelin was revealed by potentiation of afferent mechanosensitivity by a selective GHS-1R antagonist, and this was restricted to gastric afferents.

Metabotropic glutamate receptors (mGluRs) may be divided into eight molecular subtypes, which currently fall into three pharmacological and functional groups: members of group I (mGluR1 and mGluR5) are excitatory, whereas members of group II (mGluR2 and mGluR3) and group III (mGluR4, mGluR6, mGluR7 and mGluR8) are inhibitory to neuronal function. Studies in mouse and ferret indicate that group II and III receptor agonists inhibit mechanical sensitivity of vagal gastro-oesophageal afferents in a manner similar to $GABA_B$ ligands (Page et al. 2005c). A group III antagonist increased mechanosensitivity, indicating a role for endogenous glutamate. In addition, mGluR5 antagonists significantly reduce mechanosensitivity of gastro-oesophageal vagal afferents (Slattery et al. 2006; Young et al. 2007), indicating opposing excitatory and inhibitory roles for endogenous glutamate, which is probably released from the afferent endings themselves. Expression of all mGluRs in nodose ganglia has been demonstrated in several species (Page et al. 2005c), although human and ferret lack expression of mGluR3 and mGluR6 (Page et al. 2005c). Again, like $GABA_B$, there appears to be potential for mGluR targeting in the treatment of GORD, which is discussed later. The effect of mGluR agonists and antagonists in reducing signalling of spinal gastro-oesophageal afferents has not been explored, although colonic high-threshold afferents are potently inhibited by mGluR5 antagonists (Lindstrom et al. 2008).

Opioids act on three opioid receptors (μ,δ and κ). Ozaki et al. (2000) have shown that κ-opioid but not μ- or δ-opioid receptor agonists modulate vagal afferent fibres innervating the stomach. κ-opioid receptor agonists attenuated afferent fibre responses to gastric distension. This is confirmed in ferret oesophageal afferents, where the κ-opioid receptor agonist ICI 199441 reduced the response of oesophageal vagal tension receptors. However, the μ-opioid receptor agonist DAMGO also reduced the sensitivity of oesophageal tension receptors. In agreement with Ozaki et al. (2000), we found that the δ-opioid receptor agonist SNC80 has no effect on oesophageal vagal afferent mechanosensitivity (unpublished data). The effect of opioid receptor agonists on gastro-oesophageal spinal afferents is unknown, although their effects on colonic spinal afferents are comparable with the effects found by Ozaki et al. (Sengupta et al. 1996).

Somatostatin has a potent inhibitory effect on the mechanosensitivity and chemosensitivity of intestinal afferents via somatostatin 2 receptors (Booth et al. 2001), which translates to inhibition of pain in human disease by a somatostatin analogue (Schwetz et al. 2004). They may therefore have potential in treatment of oesophageal pain, but this remains to be evaluated.

2.3 Mechanosensory Ion Channels

The Deg/ENaC family of ion channels, including ASIC1, ASIC2 and ASIC3, are candidate mechanotransducers in visceral and somatic sensory neurones, although each channel may play a different role in different sensory pathways. Whereas mechanosensitivity of colonic afferents was potently reduced by the non-selective Deg/ENaC blocker benzamil, gastro-oesophageal afferents were only marginally inhibited (Page et al. 2007a). Genetic deletion of ASIC1 led to an increase in the mechanical sensitivity of all gastro-oesophageal afferents. Deletion of ASIC2 increased mechanosensitivity in mucosal receptors, yet decreased mechanosensitivity in tension receptors. In ASIC3−/− mice, tension receptors had markedly reduced mechanosensitivity, but mucosal receptors were unaffected, showing that different contributions of these channels towards mechanosensitivity occurs in different subtypes (Page et al. 2005a). Moreover, ASIC1 appears to make no positive contribution to mechanosensitivity at all (Page et al. 2004).

In addition to the roles of transient receptor potential channels in transducing acid sensitivity of afferents discussed above, there is also evidence that they may contribute to mechanosensory function. TRPV1 null mutant mice have reduced mechanosensitivity of jejunal and colonic afferents (Rong et al. 2004; Jones et al. 2005), but as yet there is no evidence for their role in gastro-oesophageal afferents. Likewise, transient receptor potential vanilloid receptor 4 makes a major contribution to colonic nociceptive afferents, but no contribution towards vagal afferent function (Brierley et al. 2008). From studies on mechanosensory ion channels it is emerging that each class of afferent fibre throughout the gastrointestinal tract has a signature of expression of a range of channels, which probably contributes significantly to their specialized mechanosensory function.

2.4 Inflammatory Pharmacology

Release of many of the excitatory substances mentioned already is increased in inflammatory conditions, and therefore their acute effects on afferents are relevant to inflammatory sensitization. There may also be chronic changes in gastro-oesophageal afferents after inflammation that may alter their sensitivity to a variety of stimuli. With use of a ferret acute oesophagitis model, it has been shown that the mechanosensitivity of vagal oesophageal mucosal receptors is significantly reduced in inflammation compared with controls (Page et al. 2000). This correlates with human data discussed later that show a lack of correlation between inflammation and symptoms. As touched upon earlier, the effects of the P2X agonist α,β-methylene ATP (α,β-meATP) on mechanosensitivity of ferret oesophageal vagal mucosal receptors is altered in inflammation. α,β-meATP had no effect on the mechanosensitivity of mucosal receptors in control animals, but significantly increased the response to mucosal stroking in the inflamed oesophagus (Page et al. 2000). In rats, both splanchnic gastric dorsal root ganglion and vagal gastric nodose ganglion neurones show an increase in excitability in gastric ulceration and inflammation (Dang et al. 2005). In addition, the proportion of gastric dorsal root ganglion and nodose ganglion neurones that responded to α,β-meATP significantly increased (Dang et al. 2005). In reflux-induced inflammation in the rat, the expression of TRPV1 in nodose ganglion and dorsal root ganglion neurones was significantly increased (Banerjee et al. 2007). Using an ovalbumin-sensitized model in guinea pig, Yu et al. (2007) showed that activation of oesophageal mast cells caused sensitization of vagal afferent responses to distension via histamine H1 receptors. There are therefore many candidates for changes in sensitivity of gastro-oesophageal vagal and spinal afferents in the clinical setting of GORD, which is discussed later.

3 Oesophageal Symptoms in Humans

3.1 Stimuli and Sensory Perception

Unlike the abdominal and pelvic viscera, the oesophagus is not generally associated with symptoms of fullness, satiety or nausea. Instead, sensations are more closely aligned with those that may be elicited from mucous membranes such as the oral cavity, such as luminal contact, burning, distension and pain, but are far less well-defined. It is clear that mechanosensory responses of oesophageal afferents reach conscious perception, because we perceive bolus transit after swallowing and balloon distension in experimental studies. Perception of chemical stimuli is chiefly to acid. How the two types of stimuli relate to one another is described below. Which pathways mediate oesophageal sensations (vagal or spinal) is difficult to determine because bilateral spinal or vagal transections in humans at the corresponding level are invariably fatal, and the basic studies described earlier do not provide clear distinctions in the adequate stimuli between pathways.

Clinically, oesophageal pain is most often caused by acid reflux from the stomach. A recent systematic epidemiological review of GORD estimated its prevalence at 10–20%, defined by occurrence of symptoms at least weekly (Dent et al. 2005), and it is therefore a major clinical problem. Different forms of pain are evoked by oesophageal acid, including heartburn and non-cardiac chest pain (NCCP). Despite the widespread nature of oesophageal pain, its cause is often difficult to ascertain. Localization of the sensation is very poor, leading to a significant number of patients with angina-like pain undergoing coronary angiography for investigation of possible cardiovascular origin of the pain (Richter 1991a, b). Approximately half of patients with chest pain in the absence of cardiac disease are diagnosed with GORD, and show symptom improvement with acid-suppressive treatment (Bautista et al. 2004). GORD may be revealed diagnostically by the positive response of patients to acid-suppressive treatment, or by reproduction of symptoms with a provocative oesophageal acid perfusion test (to mimic gastro-oesophageal acid reflux) and/or prolonged ambulatory oesophageal pH monitoring to show that excessive oesophageal acid exposure occurs (Janssens et al. 1986; Janssens and Vantrappen 1987; Hewson et al. 1989; Richter 1991a, b). The angina-like sensation that NCCP patients report is quite different from the heartburn normally associated with GORD (Janssens and Vantrappen 1987; Richter 1991b). This implies that these different sensations may be mediated by different populations of primary afferents, but we cannot yet reconcile clinical observations with basic science data. Oesophageal motor patterns may be altered by luminal acid, but are unlikely to be the cause of symptoms, or contribute to the type of pain experienced (Kjellen and Tibbling 1985). The duration of each acid exposure would appear to be closely correlated with the intensity of sensation (Smith et al. 1989). Oesophageal balloon distension may also be used as a provocative test for NCCP, and even in these cases pain is purely related to balloon volume, there being no correlation with contractions triggered secondary to inflation (Richter et al. 1986). Furthermore, pain is not necessarily correlated with muscle tension during oesophageal balloon distension (Paterson et al. 1991). This may be reflected in the finding that the edrophonium-induced oesophageal contraction test may have poor sensitivity for NCCP when used alone (Janssens and Vantrappen 1987). NCCP would therefore seem to be characterized by a multiple sensitivity of the oesophagus to stimuli acting on the epithelium and to those causing deformation of the muscle, although its primary stimulus is usually refluxed acid.

Other, less common contributors to oesophageal pain and symptoms in the clinic are discussed in detail elsewhere (Kahrilas 2000), and include achalasia, which is a disease of failed lower sphincter relaxation and aperistalsis. Diffuse oesophageal spasm, an equally rare disease, is defined by non-propagated oesophageal contractions. Non-specific motility disorders, including nutcracker oesophagus and hypertensive lower oesophageal sphincter, are more prevalent. Nutcracker oesophagus is a condition characterized by very high amplitude (more than 200 mmHg) oesophageal peristaltic contractions that give rise to pain (Agrawal et al. 2006). Recent evidence from high resolution ultrasound studies suggests specific contraction of the longitudinal muscle is most closely associated with pain episodes in many conditions (Mittal et al. 2005).

3.2 Classification of Disease According to Symptoms

In contrast to the often poor predictive value of symptoms in NCCP, patients reporting heartburn are more readily diagnosed as suffering from GORD. In GORD there is controversy as to whether or not patients undergo a sensitization of the oesophagus due to repeated acid exposure, which may relate to the performance of tests at different stages of severity of the disease. The pain associated with reflux disease has a major impact on quality of life regardless of the presence or absence of oesophageal erosions. The correlation or lack thereof of symptoms with oesophagitis has given rise to several subclassifications of disease. Thus, *functional heartburn* is characterized by heartburn in the absence of both oesophagitis and increased acid exposure (Fass and Tougas 2002). *Non-erosive reflux disease* is characterized by no oesophagitis but increased acid exposure (Fass et al. 2001). *Erosive reflux disease* is characterized by oesophagitis and increased acid exposure. NCCP may involve erosive or non-erosive reflux disease, but with a different quality to the pain than heartburn (Bautista et al. 2004). Some patients diagnosed with erosive reflux disease may have severe erosions and even metaplasia (Barrett's oesophagus) with few or no symptoms of oesophageal pain at the time of presentation (Johnson et al. 1987). These patients may indeed have oesophageal hyposensitivity, whereas many patients with non-erosive reflux disease and functional heartburn have oesophageal hypersensitivity. Interestingly, a study of the hypersensitivity seen in NCCP shows that it may be related to increased sensitivity of the afferent pathway or to hypervigilance (a central phenomenon) in two distinct subgroups of patients (Hobson et al. 2006).

3.3 Pharmacological Studies of Oesophageal Pain in Humans

Although pharmacological studies of oesophageal pain in humans are limited by which drugs can be used, some have shown that candidate mechanisms identified in basic studies have a role to play, but none have yet translated to a treatment for pain. They include NMDA receptors and prostaglandins, which specifically play a role in the development of hypersensitivity after oesophageal acid exposure (Sarkar et al. 2003; Willert et al. 2004). On the other hand, NK-1 tachykinin receptors were found not to play a role in human oesophageal hypersensitivity (Willert et al. 2007), in contrast with their important role in somatic pain models in animals (De Felipe et al. 1998). Although it is not possible to determine the site of action of these drugs in humans, they may undergo both peripheral and central sensitization after oesophageal acid perfusion (Smith et al. 1989; Willert et al. 2007).

3.4 Sensory Involvement in Motor Dysfunction

In addition to NCCP and GORD, other gastrointestinal disorders, such as dysphagia, are often characterized by increased oesophageal sensitivity (Decktor et al. 1990; Clouse et al. 1991). In the case of dysphagia, although it is classically regarded as a motor disorder, symptoms are sometimes reported in the absence of any primary peristaltic defect (Decktor et al. 1990). However, secondary (distension-induced) peristalsis is very often disturbed in patients with non-obstructive dysphagia and also in those with GORD (Schoeman and Holloway 1994, 1995). Thus, oesophageal sensory dysfunction may have more far-reaching effects than altered pain thresholds, and may lead to disturbances of motor function.

4 Origins of Gastro-oesophageal Reflux Disease

4.1 Current Treatment Does Not Relate to Cause

GORD is currently managed mainly by inhibition of acid secretion by parietal cells of the gastric epithelium using proton pump inhibitors. This is despite the fact that gastric acid secretion is actually normal in most reflux disease patients, so the problem is that acid is in the wrong place at the wrong time. Proton pump inhibitor therapy is unsuccessful in approximately 30% of patients (Fass 2007), either because of incomplete acid suppression or because of symptoms produced by non-acid or weak-acid reflux. A treatment that attacks the fundamental cause of reflux would be expected to provide a better success rate, and of course be more appropriate to the cause of the disease.

The primary cause of GORD is disordered control of the gastro-oesophageal reflux barrier. This barrier is composed of an internal lower oesophageal sphincter and an external sphincter formed by the crural diaphragm . The two sphincters briefly and simultaneously relax to allow bolus passage during oesophageal peristalsis. Brief relaxation also occurs prior to gastro-oesophageal reflux, known as transient lower oesophageal sphincter relaxation (TLOSR). TLOSRs normally allow belching to vent gas, during which some gastric acid may reflux simultaneously, but not normally enough to cause damage to the oesophageal mucosa. TLOSRs, unlike swallow-induced relaxations, are independent of oesophageal body motor activity, and have significantly longer duration (Mittal et al. 1995), from a few seconds to more than 30 s (Holloway et al. 1995). Importantly, TLOSRs are normally selective for gas reflux (Wyman et al. 1990), but the sensory mechanisms underlying selectivity remain unknown. Up to 90% of acid reflux episodes in asymptomatic controls and GORD patients are via TLOSRs (Dent et al. 1988). The development of most subtypes of GORD described above is therefore dependent upon factors that alter the rate of TLOSR and the physical (liquid vs. gas) and chemical (acid vs. neutral) composition of refluxate.

4.2 *Neural Pathways and Pharmacology of Reflux*

Early evidence from dog studies showed that TLOSRs are mediated via a vagal pathway, because they are abolished by vagal cooling (Martin et al. 1986). These authors also showed that a central mechanism was likely because of the abolition of TLOSR by anaesthesia (Cox et al. 1988), and human studies determined that they were absent during sleep (Freidin et al. 1991). TLOSRs are triggered by meals (Dent et al. 1988), but which meal components are involved and the receptor mechanisms responsible remain elusive. The trigger zone for TLOSR is localized in the proximal (cardia) portion of the stomach (Franzi et al. 1990). As discussed earlier, vagal tension receptors are located in this part of the stomach musculature. These vagal afferents have central terminals in the nucleus tractus solitarius (Young et al. 2008) where they synapse with other neurones which are believed to belong to a central programme generator (Mittal et al. 1995). There are several simultaneous outputs from the programme. First is a brief and powerful activation of vagal motor neurones (in the adjacent dorsal vagal nucleus) projecting to the lower oesophageal sphincter, which activate inhibitory motor neurones of the enteric nervous system, leading to smooth muscle relaxation. Second is a suppression of oesophageal body peristalsis (Pouderoux et al. 2003), presumably due to interruption of excitatory vagal output. Third is a suppression of motor output to the crural diaphragm leading to opening of the external striated muscle sphincter (Martin et al. 1992; Mittal et al. 1995; Mittal and Balaban 1997).

$GABA_B$ receptor agonists potently inhibit TLOSR and thus reflux in animal models (Blackshaw et al. 1999; Lehmann et al. 1999). This has provoked intense clinical and basic interest. These studies showed that a range of $GABA_B$ receptor agonists inhibited TLOSR, in some cases with complete suppression of TLOSR and thus gastro-oesophageal reflux. $GABA_B$ receptors are present at several points along the TLOSR pathway. Studies on vagal afferents described earlier indicate that these drugs act at the point of initiation of TLOSR by gastric distension. However, $GABA_B$ receptors are expressed by vagal afferent cell bodies in the nodose ganglion (Smid et al. 2001), so they may also act at their central endings in the brain stem. This results in reduced responses of brain stem neurones to gastric distension (Partosoedarso et al. 2001). $GABA_B$ receptors are also present on vagal motor neurones (McDermott et al. 2001) and influence motor outflow to the lower oesophageal sphincter directly (Blackshaw et al. 2000b; Smid and Blackshaw 2000).

Clearly there is potential for actions of $GABA_B$ receptors at numerous peripheral and central sites along the TLOSR pathway. However, the most important site of action is likely to be on the afferent pathway that triggers TLOSR, rather than the motor pathway that relaxes smooth muscle. This is evident from the fact that

$GABA_B$ receptor agonism reduces the frequency of occurrence of TLOSR, but not the depth or duration of lower oesophageal sphincter relaxation (Blackshaw et al. 1999; Lehmann et al. 1999). In humans, the $GABA_B$ agonist baclofen potently inhibits TLOSR and reflux in healthy volunteers (Lidums et al. 2000), and in reflux disease patients (Zhang et al. 2002), which may suggest its use as a treatment. However, baclofen suffers from a number of drawbacks, such as central nervous side effects and cardiovascular contraindications. Clinical trials are currently showing promise with novel $GABA_B$ receptor agonists with peripherally restricted actions. What these basic and clinical studies tell us is that vagal mechanoreceptors in the proximal stomach may now be the most important cellular target in GORD, rather than the parietal cell.

The effects of mGluR on vagal afferents in vitro described earlier have translated to corresponding responses in vivo. Group III agonists caused inhibition of TLOSR in ferrets (notably mGluR8), and group I (mGluR5) antagonists potently inhibited TLOSR in both dogs and ferrets (Frisby et al. 2005; Jensen et al. 2005). Experiments using nucleus of the tractus solitarius recordings in vivo indicate that mGluR5 effects are most likely on the peripheral endings of vagal afferents, but some central actions along excitatory pathways are evident (Young et al. 2007). These results in animal models in turn have translated to early findings in humans, which demonstrate the possibility for clinical use of mGluR5 antagonists in treatment of GORD (Addex-Pharmaceuticals 2007).

Cannabinoids are able to evoke potent inhibition of TLOSR without central nervous system side effects. This effect was not attributable to effects on vagal afferents (Lehmann et al. 2002), suggesting an action on the central programme generator for TLOSR. Although cannabinoids are promising for treatment of emesis and pain, it remains to be seen if they have potential in the treatment of GORD.

CCK receptors would appear to contribute to the triggering of TLOSR from studies in both dogs (Boulant et al. 1994, 1997) and humans (Boeckxstaens et al. 1998). These showed that a significant decrease in TLOSR occurred after CCK1 receptor antagonism. Further development of CCK1 receptor antagonists for GORD has not been evident, presumably because of their side effects on other systems relying on CCK signalling.

Nitric oxide plays an important role in lower oesophageal sphincter relaxation in a number of species. Effects of nitric oxide synthase inhibitors on TLOSR have been observed in dogs (Boulant et al. 1994) and humans (Hirsch et al. 1998), but their site of action is not yet known. It is worth noting that they do not affect the depth of lower oesophageal sphincter relaxation at the doses used in humans, and may therefore act on the trigger mechanism rather than the motor pathway, contrary to expectations. The clinical utility of nitric oxide synthase inhibitors in GORD is questionable owing to the presence of side effects on cardiovascular function and elsewhere in the gastrointestinal tract.

Other receptors, such as 5-HT, opioid, and NMDA receptors, have all been shown to play a role in the modulation of triggering of TLOSR (Rouzade et al. 1996; Penagini and Bianchi 1997; Lehmann and Branden 2001; Hirsch et al. 2002), but either the effects are marginal or the target is associated with too many side effects. The site of action to inhibit TLOSR of drugs acting on these receptors is not known, but if it were feasible to direct treatments peripherally this could improve their profile in some cases. In this context there are documented actions of 5-HT_3 and NMDA receptors at vagal afferent endings (Blackshaw and Grundy 1993b; Slattery et al. 2006) as well as in the central nervous system.

5 Conclusions

Data on the structure, function and effects of gastro-oesophageal afferents are abundant in the literature. They help to explain the way in which drug treatments inhibit the triggering of gastro-oesophageal reflux, and point towards new opportunities in this area. In this respect there is optimism for the successful treatment of oesophageal pain caused by excessive acid reflux. The mechanisms by which vagal and spinal oesophageal afferents are activated and sensitized by mechanical and chemical stimuli to give rise to pain, and which pathways or subtypes are involved remain elusive.

Acknowledgement L.A.B. is supported by a National Health and Medical Research Council of Australia Senior Research fellowship.

References

Addex-Pharmaceuticals (2007) ADX10059 may be a potential treatment for patients with gastro-esophageal reflux. Inpharma 1:10–10

Agrawal A, Hila A, Tutuian R, Mainie I, Castell DO (2006) Clinical relevance of the nutcracker esophagus: suggested revision of criteria for diagnosis. J Clin Gastroenterol 40:504–509

Baccaglini PI, Hogan PG (1983) Some rat sensory neurons in culture express characteristics of differentiated pain sensory cells. Proc Natl Acad Sci USA 80:594–598

Banerjee B, Medda BK, Lazarova Z, Bansal N, Shaker R, Sengupta JN (2007) Effect of reflux-induced inflammation on transient receptor potential vanilloid one (TRPV1) expression in primary sensory neurons innervating the oesophagus of rats. Neurogastroenterol Motil 19:681–691

Bautista J, Fullerton H, Briseno M, Cui H, Fass R (2004) The effect of an empirical trial of high-dose lansoprazole on symptom response of patients with non-cardiac chest pain – a randomized, double-blind, placebo-controlled, crossover trial. Aliment Pharmacol Ther 19:1123–1130

Berthoud HR, Powley TL (1992) Vagal afferent innervation of the rat fundic stomach: morphological characterization of the gastric tension receptor. J Comp Neurol 319:261–276

Berthoud HR, Patterson LM, Neumann F, Neuhuber WL (1997) Distribution and structure of vagal afferent intraganglionic laminar endings (IGLEs) in the rat gastrointestinal tract. Anat Embryol (Berl) 195:183–191

Beyak MJ, Vanner S (2005) Inflammation-induced hyperexcitability of nociceptive gastrointestinal DRG neurones: the role of voltage-gated ion channels. Neurogastroenterol Motil 17:175–186

Bielefeldt K (2000) Differential effects of capsaicin on rat visceral sensory neurons. Neuroscience 101:727–736

Bielefeldt K, Davis BM (2008) Differential effects of ASIC3 and TRPV1 deletion on gastroesophageal sensation in mice. Am J Physiol Gastrointest Liver Physiol 294:G130–G138

Blackshaw LA, Dent J (1997) Lower oesophageal sphincter responses to noxious oesophageal chemical stimuli in the ferret: involvement of tachykinin receptors. J Auton Nerv Syst 66:189–200

Blackshaw LA, Grundy D (1990) Effects of cholecystokinin (CCK-8) on two classes of gastroduodenal vagal afferent fibre. J Auton Nerv Syst 31:191–201

Blackshaw LA, Grundy D (1993a) Effects of 5-hydroxytryptamine (5-HT) on the discharge of vagal mechanoreceptors and motility in the upper gastrointestinal tract of the ferret. J Auton Nerv Syst 45:51–59

Blackshaw LA, Grundy D (1993b) Effects of 5-hydroxytryptamine on discharge of vagal mucosal afferent fibres from the upper gastrointestinal tract of the ferret. J Auton Nerv Syst 45:41–50

Blackshaw LA, Grundy D, Scratcherd T (1987) Vagal afferent discharge from gastric mechanoreceptors during contraction and relaxation of the ferret corpus. J Auton Nerv Syst 18:19–24

Blackshaw LA, Staunton E, Lehmann A, Dent J (1999) Inhibition of transient LES relaxations and reflux in ferrets by GABA receptor agonists. Am J Physiol 277:G867–G874

Blackshaw LA, Page AJ, Partosoedarso ER (2000a) Acute effects of capsaicin on gastrointestinal vagal afferents. Neuroscience 96:407–416

Blackshaw LA, Smid SD, O'Donnell TA, Dent J (2000b) GABA(B) receptor-mediated effects on vagal pathways to the lower oesophageal sphincter and heart. Br J Pharmacol 130:279–288

Boeckxstaens GE, Hirsch DP, Fakhry N, Holloway RH, D'Amato M, Tytgat GN (1998) Involvement of cholecystokininA receptors in transient lower esophageal sphincter relaxations triggered by gastric distension. Am J Gastroenterol 93:1823–1828

Booth CE, Kirkup AJ, Hicks GA, Humphrey PP, Grundy D (2001) Somatostatin sst(2) receptor-mediated inhibition of mesenteric afferent nerves of the jejunum in the anesthetized rat. Gastroenterology 121:358–369

Boulant J, Fioramonti J, Dapoigny M, Bommelaer G, Bueno L (1994) Cholecystokinin and nitric oxide in transient lower esophageal sphincter relaxation to gastric distention in dogs. Gastroenterology 107:1059–1066

Boulant J, Mathieu S, D'Amato M, Abergel A, Dapoigny M, Bommelaer G (1997) Cholecystokinin in transient lower oesophageal sphincter relaxation due to gastric distension in humans. Gut 40:575–581

Brierley SM, Jones RC 3rd, Gebhart GF, Blackshaw LA (2004) Splanchnic and pelvic mechanosensory afferents signal different qualities of colonic stimuli in mice. Gastroenterology 127:166–178

Brierley SM, Carter R, Jones W, Xu LJ, Robinson DR, Hicks GA, Gebhart GE, Blackshaw LA (2005) Differential chemosensory function and receptor expression of splanchnic and pelvic colonic afferents in mice. J Physiol (Lond) 567:267–281

Brierley SM, Page AJ, Hughes PA, Adam B, Liebregts T, Cooper NJ, Holtmann G, Liedtke W, Blackshaw L (2008) A selective role for TRPV4 ion channels in visceral sensory pathways. Gastroenterology 134(7):2059–2069

Broberger C, Farkas-Szallasi T, Szallasi A, Lundberg JM, Hokfelt T, Wiesenfeld-Hallin Z, Xu XJ (2000) Increased spinal cholecystokinin activity after systemic resiniferatoxin: electrophysiological and in situ hybridization studies. Pain 84:21–28

Broberger C, Holmberg K, Shi TJ, Dockray G, Hokfelt T (2001) Expression and regulation of cholecystokinin and cholecystokinin receptors in rat nodose and dorsal root ganglia. Brain Res 903:128–140

Brtva RD, Iwamoto GA, Longhurst JC (1989) Distribution of cell bodies for primary afferent fibers from the stomach of the cat. Neurosci Lett 105:287–293

Brunsden AM, Grundy D (1999) Sensitization of visceral afferents to bradykinin in rat jejunum in vitro. J Physiol 521(Pt 2):517–527

Caterina MJ, Julius D (2001) The vanilloid receptor: a molecular gateway to the pain pathway. Ann Rev Neurosci 24:487–517

Cervero F (1994) Sensory innervation of the viscera: peripheral basis of visceral pain. Physiol Rev 74:95–138

Chang HM, Liao WC, Lue JH, Wen CY, Shieh JY (2003) Upregulation of NMDA receptor and neuronal NADPH-d/NOS expression in the nodose ganglion of acute hypoxic rats. J Chem Neuroanat 25:137–147

Clerc N (1983) Afferent innervation of the lower oesophageal sphincter of the cat. An HRP study. J Auton Nerv Syst 9:623–636

Clerc N, Mazzia C (1994) Morphological relationships of choleragenoid horseradish peroxidase-labeled spinal primary afferents with myenteric ganglia and mucosal associated lymphoid tissue in the cat esophagogastric junction. J Comp Neurol 347:171–186

Clouse RE, McCord GS, Lustman PJ, Edmundowicz SA (1991) Clinical correlates of abnormal sensitivity to intraesophageal balloon distension. Dig Dis Sci 36:1040–1045

Collman PI, Tremblay L, Diamant NE (1992) The distribution of spinal and vagal sensory neurons that innervate the esophagus of the cat. Gastroenterology 103:817–822

Cook SP, Vulchanova L, Hargreaves KM, Elde R, McCleskey EW (1997) Distinct ATP receptors on pain-sensing and stretch-sensing neurons. Nature 387:505–508

Coutinho SV, Su X, Sengupta JN, Gebhart GF (2000) Role of sensitized pelvic nerve afferents from the inflamed rat colon in the maintenance of visceral hyperalgesia. Prog Brain Res 129:375–387

Cox MR, Martin CJ, Dent J, Westmore M (1988) Effect of general anaesthesia on transient lower oesophageal sphincter relaxations in the dog. Aust N Z J Surg 58:825–830

Dang K, Bielfeldt K, Lamb K, Gebhart GF (2005) Gastric ulcers evoke hyperexcitability and enhance P2X receptor function in rat gastric sensory neurons. J Neurophysiol 93:3112–3119

Date Y, Murakami N, Toshinai K, Matsukura S, Niijima A, Matsuo H, Kangawa K, Nakazato M (2002) The role of the gastric afferent vagal nerve in ghrelin-induced feeding and growth hormone secretion in rats. Gastroenterology 123:1120–1128

De Felipe C, Herrero JF, O'Brien JA, Palmer JA, Doyle CA, Smith AJ, Laird JM, Belmonte C, Cervero F, Hunt SP (1998) Altered nociception, analgesia and aggression in mice lacking the receptor for substance P. Nature 392:394–397

Decktor DL, Allen ML, Robinson M (1990) Esophageal motility, heartburn, and gastroesophageal reflux: variations in clinical presentation of esophageal dysphagia. Dysphagia 5:211–215

Dent J, Holloway RH, Toouli J, Dodds WJ (1988) Mechanisms of lower oesophageal sphincter incompetence in patients with symptomatic gastrooesophageal reflux. Gut 29:1020–1028

Dent J, El-Serag HB, Wallander MA, Johansson S (2005) Epidemiology of gastro-oesophageal reflux disease: a systematic review. Gut 54:710–717

Dutsch M, Eichhorn U, Worl J, Wank M, Berthoud HR, Neuhuber WL (1998) Vagal and spinal afferent innervation of the rat esophagus: a combined retrograde tracing and immunocytochemical study with special emphasis on calcium-binding proteins. J Comp Neurol 398:289–307

Ek M, Kurosawa M, Lundeberg T, Ericsson A (1998) Activation of vagal afferents after intravenous injection of interleukin-1beta: role of endogenous prostaglandins. J Neurosci 18:9471–9479

Fass R (2007) Proton-pump inhibitor therapy in patients with gastro-oesophageal reflux disease: putative mechanisms of failure. Drugs 67:1521–1530

Fass R, Tougas G (2002) Functional heartburn: the stimulus, the pain, and the brain. Gut 51: 885–892

Fass R, Fennerty MB, Vakil N (2001) Nonerosive reflux disease – current concepts and dilemmas. Am J Gastroenterol 96:303–314

Fong AY, Krstew EV, Barden J, Lawrence AJ (2002) Immunoreactive localisation of P2Y1 receptors within the rat and human nodose ganglia and rat brainstem: comparison with [alpha 33P]deoxyadenosine 5′-triphosphate autoradiography. Neuroscience 113:809–823

Fox EA, Phillips RJ, Martinson FA, Baronowsky EA, Powley TL (2000) Vagal afferent innervation of smooth muscle in the stomach and duodenum of the mouse: morphology and topography. J Comp Neurol 428:558–576

Franzi SJ, Martin CJ, Cox MR, Dent J (1990) Response of canine lower esophageal sphincter to gastric distension. Am J Physiol 259:G380–G385
Freidin N, Fisher MJ, Taylor W, Boyd D, Surratt P, McCallum RW, Mittal RK (1991) Sleep and nocturnal acid reflux in normal subjects and patients with reflux oesophagitis. Gut 32:1275–1279
Frisby CL, Mattsson JP, Jensen JM, Lehmann A, Dent J, Blackshaw LA (2005) Inhibition of transient lower esophageal sphincter relaxation and gastroesophageal reflux by metabotropic glutamate receptor ligands. Gastroenterology 129:995–1004
Fujino K, de la Fuente SG, Takami Y, Takahashi T, Mantyh CR (2006) Attenuation of acid induced oesophagitis in VR-1 deficient mice. Gut 55:34–40
Furness JB, Koopmans HS, Robbins HL, Lin HC (2000) Identification of intestinofugal neurons projecting to the coeliac and superior mesenteric ganglia in the rat. Auton Neurosci 83:81–85
Gold MS, Dastmalchi S, Levine JD (1996) Co-expression of nociceptor properties in dorsal root ganglion neurons from the adult rat in vitro. Neuroscience 71:265–275
Green T, Dockray GJ (1987) Calcitonin gene-related peptide and substance P in afferents to the upper gastrointestinal tract in the rat. Neurosci Lett 76:151–156
Guo A, Vulchanova L, Wang J, Li X, Elde R (1999) Immunocytochemical localization of the vanilloid receptor 1 (VR1): relationship to neuropeptides, the P2X3 purinoceptor and IB4 binding sites. Eur J Neurosci 11:946–958
Hewson EG, Sinclair JW, Dalton CB, Wu WC, Castell DO, Richter JE (1989) Acid perfusion test: does it have a role in the assessment of non cardiac chest pain? Gut 30:305–310
Hicks G, Clayton J, Gaskin P (2001) 5-HT4 receptor agonists stimulate small intestinal transit but do not have direct visceral antinociceptive effects in the rat. Gastroenterology 120:A6
Hirsch DP, Holloway RH, Tytgat GN, Boeckxstaens GE (1998) Involvement of nitric oxide in human transient lower esophageal sphincter relaxations and esophageal primary peristalsis. Gastroenterology 115:1374–1380
Hirsch DP, Tytgat GN, Boeckxstaens GE (2002) Is glutamate involved in transient lower esophageal sphincter relaxations? Dig Dis Sci 47:661–666
Hobson AR, Furlong PL, Sarkar S, Matthews PJ, Willert RP, Worthen SF, Unsworth BJ, Aziz Q (2006) Neurophysiologic assessment of esophageal sensory processing in noncardiac chest pain. Gastroenterology 130:80–88
Holloway RH, Penagini R, Ireland AC (1995) Criteria for objective definition of transient lower esophageal sphincter relaxation. Am J Physiol 268:G128–G133
Hoyer D, Martin G (1997) 5-HT receptor classification and nomenclature: towards a harmonization with the human genome. Neuropharmacology 36:419–428
Janssens J, Vantrappen G (1987) Angina-like chest pain of oesophageal origin. Baillieres Clin Gastroenterol 1:843–855
Janssens J, Vantrappen G, Ghillebert G (1986) 24-Hour recording of esophageal pressure and *p*H in patients with noncardiac chest pain. Gastroenterology 90:1978–1984
Jensen J, Lehmann A, Uvebrant A, Carlsson A, Jerndal G, Nilsson K, Frisby C, Blackshaw LA, Mattsson JP (2005) Transient lower esophageal sphincter relaxations in dogs are inhibited by a metabotropic glutamate receptor 5 antagonist. Eur J Pharmacol 519:154–157
Johnson DA, Winters C, Spurling TJ, Chobanian SJ, Cattau EL Jr (1987) Esophageal acid sensitivity in Barrett's esophagus. J Clin Gastroenterol 9:23–27
Jones RC, 3rd, Xu L, Gebhart GF (2005) The mechanosensitivity of mouse colon afferent fibers and their sensitization by inflammatory mediators require transient receptor potential vanilloid 1 and acid-sensing ion channel 3. J Neurosci 25:10981–10989
Kahrilas PJ (2000) Esophageal motility disorders: current concepts of pathogenesis and treatment. Can J Gastroenterol 14:221–231
Khurana RK, Petras JM (1991) Sensory innervation of the canine esophagus, stomach, and duodenum. Am J Anat 192:293–306

Kirkup AJ, Eastwood C, Grundy D, Chessell IP, Humphrey PP (1998) Characterization of adenosine receptors evoking excitation of mesenteric afferents in the rat. Br J Pharmacol 125:1352–1360
Kirkup AJ, Booth CE, Chessell IP, Humphrey PP, Grundy D (1999) Excitatory effect of P2X receptor activation on mesenteric afferent nerves in the anaesthetised rat. J Physiol 520(Pt 2):551–563
Kjellen G, Tibbling L (1985) Oesophageal motility during acid-provoked heartburn and chest pain. Scand J Gastroenterol 20:937–940
Kollarik M, Ru F, Undem BJ (2007) Acid-sensitive vagal sensory pathways and cough. Pulm Pharmacol Ther 20:402–411
Kressel M, Berthoud HR, Neuhuber WL (1994) Vagal innervation of the rat pylorus: an anterograde tracing study using carbocyanine dyes and laser scanning confocal microscopy. Cell Tissue Res 275:109–123
Lee KJ, Vos R, Janssens J, Tack J (2004) Differences in the sensorimotor response to distension between the proximal and distal stomach in humans. Gut 53:938–943
Lehmann A, Branden L (2001) Effects of antagonism of NMDA receptors on transient lower esophageal sphincter relaxations in the dog. Eur J Pharmacol 431:253–258
Lehmann A, Antonsson M, Bremner-Danielsen M, Flärdh M, Hansson-Branden L, Kärrberg L (1999) Activation of the GABAb receptor inhibits transient lower esophageal sphincter relaxations in dogs. Gastroenterology 117:1147–1154
Lehmann A, Blackshaw LA, Branden L, Carlsson A, Jensen J, Nygren E, Smid SD (2002) Cannabinoid receptor agonism inhibits transient lower esophageal sphincter relaxations and reflux in dogs. Gastroenterology 123:1129–1134
Lidums I, Lehmann A, Checklin H, Dent J, Holloway RH (2000) Control of transient lower esophageal sphincter relaxations and reflux by the GABA(B) agonist baclofen in normal subjects. Gastroenterology 118:7–13
Lindh B, Aldskogius H, Hokfelt T (1989) Simultaneous immunohistochemical demonstration of intra-axonally transported markers and neuropeptides in the peripheral nervous system of the guinea pig. Histochemistry 92:367–376
Lindstrom E, Brusberg M, Hughes PA, Martin CM, Brierley SM, Phillis BD, Martinsson R, Abrahamsson C, Larsson H, Martinez V, Blackshaw LA (2008) Involvement of metabotropic glutamate 5 receptor in visceral pain. Pain 137(2):295–305
Longhurst JC, Kaufman MP, Ordway GA, Musch TI (1984) Effects of bradykinin and capsaicin on endings of afferent fibers from abdominal visceral organs. Am J Physiol 247:R552–R559
Lynn PA, Blackshaw LA (1999) In vitro recordings of afferent fibres with receptive fields in the serosa, muscle and mucosa of rat colon. J Physiol 518(Pt 1):271–282
Martin CJ, Patrikios J, Dent J (1986) Abolition of gas reflux and transient lower esophageal sphincter relaxation by vagal blockade in the dog. Gastroenterology 91:890–896
Martin CJ, Dodds WJ, Liem HH, Dantas RO, layman RD, Dent J (1992) Diaphragmatic contribution to gastroesophageal competence and reflux in dogs. Am J Physiol 263:G551–G557
Matthews PJ, Aziz Q, Facer P, Davis JB, Thompson DG, Anand P (2004) Increased capsaicin receptor TRPV1 nerve fibres in the inflamed human oesophagus. Eur J Gastroenterol Hepatol 16:897–902
Mazzia C, Clerc N (1997) Ultrastructural relationships of spinal primary afferent fibres with neuronal and non-neuronal cells in the myenteric plexus of the cat oesophago-gastric junction. Neuroscience 80:925–937
McDermott CM, Abrahams TP, Partosoedarso E, Hyland N, Ekstrand J, Monroe M, Hornby PJ (2001) Site of action of GABA(B) receptor for vagal motor control of the lower esophageal sphincter in ferrets and rats. Gastroenterology 120:1749–1762
McRoberts JA, Coutinho SV, Marvizon JC, Grady EF, Tognetto M, Sengupta JN, Ennes HS, Chaban VV, Amadesi S, Creminon C, Lanthorn T, Geppetti P, Bunnett NW, Mayer EA (2001) Role of peripheral *N*-methyl-D-aspartate (NMDA) receptors in visceral nociception in rats. Gastroenterology 120:1737–1748
Medda BK, Sengupta JN, Lang IM, Shaker R (2005) Response properties of the brainstem neurons of the cat following intra-esophageal acid-pepsin infusion. Neuroscience 135:1285–1294

Mittal RK, Balaban DH (1997) The esophagogastric junction. N Engl J Med 336:924–932
Mittal RK, Holloway RH, Penagini R, Blackshaw LA, Dent J (1995) Transient lower esophageal sphincter relaxation. Gastroenterology 109:601–610
Mittal RK, Liu J, Puckett JL, Bhalla V, Bhargava V, Tipnis N, Kassab G (2005) Sensory and motor function of the esophagus: lessons from ultrasound imaging. Gastroenterology 128:487–497
Moriarty P, Dimaline R, Thompson DG, Dockray GJ (1997) Characterization of cholecystokininA and cholecystokininB receptors expressed by vagal afferent neurons. Neuroscience 79:905–913
Neuhuber WL (1987) Sensory vagal innervation of the rat esophagus and cardia: a light and electron microscopic anterograde tracing study. J Auton Nerv Syst 20:243–255
Neuhuber WL, Kressel M, Stark A, Berthoud HR (1998) Vagal efferent and afferent innervation of the rat esophagus as demonstrated by anterograde DiI and DiA tracing: focus on myenteric ganglia. J Auton Nerv Syst 70:92–102
Nicol GD, Cui M (1994) Enhancement by prostaglandin E2 of bradykinin activation of embryonic rat sensory neurones. J Physiol 480(Pt 3):485–492
Ozaki N, Gebhart GF (2001) Characterization of mechanosensitive splanchnic nerve afferent fibers innervating the rat stomach. Am J Physiol Gastrointest Liver Physiol 281:G1449–G1459
Ozaki N, Sengupta JN, Gebhart GF (2000) Differential effects of mu-, delta-, and kappa-opioid receptor agonists on mechanosensitive gastric vagal afferent fibers in the rat. J Neurophysiol 83:2209–2216
Page AJ, Blackshaw LA (1998) An in vitro study of the properties of vagal afferent fibres innervating the ferret oesophagus and stomach. J Physiol 512(Pt 3):907–916
Page AJ, Blackshaw LA (1999) GABA(B) receptors inhibit mechanosensitivity of primary afferent endings. J Neurosci 19:8597–8602
Page AJ, O'Donnell TA, Blackshaw LA (2000) P2X purinoceptor-induced sensitization of ferret vagal mechanoreceptors in oesophageal inflammation. J Physiol 523(Pt 2):403–411
Page AJ, Martin CM, Blackshaw LA (2002) Vagal mechanoreceptors and chemoreceptors in mouse stomach and esophagus. J Neurophysiol 87:2095–2103
Page AJ, Brierley SM, Martin CM, Martinez-Salgado C, Wemmie JA, Brennan TJ, Symonds E, Omari T, Lewin GR, Welsh MJ, Blackshaw LA (2004) The ion channel ASIC1 contributes to visceral but not cutaneous mechanoreceptor function. Gastroenterology 127:1739–1747
Page AJ, Brierley SM, Martin CM, Price MP, Symonds E, Butler R, Wemmie JA, Blackshaw LA (2005a) Different contributions of ASIC channels 1a, 2, and 3 in gastrointestinal mechanosensory function. Gut 54:1408–1415
Page AJ, Slattery JA, O'Donnell TA, Cooper NJ, Young RL, Blackshaw LA (2005b) Modulation of gastro-oesophageal vagal afferents by galanin in mouse and ferret. J Physiol 563:809–819
Page AJ, Young RL, Martin CM, Umaerus M, O'Donnell TA, Cooper NJ, Coldwell JR, Hulander M, Mattsson JP, Lehmann A, Blackshaw LA (2005c) Metabotropic glutamate receptors inhibit mechanosensitivity in vagal sensory neurons. Gastroenterology 128:402–410
Page AJ, Brierley SM, Martin CM, Hughes PA, Blackshaw LA (2007a) Acid sensing ion channels 2 and 3 are required for inhibition of visceral nociceptors by benzamil. Pain 133:150–160
Page AJ, O'Donnell TA, Blackshaw LA (2007b) Role of nitric oxide in peripheral control of vagal afferent mechamosensitivity. Gastroenterology 132:A155–A155
Page AJ, Slattery JA, Brierley SM, Jacoby AS, Blackshaw LA (2007c) Involvement of galanin receptors 1 and 2 in the modulation of mouse vagal afferent mechanosensitivity. J Physiol 583:675–684
Page AJ, Slattery JA, Milte C, Laker R, O'Donnell T, Dorian C, Brierley SM, Blackshaw LA (2007d) Ghrelin selectively reduces mechanosensitivity of upper gastrointestinal vagal afferents. Am J Physiol Gastrointest Liver Physiol 292:G1376–G1384
Partosoedarso ER, Blackshaw LA (1997) Vagal efferent fibre responses to gastric and oesophageal mechanical and chemical stimuli in the ferret. J Auton Nerv Syst 66:169–178
Partosoedarso ER, Young RL, Blackshaw LA (2001) GABA(B) receptors on vagal afferent pathways: peripheral and central inhibition. Am J Physiol Gastrointest Liver Physiol 280: G658–G668

Paterson WG, Selucky M, Hynna-Liepert TT (1991) Effect of intraesophageal location and muscarinic blockade on balloon distension-induced chest pain. Dig Dis Sci 36:282–288

Patterson LM, Zheng H, Ward SM, Berthoud HR (2003) Vanilloid receptor (VR1) expression in vagal afferent neurons innervating the gastrointestinal tract. Cell Tissue Res 311:277–287

Penagini R, Bianchi PA (1997) Effect of morphine on gastroesophageal reflux and transient lower esophageal sphincter relaxation. Gastroenterology 113:409–414

Phillips RJ, Powley TL (2000) Tension and stretch receptors in gastrointestinal smooth muscle: re-evaluating vagal mechanoreceptor electrophysiology. Brain Res Brain Res Rev 34:1–26

Pouderoux P, Verdier E, Kahrilas PJ (2003) Patterns of esophageal inhibition during swallowing, pharyngeal stimulation, and transient LES relaxation. Lower esophageal sphincter. Am J Physiol Gastrointest Liver Physiol 284:G242–G247

Richards W, Hillsley K, Eastwood C, Grundy D (1996) Sensitivity of vagal mucosal afferents to cholecystokinin and its role in afferent signal transduction in the rat. J Physiol 497 (Pt 2):473–481

Richter JE (1991a) Gastroesophageal reflux disease as a cause of chest pain. Med Clin North Am 75:1065–1080

Richter JE (1991b) Investigation and management of non-cardiac chest pain. Baillieres Clin Gastroenterol 5:281–306

Richter JE, Barish CF, Castell DO (1986) Abnormal sensory perception in patients with esophageal chest pain. Gastroenterology 91:845–852

Rodrigo J, Hernandez J, Vidal MA, Pedrosa JA (1975) Vegetative innervation of the esophagus. II. Intraganglionic laminar endings. Acta Anat (Basel) 92:79–100

Rong W, Hillsley K, Davis JB, Hicks G, Winchester WJ, Grundy D (2004) Jejunal afferent nerve sensitivity in wild-type and TRPV1 knockout mice. J Physiol 560:867–881

Rouzade ML, Fioramonti J, Bueno L (1996) Role of 5-HT3 receptors in the control by cholecystokinin of transient relaxations of the inferior esophageal sphincter in dogs. Gastroenterol Clin Biol 20:575–580

Ruan HZ, Burnstock G (2003) Localisation of P2Y1 and P2Y4 receptors in dorsal root, nodose and trigeminal ganglia of the rat. Histochem Cell Biol 120:415–426

Sarkar S, Hobson AR, Hughes A, Growcott J, Woolf CJ, Thompson DG, Aziz Q (2003) The prostaglandin E2 receptor-1 (EP-1) mediates acid-induced visceral pain hypersensitivity in humans. Gastroenterology 124:18–25

Schicho R, Florian W, Liebmann I, Holzer P, Lippe IT (2004) Increased expression of TRPV1 receptor in dorsal root ganglia by acid insult of the rat gastric mucosa. Eur J Neurosci 19:1811–1818

Schikowski A, Thewissen M, Mathis C, Ross HG, Enck P (2002) Serotonin type-4 receptors modulate the sensitivity of intramural mechanoreceptive afferents of the cat rectum. Neurogastroenterol Motil 14:221–227

Schoeman MN, Holloway RH (1994) Secondary oesophageal peristalsis in patients with non-obstructive dysphagia. Gut 35:1523–1528

Schoeman MN, Holloway RH (1995) Integrity and characteristics of secondary oesophageal peristalsis in patients with gastro-oesophageal reflux disease. Gut 36:499–504

Schwetz I, Naliboff B, Munakata J, Lembo T, Chang L, Matin K, Ohning G, Mayer EA (2004) Anti-hyperalgesic effect of octreotide in patients with irritable bowel syndrome. Aliment Pharmacol Ther 19:123–131

Sekizawa S, Ishikawa T, Sant'Ambrogio FB, Sant'Ambrogio G (1999) Vagal esophageal receptors in anesthetized dogs: mechanical and chemical responsiveness. J Appl Physiol 86:1231–1235

Sengupta JN, Kauvar D, Goyal RK (1989) Characteristics of vagal esophageal tension-sensitive afferent fibers in the opossum. J Neurophysiol 61:1001–1010

Sengupta JN, Saha JK, Goyal RK (1990) Stimulus-response function studies of esophageal mechanosensitive nociceptors in sympathetic afferents of opossum. J Neurophysiol 64:796–812

Sengupta JN, Saha JK, Goyal RK (1992) Differential sensitivity to bradykinin of esophageal distension-sensitive mechanoreceptors in vagal and sympathetic afferents of the opossum. J Neurophysiol 68:1053–1067

Sengupta JN, Su X, Gebhart GF (1996) Kappa, but not mu or delta, opioids attenuate responses to distention of afferent fibers innervating the rat colon. Gastroenterology 111:968–980

Sengupta JN, Medda BK, Shaker R (2002) Effect of GABA(B) receptor agonist on distension-sensitive pelvic nerve afferent fibers innervating rat colon. Am J Physiol Gastrointest Liver Physiol 283:G1343–G1351

Sengupta JN, Petersen J, Peles S, Shaker R (2004) Response properties of antral mechanosensitive afferent fibers and effects of ionotropic glutamate receptor antagonists. Neuroscience 125:711–723

Shigemoto R, Ohishi H, Nakanishi S, Mizuno N (1992) Expression of the mRNA for the rat NMDA receptor (NMDAR1) in the sensory and autonomic ganglion neurons. Neurosci Lett 144:229–232

Slattery JA, Page AJ, Dorian CL, Brierley SM, Blackshaw LA (2006) Potentiation of mouse vagal afferent mechanosensitivity by ionotropic and metabotropic glutamate receptors. J Physiol 577:295–306

Smid SD, Blackshaw LA (2000) Vagal neurotransmission to the ferret lower oesophageal sphincter: inhibition via GABA(B) receptors. Br J Pharmacol 131:624–630

Smid SD, Lynn PA, Templeman R, Blackshaw LA (1998) Activation of non-adrenergic non-cholinergic inhibitory pathways by endogenous and exogenous tachykinins in the ferret lower oesophageal sphincter. Neurogastroenterol Motil 10:149–156

Smid SD, Young RL, Cooper NJ, Blackshaw LA (2001) GABA(B)R expressed on vagal afferent neurones inhibit gastric mechanosensitivity in ferret proximal stomach. Am J Physiol Gastrointest Liver Physiol 281:G1494–G1501

Smith JL, Opekun AR, Larkai E, Graham DY (1989) Sensitivity of the esophageal mucosa to *p*H in gastroesophageal reflux disease. Gastroenterology 96:683–689

Staunton E, Smid SD, Dent J, Blackshaw LA (2000) Triggering of transient LES relaxations in ferrets: role of sympathetic pathways and effects of baclofen. Am J Physiol Gastrointest Liver Physiol 279:G157–G162

Tominaga M, Wada M, Masu M (2001) Potentiation of capsaicin receptor activity by metabotropic ATP receptors as a possible mechanism for ATP-evoked pain and hyperalgesia. Proc Natl Acad Sci USA 98:6951–6956

Uddman R, Grunditz T, Luts A, Desai H, Fernstrom G, Sundler F (1995) Distribution and origin of the peripheral innervation of rat cervical esophagus. Dysphagia 10:203–212

Wang FB, Powley TL (2000) Topographic inventories of vagal afferents in gastrointestinal muscle. J Comp Neurol 421:302–324

Wank M, Neuhuber WL (2001) Local differences in vagal afferent innervation of the rat esophagus are reflected by neurochemical differences at the level of the sensory ganglia and by different brainstem projections. J Comp Neurol 435:41–59

Willert RP, Woolf CJ, Hobson AR, Delaney C, Thompson DG, Aziz Q (2004) The development and maintenance of human visceral pain hypersensitivity is dependent on the *N*-methyl-D-aspartate receptor. Gastroenterology 126:683–692

Willert RP, Hobson AR, Delaney C, Hicks KJ, Dewit OE, Aziz Q (2007) Neurokinin-1 receptor antagonism in a human model of visceral hypersensitivity. Aliment Pharmacol Ther 25:309–316

Wyman JB, Dent J, Heddle R, Dodds WJ, Toouli J, Downton J (1990) Control of belching by the lower oesophageal sphincter. Gut 31:639–646

Young RL, Page AJ, O'Donnell TA, Cooper NJ, Blackshaw LA (2007) Peripheral versus central modulation of gastric vagal pathways by metabotropic glutamate receptor 5. Am J Physiol Gastrointest Liver Physiol 292:G501–G511

Young RL, Cooper NJ, Blackshaw LA (2008) Chemical coding and central projections of gastric vagal afferent neurons. Neurogastroenterol Motil 20(6):708–718

Yu S, Kollarik M, Ouyang A, Myers AC, Undem BJ (2007) Mast cell-mediated long-lasting increases in excitability of vagal C fibers in guinea pig esophagus. Am J Physiol Gastrointest Liver Physiol 293:G850–G856

Yu S, Undem BJ, Kollarik M (2005) Vagal afferent nerves with nociceptive properties in guinea-pig oesophagus. J Physiol 563:831–842

Zagorodnyuk VP, Brookes SJ (2000) Transduction sites of vagal mechanoreceptors in the guinea pig esophagus. J Neurosci 20:6249–6255

Zagorodnyuk VP, Chen BN, Brookes SJ (2001) Intraganglionic laminar endings are mechano-transduction sites of vagal tension receptors in the guinea-pig stomach. J Physiol 534:255–268

Zagorodnyuk VP, D'Antona G, Brookes SJ, Costa M (2002) Functional GABAB receptors are present in guinea pig nodose ganglion cell bodies but not in peripheral mechanosensitive endings. Auton Neurosci 102:20–29

Zagorodnyuk VP, Chen BN, Costa M, Brookes SJ (2003) Mechanotransduction by intraganglionic laminar endings of vagal tension receptors in the guinea-pig oesophagus. J Physiol 553:575–587

Zhang X, Dagerlind A, Elde RP, Castel MN, Broberger C, Wiesenfeld-Hallin Z, Hokfelt T (1993) Marked increase in cholecystokinin B receptor messenger RNA levels in rat dorsal root ganglia after peripheral axotomy. Neuroscience 57:227–233

Zhang Q, Lehmann A, Rigda R, Dent J, Holloway RH (2002) Control of transient lower oesophageal sphincter relaxations and reflux by the GABA(B) agonist baclofen in patients with gastro-oesophageal reflux disease. Gut 50:19–24

Part II
Cell and Molecular Mechanisms Regulating Sensory Nerve Function

Transient Receptor Potential Channels on Sensory Nerves

S.R. Eid and D.N. Cortright

Contents

Abstract The somatosensory effects of natural products such as capsaicin, mustard oil, and menthol have been long recognized. Over the last decade, the identification

S.R. Eid (✉)
Department of Pain Research, Neuroscience Drug Discovery, Merck Research Laboratories, West Point, Philadelphia, USA
samer_eid@merck.com

B.J. Canning and D. Spina (eds.), *Sensory Nerves*,
Handbook of Experimental Pharmacology 194, DOI: 10.1007/978-3-540-79090-7_8,

of transient receptor potential (TRP) channels in primary sensory neurons as the targets for these agents has led to an explosion of research into the roles of "thermoTRPs" TRPV1, TRPV2, TRPV3, TRPV4, TRPA1, and TRPM8 in nociception. In concert, through the efforts of many industrial and academic teams, a number of agonists and antagonists of these channels have been discovered, paving the way for a better understanding of sensory biology and, potentially, for novel treatments for diseases.

Keywords TRPV1, TRPV2, TRPV3, TRPV4, TRPA1, TRPM8, Pain, Nociceptors, Sensory system, Channels, Agonists, Antagonists

Abbreviations

2-APB	2-Aminoethoxydiphenyl borate
CFA	Complete Freund's adjuvant
DRG	Dorsal root ganglion
PIP_2	Phosphatidylinositol 4,5-bisphosphate
RTX	Resiniferatoxin
TRP	Transient receptor potential
TRPA1	Transient receptor potential ankyrin subfamily, member 1
TRPM8	Transient receptor potential melastatin subfamily, member 8
TRPV1	Transient receptor potential vanilloid subfamily, member 1
TRPV2	Transient receptor potential vanilloid subfamily, member 2
TRPV3	Transient receptor potential vanilloid subfamily, member 3
TRPV4	Transient receptor potential vanilloid subfamily, member 4

1 Discovery of Transient Receptor Potential Vanilloid Subfamily, Member 1: A Ticket into the Somatosensory System

The sensory nervous system is responsible for communicating information about the environment. Sensory nerve fibers originating from cells in various ganglia (trigeminal, nodose, dorsal root) constitute the initial detection apparatus of the sensory system. These sensory neurons project axons centrally to the dorsal spinal cord, and peripherally to almost all organs. In addition, the distribution of these fiber types varies by target organ; for example, Aβ fibers make up a significant percentage of the sensory innervation of the skin, whereas C fibers predominate in the urinary bladder (Meyer et al. 1994; Raja et al. 1999; Shea et al. 2000; Stucky et al. 1999).

The study of peripheral sensory fibers has been facilitated by certain natural products, such as capsaicin and mustard oil. These molecules have proven to be exquisite tools to probe the function of primary sensory neurons in a wide array of physiological processes, ranging from pain to neurogenic inflammation to airway and urinary bladder hypersensitivity. But the identification in 1997 of the capsaicin receptor as a transient receptor potential (TRP) channel (Caterina et al. 1997) provided the first evidence that TRP channels were important players in sensory biology. Since then there has been an explosion of research that has identified a number of TRP channels expressed in sensory neurons. This chapter will endeavor to summarize the key insights into the role of TRP channels in sensory neuron physiological processes, particularly in pain.

2 TRP Channels as Molecular Sensors

The activation of TRP vanilloid subfamily, member 1 (TRPV1) by the natural products capsaicin and resiniferatoxin (RTX) is but one example of TRP channel activation by natural products (Fig. 1). Other TRP channels expressed in sensory tissues are receptors for a diversity of naturally occurring substances that activate the somatosensory system (Fig. 1). Cinnamaldehyde, mustard oil, and isothiocyanate-containing plant extracts activate TRP ankyrin subfamily, member 1 (TRPA1) (Bandell et al. 2004; Jordt et al. 2004), menthol activates TRP melastatin subfamily, member 8 (TRPM8) (McKemy et al. 2002; Peier et al. 2002a), camphor activates TRP vanilloid subfamily, member 3 (TRPV3) and TRPV1 (Xu et al. 2005), and bisandrographolide A from *Andrographis paniculata* activates TRP vanilloid subfamily, member 4 (TRPV4) (Smith et al. 2006).

But sensory TRP channels are not simply natural product receptors. They are molecular sensors for an array of modalities that elicit somatosensory responses. These modalities include temperature, protein kinase activity, phospholipids, osmolarity, and pH. Moreover, sensory TRP channels can act as molecular integrators of multiple modalities, best exemplified by TRPV1 (Premkumar et al. 2000; Tominaga et al. 1998). The identification of TRP channels as the molecular transducers and integrators of a broad range of sensory modalities has provided new insights into the physiological role of sensory nerve fibers.

2.1 TRPV1

Also known as VR1, TRPV1 is the founding member of the subfamily of TRP channels expressed in sensory neurons and is the most widely studied. TRPV1 is activated by capsaicin, RTX, venoms from jellyfish and spiders, low-pH solutions, temperatures above 43°C, anandamide, arachidonic acid metabolites such as *N*-arachidonoyl dopamine, lipoxygenase products such as 12-hydroperoxyeicosatetraenoic acid, and others (Szallasi et al. 2007). As noted earlier, TRPV1 is an

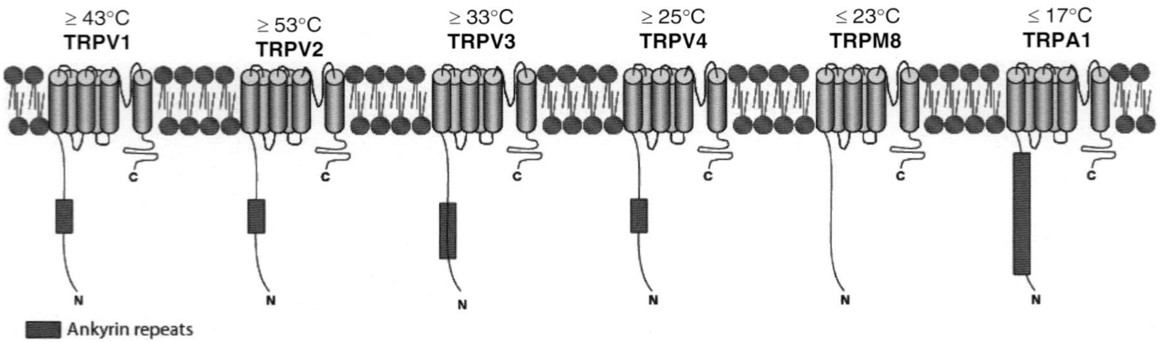

Function and activators of thermoTRP channels and their relevance to pain

Channel	Function/Phenotype	Endogenous/exogenous activators
TRPV1	Involved in noxious heat detection and mediates thermal hyperalgesia under inflammatory conditions. Decreased sensitivity to vanilloids and protons. Acute pharmacological blockade attenuates thermal hyperalgesia under inflammatory conditions.	Heat ≥ 43°C; Capsaicin; Resiniferatoxin; Piperine; Protons; Camphor; Anandamide; Arachidonic acid; 2-APB; NADA; 12-HPETE; Leukotriene B4; toxins from Jellyfish and spiders; Olvanil.
TRPV2	Responds to noxious heat in heterologous system.	Heat (≥ 53°C); 2-APB; Probenecid; Carvacrol.
TRPV3	Decreased sensitivity to innocuous and noxious heat stimulation. Diminished response to Camphor in keratinocytes from ko mice	Heat (≥ 33°C); Camphor; Carvacrol; Thymol; Eugenol; Vanillin.
TRPV4	Involved in warm temperature sensation. Controversial reports about its involvement in mediating noxious heat pain and thermal hyperalgesia	Heat (≥ 25°C); 4α-PDD; Epxoxyeicosatrienoic acids; change in osmolarity; Bisandrographolide.
TRPM8	Three independent KO studies strongly validated role of TRPM8 in mediating cold temperature sensation. Mutant mice mediates cold induced analgesia in formalin test. Reduced cold allodynia in neuropathic pain models.	Cold ≤ 23°C; Menthol; Icilin; WS-12; CPS-113; CPS-369; WS-148; WS-30; Frescolat ML; Coolact P; Cooling agent 10, WS-3; Geralniol; Linalool; Eucalyptol; Hydroxycitronellal; PIP_2
TRPA1	Involved in mustard oil-and BK-induced hyperalgesia. Reduced sensitivity to Allicin, Formalin, 15d-PGJ2, Hypochlorite, H_2O_2, and HNE; Controversial role in mechanical and noxious cold sensation. Acute pharmacological blockade attenuates mechanical hyperalgesia under inflammatory conditions.	Reactive: Mustard oil, Cinnamaldehyde; Allicin; Acrolein; Formalin; 15d-PGJ2; Hypochlorite; Tear gases; H_2O_2; HNE; Non reactive: Cold ≤ 17°C; Calcium; TNP; Hypertonicity; URB597, Icilin, FTA.

Fig. 1 Function and activators of thermo TRP channels and their relevance to pain

integrator in which each stimulus sensitizes the channel to other stimuli, the net result being that TRPV1 acts as a molecular amplifier in the sensory neuron (Crandall et al. 2002). It should be noted that phosphatidylinositol 4,5-bisphosphate (PIP_2) is a modulator of TRPV1 activity, although the specific effect of PIP_2 – activator or inhibitor – appears to be context-dependent (Lukacs et al. 2007; Prescott et al. 2003).

2.2 TRPV2

Originally described as a TRPV1-like receptor (i.e., VRL-1), TRP vanilloid subfamily, member 2 (TRPV2) exhibits a much broader tissue distribution than TRPV1, and its expression in sensory neuron subpopulations is largely distinct from that of other TRP channels (Lewinter et al. 2004, 2008). In spite of its original molecular characterization 10 years ago, TRPV2 is perhaps the most enigmatic of all sensory-neuron-expressed TRP channels in terms of its function. It is reported to be activated at very high temperatures (i.e., 52°C and higher; Caterina et al. 1999) and by aminoethoxydiphenyl borate (2-APB) (Hu et al. 2004), probenicid (Bang et al. 2007), and high concentrations of Δ^9-tetrahydrocannabinol (EC_{50} = 16–43 μM; Neeper et al. 2007). In certain cellular contexts, TRPV2's intracellular localization is affected by growth factors (Kanzaki et al. 1999); however, these observations have not been extended to sensory neurons.

2.3 TRPV3

Identified via its homology to TRPV1 and TRPV2, TRPV3 is a warm temperature (above 33°C) activated channel, which combined with its strong expression in keratinocytes supports the notion that nonneuronal cells in skin may be involved in thermal sensing. Other TRPV3 activators are 2-APB and monoterpenes, including camphor, carvacrol, and thymol, and the vanilloid compounds eugenol, vanillin, and ethyl vanillin (Hu et al. 2004; Vogt-Eisele et al. 2007; Xu et al. 2006). TRPV3 exhibits both homologous and heterologous sensitization: repeated stimulation with heat or 2-APB sensitizes the channel to subsequent application of heat or 2-APB (Chung et al. 2004; Xiao et al. 2008), a characteristic which supports its potential role as a molecular thermal nociceptor. Moreover, TRPV3 activation by 2-APB is potentiated by unsaturated fatty acids, including arachidonic acid, as well as by protein kinase activation (Hu et al. 2006).

2.4 TRPV4

Initially characterized as an osmolarity-sensitive channel, TRPV4 is also activated by temperatures above 34°C, 4α-phorbol 12,13-didecanoate, and epxoxyeicosatrienoic acids – cytochrome P450 metabolites of anandamide and arachidonic acid. Activation of TRPV4 by hypotonic solutions can be mediated via phosphorylation at Y253, a process which involves Lyn, a member of the Src tyrosine kinase family (Xu et al. 2003). Moreover, TRPV4 has been shown to complex with α2 integrin and Lyn, in sensory neurons from rats exhibiting mechanical hypersensitivity, and anti-α2 integrin antibody treatment blocks TRPV4-mediated calcium uptake in these neurons (Alessandri-Haber et al. 2008). In contrast, the interaction of TRPV4 with protein kinase C and casein kinase II substrate in neurons forms a complex in which TRPV4 activation by cell swelling and heat activation is inhibited, but 4α-phorbol 12,13-didecanoate activation is unaffected (D'Hoedt et al. 2008).

2.5 *TRPA1*

While the field awaited the identification of a channel with cold sensitivity in the noxious range, Patapoutian and colleagues (2003) identified TRPA1, distantly related to the TRP family of channels (Story et al. 2003). Although controversial, TRPA1 was originally characterized as a noxious cold-activated ion channel with a threshold of activation of about 17°C (Story et al. 2003).

This intriguing expression of TRPA1 within a subset of noxious polymodal TRPV1-expressing neurons led to the proposal that noxious cold might consist of two components: cold sensation that may be processed by TRPM8-expressing neurons and a painful component that might be brought by activation of TRPA1-expressing polymodal nociceptors (Dhaka et al. 2006). Later, several reports showed that TRPA1 can be also activated by pungent compounds and irritants such as cinnamaldehyde (cinnamon oil), isothiocyanates (such as those found in mustard oil), allicin (from garlic), acrolein (a metabolized by-product of chemotherapeutic agents and also present in tear gas and vehicle exhaust), and formalin, which can induce acute pain, hyperalgesia, or neurogenic inflammation in animals and humans (Bandell et al. 2004; Bautista et al. 2005, 2006; Macpherson et al. 2005, 2007a; McNamara et al. 2007; Namer et al. 2005; Ward et al. 1996). For example, mustard oil has been historically used as a chemical algogen resulting in neurogenic inflammation and was shown to evoke a sharp pain and hyperalgesia in human subjects (Handwerker et al. 1991; Koltzenburg et al. 1992; McMahon et al. 2006; Reeh et al. 1986). Cinnamaldehyde was shown to induce acute nociception and hyperalgesia in mice and human subjects (Bandell et al. 2004; Namer et al. 2005). More recently, the α,β-unsaturated aldehyde 4-hydroxy-2-nonenal and the electrophilic carbon-containing prostaglandin J_2 metabolite 15d-PJG(2), released in response to tissue injury, inflammation, and oxidative stress, were reported to be the first endogenous activators of TRPA1. (Macpherson et al. 2007b; Taylor-Clark et al. 2008; Trevisani et al. 2007).

The questions around the promiscuous activation of TRPA1 by structurally unrelated compounds were quickly answered by the findings that the majority of TRPA1 activators gate the channel through chemical reactivity of their electrophile groups with the nucleophilic cysteine residues at the N-terminus of the channel (Hinman et al. 2006; Macpherson et al. 2007a). In addition, it was shown that TRPA1 can be gated by calcium through another mode of activation involving its putative N-terminal EF-hand calcium binding domain. Two studies demonstrated that calcium can directly activate the channel and is a prerequisite for icilin activity on TRPA1 (Doerner et al. 2007; Zurborg et al. 2007). TRPA1 can also be activated by bradykinin and has recently been proposed as a candidate mechanically activated channel involved in hearing (Bandell et al. 2004; Corey et al. 2004). Finally, TRPA1 appears to be sensitized by NGF and proteinase-activated receptor 2 (Dai et al. 2007; Diogenes et al. 2007), both of which are known to play a role in inflammatory pain.

In addition to a role in detecting noxious chemical stimuli, there is increasing evidence to suggest that TRP channels have important roles in mechanoreception. Vertebrate TRPA1 was proposed as a candidate mechanically activated channel in hair cells (Corey et al. 2004). However, mice lacking TRPA1 function exhibit no hearing deficit, although one study showed a lower sensitivity to cutaneous mechanical stimulation (Kwan et al. 2006). Consistent with a possible role in mechanotransduction, *Caenorhabditis elegans* TRPA1 was shown to be activated (not clear if direct or indirect) by pressure in a heterologous system and to play a key role in mediating mechanosensory functions of this worm (Kindt et al. 2007).

2.6 *TRPM8*

Expression cloning in response to menthol (the natural cooling compound from the mint plant) and a bioinformatics-based cloning strategy led to the identification of TRPM8, the first TRP channel shown to be responsive to cool temperatures and menthol (McKemy et al. 2002; Peier et al. 2002a). The cloning and characterization of TRPM8 marked a milestone in understanding the molecular mechanisms underlying cold temperature transduction. TRPM8 is expressed in a subset of small-diameter dorsal root ganglion (DRG) and trigeminal neurons (McKemy et al. 2002; Peier et al. 2002a). It is a nonselective cation channel that permeates Ca^{2+}, Cs^{+}, K^{+}, and Na^{+} and can be activated by cold temperatures (threshold of 18–24°C), menthol ($EC_{50} \sim 10\ \mu M$), and icilin ($EC_{50} \sim 0.5\ \mu M$), a monoterpene synthetic supercooling compound. Activation of TRPM8 is followed by a desensitization of the channel that depends on extracellular Ca^{2+}. Several menthol-derivative agonists of TRPM8 were identified. Among the most potent are WS-12 (193 nM), CPS-113 (1.2 μM) CPS-369 (3.6 μM), WS-148 (4.1 μM), and WS-30 (5.6 μM) and with potency comparable to that of menthol are Frescolat ML, Coolact P, Cooling agent 10, and WS-3 (Behrendt et al. 2004; Bodding et al. 2007).

In analogy to the synergistic effect of capsaicin and heat on the activation of TRPV1, menthol and other agonists were shown to activate and sensitize the TRPM8 channel, rendering the channel active at higher temperatures (McKemy et al. 2002; Peier et al. 2002a). Interestingly, when compared with TRPV1, TRPM8 exhibits opposite mechanisms of activation. PIP_2 acts as an enhancer of the channel activation by cold and menthol preventing its desensitization, while protein kinase C leads to its dephosphorylation (Liu et al. 2005; Rohacs et al. 2005).

3 TRP Channels as Mediators of Pain

3.1 TRPV1

As described already, TRPV1 acts as a molecular integrator of various noxious chemical and thermal stimuli and therefore may play an important role in mediating inflammatory pain. TRPV1 is highly expressed in DRG neurons in mammals, particularly in C-fiber neurons (Caterina et al. 1997; Cortright et al. 2001; Tominaga et al. 1998), although its expression in sensory fibers appears to be somewhat different in rats and mice (Christianson et al. 2006; Rashid et al. 2003). TRPV1 is also found in discrete regions of the rat brain (Mezey et al. 2000) where it may be involved in synaptic plasticity (Gibson et al. 2008). TRPV1 protein, but not RNA, levels are increased in many pathological states that result in pain in rodents and humans (Akbar et al. 2008; Carlton et al. 2001; Facer et al. 2007; Sanchez et al. 2001).

Two independent gene-targeting studies, deleting TRPV1 alleles, conclusively showed that TRPV1 is a pivotal channel that mediates thermal hyperalgesia under inflammatory pain conditions in mice (Caterina et al. 2000; Davis et al. 2000). In addition, one study showed that TRPV1 null mice are significantly less sensitive to acute noxious heat stimulation; TRPV1−/− mice exhibit significantly larger withdrawal latencies in response to noxious heat in the hotplate assay than their wild-type littermates. The phenotype of the TRPV1 knockout mice generated tremendous interest in developing small-molecule antagonists with antihyperalgesic profile.

Studying the involvement of TRPV1 in nociception and pain has not been confined to gene-targeted deletion; other loss-of-function studies such as transgenic mice expressing TRPV1 short hairpin RNA have shown that knockdown of TRPV1 using RNA interference significantly attenuates capsaicin-induced nocifensive behavior and sensitivity toward noxious heat, a phenotype that is similar to the one observed in the TRPV1 "knockout" mice (Christoph et al. 2008). Interestingly, and unlike the TRPV1−/− mice, the TRPV1 short hairpin RNA mice did not develop mechanical hypersensitivity in the spinal nerve injury model of neuropathic pain. In addition, antisense oligonucleotides and small interfering RNAs have been reported and used to characterize the role of TRPV1 in pain (Christoph et al. 2006, 2007; Kasama et al. 2007). Surprisingly, injection of short interference RNA targeting TRPV1 significantly reduced the sensitivity of the rats to noxious heat but had no effect on the development of thermal hyperalgesia, which is highly impaired in the knockout mice and after pharmacological blockade (see Sect. 4). An antibody directed at the extracellular loop that precedes the pore domain is an antagonist in vitro, but no in vivo characterization was reported (Klionsky et al. 2006).

TRPV1 has been intensely studied in the context of pain transduction. However, recent findings point to other important roles, roles which underscore the importance of TRPV1 and sensory nerve fibers more generally in regulating physiological processes. For example, TRPV1-expressing fibers are suggested to play roles in diabetes via innervation of the pancreas (Razavi et al. 2006), regulation of cardiovascular function via innervation of the vascular system (Wang et al. 2006), and airway responses (Kollarik et al. 2004).

3.2 TRPV2

As mentioned already, TRPV2 responds to increasing temperatures with an elevated threshold of activation of 52°C, suggesting a role in detecting acute noxious temperatures (Caterina et al. 1999). Intriguingly, TRPV2 is found in myelinated sensory fibers that are mechanically sensitive, and its expression is increased in DRG in response to nerve injury and peripheral inflammation (Frederick et al. 2007; Shimosato et al. 2005). A study with TRPV2 antisense oligonucleotide provided evidence that TRPV2 mediated membrane stretch-activated currents in Chinese hamster ovary cells overexpressing TRPV2 and aortic myocytes (Muraki et al. 2003). Additionally, a TRPV2 small interfering RNA has been reported to block fMLF(N-formyl-methionyl-leucyl-phenylalanine)-activated calcium entry in a macrophage cell line (Nagasawa et al. 2007). These reagents have not been exploited as yet to probe TRPV2 function in sensory neurons. To date, no null mutant mice of TRPV2 have been reported in the peer-reviewed literature and its therapeutic potential or role in noxious stimuli detection remains to be evaluated.

3.3 TRPV3

TRPV3 is expressed in sensory neurons in humans and monkeys at levels greater than that observed in rodents, although rodents exhibit high levels of TRPV3 in keratinocytes (Peier et al. 2002b; Smith et al. 2002; Xu et al. 2002). The unusual "hysteresis" property of TRPV3 in which functional responses increase drastically upon repeated heating or exposure to other agonists suggests that this channel may play a role in nociception. Indeed, Moqrich et al. (2005) reported that TRPV3 mutant mice exhibit a deficit to noxious acute thermal stimulation at temperatures at or above 50°C (Moqrich et al. 2005). In contrast to TRPV1, TRPV3 mutant mice showed normal behavior in models of inflammatory pain.

Whether the absence of a phenotype with the TRPV3 mutant mice in models of inflammatory pain reflects the dispensable role of TRPV3 in nociception remains to be determined. Recent unpublished data suggest that acute pharmacological blockade of TRPV3 provides efficacy in models of inflammatory pain.

3.4 TRPV4

While TRPV4 is expressed in DRG neurons, it is also found at high levels in a number of other tissues, including kidney, lung, and skeletal muscle (Delany et al. 2001; Liedtke et al. 2000). Moreover, unlike TRPV3, the TRPV4 channel desensitizes in response to prolonged suprathreshold heat stimuli (Guler et al. 2002). Accordingly, it was not clear whether TRPV4 could play a role in the nociceptive pathway. However, TRPV4 null mice exhibit a higher response threshold to intense mechanical stimulation (Liedtke et al. 2003; Suzuki et al. 2003). Surprisingly, TRPV4 mutant and wild-type mice behaved similarly in the hotplate assay (latency to escape; 35–50°C) or when their paws were exposed to radiant heat, suggesting this channel is not involved in acute noxious thermal sensation (Todaka et al. 2004). In contrast, TRPV4 mutant mice exhibit higher withdrawal latency in response to heat in a tail immersion assay performed at 45–46°C (Lee et al. 2005). While the same group showed that TRPV4 mutant mice behaved normally in the temperature gradient assay after intraplantar complete Freund's adjuvant (CFA) injection, others concluded that TRPV4 plays an essential role in models of carrageenan-induced thermal hyperalgesia and inflammatory-mediator-induced mechanical hyperalgesia (Alessandri-Haber et al. 2006; Todaka et al. 2004). Furthermore, spinal administration of antisense oligodeoxynucleotides to TRPV4 abolished taxol-induced mechanical hyperalgesia in a model of chemotherapy-induced neuropathic pain (Alessandri-Haber et al. 2004).

Given the inconsistencies in these studies, the role of TRPV4 in inflammatory pain remains unclear. This discrepancy might be due to differences in the assays employed (radiant heat vs. temperature gradient and hotplate vs. tail immersion) or due to differences in irritants used to induce inflammation (CFA vs. carrageenan and inflammatory soup).

TRPV4, like TRPV1, appears to be important in physiological processes beyond pain detection. Cystometric analysis of the bladder in TRPV4−/− mice revealed a lower frequency of voiding contractions but a higher frequency of nonvoiding contractions compared with wild-type mice (Gevaert et al. 2007). In addition, the amplitude of spontaneous contractions in explanted bladder strips was significantly reduced in TRPV4−/− mice compared with their wild-type littermates (Gevaert et al. 2007), indicating that TRPV4 may play a critical role in urothelium-mediated transduction of intravesical mechanical pressure. Finally, TRPV4 is a sensor of systemic hypotonicity (Cohen 2007). These data demonstrate a role for TRPV4 in renal function.

3.5 TRPA1

TRPA1 is expressed in DRG, trigeminal, and nodose ganglia in a specific subpopulation of neurons that coexpress TRPV1, a noxious heat-activated channel (Diogenes et al. 2007; Story et al. 2003). TRPA1 was also shown to be expressed in the hair cells of the inner ear; however, a role in hearing has not been established to date (Corey et al. 2004). TRPA1 RNA expression is increased in DRG from rats ipsilateral to CFA injection corresponding with the development and maintenance of nerve-injury-induced cold hyperalgesia (Katsura et al. 2006) and ipsilateral to traumatic nerve injury (Frederick et al. 2007). Given its expression in polymodal nociceptors and activation by proalgesics and possibly noxious cold temperatures, TRPA1 is proposed to have a pivotal role in integrating nociceptive stimuli.

Two recent and independent studies disrupted TRPA1 function by gene-targeted deletion (Bautista et al. 2006; Kwan et al. 2006). Both studies validated the major role of TRPA1 in mustard oil and bradykinin induced nociception by showing that TRPA1 mutant mice do not develop acute pain and thermal and mechanical hypersensitivity after intraplantar injection of bradykinin or allylisothiocyanate (Bautista et al. 2006; Kwan et al. 2006). Strikingly, and in contrast to TRPV1 mutant mice which exhibit strong deficits in thermal hyperalgesia irrespective of the methods used to induce inflammation, TRPA1 null mice developed a robust and normal thermal and mechanical hyperalgesia upon CFA injection (Bautista et al. 2006; Petrus et al. 2007). Taken together, these results suggest that TRPA1 acts through a specific inflammatory pathway most likely involving phospholipase C activation.

In one of the two studies, TRPA1 mutant mice also showed reduced sensitivity to intense cold stimulation and a higher threshold of activation in response to painful punctuate mechanical stimulation (Bautista et al. 2006; Petrus et al. 2007). Interestingly, only females exhibited reduced sensitivity to noxious cold, possibly explaining why Bautista et al. did not observe this phenotype. In models of inflammatory and neuropathic pain, knockdown of TRPA1 by intrathecal administration of specific antisense oligodeoxynucleotides suppresses spinal nerve ligation induced and CFA-induced cold hyperalgesia (Katsura et al. 2006).

3.6 TRPM8

While in vitro data provided strong evidence of a possible role for TRPM8 in cold sensation, the validation of the role of TRPM8 in cold transduction in vivo came after three independent groups reported the behavior of TRPM8-deficient mice (Bautista et al. 2007; Colburn et al. 2007; Dhaka et al. 2007). All three groups used the two temperature preference assay and challenged the mice to choose between a preferred warm temperature (30–34°C) and a cool temperature usually avoided by mice. Strikingly, and unlike the wild-type mice, mice lacking TRPM8 function lost their preference to warm temperatures (or avoidance of cool temperatures). It is noteworthy that while two studies showed the TRPM8 knockout mice regained aversion to cold temperatures at or below 10°C (Bautista et al. 2007; Dhaka et al. 2007), one study showed that the deficit in cold temperature detection persists down to 0°C (Colburn et al. 2007). Nevertheless, all three studies indicate that TRPM8 plays a central and essential role in cold temperature transduction and perception.

Sensitivity to cold is heightened in certain inflammatory and neuropathic pain conditions. This results in the development of cold allodynia, a painful hypersensitivity to innocuous cold temperature stimulation. The role of TRPM8 in mediating cold, mechanical, and thermal hypersensitivity under pathophysiological conditions remains elusive. TRPM8 expression is increased in the ipsilateral DRG neurons after the development of neuropathic pain (Frederick et al. 2007; Proudfoot et al. 2006; Xing et al. 2007). But, different studies indicate that both agonism and antagonism of TRPM8 may be involved in mediating its analgesic effect.

It has been shown that topical or intrathecal application of TRPM8 activators (cold, menthol, or icilin), attenuates both thermal and mechanical hypersensitivity in a rodent chronic constriction injury model of neuropathic pain (Proudfoot et al. 2006). This demonstrates that central expression of TRPM8 in primary afferents innervating the dorsal horn can contribute to the analgesic effect. TRPM8 agonism was also effective in reversing both thermal and mechanical hypersensitivity in the CFA model of inflammatory pain and in the cinnamaldehyde-induced hypersensitivity (Proudfoot et al. 2006). A more recent study using a subtle modification of the formalin test elegantly showed that while wild-type mice exhibit reduced formalin-induced nocifensor behavior when placed on plates set at 17°C, mice lacking TRPM8 develop similar nociceptive responses at 17°C and room temperature (Dhaka et al. 2007).

While these studies clearly implicate TRPM8 agonism in reversing the hypersensitivity observed across a wide spectrum of pain models, recent data suggest that TRPM8 blockade may lead to an analgesic effect as well. Colburn et al. (2007) showed that TRPM8 deficient homozygous mice develop virtually no cold allodynia in both chronic constriction injury and CFA models, while tactile allodynia is not affected in both genotypes.

In summary, there is strong evidence suggesting that TRPM8 may play an important role in nociception. However, it remains unclear whether agonism or antagonism of this target should be pursued to treat clinical pain indications.

4 Pharmacology of TRP Channels

Given their expression in sensory tissues, especially sensory neuron fibers, their activation by noxious modalities, and the specific sensory deficits observed in mouse knockouts of their genes, TRPV1, TRPV3, TRPV4, TRPA1, and TRPM8 have been the focus of significant drug discovery efforts for novel pain relievers.

Because these channels are cation-permeable and ligand-gated, high-throughput assays have been readily developed to screen large compound libraries. This effort has resulted in the identification of many modulators of sensory TRP channels.

4.1 Nonselective TRP Channel Agonists and Antagonists

Some sensory TRP channel agonists found in nature are not highly selective at high concentrations. For example, menthol, a TRPM8 agonist (EC_{50} = 30 μM), also activates TRPV3 (EC_{50} ~ 20 mM) and inhibits TRPA1 (IC_{50} = 68 μM). Also, camphor is a TRPV1 agonist (EC_{50} ~ 4.5 mM) as well as a TRPV3 agonist (EC_{50} ~ 40 mM), but is a TRPA1 inhibitor (IC_{50} = 68 μM) (Macpherson et al. 2006). 2-APB is an agonist at TRPV3 (EC_{50} = 41.6 μM; Chung et al. 2004), TRPV1 (EC_{50} = 114 μM), and TRPV2 (EC_{50} = 129 μM), but is a TRPM8 antagonist (IC_{50} = 7.7 μM) (Hu et al. 2004).

Ruthenium red and certain cations, such as gadolinium and lanthanide, have been shown to inhibit the sensory TRP channels reviewed here, and many others as well. These compounds have been useful reagents to study TRP channel function in overexpressed cells or to characterize particular biophysical parameters of TRP channel activity. However, lack of selectivity limits their ability to understand physiological processes in more complex systems, e.g., in vivo.

4.2 TRPV1

The TRPV1 agonists capsaicin and RTX have long been used to probe the function of sensory fibers in a variety of physiological processes, such as the airway and urinary bladder. It has also been appreciated for some time that capsaicin and RTX treatment can result in persistent desensitization of the sensory fiber (Szallasi et al. 1999). The mechanism of desensitization likely involves both channel desensitization as well as cellular toxicity due to prolonged calcium influx (Tominaga 2007). In vivo this results in analgesia effects, which is the basis for the use of over-the-counter creams containing capsaicin as well as continued efforts to develop other capsaicin formulations for use as analgesics or for the treatment of urinary incontinence (Szallasi et al. 2007). Because capsaicin induces acute pain via activation of sensory fibers, these formulations are designed to minimize the acute effects while still driving desensitization. Other approaches include formulations of RTX and novel compounds, such as olvanil (Krause et al. 2005).

Substantial industry effort has resulted in the identification of a large number of potent and efficacious TRPV1 antagonists (Krause et al. 2005; Szallasi et al. 2007). The first reported TRPV1 antagonist of significant potency was capsazepine (Bevan et al. 1992); however, capsazepine inhibits nicotinic receptors, voltage-gated calcium channels, and TRPM8 (Behrendt et al. 2004; Krause et al. 2005). Starting in

2002, TRPV1 antagonists with greater potency and selectivity were reported (Krause et al. 2005), and the collection of novel, small-molecule inhibitors includes a wide range of structures with exquisite potency ($IC_{50} < 1$ nM in some cases; Szallasi et al. 2007). Of these inhibitors, iodoresiniferatoxin, the urea analog BCTC, and the cinnamide analog SB-366791 have been the most widely published. Within this group, iodoresiniferatoxin and SB-366791 are quite selective to TRPV1 versus other receptors and channels, whereas BCTC is an inhibitor of TRPM8 (IC_{50} = 143 nM; Weil et al. 2005). A-778317, a stereoselective, urea analog, which is a potent TRPV1 antagonist in vitro (IC_{50} = 4.9 nM), can be labeled with ^3H to yield a high-affinity radioligand with a K_D of 3.4 nM in Chinese hamster ovary cells (Bianchi et al. 2007); additional investigations of TRPV1 pharmacological effects with this radioligand have not yet been published.

Important to understanding its role in pain is defining the emerging function of TRPV1 in regulating body temperature, a role initially suggested by the observation that a urea analog TRPV1 antagonist ("Compound 41") increased core body temperature when administered to rats (Swanson et al. 2005). A subsequent study with AMG0347 suggested that TRPV1 expressed on peripheral fibers mediated the effect of a TRPV1 antagonist on core body temperature (Steiner et al. 2007), although TRPV1 antagonists (e.g., AMG8562) have recently been identified that are reported to have no effect on body temperature (Lehto et al. 2008).

TRPV1 antagonists that exhibit very limited central nervous system (CNS) exposure have been described (Cui et al. 2006; Tamayo et al. 2008). Investigations comparing very limited CNS exposure compounds (e.g., A-719614, brain-to-plasma exposure ratio 0.008) with brain-penetrant analogs (e.g., A-784168) suggest that CNS exposure improves the analgesic efficacy (Cui et al. 2006). However, rats administered compounds with very low CNS exposure exhibited core body temperature increases that were comparable to those resulting from administration of brain-penetrant compounds (Tamayo et al. 2008). These data support the hypothesis that TRPV1 expressed in the CNS (perhaps in terminals of sensory neuron projections to the spinal cord dorsal horn) are important for mediating nociception, but that TRPV1 in CNS sites such as the hypothalamus may not be involved in regulating core body temperature.

4.3 TRPA1

The first pharmacological evidence implicating the TRPA1 channel in mediating pain under inflammatory conditions came recently when it was shown that AP18, a TRPA1 small-molecule antagonist, can significantly attenuate CFA-induced inflammatory pain (Petrus et al. 2007). AP18 is a selective TRPA1 antagonist that inhibits both the mouse (IC_{50} 4.5 μM) and the human (IC_{50} 3.1 μM) receptors. Acute pharmacological inhibition of TRPA1 using intraplantar (local) injection of AP18 significantly reduced the CFA-induced mechanical hypersensitivity and cold allodynia. AP18 has no effect in TRPA1−/− mice, strongly suggesting that AP18-

induced analgesia results from on-target activities (Petrus et al. 2007). Moreover, local preadministration of AP18 in the hindpaw reversed cinnamaldehyde-induced nocifensor behavior, again indicating that AP18 acts on the TRPA1 receptors.

Another selective TRPA1 antagonist, HC-030031, has been described with an IC_{50} at the human receptor of 6.2 μM (McNamara et al. 2007). This compound was shown to significantly and dose dependently (100 and 300 mg kg^{-1}) reduce flinching in both phases of the formalin response in vivo and abolish allylisothiocyanate-induced mechanical hypersensitivity in a dose-dependent manner. Plasma or brain exposures of this compound were not reported in this study and therefore a pharmacokinetic/pharmacodynamic relationship has not been established for HC-030031.

4.4 TRPV3, TRPV4, and TRPM8

There have been no reports of small-molecule TRPV3, TRPV4, or TRPM8 selective antagonists in the peer-reviewed literature. However, several patent applications have been published which describe small-molecule inhibitors of TRPV3 that exhibit an analgesic effect in rat models of pain (WO2006/122156, WO2007/056124, and WO2008/033564). For TRPV4, many patent applications have been published to date which describe small-molecule inhibitors of TRPV4 (WO2006/029154, WO2006/029209, WO2006/029210, WO2006/105475, WO2007/082262, WO2007/098393), and one application describes TRPV4 agonists (WO2007/070865). For TRPM8, several patent applications were published reporting the discovery of TRPM8 agonists and antagonists for the treatment of urological disorders, pain, and prostate cancer (WO2005/020897, WO2006/040136, WO2007/080109, WO2007/095340 WO2007/017092, WO2007/017093, WO2007/017094, WO2007/134107).

5 Conclusions

Agents such as capsaicin, mustard oil, and menthol have provided important insights into the role of sensory neurons in diverse physiological processes such as voiding of the urinary bladder, changes in vascular permeability, and airway responsiveness and contractility. Perhaps the greatest utility of these molecules has been in probing the mechanisms by which sensory neurons transmit changes in physiological processes into pain signals, i.e., nociception. The discovery of TRP channels as mediators of chemogenic activation of sensory neurons has been an important advance in understanding the molecular underpinnings of nociception. Indeed, the high level of expression of these channels (especially TRPV1, TRPA1, and TRPM8) in sensory neurons has led many investigators to embrace the hypothesis that modulators of sensory neuron TRP channels will yield effective therapeutics for pain. This hypothesis has been extended to include all members of the so-called thermoTRP subfamily (TRPV1, TRPV2, TRPV3, TRPV4, TRPA1, TRPM8). Small-molecule antagonists of TRPV1, TRPA1, and TRPV3 have been discovered, and have been shown to exhibit efficacy in animal models of pain. Definitive evidence of human efficacy has yet to be disclosed, and the effect of thermoTRP channel inhibition on other pathophysiological conditions, such as diabetes or urinary incontinence, has not been reported. However, the availability of an ever-increasing number of potent and selective compounds should lead to a better understanding of the function of the sensory neuron and, hopefully, effective therapeutics for human disease.

References

Akbar A, Yiangou Y, Facer P, Walters JR, Anand P, Ghosh S (2008) Increased capsaicin receptor TRPV1 expressing sensory fibres in irritable bowel syndrome and their correlation with abdominal pain. Gut. doi:10.1136/gut.2007.138982

Alessandri-Haber N, Dina OA, Yeh JJ, Parada CA, Reichling DB, Levine JD (2004) Transient receptor potential vanilloid 4 is essential in chemotherapy-induced neuropathic pain in the rat. J Neurosci 24:4444–4452

Alessandri-Haber N, Dina OA, Joseph EK, Reichling D, Levine JD (2006) A transient receptor potential vanilloid 4-dependent mechanism of hyperalgesia is engaged by concerted action of inflammatory mediators. J Neurosci 26:3864–3874

Alessandri-Haber N, Dina OA, Joseph EK, Reichling DB, Levine JD (2008) Interaction of transient receptor potential vanilloid 4, integrin, and SRC tyrosine kinase in mechanical hyperalgesia. J Neurosci 28:1046–1057

Bandell M, Story GM, Hwang SW, Viswanath V, Eid SR, Petrus MJ, Earley TJ, Patapoutian A (2004) Noxious cold ion channel TRPA1 is activated by pungent compounds and bradykinin. Neuron 41:849–857

Bang S, Kim KY, Yoo S, Lee SH, Hwang SW (2007) Transient receptor potential V2 expressed in sensory neurons is activated by probenecid. Neurosci Lett 425:120–125

Bautista DM, Movahed P, Hinman A, Axelsson HE, Sterner O, Hogestatt ED, Julius D, Jordt SE, Zygmunt PM (2005) Pungent products from garlic activate the sensory ion channel TRPA1. Proc Natl Acad Sci USA 102:12248–12252

Bautista DM, Jordt SE, Nikai T, Tsuruda PR, Read AJ, Poblete J, Yamoah EN, Basbaum AI, Julius D (2006) TRPA1 mediates the inflammatory actions of environmental irritants and proalgesic agents. Cell 124:1269–1282

Bautista DM, Siemens J, Glazer JM, Tsuruda PR, Basbaum AI, Stucky CL, Jordt SE, Julius D (2007) The menthol receptor TRPM8 is the principal detector of environmental cold. Nature 448:204–208

Behrendt HJ, Germann T, Gillen C, Hatt H, Jostock R (2004) Characterization of the mouse cold-menthol receptor TRPM8 and vanilloid receptor type-1 VR1 using a fluorometric imaging plate reader (FLIPR) assay. Br J Pharmacol 141:737–745

Bevan S, Hothi S, Hughes G, James IF, Rang HP, Shah K, Walpole CS, Yeats JC (1992) Capsazepine: a competitive antagonist of the sensory neurone excitant capsaicin. Br J Pharmacol 107:544–552

Bianchi BR, El Kouhen R et al (2007) [3H]A-778317 [1-((*R*)-5-tert-butyl-indan-1-yl)-3-isoquinolin-5-yl-urea]: a novel, stereoselective, high-affinity antagonist is a useful radioligand for the human transient receptor potential vanilloid-1 (TRPV1) receptor. J Pharmacol Exp Ther 323:285–293

Bodding M, Wissenbach U, Flockerzi V (2007) Characterisation of TRPM8 as a pharmacophore receptor. Cell Calcium 42:618–628
Carlton SM, Coggeshall RE (2001) Peripheral capsaicin receptors increase in the inflamed rat hindpaw: a possible mechanism for peripheral sensitization. Neurosci Lett 310:53–56
Caterina MJ, Schumacher MA, Tominaga M, Rosen TA, Levine JD, Julius D (1997) The capsaicin receptor: a heat-activated ion channel in the pain pathway. Nature 389:816–824
Caterina MJ, Rosen TA, Tominaga M, Brake AJ, Julius D (1999) A capsaicin-receptor homologue with a high threshold for noxious heat. Nature 398:436–441
Caterina MJ, Leffler A, Malmberg AB, Martin WJ, Trafton J, Petersen-Zeitz KR, Koltzenburg M, Basbaum AI, Julius D (2000) Impaired nociception and pain sensation in mice lacking the capsaicin receptor. Science 288:306–313
Christianson JA, McIlwrath SL, Koerber HR, Davis BM (2006) Transient receptor potential vanilloid 1-immunopositive neurons in the mouse are more prevalent within colon afferents compared to skin and muscle afferents. Neuroscience 140:247–257
Christoph T, Grunweller A et al (2006) Silencing of vanilloid receptor TRPV1 by RNAi reduces neuropathic and visceral pain in vivo. Biochem Biophys Res Commun 350:238–243
Christoph T, Gillen C et al (2007) Antinociceptive effect of antisense oligonucleotides against the vanilloid receptor VR1/TRPV1. Neurochem Int 50:281–290
Christoph T, Bahrenberg G et al (2008) Investigation of TRPV1 loss-of-function phenotypes in transgenic shRNA expressing and knockout mice. Mol Cell Neurosci 37:579–589
Chung MK, Lee H, Mizuno A, Suzuki M, Caterina MJ (2004) 2-Aminoethoxydiphenyl borate activates and sensitizes the heat-gated ion channel TRPV3. J Neurosci 24:5177–5182
Cohen DM (2007) The transient receptor potential vanilloid-responsive 1 and 4 cation channels: role in neuronal osmosensing and renal physiology. Curr Opin Nephrol Hypertens 16:451–458
Colburn RW, Lubin ML et al (2007) Attenuated cold sensitivity in TRPM8 null mice. Neuron 54:379–386
Corey DP, Garcia-Anoveros J et al (2004) TRPA1 is a candidate for the mechanosensitive transduction channel of vertebrate hair cells. Nature 432:723–730
Cortright DN, Crandall M, Sanchez JF, Zou T, Krause JE, White G (2001) The tissue distribution and functional characterization of human VR1. Biochem Biophys Res Commun 281:1183–1189
Crandall M, Kwash J, Yu W, White G (2002) Activation of protein kinase C sensitizes human VR1 to capsaicin and to moderate decreases in *p*H at physiological temperatures in Xenopus oocytes. Pain 98:109–117
Cui M, Honore P et al (2006) TRPV1 receptors in the CNS play a key role in broad-spectrum analgesia of TRPV1 antagonists. J Neurosci 26:9385–9393
D'Hoedt D, Owsianik G, Prenen J, Cuajungco MP, Grimm C, Heller S, Voets T, Nilius B (2008) Stimulus-specific modulation of the cation channel TRPV4 by PACSIN 3. J Biol Chem 283:6272–6280
Dai Y, Wang S et al (2007) Sensitization of TRPA1 by PAR2 contributes to the sensation of inflammatory pain. J Clin Invest 117:1979–1987
Davis JB, Gray J et al (2000) Vanilloid receptor-1 is essential for inflammatory thermal hyperalgesia. Nature 405:183–187
Delany NS, Hurle M et al (2001) Identification and characterization of a novel human vanilloid receptor-like protein, VRL-2. Physiol Genomics 4:165–174
Dhaka A, Viswanath V, Patapoutian A (2006) TRP ion channels and temperature sensation. Annu Rev Neurosci 29:135–161
Dhaka A, Murray AN, Mathur J, Earley TJ, Petrus MJ, Patapoutian A (2007) TRPM8 is required for cold sensation in mice. Neuron 54:371–378
Diogenes A, Akopian AN, Hargreaves KM (2007) NGF up-regulates TRPA1: implications for orofacial pain. J Dent Res 86:550–555

Doerner JF, Gisselmann G, Hatt H, Wetzel CH (2007) Transient receptor potential channel A1 is directly gated by calcium ions. J Biol Chem 282:13180–13189

Facer P, Casula MA, Smith GD, Benham CD, Chessell IP, Bountra C, Sinisi M, Birch R, Anand P (2007) Differential expression of the capsaicin receptor TRPV1 and related novel receptors TRPV3, TRPV4 and TRPM8 in normal human tissues and changes in traumatic and diabetic neuropathy. BMC Neurol 7:11

Frederick J, Buck ME, Matson DJ, Cortright DN (2007) Increased TRPA1, TRPM8, and TRPV2 expression in dorsal root ganglia by nerve injury. Biochem Biophys Res Commun 358:1058–1064

Gevaert T, Vriens J et al (2007) Deletion of the transient receptor potential cation channel TRPV4 impairs murine bladder voiding. J Clin Invest 117:3453–3462

Gibson HE, Edwards JG, Page RS, Van Hook MJ, Kauer JA (2008) TRPV1 channels mediate long-term depression at synapses on hippocampal interneurons. Neuron 57:746–759

Guler AD, Lee H, Iida T, Shimizu I, Tominaga M, Caterina M (2002) Heat-evoked activation of the ion channel, TRPV4. J Neurosci 22:6408–6414

Handwerker HO, Forster C, Kirchhoff C (1991) Discharge patterns of human C-fibers induced by itching and burning stimuli. J Neurophysiol 66:307–315

Hinman A, Chuang HH, Bautista DM, Julius D (2006) TRP channel activation by reversible covalent modification. Proc Natl Acad Sci USA 103:19564–19568

Hu HZ, Gu Q, Wang C, Colton CK, Tang J, Kinoshita-Kawada M, Lee LY, Wood JD, Zhu MX (2004) 2-Aminoethoxydiphenyl borate is a common activator of TRPV1, TRPV2, and TRPV3. J Biol Chem 279:35741–35748

Hu HZ, Xiao R, Wang C, Gao N, Colton CK, Wood JD, Zhu MX (2006) Potentiation of TRPV3 channel function by unsaturated fatty acids. J Cell Physiol 208:201–212

Jordt SE, Bautista DM, Chuang HH, McKemy DD, Zygmunt PM, Hogestatt ED, Meng ID, Julius D (2004) Mustard oils and cannabinoids excite sensory nerve fibres through the TRP channel ANKTM1. Nature 427:260–265

Kanzaki M, Zhang YQ, Mashima H, Li L, Shibata H, Kojima I (1999) Translocation of a calcium-permeable cation channel induced by insulin-like growth factor-I. Nat Cell Biol 1:165–170

Kasama S, Kawakubo M, Suzuki T, Nishizawa T, Ishida A, Nakayama J (2007) RNA interference-mediated knock-down of transient receptor potential vanilloid 1 prevents forepaw inflammatory hyperalgesia in rat. Eur J Neurosci 25:2956–2963

Katsura H, Obata K et al (2006) Antisense knock down of TRPA1, but not TRPM8, alleviates cold hyperalgesia after spinal nerve ligation in rats. Exp Neurol 200:112–123

Kindt KS, Viswanath V, Macpherson L, Quast K, Hu H, Patapoutian A, Schafer WR (2007) Caenorhabditis elegans TRPA-1 functions in mechanosensation. Nat Neurosci 10:568–577

Klionsky L, Tamir R et al (2006) A polyclonal antibody to the pre-pore loop of TRPV1 blocks channel activation. J Pharmacol Exp Ther 319:192–198

Kollarik M, Undem BJ (2004) Activation of bronchopulmonary vagal afferent nerves with bradykinin, acid and vanilloid receptor agonists in wild-type and TRPV1−/− mice. J Physiol 555:115–123

Koltzenburg M, Lundberg LE, Torebjork HE (1992) Dynamic and static components of mechanical hyperalgesia in human hairy skin. Pain 51:207–219

Krause JE, Chenard BL, Cortright DN (2005) Transient receptor potential ion channels as targets for the discovery of pain therapeutics. Curr Opin Investig Drugs 6:48–57

Kwan KY, Allchorne AJ, Vollrath MA, Christensen AP, Zhang DS, Woolf CJ, Corey DP (2006) TRPA1 contributes to cold, mechanical, and chemical nociception but is not essential for hair-cell transduction. Neuron 50:277–289

Lee H, Iida T, Mizuno A, Suzuki M, Caterina MJ (2005) Altered thermal selection behavior in mice lacking transient receptor potential vanilloid 4. J Neurosci 25:1304–1310

Lehto S, Tamir R et al (2008) Antihyperalgesic effects of AMG8562, a novel vanilloid receptor TRPV1 modulator that does not cause hyperthermia in rats. J Pharmacol Exp Ther 326:218–229

Lewinter RD, Skinner K, Julius D, Basbaum AI (2004) Immunoreactive TRPV-2 (VRL-1), a capsaicin receptor homolog, in the spinal cord of the rat. J Comp Neurol 470:400–408
Lewinter RD, Scherrer G, Basbaum AI (2008) Dense transient receptor potential cation channel, vanilloid family, type 2 (TRPV2) immunoreactivity defines a subset of motoneurons in the dorsal lateral nucleus of the spinal cord, the nucleus ambiguus and the trigeminal motor nucleus in rat. Neuroscience 151:164–173
Liedtke W, Choe Y, Marti-Renom MA, Bell AM, Denis CS, Sali A, Hudspeth AJ, Friedman JM, Heller S (2000) Vanilloid receptor-related osmotically activated channel (VR-OAC), a candidate vertebrate osmoreceptor. Cell 103:525–535
Liedtke W, Friedman JM (2003) Abnormal osmotic regulation in TRPV4−/− mice. Proc Natl Acad Sci USA 100:13698–13703
Liu B, Qin F (2005) Functional control of cold- and menthol-sensitive TRPM8 ion channels by phosphatidylinositol 4,5-bisphosphate. J Neurosci 25:1674–1681
Lukacs V, Thyagarajan B, Varnai P, Balla A, Balla T, Rohacs T (2007) Dual regulation of TRPV1 by phosphoinositides. J Neurosci 27:7070–7080
Macpherson LJ, Geierstanger BH, Viswanath V, Bandell M, Eid SR, Hwang S, Patapoutian A (2005) The pungency of garlic: activation of TRPA1 and TRPV1 in response to allicin. Curr Biol 15:929–934
Macpherson LJ, Hwang SW, Miyamoto T, Dubin AE, Patapoutian A, Story GM (2006) More than cool: Promiscuous relationships of menthol and other sensory compounds. Mol Cell Neurosci 32(4):335–343
Macpherson LJ, Dubin AE, Evans MJ, Marr F, Schultz PG, Cravatt BF, Patapoutian A (2007a) Noxious compounds activate TRPA1 ion channels through covalent modification of cysteines. Nature 445:541–545
Macpherson LJ, Xiao B, Kwan KY, Petrus MJ, Dubin AE, Hwang S, Cravatt B, Corey DP, Patapoutian A (2007b) An ion channel essential for sensing chemical damage. J Neurosci 27:11412–11415
McKemy DD, Neuhausser WM, Julius D (2002) Identification of a cold receptor reveals a general role for TRP channels in thermosensation. Nature 416:52–58
McMahon SB, Wood JN (2006) Increasingly irritable and close to tears: TRPA1 in inflammatory pain. Cell 124:1123–1125
McNamara CR, Mandel-Brehm J et al (2007) TRPA1 mediates formalin-induced pain. Proc Natl Acad Sci USA 104:13525–13530
Mezey E, Toth ZE, Cortright DN, Arzubi MK, Krause JE, Elde R, Guo A, Blumberg PM, Szallasi A (2000) Distribution of mRNA for vanilloid receptor subtype 1 (VR1), and VR1-like immunoreactivity, in the central nervous system of the rat and human. Proc Natl Acad Sci USA 97:3655–3660
Meyer RA, Campbell JN, Raja SN (1994) Peripheral neural mechanisms of nociception, 4th edn, Churchill Livingstone, New York
Moqrich A, Hwang SW, Earley TJ, Petrus MJ, Murray AN, Spencer KS, Andahazy M, Story GM, Patapoutian A (2005) Impaired thermosensation in mice lacking TRPV3, a heat and camphor sensor in the skin. Science 307:1468–1472
Muraki K, Iwata Y, Katanosaka Y, Ito T, Ohya S, Shigekawa M, Imaizumi Y (2003) TRPV2 is a component of osmotically sensitive cation channels in murine aortic myocytes. Circ Res 93:829–838
Nagasawa M, Nakagawa Y, Tanaka S, Kojima I (2007) Chemotactic peptide fMetLeuPhe induces translocation of the TRPV2 channel in macrophages. J Cell Physiol 210:692–702
Namer B, Seifert F, Handwerker HO, Maihofner C (2005) TRPA1 and TRPM8 activation in humans: effects of cinnamaldehyde and menthol. Neuroreport 16:955–959
Neeper MP, Liu Y, Hutchinson TL, Wang Y, Flores CM, Qin N (2007) Activation properties of heterologously expressed mammalian TRPV2: evidence for species dependence. J Biol Chem 282:15894–15902

Peier AM, Moqrich A et al (2002a) A TRP channel that senses cold stimuli and menthol. Cell 108:705–715
Peier AM, Reeve AJ et al (2002b) A heat-sensitive TRP channel expressed in keratinocytes. Science 296:2046–2049
Petrus M, Peier AM, Bandell M, Hwang SW, Huynh T, Olney N, Jegla T, Patapoutian A (2007) A role of TRPA1 in mechanical hyperalgesia is revealed by pharmacological inhibition. Mol Pain 3:40
Patapoutian A (2007) A role of TRPA1 in mechanical hyperalgesia is revealed by pharmacological inhibition. Mol Pain 3, 40
Premkumar LS, Ahern GP (2000) Induction of vanilloid receptor channel activity by protein kinase C. Nature 408:985–990
Prescott ED, Julius D (2003) A modular PIP2 binding site as a determinant of capsaicin receptor sensitivity. Science 300:1284–1288
Proudfoot CJ, Garry EM, Cottrell DF, Rosie R, Anderson H, Robertson DC, Fleetwood-Walker SM, Mitchell R (2006) Analgesia mediated by the TRPM8 cold receptor in chronic neuropathic pain. Curr Biol 16:1591–1605
Raja SN, Meyer RA et al (1999) Peripheral neural mechanisms of nociception. In: Wall PD, Melzack R (eds) Textbook of pain. Churchill Livingston, Edinburgh
Rashid MH, Inoue M, Kondo S, Kawashima T, Bakoshi S, Ueda H (2003) Novel expression of vanilloid receptor 1 on capsaicin-insensitive fibers accounts for the analgesic effect of capsaicin cream in neuropathic pain. J Pharmacol Exp Ther 304:940–948
Razavi R, Chan Y et al (2006) TRPV1+ sensory neurons control beta cell stress and islet inflammation in autoimmune diabetes. Cell 127:1123–1135
Reeh PW, Kocher L, Jung S (1986) Does neurogenic inflammation alter the sensitivity of unmyelinated nociceptors in the rat? Brain Res 384:42–50
Rohacs T, Lopes CM, Michailidis I, Logothetis DE (2005) PI(4,5)P2 regulates the activation and desensitization of TRPM8 channels through the TRP domain. Nat Neurosci 8:626–634
Sanchez JF, Krause JE, Cortright DN (2001) The distribution and regulation of vanilloid receptor VR1 and VR1 5′ splice variant RNA expression in rat. Neuroscience 107:373–381
Shea VK, Cai R, Crepps B, Mason JL, Perl ER (2000) Sensory fibers of the pelvic nerve innervating the Rat's urinary bladder. J Neurophysiol 84:1924–1933
Shimosato G, Amaya F, Ueda M, Tanaka Y, Decosterd I, Tanaka M (2005) Peripheral inflammation induces up-regulation of TRPV2 expression in rat DRG. Pain 119:225–232
Smith GD, Gunthorpe MJ et al (2002) TRPV3 is a temperature-sensitive vanilloid receptor-like protein. Nature 418:186–190
Smith PL, Maloney KN, Pothen RG, Clardy J, Clapham DE (2006) Bisandrographolide from *Andrographis paniculata* activates TRPV4 channels. J Biol Chem 281:29897–29904
Steiner AA, Turek VF et al (2007) Nonthermal activation of transient receptor potential vanilloid-1 channels in abdominal viscera tonically inhibits autonomic cold-defense effectors. J Neurosci 27:7459–7468
Story GM, Peier AM et al (2003) ANKTM1, a TRP-like channel expressed in nociceptive neurons, is activated by cold temperatures. Cell 112:819–829
Stucky CL, Lewin GR (1999) Isolectin B(4)-positive and -negative nociceptors are functionally distinct. J Neurosci 19:6497–6505
Suzuki M, Mizuno A, Kodaira K, Imai M (2003) Impaired pressure sensation in mice lacking TRPV4. J Biol Chem 278:22664–22668
Swanson DM, Dubin AE et al (2005) Identification and biological evaluation of 4-(3-trifluoromethylpyridin-2-yl)piperazine-1-carboxylic acid (5-trifluoromethylpyridin-2-yl)amide, a high affinity TRPV1 (VR1) vanilloid receptor antagonist. J Med Chem 48:1857–1872
Szallasi A, Blumberg PM (1999) Vanilloid (Capsaicin) receptors and mechanisms. Pharmacol Rev 51:159–212
Szallasi A, Cortright DN, Blum CA, Eid SR (2007) The vanilloid receptor TRPV1: 10 years from channel cloning to antagonist proof-of-concept. Nat Rev Drug Discov 6:357–372

Tamayo N, Liao H et al (2008) Design and Synthesis of Peripherally Restricted Transient Receptor Potential Vanilloid 1 (TRPV1) Antagonists. J Med Chem 51:2744–2757
Taylor-Clark TE, Undem BJ, Macglashan DW Jr, Ghatta S, Carr MJ, McAlexander MA (2008) Prostaglandin-induced activation of nociceptive neurons via direct interaction with transient receptor potential A1 (TRPA1). Mol Pharmacol 73:274–281
Todaka H, Taniguchi J, Satoh J, Mizuno A, Suzuki M (2004) Warm temperature-sensitive transient receptor potential vanilloid 4 (TRPV4) plays an essential role in thermal hyperalgesia. J Biol Chem 279:35133–35138
Tominaga M (2007) Nociception and TRP channels. Handb Exp Pharmacol, 489–505
Tominaga M, Caterina MJ, Malmberg AB, Rosen TA, Gilbert H, Skinner K, Raumann BE, Basbaum AI, Julius D (1998) The cloned capsaicin receptor integrates multiple pain-producing stimuli. Neuron 21:531–543
Trevisani M, Siemens J et al (2007) 4-Hydroxynonenal, an endogenous aldehyde, causes pain and neurogenic inflammation through activation of the irritant receptor TRPA1. Proc Natl Acad Sci USA 104:13519–13524
Vogt-Eisele AK, Weber K, Sherkheli MA, Vielhaber G, Panten J, Gisselmann G, Hatt H (2007) Monoterpenoid agonists of TRPV3. Br J Pharmacol 151:530–540
Wang Y, Wang DH (2006) A novel mechanism contributing to development of Dahl salt-sensitive hypertension: role of the transient receptor potential vanilloid type 1. Hypertension 47:609–614
Ward L, Wright E, McMahon SB (1996) A comparison of the effects of noxious and innocuous counterstimuli on experimentally induced itch and pain. Pain 64:129–138
Weil A, Moore SE, Waite NJ, Randall A, Gunthorpe MJ (2005) Conservation of functional and pharmacological properties in the distantly related temperature sensors TRVP1 and TRPM8. Mol Pharmacol 68:518–527
Xiao R, Tang J, Wang C, Colton CK, Tian J, Zhu MX (2008) Calcium plays a central role in the sensitization of TRPV3 channel to repetitive stimulations. J Biol Chem 283:6162–6174
Xing H, Chen M, Ling J, Tan W, Gu JG (2007) TRPM8 mechanism of cold allodynia after chronic nerve injury. J Neurosci 27:13680–13690
Xu H, Ramsey IS et al (2002) TRPV3 is a calcium-permeable temperature-sensitive cation channel. Nature 418:181–186
Xu H, Zhao H, Tian W, Yoshida K, Roullet JB, Cohen DM (2003) Regulation of a transient receptor potential (TRP) channel by tyrosine phosphorylation. SRC family kinase-dependent tyrosine phosphorylation of TRPV4 on TYR-253 mediates its response to hypotonic stress. J Biol Chem 278:11520–11527
Xu H, Blair NT, Clapham DE (2005) Camphor activates and strongly desensitizes the transient receptor potential vanilloid subtype 1 channel in a vanilloid-independent mechanism. J Neurosci 25:8924–8937
Xu H, Delling M, Jun JC, Clapham DE (2006) Oregano, thyme and clove-derived flavors and skin sensitizers activate specific TRP channels. Nat Neurosci 9:628–635
Zurborg S, Yurgionas B, Jira JA, Caspani O, Heppenstall PA (2007) Direct activation of the ion channel TRPA1 by Ca^{2+}. Nat Neurosci 10:277–279

Acid-Sensitive Ion Channels and Receptors

Peter Holzer

Contents

P. Holzer
Research Unit of Translational Neurogastroenterology, Institute of Experimental and Clinical Pharmacology, Medical University of Graz, Universitätsplatz 4, 8010, Graz, Austria
peter.holzer@medunigraz.at

B.J. Canning and D. Spina (eds.), *Sensory Nerves*, Handbook of Experimental Pharmacology 194, DOI: 10.1007/978-3-540-79090-7_9,

Abstract Acidosis is a noxious condition associated with inflammation, ischaemia or defective acid containment. As a consequence, acid sensing has evolved as an important property of afferent neurons with unmyelinated and thinly myelinated nerve fibres. Protons evoke multiple currents in primary afferent neurons, which are carried by several acid-sensitive ion channels. Among these, acid-sensing ion channels (ASICs) and transient receptor potential (TRP) vanilloid-1 (TRPV1) ion channels have been most thoroughly studied. ASICs survey moderate decreases in extracellular pH, whereas TRPV1 is activated only by severe acidosis resulting in pH values below 6. Two-pore-domain K^+ (K_{2P}) channels are differentially regulated by small deviations of extra- or intracellular pH from physiological levels. Other acid-sensitive channels include TRPV4, TRPC4, TRPC5, TRPP2 (PKD2L1), ionotropic purinoceptors (P2X), inward rectifier K^+ channels, voltage-activated K^+ channels, L-type Ca^{2+} channels, hyperpolarization-activated cyclic nucleotide gated channels, gap junction channels, and Cl^- channels. In addition, acid-sensitive G protein coupled receptors have also been identified. Most of these molecular acid sensors are expressed by primary sensory neurons, although to different degrees and in various combinations. Emerging evidence indicates that many of the acid-sensitive ion channels and receptors play a role in acid sensing, acid–induced pain and acid-evoked feedback regulation of homeostatic reactions. The existence and apparent redundancy of multiple pH surveillance systems attests to the concept that acid–base regulation is a vital issue for cell and tissue homeostasis. Since upregulation and overactivity of acid sensors appear to contribute to various forms of chronic pain, acid-sensitive ion channels and receptors are considered as targets for novel analgesic drugs. This approach will only be successful if the pathological implications of acid sensors can be differentiated pharmacologically from their physiological function.

Keywords Acid surveillance, Acid-induced pain, Sour taste, Acidosis, Ischaemia, Angina pectoris, Inflammation, Acid-related gastrointestinal diseases, Cough, Bone resorption, Gastrointestinal tract, Urogenital tract, Pulmonary system, Skin, Carotid body, Proton-gated currents, Molecular acid sensors, Acid-sensing ion channels, ASIC3, TRP ion channels, TRPV1, TRPP2, Two pore domain potassium channels, TASK channels, Proton-sensing G protein coupled receptors, Ionotropic purinoceptors

1 Acid Sensing by Sensory Neurons

1.1 Acid as a Noxious Stimulus

Regulation of the acid–base balance and maintenance of pH at a narrow range around 7.4 is one of the basic principles of cellular homeostasis. This balance can be put in danger by many circumstances, including excess intake of acid, excess gastric acid secretion, defective acid containment in the gastrointestinal and urogenital tracts, metabolic acidosis and acidosis due to ischaemia (hypoxia) or inflammation. To meet with these challenges, there are not only cellular mechanisms of acid–base regulation but also systemic monitoring systems to detect harmful acidosis, to initiate appropriate emergency reactions, and thereby to limit any tissue damage that may arise. The most important systemic acid sensors are primary afferent neurons and the taste receptor cells mediating the sour taste.

It has long been known that acid can elicit pain (Steen and Reeh 1993; Steen et al. 1995), and there is plausible evidence that acidosis contributes to the pain associated with inflammation and ischaemia. Several reports summarized by Steen et al. (1992), Kress and Waldmann (2006) and Wemmie et al. (2006) indicate that interstitial pH values can fall to 4.7 in fracture-related haematomas, to 5.4 in inflammation, to 5.7 in cardiac ischaemia and to 6.2 during exhausting skeletal muscle contractions. In the lumen of the stomach, gastric acid secretion causes the pH to drop down to 1, and this acid load can only be managed by compartmentalization and a strong mucosal acid barrier in the foregut (Holzer 2007). Intrusion of acid into the mucosa of the oesophagus, stomach or duodenum contributes not only to mucosal injury but also to the pain associated with gastro-oesophageal reflux and peptic ulcer disease (Kang and Yap 1991). Acid may likewise be a factor in the pain accompanying cystitis, in which a breakdown of the uroethelial barrier exposes sensory nerve endings to the acidic and hyperosmotic urine (Chuang et al. 2003). There is now ample evidence that the pain associated with angina pectoris is due to ischaemia-induced acidosis (Sutherland et al. 2001; Yagi et al. 2006), that pulmonary acidosis is associated with asthma (Ricciardolo et al. 2004; Hunt 2006) and that acid is a stimulus to elicit the cough reflex (Kollarik et al. 2007). Acidosis also occurs in and around malignant tumours (Vaupel et al. 1989; Newell et al. 1993). Metastases in bone are particularly painful, an instance that is related to enhanced activity of osteoclasts which resorb bone by decreasing interstitial pH below 5 (Honore et al. 2000; Luger et al. 2001; Ghilardi et al. 2005; Nagae et al. 2007).

1.2 Proton-Gated Currents in Sensory Neurons

Consistent with the ability of acidosis to induce pain is its capacity to excite primary sensory neurons and to sensitize them to other noxious stimuli (Clarke and Davison 1978; Krishtal and Pidoplichko 1981; Bevan and Yeats 1991; Steen et al. 1992; Bevan and Geppetti 1994; Reeh and Kress 2001; Krishtal 2003; Kress and Waldmann 2006). The molecular basis of acid sensing was discovered when proton-activated cationic currents were described in dorsal root ganglion (DRG) neurons (Krishtal and Pidoplichko 1981; Bevan and Yeats 1991). As reviewed by Kress and Waldmann (2006), two principal types of proton-gated inward currents are observed. The first type is characterized by a fast and rapidly inactivating inward current carried by Na^+ and by a high sensitivity to H^+, threshold activation occurring at a pH of 7 and maximum activation taking place at a pH around 6 (Krishtal and Pidoplichko 1981; Konnerth et al. 1987; Davies et al. 1988). While this type of proton-gated current is seen in most DRG neurons, the second type is observed only

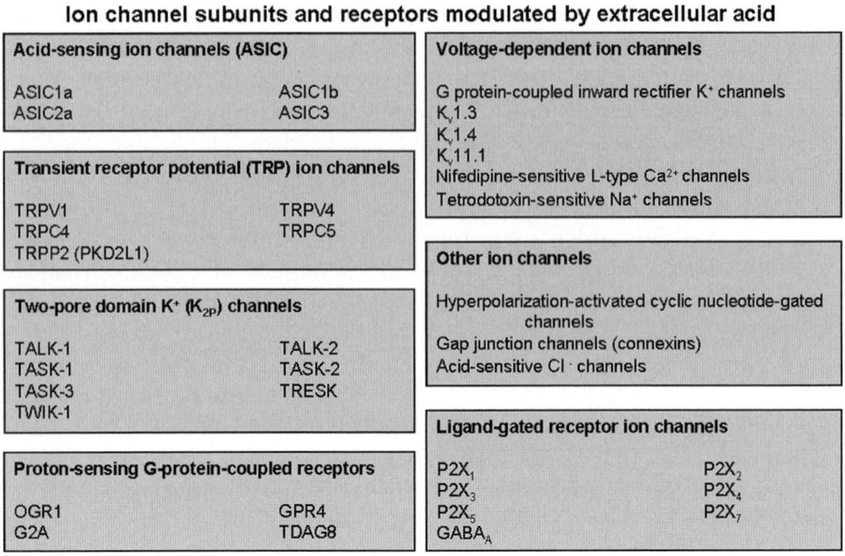
Ion channel subunits and receptors modulated by extracellular acid
Acid-sensing ion channels (ASIC)
ASIC1a
ASIC1b
ASIC2a
ASIC3
Transient receptor potential (TRP) ion channels
TRPV1
TRPV4
TRPC4
TRPC5
TRPP2 (PKD2L1)
Two-pore domain K⁺ (K2P) channels
TALK-1
TALK-2
TASK-1
TASK-2
TASK-3
TRESK
TWIK-1
Proton-sensing G-protein-coupled receptors
OGR1
GPR4
G2A
TDAG8
Voltage-dependent ion channels
G protein-coupled inward rectifier K⁺ channels
Kv1.3
Kv1.4
Kv11.1
Nifedipine-sensitive L-type Ca2+ channels
Tetrodotoxin-sensitive Na⁺ channels
Other ion channels
Hyperpolarization-activated cyclic nucleotide-gated channels
Gap junction channels (connexins)
Acid-sensitive Cl⁻ channels
Ligand-gated receptor ion channels
P2X1
P2X2
P2X3
P2X4
P2X5
P2X7
GABAA

Fig. 1 Overview of ion channel subunits and receptors that are modulated by changes in the extracellular pH (acidification) and expressed by primary afferent neurons or their associated cells. For details, see the text

in DRG neurons that are also excited by capsaicin (Bevan and Yeats 1991; Bevan and Geppetti 1994). Unlike the first type, this current is less sensitive to acidosis, activated only at pH levels below 6.2, sustained, slowly inactivating and developing tachyphylaxis on repeated activation (Bevan and Yeats 1991; Petersen and LaMotte 1993). Further studies showed that the sustained current is due to an increase in cation conductance that allows Na^+, K^+ and Ca^{2+} to pass (Bevan and Yeats 1991; Zeilhofer et al. 1996, 1997).

Molecular analysis has shown that several acid-sensitive ion channels contribute to the capacity of afferent neurons to monitor acidosis (Fig. 1). In some cases, accessory cells (such as the chemoreceptor cells in the taste buds or carotid bodies) survey the pH of their environment and transmit any aberration to adjacent sensory neurons. Among the molecular acid sensors, acid-sensing ion channels (ASICs) and transient receptor potential (TRP) vanilloid-1 (TRPV1) ion channels have been most thoroughly studied (Caterina and Julius 2001; Kress and Waldmann 2006; Wemmie et al. 2006; Diochot et al. 2007; Lingueglia 2007; Szallasi et al. 2007). While the slow proton-activated conductance in DRG neurons shares many similarities with the acidosis-evoked current through TRPV1, the fast acid-induced current resembles currents carried by ASICs (Kress and Waldmann 2006). However, the characteristics of proton-gated currents in sensory neurons are complex and subject to regional and species differences (Leffler et al. 2006; Smith et al. 2007; Sugiura et al. 2007). Accordingly, there is increasing evidence that further acid-sensitive ion channels are involved in monitoring acidosis (Fig. 1). These include TRPV4, TRPC4, TRPC5 and PKD2L1, another member of the TRP ion channel family that is relevant to the perception of the sour taste (Chandrashekar et al.

2006). Other candidates include members of the two-pore-domain K^+ (K_{2P}) channel family, inward rectifier K^+ (Kir) channels, voltage-gated K^+ channels, ionotropic purinoceptors (P2X) containing the $P2X_2$ subunit (Reeh and Kress 2001; Holzer 2003; Duprat et al. 2007) and proton-sensing G protein coupled receptors (GPCRs; Ludwig et al. 2003; Tomura et al. 2005).

The objective of this article is to give an overview of the ability of primary sensory neurons to monitor acidosis, to describe the molecular acid sensors involved (Fig. 1) and to address the physiological and pathophysiological implications of acid-sensitive ion channels and receptors in nociception with a pharmacological perspective.

2 Acid Sensors on Sensory Neurons

2.1 Acid-Sensing Ion Channels

ASICs belong to the voltage-insensitive, amiloride-sensitive epithelial Na^+ channel/degenerin family of cation channels (Waldmann and Lazdunski 1998; Kellenberger and Schild 2002; Waldmann 2001; Welsh et al. 2002). The *proton-sensitive* members of this family expressed in mammals are encoded by three different genes (*ACCN1*, *ACCN2* and *ACCN3*) which are alternatively spliced to produce five subunits: ASIC1a, ASIC1b, ASIC2a, ASIC2b and ASIC3 (Kress and Waldmann 2006; Wemmie et al. 2006; Lingueglia 2007). These subunits are characterized by two membrane-spanning helical sequences (transmembrane domains 1 and 2), a large cysteine-rich extracellular loop and short intracellular N- and C-termini (Waldmann and Lazdunski 1998; Kellenberger and Schild 2002; Welsh et al. 2002; Lingueglia 2007). With this transmembrane topology (Fig. 2), ASICs have the same structure as the ionotropic purinoceptors (P2X) but, since they lack significant sequence homology, do not seem to share a common ancestor (Kress and Waldmann 2006). The different subunits form distinct homomultimeric and heteromultimeric complexes which differ in their kinetics, external pH sensitivity, tissue distribution and pharmacological properties (Waldmann et al. 1999; Alvarez de la Rosa et al. 2002; Benson et al. 2002; Welsh et al. 2002; Kress and Waldmann 2006; Wemmie et al. 2006). Although it is not known precisely how many subunits are required to form a functional channel, there is increasing evidence that ASICs are arranged as homo- or heterotetramers (Gao et al. 2007b; Lingueglia 2007). When activated, ASICs are preferentially permeable to Na^+ but some of them can also carry other cations such as Ca^{2+} (ASIC1a) and K^+ (ASIC1b) (Kress and Waldmann 2006; Wemmie et al. 2006; Lingueglia 2007).

The functional properties of the different ASIC subunits have been characterized following heterologous expression in *Xenopous laevis* oocytes and mammalian cell lines. Mutational analyses indicate that their pH sensitivity resides in several regions of the ASIC protein, particularly with His-72 and Gly-430 in the extracellular loop (Waldmann 2001; Diochot et al. 2007). ASIC1a, ASIC1b, ASIC2a and

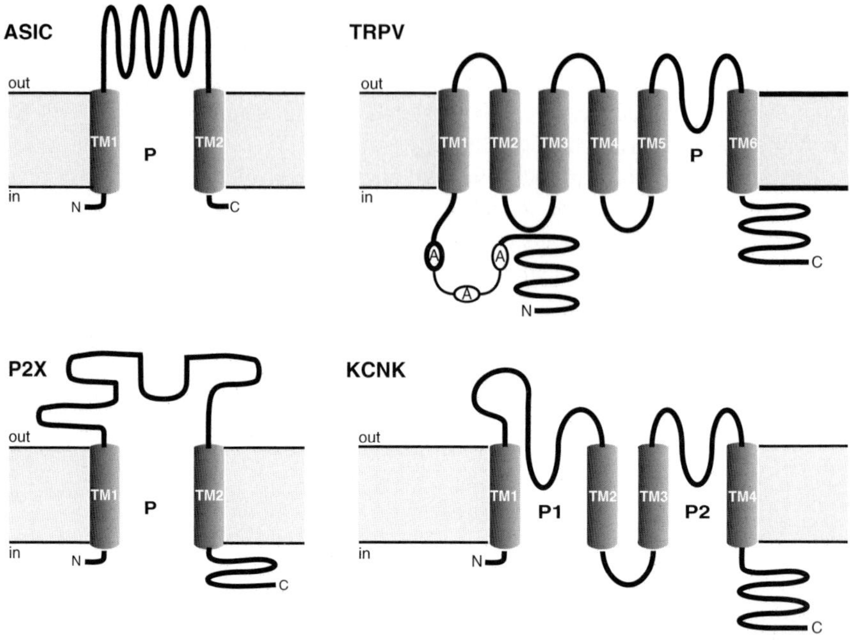

Fig. 2 Membrane topology of four classes of acid-sensitive ion channel subunits: acid-sensing ion channel (ASIC), transient receptor potential (TRP) ion channel of the vanilloid subtype (TRPV), ionotropic purinoceptor (P2X) and K_{2P} ion channel (KCNK). *A* ankyrin, *C* COOH terminal, *N* NH_2 terminal, *P* pore, *TM* transmembrane domain

ASIC3 are directly gated by protons, whereas ASIC2b does not respond to acidosis when expressed as a homomultimer but can form functional heteromultimers with other ASIC subunits, particularly ASIC3 (Kress and Waldmann 2006; Wemmie et al. 2006). ASICs are activated by changes in pH only if they occur extracellularly, the threshold for activation of ASIC3 being as low as a fall of pH to 7.2 (Kress and Waldmann 2006; Wemmie et al. 2006). The pH values required for half-maximal activation are 6.2–6.8 for ASIC1a, 5.9–6.2 for ASIC1b, around 4.9 for ASIC2a and 6.5–6.7 for ASIC3 (Benson et al. 2002; Kress and Waldmann 2006). Under physiological pH, ASIC3 is blocked by Ca^{2+} bound to a high-affinity binding site on the extracellular side of the channel pore, and protons open ASIC3 by relieving this Ca^{2+} block (Immke and McCleskey 2003).

The proton-gated ASICs are highly sensitive acid sensors as deduced from the steepness of their stimulus–response relationship. Although ASIC currents are in general fast and rapidly inactivating, there is evidence that they can also monitor prolonged acidosis. ASIC3 homomultimers and ASIC2a/ASIC3 as well as ASIC2b/ASIC3 heteromultimers produce two types of sustained current: (1) a current that occurs at low acidic or even neutral pH and is thought to result from an overlap of activation and desensitization kinetics (Benson et al. 1999; Kress and Waldmann 2006; Wemmie et al. 2006; Yagi et al. 2006), and (2) a current that is seen only at pH values below 5 (Kellenberger and Schild 2002; Kress and Waldmann 2006). In addition, persistent currents are observed when ASIC1 and ASIC3 are activated by protons in the presence of the neuropeptides neuropeptide FF or FMRFamide (Askwith et al. 2000; Catarsi et al. 2001; Deval et al. 2003).

The properties of the ASIC currents delineated above resemble the fast and rapidly inactivating inward Na^+ current that is evoked by minor acidosis in native DRG neurons (Krishtal and Pidoplichko 1981; Konnerth et al. 1987; Davies et al. 1988; Kellenberger and Schild 2002; Leffler et al. 2006; Poirot et al. 2006). The question as to which ASIC subunits contribute to the native ASIC-like current in sensory neurons has been addressed by comparing the currents carried by ASIC homo- and heteromultimers with the native currents and by analysing the expression of ASICs in sensory neurons. The pertinent studies revealed distinct regional differences, proton-gated currents being mediated by ASIC1a or ASIC3 homomultimers in some instances (Escoubas et al. 2000; Sutherland et al. 2001) and by ASIC2a/ASIC3 as well as ASIC2b/ASIC3 heteromultimers in other instances (Waldmann et al. 1999; Xie et al. 2002; Diochot et al. 2004; Yagi et al. 2006).

This heterogeneity in function is paralleled by a heterogeneity in the expression of ASIC1a, ASIC1b, ASIC2a, ASIC2b and ASIC3 by different populations of afferent neurons (Waldmann et al. 1999; Voilley et al. 2001; Alvarez de la Rosa et al. 2002; Benson et al. 2002; Mamet et al. 2002; Schicho et al. 2004; Kress and Waldmann 2006). While ASIC1a is present in both sensory neurons and neurons of the central nervous system, ASIC1b is largely confined to primary afferent neurons (Chen et al. 1998; Alvarez de la Rosa et al. 2002). In contrast, the levels of ASIC2a in sensory neurons are quite low, whereas ASIC2b occurs in both sensory and central nervous system neurons, and ASIC3 is almost exclusively expressed by sensory neurons (Lingueglia et al. 1997; Waldmann et al. 1999; Price et al. 2001; Voilley et al. 2001; Alvarez de la Rosa et al. 2002; Chen et al. 2002; Xie et al. 2002). The various ASIC subunits have been localized to primary afferent neurons of small-, medium- and large-diameter innervating skin, eye, ear, taste buds, heart, gut, skeletal muscle and bone (Kress and Waldmann 2006; Wemmie et al. 2006; Holzer 2007). Their expression has been analysed in greatest detail in the sensory innervation of the skin, in which ASIC-like immunoreactivity occurs not only in free nerve endings but, as is particularly true for ASIC2, also in specialized mechanosensitive nerve endings (Jiang et al. 2006; Kress and Waldmann 2006; Wemmie et al. 2006). ASIC1, ASIC2 and ASIC3 have also been localized to glossopharyngeal, vagal and spinal afferent neurons innervating the gut and other visceral organs (Page et al. 2005; Fukuda et al. 2006; Holzer 2007; Hughes et al. 2007), and retrograde tracing has revealed that 75% of the nodose ganglion neurons and 82% of the DRG neurons projecting to the rat stomach express ASIC3-like immunoreactivity (Schicho et al. 2004). Analysis of mouse thoracolumbar DRG has revealed that ASIC3 is expressed in 73%, ASIC2 in 47% and ASIC1 in 30% of the somata projecting to the mouse colon (Hughes et al. 2007).

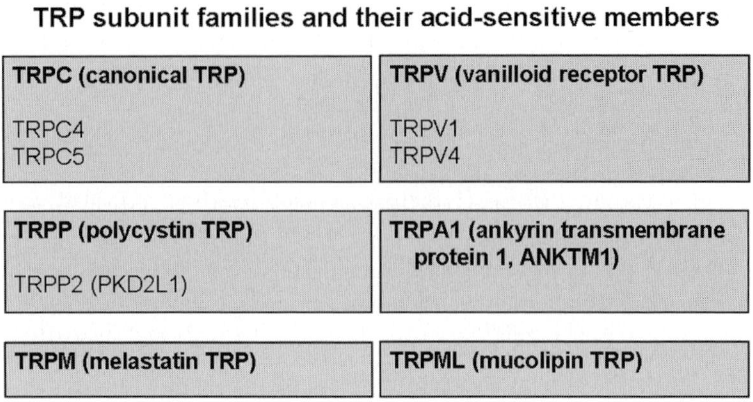

TRP subunit families and their acid-sensitive members
TRPC (canonical TRP)
TRPC4
TRPC5
TRPV (vanilloid receptor TRP)
TRPV1
TRPV4
TRPP (polycystin TRP)
TRPP2 (PKD2L1)
TRPA1 (ankyrin transmembrane protein 1, ANKTM1)
TRPM (melastatin TRP)
TRPML (mucolipin TRP)

Fig. 3 Overview of the TRP channel subfamilies and of the acid-sensitive subunit members among the TRPC, TRPP and TRPV subfamilies. For details, see the text

2.2 *TRP Ion Channels*

The TRP ion channels are named after the role these channels have in *Drosophila* phototransduction. At least 28 different TRP subunit genes have been identified in mammals (Clapham et al. 2005), comprising six subfamilies of the mammalian TRP superfamily (Fig. 3). The primary structure of the TRP channels consists of six transmembrane domains with a pore domain between transmembrane domains 5 and 6 and with both the C-teminus and the N-terminus located intracellularly (Clapham et al. 2005). This architecture (Fig. 2) is common to hundreds of ion channels but, despite the topographic similarities between the TRPs and the voltage-gated K^+ channels, the TRPs are only distantly related to these channels (Clapham et al. 2005). Since TRP channels are the subject of another chapter in this book, only TRP channels that are sensitive to pH changes (Fig. 3) are considered here.

2.2.1 TRPV1

The existence of TRPV1 (initially termed "vanilloid receptor 1", VR1), also known as the *capsaicin receptor*, has long been envisaged from the specific action of capsaicin on nociceptive afferent neurons (Jancsó 1960; Holzer 1991; Szallasi and Blumberg 1999). It is now known as a polymodal nocisensor par excellence, being receptive to noxious heat (above 43°C), capsaicin, endovanilloids and acid (Caterina et al. 1997; Tominaga et al. 1998; Jordt et al. 2000; Caterina and Julius 2001; Patapoutian et al. 2003). Assembled most likely as a homotetramer, TRPV1 is a non-selective cation channel with high permeability for Ca^{2+} (Caterina and Julius 2001; Gunthorpe et al. 2002; Patapoutian et al. 2003; García-Sanz et al. 2004). In addition, TRPV1 has also been recognized as a channel that allows protons to enter the cell in an acidic environment (Hellwig et al. 2004; Vulcu et al. 2004). The conductance of H^+ through TRPV1 results in intracellular acidification (Hellwig et al. 2004), which in turn may act on membrane channels that are sensitive to changes in intracellular pH, e.g. certain K_{2P} channels. How TRPV1 regulates an acid-sensitive Cl^- channel in Sertoli cells (Auzanneau et al. 2008) has not yet been elucidated.

The pH sensitivity of TRPV1 is fundamentally different from that of ASICs, because TRPV1 is gated open only if the extracellular pH is reduced below 6, in which case a sustained channel current is generated (Caterina et al. 1997; Tominaga et al. 1998; Jordt et al. 2000). However, mild acidosis in the range of pH 7–6 can sensitize TRPV1 to other stimuli such as capsaicin and heat (Tominaga et al. 1998; McLatchie and Bevan 2001; Ryu et al. 2003; Neelands et al. 2005). As a result, the temperature threshold for TRPV1 activation is lowered under acidotic circumstances and so this cation channel becomes active at normal body temperature (Tominaga et al. 1998). Proton-induced sensitization involves both an increase in current activation rate and a decrease in current deactivation rate (Ryu et al. 2003; Neelands et al. 2005). Besides mild acidosis, many other signalling pathways [stimulated, e.g., by inflammatory mediators such as prostaglandins, bradykinin, adenosine triphosphate (ATP), 5-hydroxytryptamine and nerve growth factor] converge on TRPV1 and enhance the probability of channel gating by protons, capsaicin and heat (Caterina and Julius 2001; Vellani et al. 2001; Gunthorpe et al. 2002; Szallasi et al. 2007).

The ability of protons to sensitize TRPV1 to heat and other stimuli, on the one hand, and to activate TRPV1 per se, on the other hand, is mediated by different amino acid residues of the channel protein. Glu-600 on the extracellular side of transmembrane segment 5 is crucial for proton-induced sensitization of TRPV1, while Val-538 in the extracellular linker between transmembrane segments 3 and 4, Thr-633 in the pore helix and Glu-648 in the linker between the selectivity filter of the pore and transmembrane segment 6 are essential for proton-induced gating of TRPV1 (Jordt et al. 2000; Ryu et al. 2007). Mutation of these amino acid residues selectively abrogates proton-evoked currents but preserves the current responses to capsaicin and heat and their potentiation by mildly acidic pH (Jordt et al. 2000; Ryu et al. 2007). Thus, the sites in the TRPV1 protein targeted by protons differ from those targeted by other stimuli (Jordt et al. 2000; Welch et al. 2000; McLatchie and Bevan 2001; Gavva et al. 2004; Ryu et al. 2007). This instance allows for the development of TRPV1 blockers that inhibit TRPV1 activation by capsaicin but not acid (Gavva et al. 2005a).

DRG neurons of TRPV1 null mice lack the slow and non-desensitizing proton-gated currents that are seen in DRG neurons of wild-type animals, whereas the fast and rapidly inactivating proton-gated currents mediated by ASICs are maintained (Caterina et al. 2000; Davis et al. 2000). The TRPV1-mediated currents due to acidification are largely confined to DRG neurons with unmyelinated fibres, whereas the ASIC-mediated currents are also found on DRG neurons with thinly myelinated axons (Leffler et al. 2006). This is consistent with the predominant expression of TRPV1 in unmyelinated primary afferent nerve fibres originating from the trigeminal ganglia, nodose ganglia and DRG, although some thinly myelinated fibres also stain for TRPV1 (Caterina et al. 1997; Guo et al. 1999; Michael and Priestley 1999; Patterson et al. 2003; Schicho et al. 2004; Szallasi et al. 2007). Of the nodose ganglion neurons that innervate the rat stomach, 42–80% stain for TRPV1, whereas 71–82% of the DRG neurons projecting to the rat stomach and mouse colon express TRPV1 (Patterson et al. 2003; Robinson et al. 2004; Schicho et al. 2004). In addition, TRPV1 is present on afferent-neuron-associated cells such as epithelial cells in the urinary bladder (Birder et al. 2001).

2.2.2 TRPV4

Much like TRPV1, TRPV4 is gated by a drop of pH to below 6 and the channel current reaches a maximum at a pH of about 4 (Suzuki et al. 2003a). TRPV4 is also activated by citrate, but not lactate (Suzuki et al. 2003a), and has turned out to play a role in mechano- and osmosensation (Güler et al. 2002; Mizuno et al. 2003; Suzuki et al. 2003a). As TRPV4 has been localized to DRG neurons with both low- and high-threshold mechanosensitive afferent nerve fibres in the skin (Suzuki et al. 2003b), a role of this TRP channel in acid sensing warrants further exploration.

2.2.3 TRPC4 and TRPC5

The TRPC subfamily, specified as *canonical* or *classical* because TRPC1 was the first member of the mammalian TRP family known to form an ion channel, can be divided into three subgroups by sequence homology and functional similarities: C1/C4/C5, C3/C6/C7 and C2 (Clapham et al. 2005). Accordingly, TRPC4 and TRPC5 are most closely related to TRPC1, which is a component of different heteromeric TRP complexes (Clapham et al. 2005). As other TRP channels, TRPC4 and TRPC5 form Ca^{2+}-permeable cation channels that are involved in receptor-mediated increases in intracellular Ca^{2+}. Their mode of activation has remained somewhat elusive, as TRPC4 and TRPC5 are activated in a phospholipase C dependent manner by an unidentified messenger.

It has recently been reported that TRPC4 and TRPC5 respond to changes in extracellular pH, given that small decreases in pH (from 7.4 to 7.0) increase both G protein activated and spontaneous TRPC5 currents (Semtner et al. 2007). TRPC4 channel activity is likewise potentiated by decreases in pH. The effects of a pH decrease on TRPC4 and TRPC5 activity are biphasic, the currents being increased by a reduction of pH down to about 6.5 but being inhibited when pH is decreased further (Semtner et al. 2007). H^+ modifies TRPC5 currents by interacting with the Gd^{3+} binding site typical of TRPC4 and TRPC5 (Semtner et al. 2007). These findings clearly indicate that TRPC4 and TRPC5 can act as acid sensors that link decreases in extracellular pH to Ca^{2+} entry and depolarization. The expression of these TRP subunits in acid-sensitive cells and their functional implications in acid monitoring await to be shown.

2.2.4 TRPP2 (PKD2L1, Polycystic Kidney Disease Like Ion Channel)

PKD2L1 is a member of the polycystin (TRPP) subfamily of TRP channels. Apart from PKD2L1 (TRPP2), the *polycystic kidney disease* (PKD) proteins or polycystins also include PKD2 (TRPP1) and PKD2L2 (TRPP3) (Clapham et al. 2005). The term "polycystin" is derived from the association of a PKD2 gene mutation with autosomal dominant PKD (Delmas 2005). Accordingly, the mouse orthologue of TRPP2 is deleted in *krd* mice which suffer from defects in the kidney and retina (Nomura et al. 1998).

PKD2L1 recently joined the network of acid-sensitive ion channels after it had been discovered to play a major role in sour taste sensing (Huang et al. 2006; Ishimaru et al. 2006; LopezJimenez et al. 2006). To form functional channels, PKD2L1 needs to associate as a heteromer with related proteins of the PKD1 family (Delmas 2005; Ishimaru et al. 2006). The PKD1 polycystins (PKD1, PKD1L1, PKD1L2, PKD1L3 and PKDREJ) are not included in the TRP channel family (Clapham et al. 2005) because they are large proteins with a very long N-terminal extracellular domain and 11 transmembrane domains that include a six-transmembrane TRP-like channel domain at the C terminus. The expression of PKD2L1 in a select class of taste chemoreceptor cells and the deleterious effect of PKD2L1 deletion on the sour taste have led to the concept that PKD2L1 is the molecular sour sensor (Huang et al. 2006; Ishimaru et al. 2006; LopezJimenez et al. 2006).

2.3 K_{2P} Channels

K_{2P} channels, encoded by the *KCNK* genes, represent one of the subfamilies of the large superfamily of K^+ channels. Defined by their membrane topology (Fig. 2), these channels possess four transmembrane domains, two pore-forming loops between transmembrane domains 1 and 2 as well as transmembrane domains 3 and 4, and a large extracellular linker region between transmembrane domain 1 and the first pore-forming loop, which forms the K^+ selectivity filter (Lesage and Lazdunski 2000; Goldstein et al. 2001; Patel and Honoré 2001; Goldstein et al. 2005; Duprat et al. 2007). Functional K_{2P} channels are made up as homo- or heterodimers (Duprat et al. 2007). Thus far, 15 human K_{2P} channel subunits (Fig. 4) have been identified and grouped into six structurally and functionally different subclasses (Goldstein et al. 2005; Duprat et al. 2007). Many of these channels are background channels that are independent of membrane voltage, constitutively active and non-inactivating. With these properties, K_{2P} channels play a key role in setting the resting membrane potential as well as membrane input resistance and, consequently, the excitability of neurons (Lesage and Lazdunski 2000; Goldstein et al. 2001; Patel and Honoré 2001; Duprat et al. 2007). In addition, many K_{2P} channels possess receptor properties, given that they are responsive to mechanical and chemical stimuli and are increasingly considered to

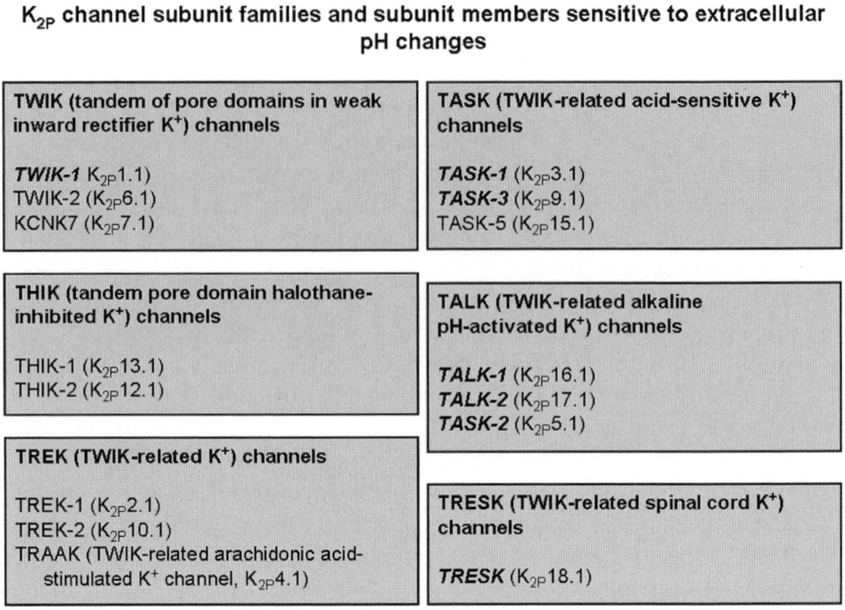
K2P channel subunit families and subunit members sensitive to extracellular pH changes
TWIK (tandem of pore domains in weak inward rectifier K+) channels
TWIK-1 K2P1.1)
TWIK-2 (K2P6.1)
KCNK7 (K2P7.1)
TASK (TWIK-related acid-sensitive K+) channels
TASK-1 (K2P3.1)
TASK-3 (K2P9.1)
TASK-5 (K2P15.1)
THIK (tandem pore domain halothane-inhibited K+) channels
THIK-1 (K2P13.1)
THIK-2 (K2P12.1)
TALK (TWIK-related alkaline pH-activated K+) channels
TALK-1 (K2P16.1)
TALK-2 (K2P17.1)
TASK-2 (K2P5.1)
TREK (TWIK-related K+) channels
TREK-1 (K2P2.1)
TREK-2 (K2P10.1)
TRAAK (TWIK-related arachidonic acid-stimulated K+ channel, K2P4.1)
TRESK (TWIK-related spinal cord K+) channels
TRESK (K2P18.1)

Fig. 4 Overview of the K_{2P} channel subunit families and of the subunit members (indicated in *bold* and *italics*) that are modulated by changes in the extracellular pH. For details, see the text

be sensors for hypoxia, hypercapnia, glucose and modifications of intra- and extracellular pH (Duprat et al. 2007). As summarized in Fig. 4, acidification or alkalinization modulates the activity of most K_{2P} subunits (Holzer 2003; Goldstein et al. 2005).

As their abbreviation for "TWIK-related acid-sensitive K^+ channels" implies, TASK channels are remarkably sensitive to variations in extracellular pH (Fig. 4). TASK-1, TASK-2 and TASK-3 homo- and heteromers are inhibited by extracellular acidification but are left unaffected by intracellular pH changes, while TASK-5 is inactive when expressed as a homomer (Duprat et al. 1997; Reyes et al. 1998; Chapman et al. 2000; Kim et al. 2000; Rajan et al. 2000; Meadows and Randall 2001; Kang and Kim 2004; Goldstein et al. 2005; Duprat et al. 2007). TASK-1 is particularly sensitive, given that only 10% of the maximal current is recorded at pH 6.7, 50% at pH 7.3 and 90% at pH 7.7 (Duprat et al. 1997). The pH sensitivity of TASK-3 is critically dependent on His-98 in the first pore-forming loop, an amino acid residue that is also present in TASK-1 but absent in TASK-2 (Kim et al. 2000; Rajan et al. 2000). In addition, His-72, Lys-73, Ile-94, Gly-95, Asp-204 and Lys-210 contribute to the acid-sensing capacity of TASK-1 and TASK-3 subunits (Kim et al. 2000; Morton et al. 2003; Yuill et al. 2004, 2007). TASK-2 differs from TASK-1 and TASK-3 not only by the amino acid residues critical to its pH sensitivity (Glu28, Lys-32, Lys-35, Lys-47 and Arg-224), but also by its property of being an alkaline-activated K_{2P} channel (Morton et al. 2005; Duprat et al. 2007; Niemeyer et al. 2007).

Acid-induced inhibition of TASK channel activity will enhance nerve excitability and hence indirectly encode the presence of acid. The high proton sensitivity of TASK subunits points to a role in surveillance of tissue acidification by ischaemia, inflammation or backdiffusion of luminal acid into the mucosa of the foregut (Lesage and Lazdunski 2000; Holzer 2003; Duprat et al. 2007). This possibility is strongly envisaged from the expression of TASK-1, TASK-2 and TASK-3 messenger RNA (mRNA) and protein in rat and human DRG neurons with nociceptive properties and in areas of the spinal cord (dorsal horn) and brainstem that receive afferent input from the periphery (Duprat et al. 1997; Bayliss et al. 2001; Medhurst et al. 2001; Talley et al. 2001; Gabriel et al. 2002; Baumann et al. 2004; Cooper et al. 2004; Rau et al. 2006).

TRESK channels are blocked by extra- and intracellular acidification and activated by extra- and intracellular alkalinization (Sano et al. 2003). TRESK is a major background K_{2P} channel in DRG neurons, and disruption of the *TRESK* gene has revealed that this channel plays a role in the regulation of DRG neuron excitability (Kang and Kim 2006; Dobler et al. 2007).

TREK-1 and TREK-2 do not respond to changes in extracellular pH but are inhibited by intracellular alkalinization and activated by intracellular acidification such that they become constitutively active (Maingret et al. 1999; Bang et al. 2000; Lesage et al. 2000; Kim et al. 2001a; Patel and Honoré 2001; Honoré et al. 2002; Miller et al. 2004). Activation of TREK-1 by intracellular acidification depends critically on protonation of Glu-306 (Honoré et al. 2002). TREK channels are also activated by a number of extracellular stimuli (including arachidonic acid, other unsaturated fatty acids, stretch, negative pressure and heat) and are inhibited by intracellular signalling cascades involving protein kinases A and C. A sensory role of TREK channels may be deduced from the expression of TREK-1 and TREK-2 in human DRG neurons as well as in neurons of the spinal cord and brainstem (Bearzatto et al. 2000; Maingret et al. 2000; Hervieu et al. 2001; Medhurst et al. 2001; Talley et al. 2001; Gu et al. 2002; Kang and Kim 2006). In the mouse DRG, TREK-1 is present in small to medium-sized primary afferent neurons (Maingret et al. 2000).

The activity of TWIK-1, but not TWIK-2, is depressed by extracellular acidification (Goldstein et al. 2005; Rajan et al. 2005), whereas intracellular acidification inhibits both TWIK-1 and TWIK-2 (Chavez et al. 1999; Patel et al. 2000). A possible role in sensory mechanisms can be envisaged from the expression of TWIK-1 and TWIK-2 mRNA in human and rat DRG neurons as well as in neurons of the spinal cord (Medhurst et al. 2001; Talley et al. 2001).

TRAAK channels are activated by intracellular alkalinization but not acidification (Lesage and Lazdunski 2000; Kim et al. 2001b; Patel and Honoré 2001). TRAAK mRNA and protein are appreciably expressed in human and rat DRG neurons as well as in the human, mouse and rat spinal cord (Bearzatto et al. 2000; Reyes et al. 2000; Medhurst et al. 2001; Talley et al. 2001; Kang and Kim 2006).

TALK-1, TALK-2 and their splice variants are blocked by extracellular acidification but are gated open by extracellular alkalinization, with Lys-224 playing a critical role in their pH sensitivity (Decher et al. 2001; Girard et al. 2001; Han et al. 2003; Duprat et al. 2005; Goldstein et al. 2005; Niemeyer et al. 2007).

Taken together, the activity of many K_{2P} channels (TASK-1, TASK-2, TASK-3, TRESK, TWIK-1, TALK-1 and TALK-2) is modified by changes in extracellular pH. Although their functional implications in acid sensing await to be explored, K_{2P} channels could play a multimodal sensory role in the peripheral and central nervous system as has been envisaged for the TASK subfamily (Duprat et al. 2007).

2.4 *Proton-Sensing GPCRs*

Proton-sensitive GPCRs are emerging as a new class of acid sensors on nociceptive afferent neurons (Fig. 1). These receptors include the ovarian cancer GPCR 1 (OGR1), GPCR 4 (GPR4), the G2 accumulation (G2A) receptor, and the T-cell death-associated gene 8 (TDAG8) receptor. Initially described as receptors for lipid molecules such as sphingosylphosphorylcholine, lysophosphatidylcholine and psychosine, some of these GPCRs have turned out to be sensors for extracellular acidosis (Ludwig et al. 2003; Tomura et al. 2005). As other GPCRs, these acid-sensitive receptors are composed of seven transmembrane domains, their signalling involving G_s, G_i, G_q and $G_{12/13}$ pathways. The sensitivity of OGR1 to extracellular pH changes resides with several histidine residues and is extremely high, given that half-maximum activation occurs at pH 7.2–7.5 and full activation occurs at pH 6.4–6.8 (Ludwig et al. 2003; Tomura et al. 2005). The transcripts of proton-sensing GPCRs are widely distributed and, importantly, also expressed by DRG neurons, particularly by small-diameter afferent neurons that are involved in nociception (Huang et al. 2007). Although the physiological and pathophysiological roles of proton-sensitive GPCRs are – for the time being – speculative, they could add significantly to the network of acid sensors of afferent neurons and their associated cells.

2.5 *Ionotropic Purinoceptors*

P2X purinoceptors are ligand-gated membrane cation channels that open when extracellular ATP is bound. They are assembled as homo- or heteromultimers (trimers or hexamers) of P2X subunits, seven of which ($P2X_1$–$P2X_7$) have been identified at the gene and protein level (Chizh and Illes 2001; Dunn et al. 2001; North 2002; Burnstock 2007). Their membrane topology (Fig. 2) is characterized by a very long extracellular polypeptide loop, which consists of about 280 amino acids and is rich in cysteine, between two transmembrane domains, with the N- and C-termini located intracellularly (Dunn et al. 2001; North 2002). Since the role of purinoceptors in sensory neuron physiology and pharmacology is the topic of another chapter in this volume, only aspects relating to the acid sensitivity of P2X purinoceptors are discussed here.

Of the various P2X subunits, $P2X_1$, $P2X_2$, $P2X_3$, $P2X_4$, $P2X_5$ and $P2X_7$ (Fig. 1) are modulated by alterations in the extracellular pH (Holzer 2003). Thus, acidification reduces the potency of ATP to gate homomultimeric $P2X_1$, $P2X_3$, $P2X_4$ and $P2X_7$ receptors usually without a change in the maximal response, while alkalinization has no effect on agonist potency and efficacy (Stoop et al. 1997; Dunn et al. 2001; Liu et al. 2001; Gerevich et al. 2007). In $P2X_5$ homomultimers, however, protons reduce both the potency and efficacy of ATP to gate the channel (Wildman et al. 2002). In contrast, acidification sensitizes homomultimeric $P2X_2$ receptors to the excitatory effect of ATP, whereas agonist potency at homomultimeric $P2X_2$ receptors is decreased at alkaline pH levels above 7.5 (Stoop et al. 1997; Ding and Sachs 1999; North 2002; Burnstock 2007). The maximal response of $P2X_2$ receptors to ATP is not altered by alkalinization or acidification. His-319 is particularly important for the effect of protons to potentiate the agonist effect of ATP on $P2X_2$ (Clyne et al. 2002), while protonation of His-206 and His-286 accounts for the inhibition of agonist-induced currents in $P2X_3$ and $P2X_4$, respectively (Clarke et al. 2000; Gerevich et al. 2007).

Acidification has a dual effect on $P2X_3$ channels in response to agonist application. While at low agonist concentrations the current amplitude is reduced owing to a decrease in the activation rate, it is enhanced at high agonist concentrations owing to a decrease in the desensitization rate (Gerevich et al. 2007). It has therefore been proposed that the effect of low ATP concentrations on $P2X_3$ channels may be attenuated during inflammatory acidosis, whereas the effects of a massive release of ATP by tissue damage may be potentiated by acidosis (Gerevich et al. 2007).

When $P2X_1$, $P2X_2$ or $P2X_3$ subunits are coexpressed with each other, the resultant heteromultimers show a pH sensitivity that is different from that of P2X homomers (Surprenant et al. 2000; Dunn et al. 2001; Liu et al. 2001; Brown et al. 2002). For instance, the potency and efficacy of ATP to gate heteromeric $P2X_{1/2}$ receptors expressed in *Xenopous* oocytes is increased under both acidic and alkaline conditions (Brown et al. 2002). While the agonist-induced currents in $P2X_{2/3}$ heteromers are less enhanced by protons than the equivalent responses in $P2X_2$ homomers (Liu et al. 2001), the ligand-induced currents in $P2X_{2/6}$ heteromers are potentiated by pH levels down to 6.5, but are inhibited by pH levels lower than 6.3 (King et al. 2000). The ATP-evoked currents in $P2X_{4/6}$ heteromers are inhibited in the presence of protons (Dunn et al. 2001), and the ligand-evoked stimulation of $P2X_{1/5}$ heteromers is inhibited by either an increase or a decrease of the extracellular pH, in terms of both potency and efficacy (Surprenant et al. 2000).

P2X receptors are expressed by many cells including primary afferent neurons. The P2X receptors on nodose ganglion neurons include predominantly homomultimeric $P2X_2$ and some heteromultimeric $P2X_{2/3}$ receptors, whereas on DRG neurons homomultimeric $P2X_3$ prevail over heteromultimeric $P2X_{2/3}$ receptors (Cockayne et al. 2000; Dunn et al. 2001; Burnstock 2007). The different P2X subunit distribution in spinal and vagal sensory neurons explains why the ATP-evoked inward currents in nodose ganglion neurons are persistent whereas those in

DRG neurons exhibit transient, persistent or biphasic components (Dunn et al. 2001). Since only $P2X_2$ homomultimers and heteromultimers involving $P2X_2$, i.e. $P2X_{1/2}$, $P2X_{2/3}$ and $P2X_{2/6}$ receptors, are sensitized by acid, it is primarily $P2X_2$-containing purinoceptors that function as indirect acid sensors. The monitoring of acidification depends on the concomitant release and/or presence of ATP or related purines whose agonist action is enhanced by a decrease of the extracellular pH. This scenario may be of functional significance, given that ATP is liberated from a number of cellular sources in response to both physiological and pathological stimuli. As a result, P2X receptors have been envisaged as potential targets in pain research because, firstly, $P2X_3$ receptors are preferentially expressed by a group of primary afferent neurons that subserve a nociceptor function and, secondly, P2X receptors on these neurons are upregulated by inflammation and nerve injury (Cockayne et al. 2000; Hamilton et al. 2001; Yiangou et al. 2001a; Xu and Huang 2002; Burnstock 2007).

2.6 Other Acid-Sensitive Ion Channels

There is an increasing network of ion channels, receptors and other membrane proteins whose activity is modified by changes in the extra- and/or intracellular pH (Fig. 1). To review these many principles is beyond the scope of the current chapter, which focuses on acid sensing as an important property of sensory neurons and associated cells. Mention needs to be made, however, of a number of mechanisms that have been discussed as contributing to the acid-monitoring capacity of chemosensory neurons both in the periphery and in the brain.

Several members of the inward rectifier K^+(Kir) channel family, such as Kir1.1, Kir4.1, Kir5.1 and Kir6.1, are highly sensitive to changes in the intra- or extracellular pH at near physiological levels. While the activity of Kir1.1, Kir4.1 and Kir5.1 channels is inhibited by a decrease in intracellular pH (Jiang et al. 1999; Claydon et al. 2000; Putnam et al. 2004; Jiang et al. 2005; Liu et al. 2005; López-López and Pérez-García 2007), Kir6.1 (K_{ATP}) channels are activated by intracellular acidosis (Xu et al. 2001; Wang et al. 2003). Similarly, G protein coupled inward rectifier K^+ channels are activated by extracellular acidification (Mao et al. 2002). The inactivation of the voltage-activated K^+ channel $K_v1.3$ is delayed when extracellular pH is lowered (Somodi et al. 2004), whereas the inactivation of $K_v1.4$ and $K_v11.1$ channels is facilitated by extracellular acidosis (Jiang et al. 1999; Claydon et al. 2000; Somodi et al. 2004; Chandrashekar et al. 2006).

Nifedipine-sensitive L-type Ca^{2+} channels can be activated by extracellular acidification (Filosa and Putnam 2003), although there are also reports that high-voltage-gated Ca^{2+} channels and tetrodotoxin-sensitive Na^+ channels are blocked by a drop of extracellular pH (Reeh and Kress 2001). Hyperpolarization-activated cyclic nucleotide gated channels (Stevens et al. 2001; Zong et al. 2001; Mistrík and Torre 2004) and gap junction channels (connexins) (Dean et al. 2002) are inhibited by intracellular acidosis. Sertoli cells express an acid-sensitive Cl^- channel which is outwardly rectifying and activated only at acidic pH in the extracellular space (Auzanneau et al. 2003, 2008). Neurotransmitter receptors other than P2X purinoceptors are likewise modulated by pH changes. This is true for $GABA_A$ receptors which can be modified by extracellular pH changes, the effect depending on the stage of development and the receptor subunit composition (Krishek and Smart 2001). Given that intracellular pH is regulated by ion pumps, it needs to be envisaged that many transporters, including Na^+/H^+ exchangers, can modify the acid sensitivity of chemosensory cells (Lyall et al. 2004; Shimokawa et al. 2005; Montrose et al. 2006).

3 Physiological and Pathophysiological Implications of Acid Sensors

In most tissues, stimulation of sensory neurons by acidosis and other noxious stimuli has two different effects: local release of neuropeptides from the peripheral nerve fibres in the tissue and induction of autonomic reflexes, sensation and pain (Holzer 1988; Holzer and Maggi 1998). By releasing peptide transmitters in the periphery, sensory nerve fibres can regulate vascular and other tissue activities embodied in the term “neurogenic inflammation”. This efferent-like mode of operation may take place independently of nociception, and it has been hypothesized that some DRG neurons are specialized in controlling peripheral effector mechanisms only, while other DRG neurons may be specialized in the afferent mode of action or both (Holzer and Maggi 1998). The neuropeptides involved in the efferent-like mode of operation include calcitonin gene-related peptide (CGRP) and the tachykinins substance P and neurokinin A. Acidosis-evoked release of CGRP, one of the most potent vasodilator peptides, has been demonstrated in a variety of tissues, including the dental pulp (Goodis et al. 2006), the gastric mucosa (Geppetti et al. 1991; Manela et al. 1995) and the myocardium (Strecker et al. 2005). Pharmacological antagonist and gene disruption studies provide increasing evidence that acid-sensitive ion channels and receptors are involved in a number of physiological and pathophysiological reactions to acidosis (Fig. 5).

3.1 Sour Taste

The detection of sour taste plays an important role in warning against ingestion of acidic (e.g. spoiled or unripe) food sources (Huang et al. 2006). Taste reception occurs at the apical tip of taste receptor cells that form taste buds composed of 50–100 taste receptor cells. After transduction of one of the five distinct taste modalities (bitter, sweet, umami, salty and sour), the taste receptor cells transmit their information to afferent neurons. Several receptors and receptor mechanisms

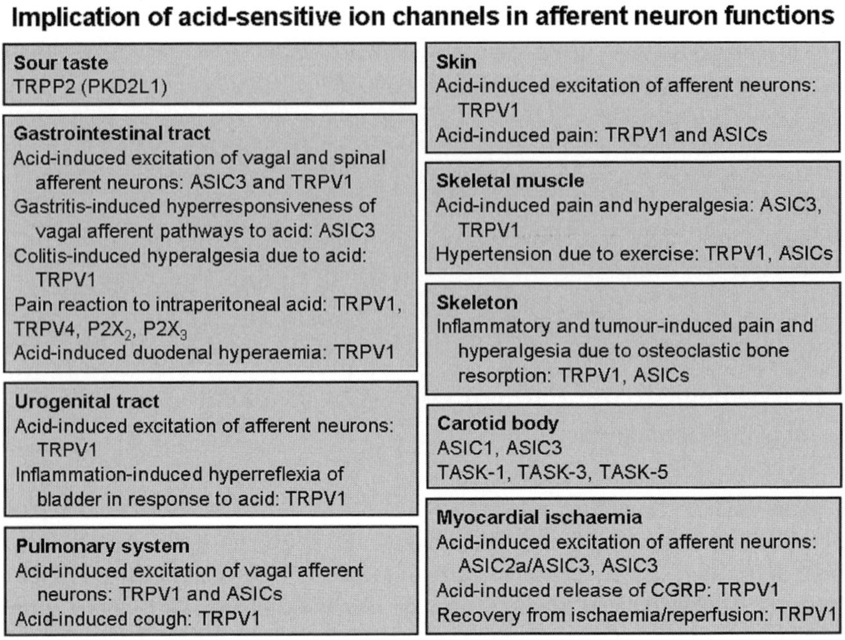
Implication of acid-sensitive ion channels in afferent neuron functions
Sour taste
TRPP2 (PKD2L1)
Gastrointestinal tract
Acid-induced excitation of vagal and spinal afferent neurons: ASIC3 and TRPV1
Gastritis-induced hyperresponsiveness of vagal afferent pathways to acid: ASIC3
Colitis-induced hyperalgesia due to acid: TRPV1
Pain reaction to intraperitoneal acid: TRPV1, TRPV4, P2X2, P2X3
Acid-induced duodenal hyperaemia: TRPV1
Urogenital tract
Acid-induced excitation of afferent neurons: TRPV1
Inflammation-induced hyperreflexia of bladder in response to acid: TRPV1
Pulmonary system
Acid-induced excitation of vagal afferent neurons: TRPV1 and ASICs
Acid-induced cough: TRPV1
Skin
Acid-induced excitation of afferent neurons: TRPV1
Acid-induced pain: TRPV1 and ASICs
Skeletal muscle
Acid-induced pain and hyperalgesia: ASIC3, TRPV1
Hypertension due to exercise: TRPV1, ASICs
Skeleton
Inflammatory and tumour-induced pain and hyperalgesia due to osteoclastic bone resorption: TRPV1, ASICs
Carotid body
ASIC1, ASIC3
TASK-1, TASK-3, TASK-5
Myocardial ischaemia
Acid-induced excitation of afferent neurons: ASIC2a/ASIC3, ASIC3
Acid-induced release of CGRP: TRPV1
Recovery from ischaemia/reperfusion: TRPV1

Fig. 5 Overview of the pathophysiological implications of acid-sensitive ion channels in afferent neuron function, based primarily on pharmacological antagonist and gene disruption studies. For details, see the text

have been proposed to mediate the sour taste (Chandrashekar et al. 2006). These include ASIC2a and ASIC2b (Ugawa et al. 2003; Shimada et al. 2006), K_{2P} channels (Lin et al. 2004; Richter et al. 2004a), Kir channels (Liu et al. 2005), proton-activated voltage-dependent Ca^{2+} channels (Chandrashekar et al. 2006), hyperpolarization-activated cyclic nucleotide gated channels (Stevens et al. 2001), Na^+/H^+ exchangers (Lyall et al. 2004) and acid-induced inactivation of K^+ channels (Chandrashekar et al. 2006). However, ASIC2 knockout mice respond normally to sour taste stimuli (Richter et al. 2004b), and there is also a lack of conclusive evidence for the other receptor mechanisms.

Histological, genetic and functional studies demonstrate that the TRP channel PKD2L1 (TRPP2) is probably the most important sour taste receptor (Huang et al. 2006; Ishimaru et al. 2006; LopezJimenez et al. 2006; Kataoka et al. 2008). PKD2L1 and the related PKD1L3 are selectively coexpressed in a population of taste receptor cells distinct from those mediating sweet, umami and bitter tastes (Huang et al. 2006; Ishimaru et al. 2006; LopezJimenez et al. 2006). PKD2L1 is accumulated at the taste pore region where taste chemicals are detected, and coexpression of PKD2L1 and PKD1L3 is necessary for their functional cell surface expression (Ishimaru et al. 2006). In addition, PKD2L1 and PKD1L3 are activated by various acids when coexpressed in heterologous cells but not by other classes of tastants (Ishimaru et al. 2006). Targeted ablation of PKD2L1-expressing taste receptor cells results in a specific and total loss of the sour taste, whereas responses to sweet, umami, bitter or salty tastants remain indistinguishable from those in wild-type animals (Huang et al. 2006). These findings firmly establish PKD2L1-expressing cells as specific sour taste receptors. Since PKD2L1 is expressed in neurons surrounding the central canal of the spinal cord, this channel has also been suggested to serve as a chemoreceptor monitoring the acidity of the cerebrospinal fluid (Huang et al. 2006).

3.2 Acidosis in the Gastrointestinal Tract

3.2.1 Acidity and Acidosis in the Gastrointestinal Tract

The stomach is the most productive source of acid in the body. The gastric parietal cells can secrete hydrochloric acid (HCl) to yield a H^+ concentration in the gastric lumen that – with an average diurnal pH of 1.5 – is 6 orders of magnitude higher than in the interstitial space of the gastric lamina propria (Holzer 2007). Most tissues would rapidly disintegrate if exposed to acid of this pH, yet gastric acid is essential for the digestive breakdown of food and elimination of ingested pathogens. The autoaggressive potential of HCl is kept in check by an elaborate network of mucosal defence mechanisms and by the functional compartmentalization of the oesophagogastroduodenal region (Holzer 2007). Both strategies require an acid surveillance system, among which acid-sensitive afferent neurons play an important role. If the pathophysiological impact of gastric acid gets out of control, acid-related diseases including gastritis, gastroduodenal ulceration, dyspepsia and gastro-oesophageal reflux disease may ensue.

Acid sensors are not only relevant for control of the secretion and actions of gastric acid but also for the detection of tissue acidosis resulting from ischaemia, inflammation, microbial activity, malignant tumour growth and gastrointestinal motor stasis. The pH profile in the gastrointestinal lumen of healthy subjects shows a distinct shape (Fallingborg 1999; Nugent et al. 2001), with peaks of acidity in the stomach and proximal large bowel. While HCl and bicarbonate (HCO_3^-) secretion are the major determinants of luminal pH in the foregut, luminal pH in the colon depends on mucosal HCO_3^- and lactate production as well as on microbial transformation of carbohydrates to short chain fatty acids and formation of ammonia. This pH profile can be changed by surgical interventions and in inflammatory bowel disease (Nugent et al. 2001; Holzer 2007).

3.2.2 Acid Sensing as a Feedback in the Control of Foregut Homeostasis

The secretion of gastric acid at highly toxic concentrations requires a tight control of its production according to need. The major inhibitory regulator is an increase in intragastric acidity, given that a decrease of luminal pH below 3 has a concentration-dependent inhibitory influence on HCl and gastrin secretion, and at pH 1 further acid output is abolished (Shulkes et al. 2006). The major mediator of this feedback inhibition is somatostatin, which via paracrine and endocrine pathways inhibits parietal cell function both directly and indirectly via reduction of gastrin secretion. The activity of D cells is in part regulated by acid-sensitive primary afferent neurons in the gastric mucosa which following luminal acidification release CGRP to stimulate D cells (Manela et al. 1995; Holzer 1998). The acid sensors of the somatostatin-releasing D cells and of other endocrine cells in the gastrointestinal mucosa await to be explored. Excess acid causes release of 5-hydroxytryptamine from enterochromaffin cells in the rat gastric mucosa (Wachter et al. 1998). Enterochromaffin cells are often called the "taste buds" of the gut, but whether they monitor intraluminal pH is not known.

Exposure of the oesophageal, gastric and duodenal mucosa to excess acid elicits protective mechanisms, including an increase in mucus gel thickness, HCO_3^- secretion and mucosal blood flow (Holzer 1998; Aihara et al. 2005; Akiba et al. 2006b; Montrose et al. 2006). These reactions are initiated in part by epithelial cells and their acid-sensing mechanisms and in part by capsaicin-sensitive afferent nerve fibres. Since these nerve fibres reside in the lamina propria behind the epithelium, the mucosal acid signal must be transduced across the epithelium. In the duodenum, this seems to be achieved by diffusion of CO_2 into the epithelial cells, hydration to H^+ and HCO_3^-, intracellular acidification and exit of H^+ via the basolateral Na^+/H^+ exchanger of type 1 (Akiba et al. 2006b; Montrose et al. 2006). As a result, interstitial pH is lowered, which activates sensory nerve terminals that release the vasodilator peptide CGRP (Akiba et al. 2006b). TRPV1 is involved in the duodenal hyperaemia evoked by luminal acid exposure, since it is attenuated by the TRPV1 blocker capsazepine (Akiba et al. 2006b), whereas the gastric hyperaemia is left unaltered by capsazepine (Tashima et al. 2002). The acid-evoked secretion of gastric and duodenal HCO_3^- also remains unchanged by capsazepine (Kagawa et al. 2003; Aihara et al. 2005).

The injurious potential of gastric acid is, in addition, kept in check by compartmentalization of the oesophagogastroduodenal region. This strategy is to restrict the presence of high acid concentrations to the stomach, the mucosa of which is most resistant to intrusion by H^+, and to precisely control H^+ passage from the stomach to the duodenum through coordinated activity of the lower oesophageal and pyloric sphincters. Both sphincters are under the control of neural reflexes involving acid-sensitive neurons which adjust the tone of these sphincters to balance the levels of acid present in the oesophagus, stomach and duodenum with the mucosal defence mechanisms in these compartments (Forster et al. 1990; Lu and Owyang 1999; Holzer et al. 2003; Holzer 2007). The molecular acid sensors and sensory neurons involved in the control of oesophagogastroduodenal motor activity await full exploration (Holzer 2007). Apart from extrinsic sensory neurons, it is likely that intrinsic primary afferent neurons of the enteric nervous system are involved, given that they have been found to respond to acidosis (Bertrand et al. 1997; Schicho et al. 2003).

Paradoxically, knockout of TRPV1 has been reported to ameliorate acid-induced injury in the oesophagus and stomach (Akiba et al. 2006a; Fujino et al. 2006). Analysis of this unexpected observation in the stomach has revealed that disruption of the *TRPV1* gene causes a compensatory upregulation of other protective mechanisms in the gastric mucosa (Akiba et al. 2006a). Thus, experiments with selective TRPV1 blockers are needed to unveil the precise role of TRPV1 in acid-induced mucosal injury in the foregut.

3.2.3 Acid as a Factor in Abdominal Pain

Acid is not only a factor in gastrointestinal tissue injury but also in gastrointestinal pain, contributing to the symptoms of gastro-oesophageal reflux disease and peptic ulcer (Kang and Yap 1991). Whether acid also plays a role in the pain associated with functional gastrointestinal disorders such as non-cardiac chest pain, functional dyspepsia, irritable bowel syndrome and functional abdominal pain syndrome is less well understood (Holzer 2007). Whole-cell voltage-clamp recordings from DRG and nodose ganglion neurons innervating the rat stomach and mouse colon have shown that acidosis induces currents that can to a variable degree be attributed to the gating of ASICs and TRPV1 (Sugiura et al. 2005, 2007). The pH sensitivity and kinetics of these currents are distinctly altered after experimental induction of gastric ulcers (Sugiura et al. 2005).

Intramucosal acidosis induced by exposure of the rat or mouse gastric lumen to supraphysiological HCl concentrations (above 0.15 M) elicits a visceromotor response indicative of pain (Lamb et al. 2003) and causes many neurons in the nucleus of the solitary tract in the brainstem to express c-Fos, a marker of neuronal excitation (Schuligoi et al. 1998; Danzer et al. 2004; Wultsch et al. 2008). The gastric HCl evoked visceromotor reaction and medullary c-Fos response are suppressed by vagotomy, but not transection of the sympathetic nerve supply to the stomach, which indicates that gastric HCl evoked nociception depends critically on the integrity of the vagal afferent innervation (Schuligoi et al. 1998; Lamb et al. 2003). Apart from eliciting pain, acid causes sensitization of mechanosensitive afferent pathways from the oesophagus, stomach and colon (Coffin et al. 2001; Medda et al. 2005). Experimentally induced gastritis and gastric ulceration enhance the gastric HCl evoked visceromotor reaction and medullary c-Fos response (Lamb et al. 2003; Holzer et al. 2007; Wultsch et al. 2008).

The gastric HCl evoked visceromotor reaction is inhibited by pretreatment of rats with a neurotoxic dose of capsaicin (Lamb et al. 2003). In contrast, the medullary c-Fos response to gastric acid challenge is neither altered by pretreatment with capsaicin (Schuligoi et al. 1998) nor by deletion of the *TRPV1* gene (Peter Holzer, Thomas Wultsch and Peter W. Reeh, unpublished observation). While afferent acid signalling from the normal stomach to the brainstem is preserved in ASIC3 knockout mice, the effect of gastritis to enhance the gastric acid evoked expression of c-Fos in the brainstem is abolished by disruption of the *ASIC3* gene (Wultsch et al. 2008). ASIC3 thus seems to play a major role in the inflammatory hyperresponsiveness of the vagal afferent–brainstem axis to gastric acid. Conversely, *ASIC2* gene knockout does not alter inflammatory hyperresponsiveness but enhances the medullary c-Fos response to gastric acid challenge of the normal stomach (Wultsch et al. 2008). Although this finding suggests that ASIC2 may normally dampen acid-induced afferent input, it must not be forgotten that compensatory changes in germline knockout mice may obscure the functional implication of the disrupted gene.

Activation of TRPV1 on abdominal afferent neurons by capsaicin elicits visceral pain in animals and humans (Drewes et al. 2003; Holzer 2004a; Schmidt et al. 2004). The stimulant effect of luminal acidification on gastric and oesophageal vagal afferent nerve fibres is ablated in both TRPV1 null and ASIC3 null mice (Bielefeldt and Davis 2008). Similarly, disruption of the *TRPV1* gene and blockade of TRPV1 by capsazepine depress the acid-evoked stimulation of afferent nerve fibres supplying the mouse jejunum (Rong et al. 2004) and the acid-evoked currents in thoracolumbar and lumbosacral DRG neurons innervating the mouse colon (Sugiura et al. 2007). Experimental colitis induced by trinitrobenzene sulfonic acid is associated with an increase in TRPV1 expression in thoracolumbar and lumbosacral DRG neurons and in the visceromotor response to intracolonic acid administration (Miranda et al. 2007). The effects of trinitrobenzene sulfonic acid to induce colitis, TRPV1 overexpression and hyperalgesia in response to acid challenge are counteracted by the TRPV1 blocker JYL1421 (Miranda et al. 2007).

Pharmacological blockade of TRPV1 with SDZ 249-665, a vanilloid compound causing desensitization of sensory neurons to capsaicin, attenuates the behavioural pain response to intraperitoneal administration of acetic acid in rats (Urban et al. 2000). This pain reaction may indeed reflect a response to acidosis because the writhing response to intraperitoneal injection of acetic, lactic and propionic acid is attenuated by capsazepine, whereas that to phenylbenzoquinone is not (Ikeda et al. 2001). An involvement of TRPV1 in acetic acid induced writhing is further corroborated by the ability of various TRPV1 blockers to reduce the abdominal muscle contractions caused by intraperitoneal injection of acetic acid (Rigoni et al. 2003; Tang et al. 2007). Likewise, mice lacking TRPV4 are hyporesponsive to intraperitoneal injection of acetic acid (Suzuki et al. 2003a). Overexpression of a dominant-negative ASIC3 subunit has been found to increase the writhing response to intraperitoneal acetic acid (Mogil et al. 2005), a change that paradoxically is also seen in ASIC3 null mice (Chen et al. 2002). Whether this finding is the result of a change in the kinetics of ASIC1 and ASIC2 after knockout of ASIC3 (Kress and Waldmann 2006) or of a compensatory upregulation of acid sensors other than ASIC3 is not known.

The available information points to a role of TRPV1 and ASIC3 in acid sensing within the gastrointestinal tract as well as in ulceration- and inflammation-evoked sensitization of afferent neurons (Fig. 5). This inference is consistent with a number of findings that show that abdominal hyperalgesia is associated with an upregulation in acid sensor expression and/or function. For instance, acute exposure of the rat gastric mucosa to a noxious HCl concentration leads to a rise of TRPV1 immunoreactivity, but not TRPV1 mRNA, in DRG neurons innervating the stomach

(Schicho et al. 2004). TRPV1 in vagal and spinal afferent neurons is upregulated in acid-evoked oesophagitis as well as in trinitrobenzene sulfonic acid induced pancreatitis and colitis (Banerjee et al. 2007; Miranda et al. 2007; Xu et al. 2007). Similarly, the expression of TRPV1 and ASIC3, but not ASIC1 and ASIC2, is enhanced in the colonic mucosa of patients with inflammatory bowel disease (Yiangou et al. 2001b, c). TRPV1-like immunoreactivity is likewise increased in oesophagitis (Matthews et al. 2004), non-erosive reflux disease (Bhat and Bielefeldt 2006), rectal hypersensitivity and faecal urgency (Chan et al. 2003).

There is some evidence that P2X receptors are involved in gastrointestinal sensation and pain related to acidosis. Protons potentiate the ATP-evoked stimulation of nodose ganglion and DRG cells (Li et al. 1996, 1997; Dunn et al. 2001; Zhong et al. 2001). The writhing behaviour elicited by intraperitoneal injection of acetic acid is inhibited by trinitrophenyl-ATP (a $P2X_1$, $P2X_3$ and $P2X_{2/3}$ receptor blocker) and A-317491 (a $P2X_3$ and $P2X_{2/3}$ receptor antagonist), whereas the $P2X_1$ channel blocker diinosine pentaphosphate is ineffective (Honore et al. 2002; Jarvis et al. 2002). Distension of the gut is thought to release ATP from the intestinal mucosa, which subsequently excites afferent neurons expressing P2X receptors. This mode of mechanosensory transduction via $P2X_3$ receptors is enhanced by experimental colitis in the rat (Wynn et al. 2004) and may, conceivably, involve inflammation-associated acidosis and/or upregulation of $P2X_3$ purinoceptors as has been observed in the colonic mucosa of patients with inflammatory bowel disease (Yiangou et al. 2001a).

3.3 *Acidosis in the Urogenital Tract*

The sensory innervation of the urogenital tract is of paramount relevance to the regulation of urine storage and voiding. Given that the urine is usually acidic and hyperosmotic, nerve endings behind the urothelium are likely to be exposed to excess acid if the urothelial barrier is disrupted (Chuang et al. 2003). This scenario is likely to occur under the conditions of irritable bladder and cystitis in which there is evidence for sensitization of afferent neurons, at least to mechanical stimuli. As a result, bladder hyperactivity, bladder hyperreflexia and pain may occur. The plausibility of this concept receives support from the finding that both populations of afferent neurons innervating the bladder, thoracolumbar and lumbosacral DRG neurons, are excited by acidification and exhibit proton-evoked currents with different inactivation kinetics (Dang et al. 2005; Daly et al. 2007). Furthermore, there is emerging evidence that acid sensors on afferent neurons such as TRPV1 play an appreciable role in diseases of the urogenital tract (Fig. 5).

An implication of TRPV1 in bladder overactivity and pain has been proved by both experimental and clinical evidence. Thus, chronic intravesical administration of capsaicin or resiniferatoxin to desensitize the sensory innervation of the bladder is beneficial in patients with urinary bladder pain and hyperreflexia (Bley 2004; Brady et al. 2004; Avelino and Cruz 2006; Cruz and Dinis 2007). This finding is consistent with the finding that TRPV1-like immunoreactivity is upregulated in neurogenic bladder overactivity (Brady et al. 2004). The symptoms of women with sensory urgency, but not idiopathic detrusor overactivity, have been associated with increased expression of TRPV1 mRNA in the trigonal mucosa (Liu et al. 2007). A contribution of TRPV1 to bladder function has been confirmed experimentally by genetic and pharmacological studies. Knockout of the *TRPV1* gene blunts the responsiveness of bladder afferent neurons to intravesical administration of HCl and capsaicin as well as to bladder distension and impairs the function of low-threshold afferents (Birder et al. 2002; Daly et al. 2007).

There is ample evidence that $P2X_2$ and $P2X_3$ purinoceptors are involved in the physiological and pathophysiological processes of urinary bladder voiding (Cockayne et al. 2000, 2005; Burnstock 2007), but it is not known whether they contribute to acid sensing in the urogenital tract.

3.4 Acidosis in the Pulmonary System

DRG and nodose ganglion neurons projecting to the lung and pleura express TRPV1 and ASICs (Groth et al. 2006; Jia and Lee 2007; Kollarik et al. 2007). Accordingly, vagal afferent neurons supplying the rat and guinea-pig lung display proton-induced currents with rapid and slow inactivation currents that appear to be carried by ASICs and TRPV1 as they are inhibited by amiloride and capsazepine, respectively (Kollarik and Undem 2002; Gu and Lee 2006). Acidosis in the airways can be the result of several processes, including inflammation, ischaemia or aspiration of refluxing gastric contents, and exhaled breath condensate studies indicate that acidosis is associated with obstructive airway diseases such as asthma (Ricciardolo et al. 2004; Hunt 2006). The functional implications of acidosis in the airways are manifold and include local effects on airway muscle tone and inflammatory processes as well as effects involving the central nervous system: cough, discomfort and pain (Jia and Lee 2007). In the guinea-pig isolated trachea acidosis has a differential effect on basal airway muscle tone and muscle responsiveness to contractile stimuli (Faisy et al. 2007). The acid-induced airway relaxation seems to be independent of sensory neurons and mediated by ASICs on smooth muscle cells, whereas the acid-evoked muscle hyperresponsiveness to acetylcholine involves sensory neurons expressing ASICs and TRPV1 (Faisy et al. 2007).

There is increasing evidence that acid is an important mediator in the pathogenesis of cough, given that inhalation of exogenous acid triggers cough, and acidosis accompanies a variety of respiratory diseases (Jia and Lee 2007; Kollarik et al. 2007). Following local generation, inhalation or aspiration, acid can directly stimulate vagal bronchopulmonary sensory nerve fibres involved in the cough reflex, Aδ-fibre nociceptors in the large airways being most efficiently stimulated by rapid acidification (Kollarik et al. 2007). In contrast, C-fibre nociceptors expressing TRPV1 are able to continuously monitor the pH in the tracheopulmonary tissue and thus to react to persistent acidosis as it occurs in inflammation. In addition, acid is the single most important mediator of cough due to gastro-oesophageal reflux, given that acid-sensitive oesophageal afferent neurons sensitize the neural pathways underlying the cough reflex (Kollarik et al. 2007).

The sensors of vagal afferent neurons involved in acid surveillance and the cough reflex include TRPV1 and other probes (Fig. 5). Accordingly, the TRPV1 blockers iodoresiniferatoxin, JNJ17203212 and V112220 are able to attenuate cough induced by citric acid inhalation in guinea pigs (Trevisani et al. 2004; Bhattacharya et al. 2007; Leung et al. 2007). It is not yet known whether ASICs account in full for the TRPV1-independent mechanisms of acid sensing in the airways (Canning et al. 2006; Kollarik et al. 2007; Leung et al. 2007). There is evidence that a TREK-like K_{2P} channel, which is sensitive to intracellular pH changes, could contribute to the function of intrapulmonary chemoreceptors (Bina and Hempleman 2007).

3.5 Acidosis in the Skin

DRG neurons innervating the skin express many of the known acid-sensitive ion channels, including TRPV1, ASICs and P2X. ASICs, for instance, are expressed by nociceptive and non-nociceptive afferent neurons innervating glabrous and hairy skin (Jiang et al. 2006). While intracutaneous perfusion of acid in human volunteers induces long-lasting non-adapting pain (Steen and Reeh 1993; Steen et al. 1995), transdermal iontophoresis of protons elicits transient pain that subsides within 5 min despite extended acid application (Jones et al. 2004; Cadiou et al. 2007). Intracutaneous injection of protons evokes an even shorter pain sensation that declines within 100 s (Rukwied et al. 2007). The route-dependent time course of proton-evoked cutaneous pain is probably due to differences in the kinetics of acid exposure as well as in the activation/inactivation kinetics of the acid-sensitive ion channels involved (Kress and Waldmann 2006).

Intracutaneous coinjection of prostaglandin E_2 and acid enabled Rukwied et al. (2007) to differentiate an early and a late phase of proton-evoked pain. The late phase is thought to be mediated by TRPV1, because it is selectively potentiated by prostaglandin E_2 (Rukwied et al. 2007). Indeed, disruption of the *TRPV1* gene prevents acid from stimulating unmyelinated afferent nerve fibres in a mouse skin-nerve preparation, whereas the proton-induced excitation of thinly myelinated nerve fibres persists (Caterina et al. 2000). Similarly, the effect of strong acidosis (pH 5.2) to cause release of CGRP from rat sciatic nerve axons is attenuated by capsazepine, whereas the peptide release evoked by mild acidosis (pH 6.1) is left unaltered (Fischer et al. 2003). Inflammation leads to upregulation of TRPV1 expression and function in afferent neurons supplying the skin and to an increase in the proton sensitivity of isolectin B_4 positive C-fibres (Carlton and Coggeshall 2001; Ji et al. 2002; Breese et al. 2005).

Other studies attribute an important role to ASICs (Fig. 5). Nitric oxide donors potentiate acid-induced currents in ASIC1, ASIC2 and ASIC3 homomeric channels and increase acid-evoked pain in the human skin (Cadiou et al. 2007). Acid-evoked pain is attenuated by nonsteroidal anti-inflammatory drugs (NSAIDs), which are known to interfere with ASIC expression and function, but is left unaffected by the TRPV1 blocker capsazepine or desensitization to capsaicin (Steen et al. 1995; Voilley et al. 2001; Ugawa et al. 2002; Jones et al. 2004). These findings suggest that part of the analgesic effect of NSAIDs could be due to interference with ASICs, a conjecture that is consistent with the upregulation of ASICs in DRG neurons by cutaneous inflammation due to Freund's adjuvant (Voilley et al. 2001). An implication of ASICs is further supported by the ability of amiloride to reduce acid-induced pain in the skin but to spare capsaicin-induced pain (Ugawa et al. 2002; Jones et al. 2004). Postoperative pain due to skin incision in rats is attenuated by A-317567, a blocker of ASIC1, ASIC2 and ASIC3 subunits (Dubé et al. 2005).

Studies with ASIC knockout mice have yielded ambiguous results, which is not totally unexpected in view of the redundancy of acid sensors present on sensory neurons and the likelihood of compensatory changes that occur during the development of ASIC null mice. In the isolated skin-nerve preparation, the response of mechanoheat-sensitive C-fibres to acid is reduced in ASIC3 null mice (Price et al. 2001). Paradoxically, however, the behavioural licking response to acetic acid injection into the paw is preserved in ASIC3 knockout animals (Price et al. 2001). It awaits to be explored whether other acid sensors, e.g., K_{2P} channels and P2X purinoceptors, contribute to acidosis-evoked pain in the skin.

3.6 Acid Sensors in the Carotid Body

Detection of blood pH and systemic acidosis is important for feedback regulation of respiration and cardiovascular function. To this end, O_2-, CO_2- and pH-sensitive chemoreceptors are present both in the carotid bodies and in the brain (López-López and Pérez-García 2007). The acid sensors operating in the chemoreceptor (glomus type I) cells of the carotid body (Fig. 5) include Kir channels (Putnam et al. 2004), K_{2P} channels containing the TASK-1, TASK-3 and/or TASK-5 subunits (Buckler 2007; Duprat et al. 2007), inwardly rectifying Cl^- channels (Petheo et al. 2001) and ASICs made up of ASIC1 and ASIC3 (Tan et al. 2007). It is thus emerging that there is a parallel processing of O_2, CO_2 and pH signals in carotid body chemoreceptor cells, the resulting depolarization causing release of transmitters (ATP, acetylcholine and dopamine) from the chemoreceptor cells and subsequent excitation of afferent nerve endings (Rong et al. 2003; Zhang and Nurse 2004; López-López and Pérez-García 2007; Tan et al. 2007).

Apart from acting on glomus type I cells, acidosis could also directly modify sensory neurons in the glossopharyngeal nerve, given that these neurons display a background K^+ conductance resembling that of THIK-1 which is weakly inhibited by extracellular acidosis (Campanucci et al. 2003). Acidosis enhances the ATP-induced whole cell current of petrosal ganglion afferents, which suggests that increased sensitivity of P2X receptors on afferent nerve fibres contributes to the transmission of acidosis in the carotid body (Zhang and Nurse 2004). Genetic disruption of the *P2X*$_2$ gene blunts the hyperventilatory response to hypoxia, which is consistent with the release of ATP from the glomus cells and the expression of P2X purinoceptors containing the acid-sensitive $P2X_2$ subunit by afferent neurons in the carotid sinus nerves (Rong et al. 2003). The ability of compounds such as halothane and isoflurane to activate TASK-3 channels in the carotid body is likely to have a direct bearing on their property to depress the hypoxic ventilatory drive when used for anaesthesia (Buckler 2007; Duprat et al. 2007).

3.7 Acidosis Due To Myocardial Ischaemia

There is emerging evidence that ASICs account for the anginal pain associated with myocardial ischaemia, with lactate as a factor involved in channel activation. ASIC3 is highly expressed by sensory neurons innervating the rat heart (Benson et al. 1999; Sutherland et al. 2001; Yagi et al. 2006). Patch-clamp analysis of rat ASIC3 homomers and ASIC2a/ASIC3 heteromers shows that both channel complexes generate persistent inward currents at the modest extracellular pH changes typical of muscle ischaemia, the currents produced by the ASIC2a/ASIC3 heteromers being much larger than those produced by ASIC3 homomers (Yagi et al. 2006). The sustained current is caused by a region of pH where there is overlap between inactivation and activation of the channel (Yagi et al. 2006). Lactate causes the current to activate at slightly more basic pH values. The currents produced by the heterologously expressed ASIC3 and ASIC2a/ASIC3 complexes are in keeping with the sustained currents that changes of pH from 7.4 to 7.0 produce in somata of DRG neurons innervating the rat heart (Yagi et al. 2006). These observations indicate that ASIC3 homo- and heteromers may play a major role in detecting sustained myocardial ischaemia and in mediating prolonged anginal pain (Fig. 5).

In contrast, the acidosis-evoked release of CGRP from sensory nerve fibres within the mouse heart appears to be mediated by TRPV1, since the response is absent in TRPV1 null mice but is left unaltered in ASIC3 knockout animals (Strecker et al. 2005). Given that the neuropeptides (CGRP and substance P) released from afferent nerve fibres in the tissue are potent vasodilators, the TRPV1-mediated release of these peptides in myocardial ischaemia is likely to have a local cardioprotective effect (Wang and Wang 2005; Zhong and Wang 2007). This concept is supported by the finding that the recovery of cardiac function after exposure to ischaemia/reperfusion is impaired by capsazepine and disruption of the *TRPV1* gene (Wang and Wang 2005). The beneficial effect of preconditioning against cardiac injury induced by ischaemia/reperfusion is likewise attenuated in TRPV1 null mice (Zhong and Wang 2007).

3.8 Acidosis in the Skeletal Muscle

Unmyelinated afferent neurons innervating the skeletal muscle are excited by acidosis (Hoheisel et al. 2004), and injection of acid into the anterior tibial muscle of humans elicits a biphasic but short-lasting pain response (Rukwied et al. 2007). The second phase is suggested to involve TRPV1, because it is selectively potentiated by prostaglandin E_2 (Rukwied et al. 2007). Other studies provide evidence that ASIC3 is relevant to sensing acidosis in skeletal muscle. Thus, repeated intramuscular injection of acidic saline induces mechanical hyperalgesia, a response that is blunted by amiloride and knockout of the *ASIC3* gene (Fig. 5), but not by deletion of ASIC1a (Price et al. 2001; Sluka et al. 2003). Furthermore, ASIC3 is involved in the mechanical hyperalgesia that is associated with muscle inflammation (Sluka et al. 2007). Thus, ASIC3-deficient mice fail to develop mechanical hyperalgesia following experimental inflammation by injection of carrageenan into the muscle, whereas injection of a recombinant herpes virus vector to express ASIC3 in the muscle of ASIC3 knockout mice rescues the hyperalgesia phenotype (Sluka et al. 2007).

Analogously to the situation in the myocardium (Benson et al. 1999; Sutherland et al. 2001; Yagi et al. 2006), there is good reason to assume that lactic acid is a factor relevant to acidosis-evoked muscle pain. Lactate is formed under limited oxygen availability in the muscle and causes acidification of the extracellular space. In addition, lactate is able to sensitize ASIC3 to acid by decreasing the extracellular concentration of Ca^{2+} (Immke and McCleskey 2001). Lactic acid accumulation and activation of acid-sensitive afferent neurons in skeletal muscle contribute to the reflex hypertension and tachycardia that is evoked by exercise. A participation of ASICs is deduced from the ability of a low dose of amiloride (0.5 $\mu g\ kg^{-1}$) to selectively block the hypertensive response to muscle exercise (Fig. 5), whereas the response to capsaicin or muscle stretch is spared (Li et al. 2004; Hayes et al. 2007). In addition, P2X receptors and – at more pronounced acidity – TRPV1 also come into play (Gao et al. 2007a). Another factor contributing to the muscle pressor reflex is thought to be diprotonated phosphate ($H_2PO_4^-$), whose excitatory action on afferent neurons involves both TRPV1 and ASICs as deduced from the inhibitory effects of capsazepine and amiloride, respectively (Gao et al. 2006).

3.9 Acidosis in the Skeleton

ASICs are expressed not only by sensory neurons innervating bone but also by cells of the skeleton. ASIC1, ASIC2 and ASIC3 are found in the skeleton, with ASIC1 prevailing in chondrocytes, and ASIC2 and ASIC3 predominating in osteoclasts and osteoblasts (Jahr et al. 2005). These findings carry two important perspectives, because osteoclasts actively secrete acid when they resorb bone and because bone disorders with increased bone resorption by osteoclasts are frequently associated with pain. Osteoclasts degrade bone by secreting protons through a vacuolar H^+-ATPase, thereby creating an acidic microenvironment. Inflammation-induced mineral resorption in metatarsal bones of the rat is associated with hyperalgesia, increased expression of ASIC1a, ASIC1b and ASIC3 in DRG neurons and enhanced c-Fos expression in the dorsal horn of the spinal cord (Nagae et al. 2006). The inflammation-induced hyperalgesia and upregulation of ASICs are reversed by bisphosphonate zoledronic acid, which inhibits osteoclastic bone resoption, and by bafilomycin A1, an inhibitor of vacuolar H^+-ATPase (Nagae et al. 2006). Since amiloride is also beneficial (Nagae et al. 2006), it would seem that ASICs play a role in bone pain associated with osteoclastic mineral resorption (Fig. 5).

Bone pain is one of the most common complications in cancer patients with bone metastases. Experimental evidence indicates that this type of bone pain is also related to bone degradation by osteoclasts and the acidic microenvironment to which afferent neurons in the bone matrix are exposed (Honore et al. 2000; Luger et al. 2001). Afferent neurons expressing TRPV1 innervate the mouse femur, and both genetic and pharmacological studies indicate that TRPV1 contributes to the hyperalgesia associated with an in vivo bone cancer model (Fig. 5), given that disruption of the *TRPV1* gene or treatment with the TRPV1 blocker capsazepine attenuates both ongoing and movement-evoked nocifensive behaviours (Ghilardi et al. 2005). In a model of bone cancer pain in the rat tibia, hyperalgesia is associated with an upregulation of mRNA for ASIC1a and ASIC1b, but not ASIC3 and TRPV1, in DRG neurons (Nagae et al. 2007). Although the findings in the rat and mouse have not yet been reconciled with each other, it is envisaged that both TRPV1 and ASICs participate in bone cancer pain.

Another line of investigation ascribes a role to ASICs in the pain arising from vertebral disc herniation. The vertebral discs are innervated by primary afferent neurons (Ohtori et al. 2007), and an experimental model of lumbar disc herniation produced by application of nucleus pulposus to, and pinching of, L5 nerve roots is associated with mechanical allodynia and an upregulation of ASIC3 in the respective DRG (Ohtori et al. 2006). Local administration of lidocaine has been found to reverse both mechanical allodynia and ASIC3 upregulation (Ohtori et al. 2006), which makes a case for ASIC3 being involved in radicular pain. In this context it need be considered that ASIC3 is present on nucleus pulposus cells of the intervertebral discs and that ASIC3 expression by these cells is under the control of nerve growth factor (Uchiyama et al. 2007). In a functional perspective it would seem that ASIC3 is required for adaptation of nucleus pulposus cells to the acidic and hyperosmotic microenvironment of the intervertebral disc (Uchiyama et al. 2007).

4 Pharmacological Interference with Acid Sensors

From the pertinent studies it is clear that no single molecular sensor alone accounts for the acid sensitivity of afferent neurons. Neuroanatomical analyses and recordings from DRG and nodose ganglion neurons have shown that acidosis induces currents that can to a variable degree be attributed to the gating of ASICs, TRPV1 and other acid sensors, because these probes are differentially expressed by different subpopulations of sensory neurons (Liu et al. 2004; Dang et al. 2005; Sugiura et al. 2005; Ugawa et al. 2005; Leffler et al. 2006; Poirot et al. 2006; Smith et al. 2007; Sugiura et al. 2007). Although ASICs and TRPV1 survey different spectra of acidic pH, it is obvious that there is a redundancy of molecular acid sensors, which signifies that early detection of acidosis is physiologically so important that multiple mechanisms of acid sensing have evolved.

Acid sensors can be considered as drug targets in more than one respect. Many of the acid-sensitive ion channels are highly regulated by a number of endogenous factors as well as pharmacological agents. This is true, e.g., for NSAIDs regulating the expression and function of ASICs, proinflammatory mediators causing sensitization of TRPV1, and anaesthetics and other neuroactive drugs controlling the activity of K_{2P} channels. A number of acid-sensitive ion channels and receptors, including ASICs, TRPV1 and P2X, are upregulated by inflammation and nerve injury and appear to contribute to the hyperalgesia associated with these conditions. If so, drugs targeting peripheral acid sensors may evolve as novel therapies of chronic inflammation and pain. This concept is attractive for a number of reasons, particularly because it offers the opportunity to develop antinociceptive drugs with a peripherally restricted site of action, avoiding unwanted effects on the central nervous system. However, interfering with molecular probes that are physiologically so important poses a serious threat to homeostasis unless selective inhibition of "excess" acid sensors can be achieved while their physiological function is preserved.

With these considerations in mind, some of the attempts and developments to pharmacologically modulate acid sensors are discussed in the following sections, along with the rationale behind their design and emerging information on their utility and limitations.

4.1 Acid-Sensing Ion Channels

There is emerging evidence that ASIC expression is altered following inflammation and nerve injury (Voilley et al. 2001; Yiangou et al. 2001c; Mamet et al. 2002; Ohtori et al. 2006; Poirot et al. 2006; Nagae et al. 2007). These pathological implications of ASICs in pain and hyperalgesia suggest that ASIC blockade could be a novel avenue in pain therapy.

The pharmacological aspects of specific ASIC-targeting drugs is just emerging. Most ASIC currents are blocked by the diuretic drug amiloride and its derivatives (e.g. benzamil) which, at the concentrations needed to inhibit ASIC activity, also suppress other ion channels and ion exchangers (Kress and Waldmann 2006; Page et al. 2007). As a consequence, the use of amiloride as a probe for the functional implications of ASICs is a pharmacological approach with limited specificity. In contrast, the peptide psalmotoxin 1 (PcTx1) isolated from the venom of the South American tarantula *Psalmopoeus cambridgei* is a highly selective ASIC blocker as it inhibits ASIC1a homomers with an affinity of 0.7 nM (IC_{50}) but does not affect ASIC1a-containing heteromers (Escoubas et al. 2000). It modifies ASIC1a gating by shifting the channel from the resting to an inactivated state (Escoubas et al. 2000; Diochot et al. 2007; Mazzuca et al. 2007). Another selective ASIC blocker, APETx2, has been isolated from the venom of the sea anemone *Anthopleura elegantissima*. This peptide toxin inhibits several ASIC3-containing channels with IC_{50} values between 63 nM and 2 μM, while its mode of action awaits to be elucidated (Diochot et al. 2004, 2007). The first synthetic ASIC inhibitor different from amiloride is A-317567, a compound that blocks proton-evoked currents through ASIC1, ASIC2 and ASIC3 channels as well as the sustained phase of the ASIC3-like current in DRG neurons (Dubé et al. 2005).

A number of drugs interfere with ASIC function in a nonselective manner. This is in particular true for NSAIDs, which counteract the upregulation of ASICs caused by experimental inflammation and inhibit proton-evoked ASIC currents in afferent neurons (Voilley et al. 2001; Mamet et al. 2002). Ibuprofen and flurbiprofen inhibit homomultimeric ASIC1a channels, whereas salicylic acid, aspirin and diclofenac block the sustained currents of ASIC3 and ASIC2b/ASIC3 channels (Voilley et al. 2001). Although it remains to be established whether the effects of NSAIDs on ASICs are relevant to their anti-inflammatory and analgesic action, it appears conceivable that ASICs participate in inflammatory hyperalgesia. This inference is supported by the ability of proinflammatory mediators such as nerve growth factor, 5-hydroxytryptamine, interleukin-1 and bradykinin to promote the transcription of ASIC3 in sensory neurons, 5-hydroxytryptamine and nerve growth factor interacting directly with the promoter region of the *ASIC3* gene (Mamet et al. 2002). Another proinflammatory mediator, arachidonic acid, is able to potentiate proton-evoked currents in heterologously expressed ASIC1a, ASIC2a and ASIC3 by a direct action on the channel protein (Smith et al. 2007).

Peripheral inflammation causes upregulation of FMRFamide-like peptides, including neuropeptide FF and neuropeptide FF-R2 in DRG neurons and the spinal cord, and both neuropeptide FF and FMRFamide are able to potentiate H^+-gated currents in cultured sensory neurons and heterologously expressed ASIC1 and ASIC3 channels (Askwith et al. 2000; Catarsi et al. 2001; Deval et al. 2003; Yang et al. 2008). This action appears to result from a delay in current inactivation or from enhancement of a sustained and slowly inactivating current. ASICs are modulated by a number of other factors, some of which may be generated or released during inflammation and acidosis. Nitric oxide, for instance, is able to potentiate acid-induced currents in ASIC1, ASIC2 and ASIC3 homomeric channels (Cadiou et al. 2007). Serine proteases modulate the pH sensitivity of ASIC1a and ASIC1b, probably by proteolytic cleavage of the long extracellular loop (Poirot et al. 2004).

An approach to reduce excess ASIC expression and function could be the interference with ASIC translocation to the cell membrane, integration in the cell membrane and phosphorylation. As other membrane proteins, ASICs appear to form macromolecular complexes with other proteins that may control the trafficking, function and turnover of ASIC subunits (Kress and Waldmann 2006; Wemmie et al. 2006) and may be future targets for pharmacological intervention.

ASICs do not only play a role in pain owing to their peripheral nocisensor function but also in the spinal transmission of pain impulses. ASIC1a is prominently expressed by neurons in the dorsal horn of the spinal cord, and downregulation of these ASIC1a channels by antisense oligonucleotides attenuates thermal and mechanical hypersensitivity induced by peripheral administration of complete Freund's adjuvant (Duan et al. 2007). ASIC1a participates in two forms of central sensitization in the spinal cord: C-fibre-induced "wind-up" and inflammation-evoked hypersensitivity of dorsal horn neurons (Duan et al. 2007). On the basis of these observations it has been proposed that specific blockade of Ca^{2+}-permeable ASIC1a channels may have an antinociceptive effect by reducing or preventing the development of central sensitization due to inflammation (Duan et al. 2007). ASIC1a in the brain emerges as being involved in cell damage after ischaemic stroke (Wemmie et al. 2006; Friese et al. 2007), and blockade of this Ca^{2+}-permeable channel has been proposed to offer a 5-h therapeutic time window following a cerebral vascular insult (Xiong et al. 2006).

4.2 TRPV Channels

Recognition of TRPV1 as a multimodal nocisensor, its sensitization by a number of proalgesic pathways and its upregulation under conditions of hyperalgesia have made this ion channel an attractive target for novel antinociceptive drugs. TRPV1 function can be counteracted by both desensitizing TRPV1 agonists as well as TRPV1 antagonists, and the current patent literature discloses more than 1,000 natural and synthetic compounds as TRPV1 activators or blockers (Gharat and Szallasi 2008). It is important to consider that uses of TRPV1 agonists and antagonists are not equivalent approaches (Holzer 1991; Szallasi et al. 2007). Capsaicin-sensitive afferent neurons express a plethora of different nocisensors, and desensitizing TRPV1 agonists do not only inactivate this nocisensor alone but defunctionalize the whole afferent neuron expressing TRPV1. In contrast, TRPV1 blockers selectively target this nocisensor and prevent its function. Resiniferatoxin and other compounds such as SDZ 249-665 are examples of TRPV1 agonists whose action manifests itself primarily in a defunctionalization of nociceptive neurons. Intravesical resiniferatoxin has been shown to be beneficial in patients with neurogenic bladder disorders (Avelino and Cruz 2006; Cruz and Dinis 2007) in which activation of afferent neurons by acidic urine penetrating through a leaky urothelium may play a role. SDZ 249-665 is able to attenuate acid-induced nociception arising from the peritoneal cavity of rats (Urban et al. 2000).

Most efforts have been directed at developing compounds that block TRPV1 activation in a competitive or non-competitive manner. The first of this kind, capsazepine, has been extensively used in the exploration of the pathophysiological implications of TRPV1. However, the results obtained with this compound need to be judged with caution because the selectivity of capsazepine as a TRPV1 blocker is limited by its inhibitory action on nicotinic acetylcholine receptors, voltage-activated Ca^{2+} channels and other TRP channels such as TRPM8 (Docherty et al. 1997; Liu and Simon 1997; Behrendt et al. 2004). Since TRPV1 is activated by multiple stimuli that interact with different domains of the channel protein, not all TRPV1 blockers prevent acid from gating TRPV1 (Gavva et al. 2005a). For instance, AMG-0610 and SB-366791 inhibit the activation of rat TRPV1 by capsaicin but not acid, whereas iodoresiniferatoxin, BCTC, AMG-6880, AMG-7472, AMG-9810 and A-425619 are TRPV1 antagonists that do not differentiate between capsaicin and protons (Seabrook et al. 2002; Gavva et al. 2004, 2005a, b; Neelands et al. 2005). In addition, there are species differences in the stimulus selectivity of TRPV1 blockers as, e.g., capsazepine and SB-366791 are more effective in blocking proton-induced gating of human TRPV1 than of rat TRPV1 (Gunthorpe et al. 2004; Gavva et al. 2005a).

While the vast list of emerging TRPV1 blockers attests to the antinociceptive potential that is attributed to this class of pharmacological agent, it is important to be aware of the likely drawbacks these compounds may have. It has repeatedly been argued that TRPV1 subserves important homeostatic functions, and that the challenge for an effective and safe therapy with TRPV1 blockers will be to suppress the pathological contribution of "excess" TRPV1 while preserving its physiological role (Holzer 2004b; Hicks 2006; Szallasi et al. 2007). TRPV1 is emerging as an important heat sensor involved in thermoregulation, given that most TRPV1 blockers cause hyperthermia in rats, dogs, monkeys and humans by a peripheral site of action (Gavva et al. 2007, 2008; Lehto et al. 2008). This hyperthermic action is unrelated to the ability of TRPV1 antagonists to block proton-induced activation of TRPV1 (Gavva et al. 2007). Hyperthermia is a serious adverse effect of TRPV1 blockade that went unnoticed after disruption of the *TRPV1* gene (Szelényi et al. 2004; Woodbury et al. 2004), most probably because of developmental compensations in heat sensing.

One possible approach to differentiate between the pathological and physiological implications of TRPV1 is the development of uncompetitive blockers that preferentially bind to the active, open state of the channel and therefore will predominantly silence overactive TRPV1 (García-Martínez et al. 2006). Another approach that appears increasingly feasible is interference with the intracellular trafficking of TRPV1 to the cell membrane, which will result in a reduction of TRPV1 channels on the cell surface (Morenilla-Palao et al. 2004; Planells-Cases et al. 2005). Sensitization of TRPV1 is due not only to an enhancement of channel currents but also to a rapid translocation of TRPV1 from the cytosol to the plasma membrane (Morenilla-Palao et al. 2004; Van Buren et al. 2005; Zhang et al. 2005). The trafficking of TRPV1 (and other channels) to the cell surface is blocked by botulinum neurotoxin A (Morenilla-Palao et al. 2004), which may explain why intradetrusor injection of botulinum neurotoxin A in patients with urinary bladder overactivity reduces TRPV1- and $P2X_3$-like immunoreactivity in the detrusor muscle and causes improvement of clinical and urodynamic parameters (Apostolidis et al. 2005). Intravesical administration of botulinum toxin likewise counteracts acetic acid evoked bladder overactivity in rats (Chuang et al. 2004).

4.3 K_{2P} Channels

Blockade of K_{2P} channels contributes to proton-evoked depolarization of DRG neurons from humans with neuropathic pain (Baumann et al. 2004), which makes it worthwhile to elucidate the role of these background channels in health and disease. Apart from the targeted design of drugs specifically acting at K_{2P} channels, it is important to realize that many endogenous and exogenous factors modify and regulate the activity of these channels (Duprat et al. 2007; Mathie 2007). For instance, K_{2P} channels of the TASK subfamily are regulated by a number of different GPCR pathways (Duprat et al. 2007; Mathie 2007). Along these lines, TASK-1 and TASK-3 are inhibited by the endocannabinoid anandamide (Maingret et al. 2001; Duprat et al. 2007). Another interaction that is of clinical relevance relates to the effect of anaesthetics on K_{2P} channels. TASK-1 activity is stimulated by halothane and partially inhibited by isoflurane, whereas TASK-3 channel activity is enhanced by halothane as well as isoflurane (Duprat et al. 2007). In addition, the activity of both TASK-1 and TASK-3 is inhibited by bupivacaine (Duprat et al. 2007).

5 Conclusions

Acidosis is a noxious condition associated with many pathological changes such as inflammation, ischaemia or mucosal defects in the upper gastrointestinal tract. To monitor these challenges of homeostasis, chemonociceptive afferent neurons express several acid sensors with distinct and overlapping properties. ASICs and TRPV1 have been most thoroughly studied, given that their proton sensitivities cover a complementary range of pH aberrations. While ASICs survey moderate decreases in extracellular pH, TRPV1 is activated only by severe acidosis resulting in pH values below 6. Acidosis, however, can sensitize TRPV1 to stimuli that are known to participate in inflammatory hyperalgesia. Emerging evidence indicates that other TRP channels such as TRPV4, TRPC4, TRPC5 and TRPP2, P2X purinoceptors, K_{2P} channels, Kir channels, voltage-activated K^+ channels, L-type Ca^{2+} channels, hyperpolarization-activated cyclic nucleotide gated channels, gap junction channels, Cl^- channels and acid-sensitive GPCRs also contribute to the acid sensitivity of afferent neurons. This redundancy of pH surveillance systems testifies that the maintenance of interstitial and intracellular pH within a narrow range is of paramount physiological importance. Since acid-sensitive ion channels and receptors have been found to be overactive and/or upregulated in chronic pain conditions and to play a role in chemonociception, they represent worthwhile targets for novel analgesic drugs. The pharmacological challenge in pursuing this goal is to differentiate between the pathological implications of acid sensors, which should be suppressed, and their physiological functions, which should be preserved.

Acknowledgements Work performed in the author's laboratory was supported by the Zukunftsfonds Steiermark (grant 262), the Austrian Scientific Research Funds (FWF grant L25-B05), the Jubilee Foundation of the Austrian National Bank (grant 9858) and the Austrian Federal Ministry of Science and Research. Evelin Painsipp is acknowledged for drawing Fig. 2.

References

Aihara E, Hayashi M, Sasaki Y, Kobata A, Takeuchi K (2005) Mechanisms underlying capsaicin-stimulated secretion in the stomach: comparison with mucosal acidification. J Pharmacol Exp Ther 315:423–432

Akiba Y, Takeuchi T, Mizumori M, Guth PH, Engel E, Kaunitz JD (2006a) TRPV-1 knockout paradoxically protects mouse gastric mucosa from acid/ethanol-induced injury by upregulating compensatory protective mechanisms. Gastroenterology 130(Suppl 2):A–106

Akiba Y, Ghayouri S, Takeuchi T, Mizumori M, Guth PH, Engel E, Swenson ER, Kaunitz JD (2006b) Carbonic anhydrases and mucosal vanilloid receptors help mediate the hyperemic response to luminal CO_2 in rat duodenum. Gastroenterology 131:142–152

Alvarez de la Rosa D, Zhang P, Shao D, White F, Canessa CM (2002) Functional implications of the localization and activity of acid-sensitive channels in rat peripheral nervous system. Proc Natl Acad Sci USA 99:2326–2331

Apostolidis A, Popat R, Yiangou Y, Cockayne D, Ford AP, Davis JB, Dasgupta P, Fowler CJ, Anand P (2005) Decreased sensory receptors $P2X_3$ and TRPV1 in suburothelial nerve fibers following intradetrusor injections of botulinum toxin for human detrusor overactivity. J Urol 174:977–982

Askwith CC, Cheng C, Ikuma M, Benson C, Price MP, Welsh MJ (2000) Neuropeptide FF and FMRFamide potentiate acid-evoked currents from sensory neurons and proton-gated DEG/ENaC channels. Neuron 26:133–141

Auzanneau C, Thoreau V, Kitzis A, Becq F (2003) A novel voltage-dependent chloride current activated by extracellular acidic *p*H in cultured rat Sertoli cells. J Biol Chem 278:19230–19236

Auzanneau C, Norez C, Antigny F, Thoreau V, Jougla C, Cantereau A, Becq F, Vandebrouck C (2008) Transient receptor potential vanilloid 1 (TRPV1) channels in cultured rat Sertoli cells regulate an acid sensing chloride channel. Biochem Pharmacol 75:476–483

Avelino A, Cruz F (2006) TRPV1 (vanilloid receptor) in the urinary tract: expression, function and clinical applications. Naunyn Schmiedebergs Arch Pharmacol 373:287–299

Banerjee B, Medda BK, Lazarova Z, Bansal N, Shaker R, Sengupta JN (2007) Effect of reflux-induced inflammation on transient receptor potential vanilloid one (TRPV1) expression in primary sensory neurons innervating the oesophagus of rats. Neurogastroenterol Motil 19:681–691

Bang H, Kim Y, Kim D (2000) TREK-2, a new member of the mechanosensitive tandem-pore K^+ channel family. J Biol Chem 275:17412–17419

Baumann TK, Chaudhary P, Martenson ME (2004) Background potassium channel block and TRPV1 activation contribute to proton depolarization of sensory neurons from humans with neuropathic pain. Eur J Neurosci 19:1343–1351
Bayliss DA, Talley EM, Sirois JE, Lei Q (2001) TASK-1 is a highly modulated *p*H-sensitive 'leak' K^+ channel expressed in brainstem respiratory neurons. Respir Physiol 129:159–174
Bearzatto B, Lesage F, Reyes R, Lazdunski M, Laduron PM (2000) Axonal transport of TREK and TRAAK potassium channels in rat sciatic nerves. Neuroreport 11:927–930
Behrendt HJ, Germann T, Gillen C, Hatt H, Jostock R (2004) Characterization of the mouse cold-menthol receptor TRPM8 and vanilloid receptor type-1 VR1 using a fluorometric imaging plate reader (FLIPR) assay. Br J Pharmacol 141:737–745
Benson CJ, Eckert SP, McCleskey EW (1999) Acid-evoked currents in cardiac sensory neurons: a possible mediator of myocardial ischemic sensation. Circ Res 84:921–928
Benson CJ, Xie J, Wemmie JA, Price MP, Henss JM, Welsh MJ, Snyder PM (2002) Heteromultimers of DEG/ENaC subunits form H^+-gated channels in mouse sensory neurons. Proc Natl Acad Sci USA 99:2338–2343
Bertrand PP, Kunze WA, Bornstein JC, Furness JB, Smith ML (1997) Analysis of the responses of myenteric neurons in the small intestine to chemical stimulation of the mucosa. Am J Physiol 273:G422–G435
Bevan S, Geppetti P (1994) Protons: small stimulants of capsaicin-sensitive sensory nerves. Trends Neurosci 17:509–512
Bevan S, Yeats J (1991) Protons activate a cation conductance in a sub-population of rat dorsal root ganglion neurones. J Physiol (Lond) 433:145–161
Bhat YM, Bielefeldt K (2006) Capsaicin receptor (TRPV1) and non-erosive reflux disease. Eur J Gastroenterol Hepatol 18:263–270
Bhattacharya A, Scott BP, Nasser N, Ao H, Maher MP, Dubin AE, Swanson DM, Shankley NP, Wickenden AD, Chaplan SR (2007) Pharmacology and antitussive efficacy of 4-(3-trifluoromethyl-pyridin-2-yl)-piperazine-1-carboxylic acid (5-trifluoromethyl-pyridin-2-yl)-amide (JNJ17203212), a transient receptor potential vanilloid 1 antagonist in guinea pigs. J Pharmacol Exp Ther 323:665–674
Bielefeldt K, Davis BM (2008) Differential effects of ASIC3 and TRPV1 deletion on gastroesophageal sensation in mice. Am J Physiol 294:G130–G138
Bina RW, Hempleman SC (2007) Evidence for TREK-like tandem-pore domain channels in intrapulmonary chemoreceptor chemotransduction. Respir Physiol Neurobiol 156:120–131
Birder LA, Kanai AJ, de Groat WC, Kiss S, Nealen ML, Burke NE, Dineley KE, Watkins S, Reynolds IJ, Caterina MJ (2001) Vanilloid receptor expression suggests a sensory role for urinary bladder epithelial cells. Proc Natl Acad Sci USA 98:13396–13401
Birder LA, Nakamura Y, Kiss S, Nealen ML, Barrick S, Kanai AJ, Wang E, Ruiz G, De Groat WC, Apodaca G, Watkins S, Caterina MJ (2002) Altered urinary bladder function in mice lacking the vanilloid receptor TRPV1. Nat Neurosci 5:856–860
Bley KR (2004) Recent developments in transient receptor potential vanilloid receptor 1 agonist-based therapies. Expert Opin Investig Drugs 13:1445–1456
Brady CM, Apostolidis AN, Harper M, Yiangou Y, Beckett A, Jacques TS, Freeman A, Scaravilli F, Fowler CJ, Anand P (2004) Parallel changes in bladder suburothelial vanilloid receptor TRPV1 and pan-neuronal marker PGP9.5 immunoreactivity in patients with neurogenic detrusor overactivity after intravesical resiniferatoxin treatment. BJU Int 93:770–776
Breese NM, George AC, Pauers LE, Stucky CL (2005) Peripheral inflammation selectively increases TRPV1 function in IB_4-positive sensory neurons from adult mouse. Pain 115:37–49
Brown SG, Townsend-Nicholson A, Jacobson KA, Burnstock G, King BF (2002) Heteromultimeric $P2X_{1/2}$ receptors show a novel sensitivity to extracellular *p*H. J Pharmacol Exp Ther 300:673–680
Buckler KJ (2007) TASK-like potassium channels and oxygen sensing in the carotid body. Respir Physiol Neurobiol 157:55–64

Burnstock G (2007) Physiology and pathophysiology of purinergic neurotransmission. Physiol Rev 87:659–797

Cadiou H, Studer M, Jones NG, Smith ES, Ballard A, McMahon SB, McNaughton PA (2007) Modulation of acid-sensing ion channel activity by nitric oxide. J Neurosci 27:13251–13260

Campanucci VA, Fearon IM, Nurse CA (2003) A novel O_2-sensing mechanism in rat glossopharyngeal neurones mediated by a halothane-inhibitable background K^+ conductance. J Physiol (Lond) 548:731–743

Canning BJ, Farmer DG, Mori N (2006) Mechanistic studies of acid-evoked coughing in anesthetized guinea pigs. Am J Physiol 291:R454–R463

Carlton SM, Coggeshall RE (2001) Peripheral capsaicin receptors increase in the inflamed rat hindpaw: a possible mechanism for peripheral sensitization. Neurosci Lett 310:53–56

Catarsi S, Babinski K, Séguéla P (2001) Selective modulation of heteromeric ASIC proton-gated channels by neuropeptide FF. Neuropharmacology 41:592–600

Caterina MJ, Julius D (2001) The vanilloid receptor: a molecular gateway to the pain pathway. Annu Rev Neurosci 24:487–517

Caterina MJ, Schumacher MA, Tominaga M, Rosen TA, Levine JD, Julius D (1997) The capsaicin receptor: a heat-activated ion channel in the pain pathway. Nature 389:816–824

Caterina MJ, Leffler A, Malmberg AB, Martin WJ, Trafton J, Petersen-Zeitz KR, Koltzenburg M, Basbaum AI, Julius D (2000) Impaired nociception and pain sensation in mice lacking the capsaicin receptor. Science 288:306–313

Chan CL, Facer P, Davis JB, Smith GD, Egerton J, Bountra C, Williams NS, Anand P (2003) Sensory fibres expressing capsaicin receptor TRPV1 in patients with rectal hypersensitivity and faecal urgency. Lancet 361:385–391

Chandrashekar J, Hoon MA, Ryba NJ, Zuker CS (2006) The receptors and cells for mammalian taste. Nature 444:288–294

Chapman CG, Meadows HJ, Godden RJ, Campbell DA, Duckworth M, Kelsell RE, Murdock PR, Randall AD, Rennie GI, Gloger IS (2000) Cloning, localisation and functional expression of a novel human, cerebellum specific, two pore domain potassium channel. Mol Brain Res 82:74–83

Chavez RA, Gray AT, Zhao BB, Kindler CH, Mazurek MJ, Mehta Y, Forsayeth JR, Yost CS (1999) TWIK-2, a new weak inward rectifying member of the tandem pore domain potassium channel family. J Biol Chem 274:7887–7892

Chen CC, England S, Akopian AN, Wood JN (1998) A sensory neuron-specific, proton-gated ion channel. Proc Natl Acad Sci USA 95:10240–10245

Chen CC, Zimmer A, Sun WH, Hall J, Brownstein MJ, Zimmer A (2002) A role for ASIC3 in the modulation of high-intensity pain stimuli. Proc Natl Acad Sci USA 99:8992–8997

Chizh BA, Illes P (2001) P2X receptors and nociception. Pharmacol Rev 53:553–568

Chuang YC, Chancellor MB, Seki S, Yoshimura N, Tyagi P, Huang L, Lavelle JP, De Groat WC, Fraser MO (2003) Intravesical protamine sulfate and potassium chloride as a model for bladder hyperactivity. Urology 61:664–670

Chuang YC, Yoshimura N, Huang CC, Chiang PH, Chancellor MB (2004) Intravesical botulinum toxin a administration produces analgesia against acetic acid induced bladder pain responses in rats. J Urol 172:1529–1532

Clapham DE, Julius D, Montell C, Schultz G (2005) International Union of Pharmacology. XLIX. Nomenclature and structure-function relationships of transient receptor potential channels. Pharmacol Rev 57:427–450

Clarke GD, Davison JS (1978) Mucosal receptors in the gastric antrum and small intestine of the rat with afferent fibres in the cervical vagus. J Physiol (Lond) 284:55–67

Clarke CE, Benham CD, Bridges A, George AR, Meadows HJ (2000) Mutation of histidine 286 of the human $P2X_4$ purinoceptor removes extracellular *p*H sensitivity. J Physiol (Lond) 523:697–703

Claydon TW, Boyett MR, Sivaprasadarao A, Orchard CH (2000) Two pore residues mediate acidosis-induced enhancement of C-type inactivation of the $K_v1.4$ K^+ channel. Am J Physiol 283:C1114–C1121

Clyne JD, LaPointe LD, Hume RI (2002) The role of histidine residues in modulation of the rat $P2X_2$ purinoceptor by zinc and *p*H. J Physiol (Lond) 539:347–359

Cockayne DA, Hamilton SG, Zhu QM, Dunn PM, Zhong Y, Novakovic S, Malmberg AB, Cain G, Berson A, Kassotakis L, Hedley L, Lachnit WG, Burnstock G, McMahon SB, Ford AP (2000) Urinary bladder hyporeflexia and reduced pain-related behaviour in $P2X_3$-deficient mice. Nature 407:1011–1015

Cockayne DA, Dunn PM, Zhong Y, Rong W, Hamilton SG, Knight GE, Ruan HZ, Ma B, Yip P, Nunn P, McMahon SB, Burnstock G, Ford AP (2005) $P2X_2$ knockout mice and $P2X_2/P2X_3$ double knockout mice reveal a role for the $P2X_2$ receptor subunit in mediating multiple sensory effects of ATP. J Physiol (2005) 567:621–639

Coffin B, Chollet R, Flourie B, Lemann M, Franchisseur C, Rambaud JC, Jian R (2001) Intraluminal modulation of gastric sensitivity to distension: effects of hydrochloric acid and meal. Am J Physiol 280:G904–G909

Cooper BY, Johnson RD, Rau KK (2004) Characterization and function of TWIK-related acid sensing K^+ channels in a rat nociceptive cell. Neuroscience 129:209–224

Cruz F, Dinis P (2007) Resiniferatoxin and botulinum toxin type A for treatment of lower urinary tract symptoms. Neurourol Urodyn 26(6 suppl):920–927

Daly D, Rong W, Chess-Williams R, Chapple C, Grundy D (2007) Bladder afferent sensitivity in wild-type and TRPV1 knockout mice. J Physiol (Lond) 583:663–674

Dang K, Bielefeldt K, Gebhart GF (2005) Differential responses of bladder lumbosacral and thoracolumbar dorsal root ganglion neurons to purinergic agonists, protons, and capsaicin. J Neurosci 25:3973–3984

Danzer M, Jocic M, Samberger C, Painsipp E, Bock E, Pabst MA, Crailsheim K, Schicho R, Lippe IT, Holzer P (2004) Stomach-brain communication by vagal afferents in response to luminal acid backdiffusion, gastrin, and gastric acid secretion. Am J Physiol 286:G403–G411

Davies NW, Lux HD, Morad M (1988) Site and mechanism of activation of proton-induced sodium current in chick dorsal root ganglion neurones. J Physiol (Lond) 400:159–187

Davis JB, Gray J, Gunthorpe MJ, Hatcher JP, Davey PT, Overend P, Harries MH, Latcham J, Clapham C, Atkinson K, Hughes SA, Rance K, Grau E, Harper AJ, Pugh PL, Rogers DC, Bingham S, Randall A, Sheardown SA (2000) Vanilloid receptor-1 is essential for inflammatory thermal hyperalgesia. Nature 405:183–187

Delmas P (2005) Polycystins: polymodal receptor/ion-channel cellular sensors. Pflügers Arch 451:264–276

Dean JB, Ballantyne D, Cardone DL, Erlichman JS, Solomon IC (2002) Role of gap junctions in CO_2 chemoreception and respiratory control. Am J Physiol 283:L665–L670

Decher N, Maier M, Dittrich W, Gassenhuber J, Bruggemann A, Busch AE, Steinmeyer K (2001) Characterization of TASK-4, a novel member of the *p*H-sensitive, two-pore domain potassium channel family. FEBS Lett 492:84–89

Deval E, Baron A, Lingueglia E, Mazarguil H, Zajac JM, Lazdunski M (2003) Effects of neuropeptide SF and related peptides on acid sensing ion channel 3 and sensory neuron excitability. Neuropharmacology 44:662–671

Ding S, Sachs F (1999) Single channel properties of $P2X_2$ purinoceptors. J Gen Physiol 113:695–720

Diochot S, Baron A, Rash LD, Deval E, Escoubas P, Scarzello S, Salinas M, Lazdunski M (2004) A new sea anemone peptide, APETx2, inhibits ASIC3, a major acid-sensitive channel in sensory neurons. EMBO J 23:1516–1525

Diochot S, Salinas M, Baron A, Escoubas P, Lazdunski M (2007) Peptides inhibitors of acid-sensing ion channels. Toxicon 49:271–284

Dobler T, Springauf A, Tovornik S, Weber M, Schmitt A, Sedlmeier R, Wischmeyer E, Döring F (2007) TRESK two-pore-domain K^+ channels constitute a significant component of background potassium currents in murine dorsal root ganglion neurones. J Physiol (Lond) 585:867–879

Docherty RJ, Yeats JC, Piper AS (1997) Capsazepine block of voltage-activated calcium channels in adult rat dorsal root ganglion neurones in culture. Br J Pharmacol 121:1461–1467

Drewes AM, Schipper KP, Dimcevski G, Petersen P, Gregersen H, Funch-Jensen P, Arendt-Nielsen L (2003) Gut pain and hyperalgesia induced by capsaicin: a human experimental model. Pain 104:333–341

Duan B, Wu LJ, Yu YQ, Ding Y, Jing L, Xu L, Chen J, Xu TL (2007) Upregulation of acid-sensing ion channel ASIC1a in spinal dorsal horn neurons contributes to inflammatory pain hypersensitivity. J Neurosci 27:11139–11148

Dubé GR, Lehto SG, Breese NM, Baker SJ, Wang X, Matulenko MA, Honoré P, Stewart AO, Moreland RB, Brioni JD (2005) Electrophysiological and in vivo characterization of A-317567, a novel blocker of acid sensing ion channels. Pain 117:88–96

Dunn PM, Zhong Y, Burnstock G (2001) P2X receptors in peripheral neurons. Prog Neurobiol 65:107–134

Duprat F, Lesage F, Fink M, Reyes R, Heurteaux C, Lazdunski M (1997) TASK, a human background K^+ channel to sense external *p*H variations near physiological *p*H. EMBO J 16:5464–5471

Duprat F, Girard C, Jarretou G, Lazdunski M (2005) Pancreatic two P domain K^+ channels TALK-1 and TALK-2 are activated by nitric oxide and reactive oxygen species. J Physiol (Lond) 562:235–244

Duprat F, Lauritzen I, Patel A, Honoré E (2007) The TASK background K2P channels: chemo- and nutrient sensors. Trends Neurosci 30:573–580

Escoubas P, De Weille JR, Lecoq A, Diochot S, Waldmann R, Champigny G, Moinier D, Menez A, Lazdunski M (2000) Isolation of a tarantula toxin specific for a class of proton-gated Na^+ channels. J Biol Chem 275:25116–25121

Faisy C, Planquette B, Naline E, Risse PA, Frossard N, Fagon JY, Advenier C, Devillier P (2007) Acid-induced modulation of airway basal tone and contractility: role of acid-sensing ion channels (ASICs) and TRPV1 receptor. Life Sci 81:1094–1102

Fallingborg J (1999) Intraluminal *p*H of the human gastrointestinal tract. Dan Med Bull 46:183–196

Filosa JA, Putnam RW (2003) Multiple targets of chemosensitive signaling in locus coeruleus neurons: role of K^+ and Ca^{2+} channels. Am J Physiol 284:C145–C155

Fischer MJ, Reeh PW, Sauer SK (2003) Proton-induced calcitonin gene-related peptide release from rat sciatic nerve axons, in vitro, involving TRPV1. Eur J Neurosci 18:803–810

Forster ER, Green T, Elliot M, Bremner A, Dockray GJ (1990) Gastric emptying in rats: role of afferent neurons and cholecystokinin. Am J Physiol 258:G552–G556

Friese MA, Craner MJ, Etzensperger R, Vergo S, Wemmie JA, Welsh MJ, Vincent A, Fugger L (2007) Acid-sensing ion channel-1 contributes to axonal degeneration in autoimmune inflammation of the central nervous system. Nat Med 13:1483–1489

Fujino K, de la Fuente SG, Takami Y, Takahashi T, Mantyh CR (2006) Attenuation of acid induced oesophagitis in VR-1 deficient mice. Gut 55:34–40

Fukuda T, Ichikawa H, Terayama R, Yamaai T, Kuboki T, Sugimoto T (2006) ASIC3-immunoreactive neurons in the rat vagal and glossopharyngeal sensory ganglia. Brain Res 1081:150–155

Gabriel A, Abdallah M, Yost CS, Winegar BD, Kindler CH (2002) Localization of the tandem pore domain K^+ channel KCNK5 (TASK-2) in the rat central nervous system. Mol Brain Res 98:153–163

Gao Z, Henig O, Kehoe V, Sinoway LI, Li J (2006) Vanilloid type 1 receptor and the acid-sensing ion channel mediate acid phosphate activation of muscle afferent nerves in rats. J Appl Physiol 100:421–426

Gao Z, Li JD, Sinoway LI, Li J (2007a) Effect of muscle interstitial *p*H on P2X and TRPV1 receptor-mediated pressor response. J Appl Physiol 102:2288–2293

Gao Y, Liu SS, Qiu S, Cheng W, Zheng J, Luo JH (2007b) Fluorescence resonance energy transfer analysis of subunit assembly of the ASIC channel. Biochem Biophys Res Commun 359:143–150

García-Martínez C, Fernández-Carvajal A, Valenzuela B, Gomis A, Van Den Nest W, Ferroni S, Carreño C, Belmonte C, Ferrer-Montiel A (2006) Design and characterization of a noncompetitive antagonist of the transient receptor potential vanilloid subunit 1 channel with in vivo analgesic and anti-inflammatory activity. J Pain 7:735–746

García-Sanz N, Fernández-Carvajal A, Morenilla-Palao C, Planells-Cases R, Fajardo-Sánchez E, Fernández-Ballester G, Ferrer-Montiel A (2004) Identification of a tetramerization domain in the C terminus of the vanilloid receptor. J Neurosci 24:5307–5314

Gavva NR, Klionsky L, Qu Y, Shi L, Tamir R, Edenson S, Zhang TJ, Viswanadhan VN, Toth A, Pearce LV, Vanderah TW, Porreca F, Blumberg PM, Lile J, Sun Y, Wild K, Louis JC, Treanor JJ (2004) Molecular determinants of vanilloid sensitivity in TRPV1. J Biol Chem 279:20283–20295

Gavva NR, Tamir R, Klionsky L, Norman MH, Louis JC, Wild KD, Treanor JJ (2005a) Proton activation does not alter antagonist interaction with the capsaicin-binding pocket of TRPV1. Mol Pharmacol 68:1524–1533

Gavva NR, Tamir R, Qu Y, Klionsky L, Zhang TJ, Immke D, Wang J, Zhu D, Vanderah TW, Porreca F, Doherty EM, Norman MH, Wild KD, Bannon AW, Louis JC, Treanor JJ (2005b) AMG 9810 [(*E*)-3-(4-t-butylphenyl)-*N*-(2,3-dihydrobenzo[b][1,4] dioxin-6-yl)acrylamide], a novel vanilloid receptor 1 (TRPV1) antagonist with antihyperalgesic properties. J Pharmacol Exp Ther 313:474–484

Gavva NR, Bannon AW, Surapaneni S, Hovland DN Jr, Lehto SG, Gore A, Juan T, Deng H, Han B, Klionsky L, Kuang R, Le A, Tamir R, Wang J, Youngblood B, Zhu D, Norman MH, Magal E, Treanor JJ, Louis JC (2007) The vanilloid receptor TRPV1 is tonically activated in vivo and involved in body temperature regulation. J Neurosci 27:3366–3374

Gavva NR, Treanor JJ, Garami A, Fang L, Surapaneni S, Akrami A, Alvarez F, Bak A, Darling M, Gore A, Jang GR, Kesslak JP, Ni L, Norman MH, Palluconi G, Rose MJ, Salfi M, Tan E, Romanovsky AA, Banfield C, Davar G (2008) Pharmacological blockade of the vanilloid receptor TRPV1 elicits marked hyperthermia in humans. Pain 136:202–210

Geppetti P, Tramontana M, Evangelista S, Renzi D, Maggi CA, Fusco BM, Del Bianco E (1991) Differential effect on neuropeptide release of different concentrations of hydrogen ions on afferent and intrinsic neurons of the rat stomach. Gastroenterology 101:1505–1511

Gerevich Z, Zadori ZS, Köles L, Kopp L, Milius D, Wirkner K, Gyires K, Illes P (2007) Dual effect of acid *p*H on purinergic P2X3 receptors depends on the histidine 206 residue. J Biol Chem 282:33949–33957

Gharat LA, Szallasi A (2008) Advances in the design and therapeutic use of capsaicin receptor TRPV1 agonists and antagonists. Expert Opin Ther Patents 18:159–209

Ghilardi JR, Röhrich H, Lindsay TH, Sevcik MA, Schwei MJ, Kubota K, Halvorson KG, Poblete J, Chaplan SR, Dubin AE, Carruthers NI, Swanson D, Kuskowski M, Flores CM, Julius D, Mantyh PW (2005) Selective blockade of the capsaicin receptor TRPV1 attenuates bone cancer pain. J Neurosci 25:3126–3131

Girard C, Duprat F, Terrenoire C, Tinel N, Fosset M, Romey G, Lazdunski M, Lesage F (2001) Genomic and functional characteristics of novel human pancreatic 2P domain K^+ channels. Biochem Biophys Res Commun 282:249–256

Goldstein SA, Bockenhauer D, O'Kelly I, Zilberberg N (2001) Potassium leak channels and the KCNK family of two-P-domain subunits. Nat Rev Neurosci 2:175–184

Goldstein SA, Bayliss DA, Kim D, Lesage F, Plant LD, Rajan S (2005) International Union of Pharmacology. LV. Nomenclature and molecular relationships of two-P potassium channels. Pharmacol Rev 57:527–540

Goodis HE, Poon A, Hargreaves KM (2006) Tissue *p*H and temperature regulate pulpal nociceptors. J Dent Res 85:1046–1049

Groth M, Helbig T, Grau V, Kummer W, Haberberger RV (2006) Spinal afferent neurons projecting to the rat lung and pleura express acid sensitive channels. Respir Res 7:96

Gu Q, Lee LY (2006) Characterization of acid signaling in rat vagal pulmonary sensory neurons. Am J Physiol 291:L58–L65

Gu W, Schlichthörl G, Hirsch JR, Engels H, Karschin C, Karschin A, Derst C, Steinlein OK, Daut J (2002) Expression pattern and functional characteristics of two novel splice variants of the two-pore-domain potassium channel TREK-2. J Physiol (Lond) 539:657–668

Güler AD, Lee H, Iida T, Shimizu I, Tominaga M, Caterina M (2002) Heat-evoked activation of the ion channel, TRPV4. J Neurosci 22:6408–6414

Gunthorpe MJ, Benham CD, Randall A, Davis JB (2002) The diversity in the vanilloid (TRPV) receptor family of ion channels. Trends Pharmacol Sci 23:183–191

Gunthorpe MJ, Rami HK, Jerman JC, Smart D, Gill CH, Soffin EM, Luis Hannan S, Lappin SC, Egerton J, Smith GD, Worby A, Howett L, Owen D, Nasir S, Davies CH, Thompson M, Wyman PA, Randall AD, Davis JB (2004) Identification and characterisation of SB-366791, a potent and selective vanilloid receptor (VR1/TRPV1) antagonist. Neuropharmacology 46:133–149

Guo A, Vulchanova L, Wang J, Li X, Elde R (1999) Immunocytochemical localization of the vanilloid receptor 1 (VR1): relationship to neuropeptides, the $P2X_3$ purinoceptor and IB_4 binding sites. Eur J Neurosci 11:946–958

Hamilton SG, McMahon SB, Lewin GR (2001) Selective activation of nociceptors by P2X receptor agonists in normal and inflamed rat skin. J Physiol (Lond) 534:437–445

Han J, Kang D, Kim D (2003) Functional properties of four splice variants of a human pancreatic tandem-pore K^+ channel, TALK-1. Am J Physiol 285:C529–C538

Hayes SG, Kindig AE, Kaufman MP (2007) Blockade of acid sensing ion channels attenuates the exercise pressor reflex in cats. J Physiol 581:1271–1282

Hellwig N, Plant TD, Janson W, Schäfer M, Schultz G, Schaefer M (2004) TRPV1 acts as proton channel to induce acidification in nociceptive neurons. J Biol Chem 279:34553–34561

Hervieu GJ, Cluderay JE, Gray CW, Green PJ, Ranson JL, Randall AD, Meadows HJ (2001) Distribution and expression of TREK-1, a two-pore-domain potassium channel, in the adult rat CNS. Neuroscience 103:899–919

Hicks GA (2006) TRP channels as therapeutic targets: hot property, or time to cool down? Neurogastroenterol Motil 18:590–594

Hoheisel U, Reinöhl J, Unger T, Mense S (2004) Acidic *p*H and capsaicin activate mechanosensitive group IV muscle receptors in the rat. Pain 110:149–157

Holzer P (1988) Local effector functions of capsaicin-sensitive sensory nerve endings: involvement of tachykinins, calcitonin gene-related peptide and other neuropeptides Neuroscience 24:739–768

Holzer P (1991) Capsaicin: cellular targets, mechanisms of action, and selectivity for thin sensory neurons. Pharmacol Rev 43:143–201

Holzer P (1998) Neural emergency system in the stomach. Gastroenterology 114:823–839

Holzer P (2003) Acid-sensitive ion channels in gastrointestinal function. Curr Opin Pharmacol 3:618–625

Holzer P (2004a) TRPV1 and the gut: from a tasty receptor for a painful vanilloid to a key player in hyperalgesia. Eur J Pharmacol 500:231–241

Holzer P (2004b) Vanilloid receptor TRPV1: hot on the tongue and inflaming the colon. Neurogastroenterol Motil 16:697–699

Holzer P (2007) Taste receptors in the gastrointestinal tract. V. Acid sensing in the gastrointestinal tract. Am J Physiol 292:G699–G705

Holzer P, Maggi CA (1998) Dissociation of dorsal root ganglion neurons into afferent and efferent-like neurons. Neuroscience 86:389–398

Holzer P, Painsipp E, Jocic M, Heinemann A (2003) Acid challenge delays gastric pressure adaptation, blocks gastric emptying and stimulates gastric fluid secretion in the rat. Neurogastroenterol Motil 15:45–55

Holzer P, Wultsch T, Edelsbrunner M, Mitrovic M, Shahbazian A, Painsipp E, Bock E, Pabst MA (2007) Increase in gastric acid-induced afferent input to the brainstem in mice with gastritis. Neuroscience 145:1108–1119

Honore P, Luger NM, Sabino MA, Schwei MJ, Rogers SD, Mach DB, O'Keefe PF, Ramnaraine ML, Clohisy DR, Mantyh PW (2000) Osteoprotegerin blocks bone cancer-induced skeletal destruction, skeletal pain and pain-related neurochemical reorganization of the spinal cord. Nat Med 6:521–528

Honore P, Mikusa J, Bianchi B, McDonald H, Cartmell J, Faltynek C, Jarvis MF (2002) TNP-ATP, a potent $P2X_3$ receptor antagonist, blocks acetic acid-induced abdominal constriction in mice: comparison with reference analgesics. Pain 96:99–105

Honoré E, Maingret F, Lazdunski M, Patel AJ (2002) An intracellular proton sensor commands lipid- and mechano-gating of the K^+ channel TREK-1. EMBO J 21:2968–2976

Huang AL, Chen X, Hoon MA, Chandrashekar J, Guo W, Tränkner D, Ryba NJ, Zuker CS (2006) The cells and logic for mammalian sour taste detection. Nature 442:934–938

Huang CW, Tzeng JN, Chen YJ, Tsai WF, Chen CC, Sun WH (2007) Nociceptors of dorsal root ganglion express proton-sensing G-protein-coupled receptors. Mol Cell Neurosci 36:195–210

Hughes PA, Brierley SM, Young RL, Blackshaw LA (2007) Localization and comparative analysis of acid-sensing ion channel (ASIC1, 2, and 3) mRNA expression in mouse colonic sensory neurons within thoracolumbar dorsal root ganglia. J Comp Neurol 500:863–875

Hunt J (2006) Exhaled breath condensate *p*H: reflecting acidification of the airway at all levels. Am J Respir Crit Care Med 173:366–367

Ikeda Y, Ueno A, Naraba H, Oh-ishi S (2001) Involvement of vanilloid receptor VR1 and prostanoids in the acid-induced writhing responses of mice. Life Sci 69:2911–2919

Immke DC, McCleskey EW (2001) Lactate enhances the acid-sensing Na^+ channel on ischemia-sensing neurons. Nat Neurosci 4:869–870

Immke DC, McCleskey EW (2003) Protons open acid-sensing ion channels by catalyzing relief of Ca^{2+} blockade. Neuron 37:75–84

Ishimaru Y, Inada H, Kubota M, Zhuang H, Tominaga M, Matsunami H (2006) Transient receptor potential family members PKD1L3 and PKD2L1 form a candidate sour taste receptor. Proc Natl Acad Sci USA 103:12569–12574

Jahr H, van Driel M, van Osch GJ, Weinans H, van Leeuwen JP (2005) Identification of acid-sensing ion channels in bone. Biochem Biophys Res Commun 337:349–354

Jancsó N (1960) Role of the nerve terminals in the mechanism of inflammatory reactions. Bull Millard Fillmore Hosp 7:53–77

Jarvis MF, Burgard EC, McGaraughty S, Honore P, Lynch K, Brennan TJ, Subieta A, Van Biesen T, Cartmell J, Bianchi B, Niforatos W, Kage K, Yu H, Mikusa J, Wismer CT, Zhu CZ, Chu K, Lee CH, Stewart AO, Polakowski J, Cox BF, Kowaluk E, Williams M, Sullivan J, Faltynek C (2002) A-317491, a novel potent and selective non-nucleotide antagonist of $P2X_3$ and $P2X_{2/3}$ receptors, reduces chronic inflammatory and neuropathic pain in the rat. Proc Natl Acad Sci USA 99:17179–17184

Ji RR, Samad TA, Jin SX, Schmoll R, Woolf CJ (2002) p38 MAPK activation by NGF in primary sensory neurons after inflammation increases TRPV1 levels and maintains heat hyperalgesia. Neuron 36:57–68

Jia Y, Lee LY (2007) Role of TRPV receptors in respiratory diseases. Biochim Biophys Acta 1772:915–927

Jiang M, Dun W, Tseng GN (1999) Mechanism for the effects of extracellular acidification on HERG-channel function. Am J Physiol 277:H1283–H1292

Jiang C, Rojas A, Wang R, Wang X (2005) CO_2 central chemosensitivity: why are there so many sensing molecules? Respir Physiol Neurobiol 145:115–126

Jiang N, Rau KK, Johnson RD, Cooper BY (2006) Proton sensitivity Ca^{2+} permeability and molecular basis of acid-sensing ion channels expressed in glabrous and hairy skin afferents. J Neurophysiol 95:2466–2478

Jones NG, Slater R, Cadiou H, McNaughton P, McMahon SB (2004) Acid-induced pain and its modulation in humans. J Neurosci 24:10974–10979

Jordt SE, Tominaga M, Julius D (2000) Acid potentiation of the capsaicin receptor determined by a key extracellular site. Proc Natl Acad Sci USA 97:8134–8139

Kagawa S, Aoi M, Kubo Y, Kotani T, and Takeuchi K (2003) Stimulation by capsaicin of duodenal HCO_3^- secretion via afferent neurons and vanilloid receptors in rats: comparison with acid-induced HCO_3^- response. Dig Dis Sci 48:1850–1856

Kang D, Kim D (2004) Single-channel properties and *p*H sensitivity of two-pore domain K^+ channels of the TALK family. Biochem Biophys Res Commun 315:836–844

Kang D, Kim D (2006) TREK-2 (K2P10.1) and TRESK (K2P18.1) are major background K^+ channels in dorsal root ganglion neurons. Am J Physiol 291:C138–C146

Kang JY, Yap I (1991) Acid and gastric ulcer pain. J Clin Gastroenterol 13:514–516

Kataoka S, Yang R, Ishimaru Y, Matsunami H, Sévigny J, Kinnamon JC, Finger TE (2008) The candidate sour taste receptor, PKD2L1, is expressed by type III taste cells in the mouse. Chem Senses 33:243–254

Kellenberger S, Schild L (2002) Epithelial sodium channel/degenerin family of ion channels: a variety of functions for a shared structure. Physiol Rev 82:735–767

Kim Y, Bang H, Kim D (2000) TASK-3, a new member of the tandem pore K^+ channel family. J Biol Chem 275:9340–9347

Kim Y, Gnatenco C, Bang H, Kim D (2001a) Localization of TREK-2 K^+ channel domains that regulate channel kinetics and sensitivity to pressure, fatty acids and *p*Hi. Pflügers Arch 442:952–960

Kim Y, Bang H, Gnatenco C, Kim D (2001b) Synergistic interaction and the role of C-terminus in the activation of TRAAK K^+ channels by pressure, free fatty acids and alkali. Pflügers Arch 442:64–72

King BF, Townsend-Nicholson A, Wildman SS, Thomas T, Spyer KM, Burnstock G (2000) Coexpression of rat $P2X_2$ and $P2X_6$ subunits in Xenopus oocytes. J Neurosci 20:4871–4877

Kollarik M, Undem BJ (2002) Mechanisms of acid-induced activation of airway afferent nerve fibres in guinea-pig. J Physiol 543:591–600

Kollarik M, Fei Ru F, Undem BJ (2007) Acid-sensitive vagal sensory pathways and cough. Pulm Pharmacol Ther 20:402–411

Konnerth A, Lux HD, Morad M (1987) Proton-induced transformation of calcium channel in chick dorsal root ganglion cells. J Physiol (Lond) 386:603–633

Kress M, Waldmann R (2006) Acid sensing ionic channels. Curr Top Membr 57:241–276

Krishek BJ, Smart TG (2001) Proton sensitivity of rat cerebellar granule cell $GABA_A$ receptors: dependence on neuronal development. J Physiol (Lond) 530:219–233

Krishtal O (2003) The ASICs: signaling molecules? Modulators? Trends Neurosci 26:477–483

Krishtal OA, Pidoplichko VI (1981) A receptor for protons in the membrane of sensory neurons may participate in nociception. Neuroscience 6:2599–2601

Lamb K, Kang YM, Gebhart GF, Bielefeldt K (2003) Gastric inflammation triggers hypersensitivity to acid in awake rats. Gastroenterology 125:1410–1418

Leffler A, Mönter B, Koltzenburg M (2006) The role of the capsaicin receptor TRPV1 and acid-sensing ion channels ASICs in proton sensitivity of subpopulations of primary nociceptive neurons in rats and mice. Neuroscience 139:699–709

Lehto SG, Tamir R, Deng H, Klionsky L, Kuang R, Le A, Lee D, Louis JC, Magal E, Manning BH, Rubino J, Surapaneni S, Tamayo N, Wang T, Wang J, Wang J, Wang W, Youngblood B, Zhang M, Zhu D, Norman MH, Gavva NR (2008) Antihyperalgesic effects of AMG8562, a novel vanilloid receptor TRPV1 modulator that does not cause hyperthermia in rats. J Pharmacol Exp Ther 326:218–229

Lesage F, Lazdunski M (2000) Molecular and functional properties of two-pore-domain potassium channels. Am J Physiol 279:F793–F801

Lesage F, Terrenoire C, Romey G, Lazdunski M (2000) Human TREK2, a 2P domain mechano-sensitive K^+ channel with multiple regulations by polyunsaturated fatty acids, lysophospholipids, and Gs, Gi, and Gq protein-coupled receptors. J Biol Chem 275:28398–28405

Leung SY, Niimi A, Williams AS, Nath P, Blanc FX, Dinh QT, Chung KF (2007) Inhibition of citric acid- and capsaicin-induced cough by novel TRPV-1 antagonist, V112220, in guinea-pig. Cough 3:10

Li C, Peoples RW, Weight FF (1996) Proton potentiation of ATP-gated ion channel responses to ATP and Zn^{2+} in rat nodose ganglion neurons. J Neurophysiol 76:3048–3058

Li C, Peoples RW, Weight FF (1997) Enhancement of ATP-activated current by protons in dorsal root ganglion neurons. Pflügers Arch 433:446–454

Li J, Maile MD, Sinoway AN, Sinoway LI (2004) Muscle pressor reflex: potential role of vanilloid type 1 receptor and acid-sensing ion channel. J Appl Physiol 97:1709–1714

Lin W, Burks CA, Hansen DR, Kinnamon SC, Gilbertson TA (2004) Taste receptor cells express *p*H-sensitive leak K^+ channels. J Neurophysiol 92:2909–2919

Lingueglia E (2007) Acid-sensing ion channels in sensory perception. J Biol Chem 282:17325–17329

Lingueglia E, de Weille JR, Bassilana F, Heurteaux C, Sakai H, Waldmann R, Lazdunski M (1997) A modulatory subunit of acid sensing ion channels in brain and dorsal root ganglion cells. J Biol Chem 272:29778–29783

Liu L, Simon SA (1997) Capsazepine, a vanilloid receptor antagonist, inhibits nicotinic acetylcholine receptors in rat trigeminal ganglia. Neurosci Lett 228:29–32

Liu M, King BF, Dunn PM, Rong W, Townsend-Nicholson A, Burnstock G (2001) Coexpression of $P2X_3$ and $P2X_2$ receptor subunits in varying amounts generates heterogeneous populations of P2X receptors that evoke a spectrum of agonist responses comparable to that seen in sensory neurons. J Pharmacol Exp Ther 296:1043–1050

Liu M, Willmott NJ, Michael GJ, Priestley JV (2004) Differential *p*H and capsaicin responses of Griffonia simplicifolia IB4 (IB4)-positive and IB4-negative small sensory neurons. Neuroscience 127:659–672

Liu L, Hansen DR, Kim I, Gilbertson TA (2005) Expression and characterization of delayed rectifying K^+ channels in anterior rat taste buds. Am J Physiol 289:C868–C880

Liu L, Mansfield KJ, Kristiana I, Vaux KJ, Millard RJ, Burcher E (2007) The molecular basis of urgency: regional difference of vanilloid receptor expression in the human urinary bladder. Neurourol Urodyn 26:433–438

LopezJimenez ND, Cavenagh MM, Sainz E, Cruz-Ithier MA, Battey JF, Sullivan SL (2006) Two members of the TRPP family of ion channels, Pkd1l3 and Pkd2l1, are co-expressed in a subset of taste receptor cells. J Neurochem 98:68–77

López-López JR, Pérez-García MT (2007) An ASIC channel for acid chemotransduction. Circ Res 101:965–967

Lu YX, Owyang C (1999) Duodenal acid-induced gastric relaxation is mediated by multiple pathways. Am J Physiol 276:G1501–G1506

Ludwig MG, Vanek M, Guerini D, Gasser JA, Jones CE, Junker U, Hofstetter H, Wolf RM, Seuwen K (2003) Proton-sensing G-protein-coupled receptors. Nature 425:93–98

Luger NM, Honore P, Sabino MA, Schwei MJ, Rogers SD, Mach DB, Clohisy DR, Mantyh PW (2001) Osteoprotegerin diminishes advanced bone cancer pain. Cancer Res 61:4038–4047

Lyall V, Alam RI, Malik SA, Phan TH, Vinnikova AK, Heck GL, DeSimone JA (2004) Basolateral Na^+-H^+ exchanger-1 in rat taste receptor cells is involved in neural adaptation to acidic stimuli. J Physiol (Lond) 556:159–173

Maingret F, Patel AJ, Lesage F, Lazdunski M, Honoré E (1999) Mechano- or acid stimulation, two interactive modes of activation of the TREK-1 potassium channel. J Biol Chem 274:26691–26696

Maingret F, Lauritzen I, Patel AJ, Heurteaux C, Reyes R, Lesage F, Lazdunski M, Honoré E (2000) TREK-1 is a heat-activated background K^+ channel. EMBO J 19:2483–2491

Maingret F, Patel AJ, Lazdunski M, Honoré E (2001) The endocannabinoid anandamide is a direct and selective blocker of the background K^+ channel TASK-1. EMBO J 20:47–54

Mamet J, Baron A, Lazdunski M, Voilley N (2002) Proinflammatory mediators, stimulators of sensory neuron excitability via the expression of acid-sensing ion channels. J Neurosci 22:10662–10670

Manela FD, Ren J, Gao J, McGuigan JE, Harty RF (1995) Calcitonin gene-related peptide modulates acid-mediated regulation of somatostatin and gastrin release from rat antrum. Gastroenterology 109:701–706

Mao J, Li L, McManus M, Wu J, Cui N, Jiang C (2002) Molecular determinants for activation of G-protein-coupled inward rectifier K^+ (GIRK) channels by extracellular acidosis. J Biol Chem 277:46166–46171

Mathie A (2007) Neuronal two-pore-domain potassium channels and their regulation by G protein-coupled receptors. J Physiol (Lond) 578:377–385

Matthews PJ, Aziz Q, Facer P, Davis JB, Thompson DG, Anand P (2004) Increased capsaicin receptor TRPV1 nerve fibres in the inflamed human oesophagus. Eur J Gastroenterol Hepatol 16:897–902

Mazzuca M, Heurteaux C, Alloui A, Diochot S, Baron A, Voilley N, Blondeau N, Escoubas P, Gélot A, Cupo A, Zimmer A, Zimmer AM, Eschalier A, Lazdunski M (2007) A tarantula peptide against pain via ASIC1a channels and opioid mechanisms. Nat Neurosci 10:943–945

McLatchie LM, Bevan S (2001) The effects of *p*H on the interaction between capsaicin and the vanilloid receptor in rat dorsal root ganglia neurons. Br J Pharmacol 132:899–908

Meadows HJ, Randall AD (2001) Functional characterisation of human TASK-3, an acid-sensitive two-pore domain potassium channel. Neuropharmacology 40:551–559

Medda BK, Sengupta JN, Lang IM, Shaker R (2005) Response properties of the brainstem neurons of the cat following intra-esophageal acid-pepsin infusion. Neuroscience 135:1285–1294

Medhurst AD, Rennie G, Chapman CG, Meadows H, Duckworth MD, Kelsell RE, Gloger II, Pangalos MN (2001) Distribution analysis of human two pore domain potassium channels in tissues of the central nervous system and periphery. Mol Brain Res 86:101–114

Michael GJ, Priestley JV (1999) Differential expression of the mRNA for the vanilloid receptor subtype 1 in cells of the adult rat dorsal root and nodose ganglia and its downregulation by axotomy. J Neurosci 19:1844–1854

Miller P, Peers C, Kemp PJ (2004) Polymodal regulation of hTREK1 by *p*H, arachidonic acid, and hypoxia: physiological impact in acidosis and alkalosis. Am J Physiol 286:C272–C282

Miranda A, Nordstrom E, Mannem A, Smith C, Banerjee B, Sengupta JN (2007) The role of transient receptor potential vanilloid 1 in mechanical and chemical visceral hyperalgesia following experimental colitis. Neuroscience 148:1021–1032

Mistrík P, Torre V (2004) Histidine 518 in the S6-CNBD linker controls *p*H dependence and gating of HCN channel from sea-urchin sperm. Pflugers Arch 448:76–84

Mizuno A, Matsumoto N, Imai M, Suzuki M (2003) Impaired osmotic sensation in mice lacking TRPV4. Am J Physiol 285:C96–C101

Mogil JS, Breese NM, Witty MF, Ritchie J, Rainville ML, Ase A, Abbadi N, Stucky CL, Seguela P (2005) Transgenic expression of a dominant-negative ASIC3 subunit leads to increased sensitivity to mechanical and inflammatory stimuli. J Neurosci 25:9893–9901

Montrose MH, Akiba Y, Takeuchi K, Kaunitz JD (2006) Gastroduodenal mucosal defense. In: Johnson LR (ed) Physiology of the gastrointestinal tract, 4th edn. Academic, San Diego, pp 1259–1291

Morenilla-Palao C, Planells-Cases R, García-Sanz N, Ferrer-Montiel A (2004) Regulated exocytosis contributes to protein kinase C potentiation of vanilloid receptor activity. J Biol Chem 279:25665–25672

Morton MJ, O'Connell AD, Sivaprasadarao A, Hunter M (2003) Determinants of *p*H sensing in the two-pore domain K^+ channels TASK-1 and -2. Pflügers Arch 445:577–583

Morton MJ, Abohamed A, Sivaprasadarao A, Hunter M (2005) *p*H sensing in the two-pore domain K^+ channel, TASK2. Proc Natl Acad Sci USA 102:16102–16106

Nagae M, Hiraga T, Wakabayashi H, Wang L, Iwata K, Yoneda T (2006) Osteoclasts play a part in pain due to the inflammation adjacent to bone. Bone 39:1107–1115

Nagae M, Hiraga T, Yoneda T (2007) Acidic microenvironment created by osteoclasts causes bone pain associated with tumor colonization. J Bone Miner Metab 25:99–104

Neelands TR, Jarvis MF, Han P, Faltynek CR, Surowy CS (2005) Acidification of rat TRPV1 alters the kinetics of capsaicin responses. Mol Pain 1:28

Newell K, Franchi A, Pouysségur J, Tannock I (1993) Studies with glycolysis-deficient cells suggest that production of lactic acid is not the only cause of tumor acidity. Proc Natl Acad Sci USA 90:1127–1131

Niemeyer MI, González-Nilo FD, Zúñiga L, González W, Cid LP, Sepúlveda FV (2007) Neutralization of a single arginine residue gates open a two-pore domain, alkali-activated K^+ channel. Proc Natl Acad Sci USA 104:666–671

Nomura H, Turco AE, Pei Y, Kalaydjieva L, Schiavello T, Weremowicz S, Ji W, Morton CC, Meisler M, Reeders ST, Zhou J (1998) Identification of PKDL, a novel polycystic kidney disease 2-like gene whose murine homologue is deleted in mice with kidney and retinal defects. J Biol Chem 273:25967–25973

North RA (2002) Molecular physiology of P2X receptors. Physiol Rev 82:1013–1067

Nugent SG, Kumar D, Rampton DS, Evans DF (2001) Intestinal luminal *p*H in inflammatory bowel disease: possible determinants and implications for therapy with aminosalicylates and other drugs. Gut 48:71–577

Ohtori S, Inoue G, Koshi T, Ito T, Doya H, Saito T, Moriya H, Takahashi K (2006) Up-regulation of acid-sensing ion channel 3 in dorsal root ganglion neurons following application of nucleus pulposus on nerve root in rats. Spine 31:2048–2052

Ohtori S, Inoue G, Koshi T, Ito T, Watanabe T, Yamashita M, Yamauchi K, Suzuki M, Doya H, Moriya H, Takahashi Y, Takahashi K (2007) Sensory innervation of lumbar vertebral bodies in rats. Spine 32:1498–1502

Page AJ, Brierley SM, Martin CM, Price MP, Symonds E, Butler R, Wemmie JA, Blackshaw LA (2005) Different contributions of ASIC channels 1a, 2, and 3 in gastrointestinal mechanosensory function. Gut 54:1408–1415

Page AJ, Brierley SM, Martin CM, Hughes PA, Blackshaw LA (2007) Acid sensing ion channels 2 and 3 are required for inhibition of visceral nociceptors by benzamil. Pain 133:150–160

Patapoutian A, Peier AM, Story GM, Viswanath V (2003) ThermoTRP channels and beyond: mechanisms of temperature sensation. Nat Rev Neurosci 4:529–539

Patel AJ, Honoré E (2001) Properties and modulation of mammalian 2P domain K^+ channels. Trends Neurosci 24:339–346

Patel AJ, Maingret F, Magnone V, Fosset M, Lazdunski M, Honoré E (2000) TWIK-2, an inactivating 2P domain K^+ channel. J Biol Chem 275:28722–28730

Patterson LM, Zheng H, Ward SM, Berthoud HR (2003) Vanilloid receptor (VR1) expression in vagal afferent neurons innervating the gastrointestinal tract. Cell Tissue Res 311:277–287

Petersen M, LaMotte RH (1993) Effect of protons on the inward current evoked by capsaicin in isolated dorsal root ganglion cells. Pain 54:37–42

Petheo GL, Molnár Z, Róka A, Makara JK, Spät A (2001) A *p*H-sensitive chloride current in the chemoreceptor cell of rat carotid body. J Physiol (Lond) 535:95–106

Planells-Cases R, Garcìa-Sanz N, Morenilla-Palao C, Ferrer-Montiel A (2005) Functional aspects and mechanisms of TRPV1 involvement in neurogenic inflammation that leads to thermal hyperalgesia. Pflügers Arch 451:151–159

Poirot O, Vukicevic M, Boesch A, Kellenberger S (2004) Selective regulation of acid-sensing ion channel 1 by serine proteases. J Biol Chem 279:38448–38457

Poirot O, Berta T, Decosterd I, Kellenberger S (2006) Distinct ASIC currents are expressed in rat putative nociceptors and are modulated by nerve injury. J Physiol (Lond) 576:215–234

Price MP, McIlwrath SL, Xie J, Cheng C, Qiao J, Tarr DE, Sluka KA, Brennan TJ, Lewin GR, Welsh MJ (2001) The DRASIC cation channel contributes to the detection of cutaneous touch and acid stimuli in mice. Neuron 32:1071–1083

Putnam RW, Filosa JA, Ritucci NA (2004) Cellular mechanisms involved in CO_2 and acid signaling in chemosensitive neurons. Am J Physiol 287:C1493–C1526

Rajan S, Wischmeyer E, Xin Liu G, Preisig-Müller R, Daut J, Karschin A, Derst C (2000) TASK-3, a novel tandem pore domain acid-sensitive K^+ channel. An extracellular histidine as *p*H sensor. J Biol Chem 275:16650–16657

Rajan S, Plant LD, Rabin ML, Butler MH, Goldstein SA (2005) Sumoylation silences the plasma membrane leak K^+ channel $K_{2P}1$. Cell 121:37–47

Rau KK, Cooper BY, Johnson RD (2006) Expression of TWIK-related acid sensitive K^+ channels in capsaicin sensitive and insensitive cells of rat dorsal root ganglia. Neuroscience 141:955–963

Reeh PW, Kress M (2001) Molecular physiology of proton transduction in nociceptors. Curr Opin Pharmacol 1:45–51

Reyes R, Duprat F, Lesage F, Fink M, Salinas M, Farman N, Lazdunski M (1998) Cloning and expression of a novel *p*H-sensitive two pore domain K^+ channel from human kidney. J Biol Chem 273:30863–30869

Reyes R, Lauritzen I, Lesage F, Ettaiche M, Fosset M, Lazdunski M (2000) Immunolocalization of the arachidonic acid and mechanosensitive baseline TRAAK potassium channel in the nervous system. Neuroscience 95:893–901

Ricciardolo FL, Gaston B, Hunt J (2004) Acid stress in the pathology of asthma. J Allergy Clin Immunol 113:610–619

Richter TA, Dvoryanchikov GA, Chaudhari N, Roper SD (2004a) Acid-sensitive two-pore domain potassium (K_{2P}) channels in mouse taste buds. J Neurophysiol 92:1928–1936

Richter TA, Dvoryanchikov GA, Roper SD, Chaudhari N (2004b) Acid-sensing ion channel-2 is not necessary for sour taste in mice. J Neurosci 24:4088–4091

Rigoni M, Trevisani M, Gazzieri D, Nadaletto R, Tognetto M, Creminon C, Davis JB, Campi B, Amadesi S, Geppetti P, Harrison S (2003) Neurogenic responses mediated by vanilloid receptor-1 (TRPV1) are blocked by the high affinity antagonist, iodo-resiniferatoxin. Br J Pharmacol 138:977–985

Robinson DR, McNaughton PA, Evans ML, Hicks GA (2004) Characterization of the primary spinal afferent innervation of the mouse colon using retrograde labelling. Neurogastroenterol Motil 16:113–124

Rong W, Gourine AV, Cockayne DA, Xiang Z, Ford AP, Spyer KM, Burnstock G (2003) Pivotal role of nucleotide $P2X_2$ receptor subunit of the ATP-gated ion channel mediating ventilatory responses to hypoxia. J Neurosci 23:11315–11321

Rong W, Hillsley K, Davis JB, Hicks G, Winchester WJ, Grundy D (2004) Jejunal afferent nerve sensitivity in wild-type and TRPV1 knockout mice. J Physiol (Lond) 560:867–881

Rukwied R, Chizh BA, Lorenz U, Obreja O, Margarit S, Schley M, Schmelz M (2007) Potentiation of nociceptive responses to low *p*H injections in humans by prostaglandin E_2. J Pain 8:443–451

Ryu S, Liu B, Qin F (2003) Low *p*H potentiates both capsaicin binding and channel gating of VR1 receptors. J Gen Physiol 122:45–61

Ryu S, Liu B, Yao J, Fu Q, Qin F (2007) Uncoupling proton activation of vanilloid receptor TRPV1. J Neurosci 27:12797–12807

Sano Y, Inamura K, Miyake A, Mochizuki S, Kitada C, Yokoi H, Nozawa K, Okada H, Matsushime H, Furuichi K (2003) A novel two-pore domain K^+ channel, TRESK, is localized in the spinal cord. J Biol Chem 278:27406–27412

Schicho R, Schemann M, Pabst MA, Holzer P, Lippe IT (2003) Capsaicin-sensitive extrinsic afferents are involved in acid-induced activation of distinct myenteric neurons in the rat stomach. Neurogastroenterol Motil 15:33–44

Schicho R, Florian W, Liebmann I, Holzer P, Lippe IT (2004) Increased expression of TRPV1 receptor in dorsal root ganglia by acid insult of the rat gastric mucosa. Eur J Neurosci 19:1811–1818

Schmidt B, Hammer J, Holzer P, Hammer HF (2004) Chemical nociception in the jejunum induced by capsaicin. Gut 53:1109–1116

Schuligoi R, Jocic M, Heinemann A, Schöninkle E, Pabst MA, Holzer P (1998) Gastric acid-evoked c-fos messenger RNA expression in rat brainstem is signaled by capsaicin-resistant vagal afferents. Gastroenterology 115:649–660

Seabrook GR, Sutton KG, Jarolimek W, Hollingworth GJ, Teague S, Webb J, Clark N, Boyce S, Kerby J, Ali Z, Chou M, Middleton R, Kaczorowski G, Jones AB (2002) Functional properties of the high-affinity TRPV1 (VR1) vanilloid receptor antagonist (4-hydroxy-5-iodo-3-methoxyphenylacetate ester) iodo-resiniferatoxin. J Pharmacol Exp Ther 303:1052–1060

Semtner M, Schaefer M, Pinkenburg O, Plant TD (2007) Potentiation of TRPC5 by protons. J Biol Chem 282:33868–33878

Shimada S, Ueda T, Ishida Y, Yamamoto T, Ugawa S (2006) Acid-sensing ion channels in taste buds. Arch Histol Cytol 69:227–231

Shimokawa N, Dikic I, Sugama S, Koibuchi N (2005) Molecular responses to acidosis of central chemosensitive neurons in brain. Cell Signal 17:799–808

Shulkes A, Baldwin GS, Giraud AS (2006) Regulation of gastric acid secretion. In: Johnson LR (ed) Physiology of the gastrointestinal tract, 4th edn. Academic, San Diego, pp 1223–1258

Sluka KA, Price MP, Breese NA, Stucky CL, Wemmie JA, Welsh MJ (2003) Chronic hyperalgesia induced by repeated acid injections in muscle is abolished by the loss of ASIC3, but not ASIC1. Pain 106:229–239

Sluka KA, Radhakrishnan R, Benson CJ, Eshcol JO, Price MP, Babinski K, Audette KM, Yeomans DC, Wilson SP (2007) ASIC3 in muscle mediates mechanical, but not heat, hyperalgesia associated with muscle inflammation. Pain 129:102–112

Smith ES, Cadiou H, McNaughton PA (2007) Arachidonic acid potentiates acid-sensing ion channels in rat sensory neurons by a direct action. Neuroscience 145:686–698

Somodi S, Varga Z, Hajdu P, Starkus JG, Levy DI, Gáspár R, Panyi G (2004) *p*H-dependent modulation of $K_v1.3$ inactivation: role of His399. Am J Physiol 287:C1067–C1076

Steen KH, Reeh PW (1993) Sustained graded pain and hyperalgesia from harmless experimental tissue acidosis in human skin. Neurosci Lett 154:113–116

Steen KH, Reeh PW, Anton F, Handwerker HO (1992) Protons selectively induce lasting excitation and sensitization to mechanical stimulation of nociceptors in rat skin, in vitro. J Neurosci 12:86–95

Steen KH, Reeh PW, Kreysel HW (1995) Topical acetylsalicylic, salicylic acid and indomethacin suppress pain from experimental tissue acidosis in human skin. Pain 62:339–347

Stevens DR, Seifert R, Bufe B, Müller F, Kremmer E, Gauss R, Meyerhof W, Kaupp UB, Lindemann B (2001) Hyperpolarization-activated channels HCN1 and HCN4 mediate responses to sour stimuli. Nature 413:631–635

Stoop R, Surprenant A, North RA (1997) Different sensitivities to *p*H of ATP-induced currents at four cloned P2X receptors. J Neurophysiol 78:1837–1840

Strecker T, Messlinger K, Weyand M, Reeh PW (2005) Role of different proton-sensitive channels in releasing calcitonin gene-related peptide from isolated hearts of mutant mice. Cardiovasc Res 65:405–410

Sugiura T, Dang K, Lamb K, Bielefeldt K, Gebhart GF (2005) Acid-sensing properties in rat gastric sensory neurons from normal and ulcerated stomach. J Neurosci 25:2617–2627

Sugiura T, Bielefeldt K, Gebhart GF (2007) Mouse colon sensory neurons detect extracellular acidosis via TRPV1. Am J Physiol 292:C1768–C1774

Surprenant A, Schneider DA, Wilson HL, Galligan JJ, North RA (2000) Functional properties of heteromeric $P2X_{1/5}$ receptors expressed in HEK cells and excitatory junction potentials in guinea-pig submucosal arterioles. J Auton Nerv Syst 81:249–263

Sutherland SP, Benson CJ, Adelman JP, McCleskey EW (2001) Acid-sensing ion channel 3 matches the acid-gated current in cardiac ischemia-sensing neurons. Proc Natl Acad Aci USA 98:711–716

Suzuki M, Mizuno A, Kodaira K, Imai M (2003a) Impaired pressure sensation in mice lacking TRPV4. J Biol Chem 278:22664–22668

Suzuki M, Watanabe Y, Oyama Y, Mizuno A, Kusano E, Hirao A, Ookawara S (2003b) Localization of mechanosensitive channel TRPV4 in mouse skin. Neurosci Lett 353:189–192

Szallasi A, Blumberg PM (1999) Vanilloid (capsaicin) receptors and mechanisms. Pharmacol Rev 51:159–212

Szallasi A, Cortright DN, Blum CA, Eid SR (2007) The vanilloid receptor TRPV1: 10 years from channel cloning to antagonist proof-of-concept. Nat Rev Drug Discov 6:357–372

Szelényi Z, Hummel Z, Szolcsányi J, Davis JB (2004) Daily body temperature rhythm and heat tolerance in TRPV1 knockout and capsaicin pretreated mice. Eur J Neurosci 19:1421–1424

Talley EM, Solorzano G, Lei Q, Kim D, Bayliss DA (2001) CNS distribution of members of the two-pore-domain (KCNK) potassium channel family. J Neurosci 21:7491–7505

Tan ZY, Lu Y, Whiteis CA, Benson CJ, Chapleau MW, Abboud FM (2007) Acid-sensing ion channels contribute to transduction of extracellular acidosis in rat carotid body glomus cells. Circ Res 101:1009–1019

Tang L, Chen Y, Chen Z, Blumberg PM, Kozikowski AP, Wang ZJ (2007) Antinociceptive pharmacology of *N*-(4-chlorobenzyl)-*N*′-(4-hydroxy-3-iodo-5-methoxybenzyl) thiourea, a high-affinity competitive antagonist of the transient receptor potential vanilloid 1 receptor. J Pharmacol Exp Ther 321:791–798

Tashima K, Nakashima M, Kagawa S, Kato S, Takeuchi K (2002) Gastric hyperemic response induced by acid back-diffusion in rat stomachs following barrier disruption – relation to vanilloid type-1 receptors. Med Sci Monit 8:BR157–BR163

Tominaga M, Caterina M, Malmberg AB, Rosen TA, Gilbert H, Skinner K, Raumann BE, Basbaum AI, Julius D (1998) The cloned capsaicin receptor integrates multiple pain-producing stimuli. Neuron 21:531–543

Tomura H, Mogi C, Sato K, Okajima F (2005) Proton-sensing and lysolipid-sensitive G-protein-coupled receptors: a novel type of multi-functional receptors. Cell Signal 17:1466–1476

Trevisani M, Milan A, Gatti R, Zanasi A, Harrison S, Fontana G, Morice AH, Geppetti P (2004) Antitussive activity of iodo-resiniferatoxin in guinea pigs. Thorax 59:769–772

Uchiyama Y, Cheng CC, Danielson KG, Mochida J, Albert TJ, Shapiro IM, Risbud MV (2007) Expression of acid-sensing ion channel 3 (ASIC3) in nucleus pulposus cells of the intervertebral disc is regulated by p75NTR and ERK signaling. J Bone Miner Res 22:1996–2006

Ugawa S, Ueda T, Ishida Y, Nishigaki M, Shibata Y, Shimada S (2002) Amiloride-blockable acid-sensing ion channels are leading acid sensors expressed in human nociceptors. J Clin Invest 110:1185–1190

Ugawa S, Yamamoto T, Ueda T, Ishida Y, Inagaki A, Nishigaki M, Shimada S (2003) Amiloride-insensitive currents of the acid-sensing ion channel-2a (ASIC2a)/ASIC2b heteromeric sour-taste receptor channel. J Neurosci 23:3616–3622

Ugawa S, Ueda T, Yamamura H, Shimada S (2005) In situ hybridization evidence for the coexistence of ASIC and TRPV1 within rat single sensory neurons. Mol Brain Res 136:125–133

Urban L, Campbell EA, Panesar M, Patel S, Chaudhry N, Kane S, Buchheit K, Sandells B, James IF (2000) In vivo pharmacology of SDZ 249-665, a novel, non-pungent capsaicin analogue. Pain 89:65–74

Van Buren JJ, Bhat S, Rotello R, Pauza ME, Premkumar LS (2005) Sensitization and translocation of TRPV1 by insulin and IGF-I. Mol Pain 1:17

Vaupel P, Kallinowski F, Okunieff P (1989) Blood flow, oxygen and nutrient supply, and metabolic microenvironment of human tumors: a review. Cancer Res 49:6449–6465

Vellani V, Mapplebeck S, Moriondo A, Davis JB, McNaughton PA (2001) Protein kinase C activation potentiates gating of the vanilloid receptor VR1 by capsaicin, protons, heat and anandamide. J Physiol 534:813–825

Voilley N, de Weille J, Mamet J, Lazdunski M (2001) Nonsteroid anti-inflammatory drugs inhibit both the activity and the inflammation-induced expression of acid-sensing ion channels in nociceptors. J Neurosci 21:8026–8033

Vulcu SD, Liewald JF, Gillen C, Rupp J, Nawrath H (2004) Proton conductance of human transient receptor potential-vanilloid type-1 expressed in oocytes of Xenopus laevis and in Chinese hamster ovary cells. Neuroscience 125:861–866

Wachter CH, Heinemann A, Donnerer J, Pabst MA, Holzer P (1998) Mediation by 5-hydroxytryptamine of the femoral vasoconstriction induced by acid challenge of the rat gastric mucosa. J Physiol (Lond) 509:541–550

Waldmann R (2001) Proton-gated cation channels – neuronal acid sensors in the central and peripheral nervous system. Adv Exp Med Biol 502:293–304

Waldmann R, Lazdunski M (1998) H^+-gated cation channels: neuronal acid sensors in the NaC/DEG family of ion channels. Curr Opin Neurobiol 8:418–424

Waldmann R, Champigny G, Lingueglia E, De Weille JR, Heurteaux C, Lazdunski M (1999) H^+-gated cation channels. Ann N Y Acad Sci 868:67–76

Wang L, Wang DH (2005) *TRPV1* gene knockout impairs postischemic recovery in isolated perfused heart in mice. Circulation 112:3617–3623

Wang X, Wu J, Li L, Chen F, Wang R, Jiang C (2003) Hypercapnic acidosis activates K_{ATP} channels in vascular smooth muscles. Circ Res 92:1225–1232

Welch JM, Simon SA, Reinhart PH (2000) The activation mechanism of rat vanilloid receptor 1 by capsaicin involves the pore domain and differs from the activation by either acid or heat. Proc Natl Acad Sci USA 97:13889–13894

Welsh MJ, Price MP, Xie J (2002) Biochemical basis of touch perception: mechanosensory function of degenerin/epithelial Na^+ channels. J Biol Chem 277:2369–2372

Wemmie JA, Price MP, Welsh MJ (2006) Acid-sensing ion channels: advances, questions and therapeutic opportunities. Trends Neurosci 29:578–586

Wildman SS, Brown SG, Rahman M, Noel CA, Churchill L, Burnstock G, Unwin RJ, King BF (2002) Sensitization by extracellular Ca^{2+} of rat $P2X_5$ receptor and its pharmacological properties compared with rat $P2X_1$. Mol Pharmacol 62:957–966

Woodbury CJ, Zwick M, Wang S, Lawson JJ, Caterina MJ, Koltzenburg M, Albers KM, Koerber HR, Davis BM (2004) Nociceptors lacking TRPV1 and TRPV2 have normal heat responses. J Neurosci 24:6410–6415

Wultsch T, Painsipp E, Shahbazian A, Mitrovic M, Edelsbrunner M, Waldmann R, Lazdunski M, Holzer P (2008) Deletion of the acid-sensing ion channel ASIC3 prevents gastritis-induced acid hyperresponsiveness of the stomach-brainstem axis. Pain 134:245–253

Wynn G, Ma B, Ruan HZ, Burnstock G (2004) Purinergic component of mechanosensory transduction is increased in a rat model of colitis. Am J Physiol 287:G647–G657

Xie J, Price MP, Berger AL, Welsh MJ (2002) DRASIC contributes to *p*H-gated currents in large dorsal root ganglion sensory neurons by forming heteromultimeric channels. J Neurophysiol 87:2835–2843

Xiong ZG, Chu XP, Simon RP (2006) Ca^{2+}-permeable acid-sensing ion channels and ischemic brain injury. J Membr Biol 209:59–68

Xu GY, Huang LY (2002) Peripheral inflammation sensitizes P2X receptor-mediated responses in rat dorsal root ganglion neurons. J Neurosci 22:93–102

Xu GY, Winston JH, Shenoy M, Yin H, Pendyala S, Pasricha PJ (2007) Transient receptor potential vanilloid 1 mediates hyperalgesia and is up-regulated in rats with chronic pancreatitis. Gastroenterology 133:1282–1292

Xu H, Cui N, Yang Z, Wu J, Giwa LR, Abdulkadir L, Sharma P, Jiang C (2001) Direct activation of cloned K_{ATP} channels by intracellular acidosis. J Biol Chem 276:12898–12902

Yagi J, Wenk HN, Naves LA, McCleskey EW (2006) Sustained currents through ASIC3 ion channels at the modest *p*H changes that occur during myocardial ischemia. Circ Res 99:501–509

Yang HYT, Tao T, Iadarola MJ (2008) Modulatory role of neuropeptide FF system in nociception and opiate analgesia. Neuropeptides 42:1–18

Yiangou Y, Facer P, Baecker PA, Ford AP, Knowles CH, Chan CL, Williams NS, Anand P (2001a) ATP-gated ion channel $P2X_3$ is increased in human inflammatory bowel disease. Neurogastroenterol Motil 13:365–369

Purines and Sensory Nerves

Geoffrey Burnstock

Contents

G. Burnstock
Autonomic Neuroscience Centre, Royal Free and University College Medical School, Rowland Hill Street, London, NW3 2PF, UK
g.burnstock@ucl.ac.uk

B.J. Canning and D. Spina (eds.), *Sensory Nerves*,
Handbook of Experimental Pharmacology 194, DOI: 10.1007/978-3-540-79090-7_10,

Abstract P2X and P2Y nucleotide receptors are described on sensory neurons and their peripheral and central terminals in dorsal root, nodose, trigeminal, petrosal, retinal and enteric ganglia. Peripheral terminals are activated by ATP released from local cells by mechanical deformation, hypoxia or various local agents in the carotid body, lung, gut, bladder, inner ear, eye, nasal organ, taste buds, skin, muscle and joints mediating reflex responses and nociception. Purinergic receptors on fibres in the dorsal spinal cord and brain stem are involved in reflex control of visceral and cardiovascular activity, as well as relaying nociceptive impulses to pain centres. Purinergic mechanisms are enhanced in inflammatory conditions and may be involved in migraine, pain, diseases of the special senses, bladder and gut, and the possibility that they are also implicated in arthritis, respiratory disorders and some central nervous system disorders is discussed. Finally, the development and evolution of purinergic sensory mechanisms are considered.

Keywords Bladder, Brain stem, Carotid body, Ganglion, Gut

1 Introduction

Review articles have been published concerned with P2X and P2Y receptors in sensory neurons (Burnstock 2000, 2007; Tsuda and Inoue 2006), purinergic sensory-motor neurotransmission (Rubino and Burnstock 1996) and purine-mediated signalling in pain (Burnstock and Wood 1996; Burnstock1996b, 2001a, 2006; McGaraughty and Jarvis 2006; Shieh et al. 2006; Inoue 2007).

The first hint that ATP might be a neurotransmitter arose when it was proposed that ATP released from sensory nerve collaterals during antidromic nerve stimulation of the great auricular nerve caused vasodilatation of the rabbit ear artery (Holton 1959). ATP was shown early to excite mammalian dorsal root ganglia (DRG) neurons and some neurons in the dorsal horn of the spinal cord (Jahr and Jessell 1983; Krishtal et al. 1983). Extracellular ATP was reported early to produce pain sensation in humans (Collier et al. 1966; Bleehen and Keele 1977) and to participate in pain pathways in the spinal cord (Fyffe and Perl 1984; Salter and Henry 1985).

Recent reviews about the current status of and pharmacological characterization of subtypes of receptors for purines and pyrimidines are available, including four subtypes of P1 (adenosine), seven subtypes of P2X ionotropic and eight subtypes of P2Y metabotropic receptors (North 2002; Abbracchio et al. 2006). A landmark discovery related to this chapter was the cloning of $P2X_3$ receptors and their localization on sensory nerves in 1995 (Chen et al. 1995b; Lewis et al. 1995). All P2X subtypes, except $P2X_7$, are found in sensory neurons, although the $P2X_3$ receptor has the highest level of expression [in terms of both messenger RNA (mRNA) and protein] and $P2X_{2/3}$ heteromultimers are particularly prominent in the nodose ganglion. $P2X_3$ and $P2X_{2/3}$ receptors are expressed on isolectin B4 (IB_4) binding subpopulations of small nociceptive neurons (Bradbury et al. 1998). P2Y receptors are also present on sensory neurons sometimes coexpressed with $P2X_3$ receptors (Burnstock 2007). It has been suggested that while $P2X_3$ receptor activation leads to increased firing of DRG neurons and subsequently to increased release of sensory transmitter from their central processes, $P2Y_1$ receptor activation may decrease the release of sensory transmitter onto spinal cord neurons and may thereby partly counterbalance the excitatory effect of ATP.

2 Peripheral Sensory Ganglionic Neurons

There have been many reports characterizing the native P2X receptors in sensory neurons, including those from DRG, trigeminal, nodose, petrosal and enteric ganglia (Burnstock 2000, 2007; Dunn et al. 2001). DRG and trigeminal ganglia contain primary somatosensory neurons, receiving nociceptive, mechanical and proprioceptive inputs. Nodose and petrosal ganglia, on the other hand, contain cell bodies of afferents to visceral organs.

All P2X subtypes, except $P2X_7$, are found in sensory neurons, and most prominent is the $P2X_3$ receptor. $P2Y_1$, $P2Y_2$, $P2Y_4$ and $P2Y_6$ receptors have also been described in sensory neurons (Burnstock and Knight 2004).

It has been shown that the sensory neurons have the machinery to form purinergic synapses on each other when placed in short-term tissue culture (Zarei et al. 2004). The resulting neurotransmitter release is calcium-dependent and uses synaptotagmin-containing vesicles; the postsynaptic receptor involved is a P2X subtype.

2.1 Dorsal Root Ganglia

The $P2X_3$ receptor subunit that was first cloned using a complementary DNA library from neonatal rat DRG neurons shows a selectively high level of expression in a subset of sensory neurons, including those in DRG. In DRG, the level of $P2X_3$ transcript is the highest, although mRNA transcripts of $P2X_{1-6}$ have been detected. In DRG, intensive $P2X_3$ immunoreactivity is found predominantly in a subset of small- and medium-diameter neurons, although it was absent from most large neurons. The $P2X_3$ subunit is predominantly located in the non-peptidergic subpopulation of nociceptors that binds IB_4, and is greatly reduced by neonatal capsaicin treatment. The $P2X_3$ subunit is present in an approximately equal number of neurons projecting to skin and viscera, but in very few of those innervating skeletal muscle (Bradbury et al. 1998). $P2X_2$ receptor immunoreactivity is observed in many small and large DRG neurons, although the level is lower than that of $P2X_3$. Some neurons show both $P2X_2$ and $P2X_3$ immunoreactivity, probably indicating a $P2X_{2/3}$ heteromultimer receptor. Variable levels of immunoreactivity for $P2X_1$, $P2X_2$, $P2X_4$, $P2X_5$ and $P2X_6$ receptors have also been detected in DRG neurons.

Both transient and sustained responses to P2 receptor agonists occur in DRG neurons (Dunn et al. 2001). The transient response in DRG neurons is activated by ATP, α,β-methylene-ATP (α,β-meATP) and 2-methylthio-ATP (2-MeSATP). The pharmacological evidence to date is generally for homomeric $P2X_3$ receptors. P2X receptors on the cell bodies of the sensory neurons have been studied extensively using voltage-clamp recordings from dissociated neurons of the DRG (Fig. 1a–c). Rapid application of ATP evokes action potentials and under voltage clamp, a fast-activating inward current (mediated by $P2X_3$ receptors), a sustained response (mediated by $P2X_2$ receptors) and a rapid response, followed by slow responses (mediated by $P2X_{2/3}$ receptors), as well as depolarization and an increase in intracellular Ca^{2+} concentration. Rapid reduction of the excitatory action of ATP on DRG neurons by GABA, probably via $GABA_A$ anionic receptors, and slow inhibition of ATP currents via metabotropic $GABA_B$ receptors appear to be additional mechanisms of sensory information processing. Oxytocin and 17β-oestradiol attenuate ATP-activated currents in DRG neurons. In contrast, neurokinin B potentiates ATP-activated currents in DRG neurons. Ω-Conotoxin GVIA, known as a selective blocker of N-type calcium channels, potently inhibits the currents mediated by P2X receptors in rat DRG neurons. There are species differences in the responses of DRG neurons to ATP. Transient responses are the predominant type evoked by P2X agonists from DRG neurons of rat and mouse, with persistent and biphasic types seen less frequently. In contrast, only sustained inward currents have been reported on DRG neurons from bullfrog. It has been claimed that release of ATP from neuronal cell bodies in DRG triggers neuron-satellite glial cell communication via $P2X_7$ receptors (Zhang et al. 2007b).

Neurons and glial cells differentially express P2Y receptor subtype mRNA in rat DRG (Kobayashi et al. 2006). $P2Y_1$ and $P2Y_2$ receptor mRNA was expressed in

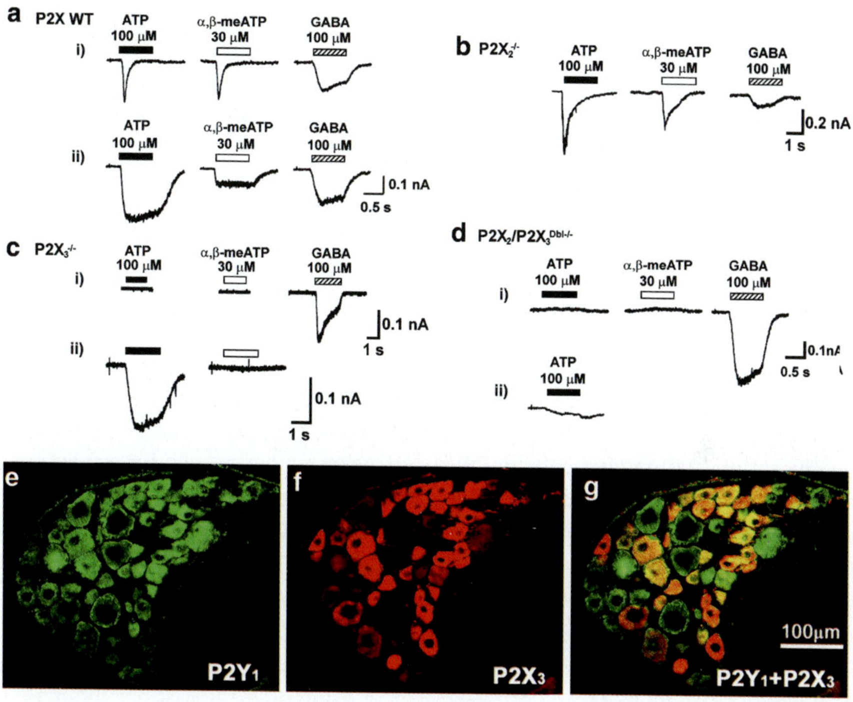

Fig. 1 Dorsal root ganglion (DRG). (**a–d**) Whole-cell patch-clamp recordings of DRG neurons from $P2X_2^{-/-}$, $P2X_3^{-/-}$ and $P2X_2/P2X_3^{Dbl-/-}$ mice in response to P2X agonists. (**a**) Wild-type DRG neurons responded to ATP and α,β-methylene-ATP (α,β-meATP) with either rapidly desensitizing (*i*) or sustained (*ii*) responses; a composite response having both rapidly and slowly desensitizing components was also observed in some neurons (data not shown). All DRG neurons examined responded to 100 μM GABA with a sustained inward current. (**b**) In $P2X_2^{-/-}$ mice, DRG neurons all responded to ATP and α,β-meATP with rapidly desensitizing transient responses. (**c**) In $P2X_3^{-/-}$ mice, many DRG neurons failed to respond to either ATP or α,β-meATP, but did respond to 100 μM GABA (*i*). Other $P2X_3^{-/-}$ neurons responded to ATP with a sustained inward current, but failed to respond to α,β-meATP (*ii*). (**d**) In $P2X_2/P2X_3^{Dbl-/-}$ mice, most DRG neurons failed to respond to ATP or α,β-meATP, but did respond to 100 μM GABA (*i*). A small percentage of neurons in double knockout mice gave small, very low amplitude responses to ATP (*ii*), but did not respond to α,β-meATP. (**e–g**) Colocalization (**g**) (*yellow/orange*) of $P2Y_1$ receptor immunoreactivity (**e**) (*green*) with $P2X_3$ receptor immunoreactivity (**f**) (*red*) in rat DRG. Examples of double-labelled neurons, $P2X_3$ receptor positive cells that are not double labelled and $P2Y_1$ receptor positive cells that are not $P2X_3$ receptor immunoreactive are shown in **g**. (**a–d** Reproduced from Cockayne et al. 2005, with permission from Blackwell Publishing; **e–g** reproduced from Ruan and Burnstock 2003, with kind permission from Springer Science and Business Media)

about 20% of neurons; Schwann cells expressed $P2Y_2$ mRNA and non-neuronal satellite cells expressed $P2Y_{12}$ and $P2Y_{14}$ mRNA. ATP and UTP produce slow and sustained excitation of sensory neurons in DRG via $P2Y_2$ receptors. $P2Y_1$, $P2Y_2$, $P2Y_4$ and $P2Y_6$ mRNA is expressed on neurons of rat DRG and receptor protein for $P2Y_1$ is localized on over 80% of mostly small neurons (Ruan and Burnstock 2003). Double immunolabelling showed that 73–84% of $P2X_3$ receptor positive neurons also stained for the $P2Y_1$ receptor (Fig. 1e–g), while 25–35% also stained for the $P2Y_4$ receptor. The findings of patch-clamp studies of cultured neurons from DRG were consistent with both $P2X_3$ and $P2Y_1$ receptors being present in a subpopulation of DRG neurons. Inhibition of N-type voltage-activated calcium channels in DRG neurons by P2Y receptors has been proposed as a mechanism of ADP-induced analgesia. $P2Y_2$ and $P2Y_4$ receptors were strongly expressed in DRG of the cat, as were $P2X_3$ receptors (Ruan et al. 2005). However, there was low expression of $P2Y_1$ receptors compared with more than 80% of $P2Y_1$ receptor positive neurons in rat DRG. Green fluorescent protein studies have shown that there is ADP-induced endocytosis and internalization of P2Y receptors in DRG neurons (Wang et al. 2006).

Adenosine 5′-*O*-(3-thiotriphosphate) enhances nerve growth factor (NGF)-promoted neurite formation in DRG neurons, perhaps via its ability to increase NGF-promoted TrkA activation (Arthur et al. 2005). NTPDase2 has been shown to be present in satellite glial cells in DRG, consistent with evidence for a functional role for ATP in satellite glial cells. Functional expression of $P2X_7$ receptors on non-neuronal glial cells, but not on small-diameter neurons from rat DRG, has been reported.

2.2 *Nodose Ganglia*

$P2X_2$ and $P2X_3$ receptors are expressed in rat nodose ganglia. ATP, α,β-meATP and 2-MeSATP evoke sustained currents in rat nodose neurons. These responses are inhibited by suramin, pyridoxal phosphate-6-azopheyl-2′,4′-disulphonic acid (PPADS), Cibacron blue and trinitrophenyl ATP (TNP-ATP), but not by diinosine pentaphosphate. Therefore, the α,β-meATP-sensitive persistent responses in nodose neurons resemble the recombinant $P2X_{2/3}$ receptors. Neurons of the mouse nodose ganglion give persistent responses to both ATP and α,β-meATP similar to those seen in the rat and guinea pig. In $P2X_3$ receptor-deficient mice, no nodose neurons respond to α,β-meATP at concentrations up to 100 μM, while the response to ATP is significantly reduced. The residual persistent responses to ATP have all the characteristics of recombinant $P2X_2$ homomers. Thus, the pharmacological evidence is consistent with the notion that both heteromeric $P2X_{2/3}$ and homomeric $P2X_2$ receptors are present in significant amounts in nodose neurons, although the proportions may vary from cell to cell (Cockayne et al. 2005). Subpopulations of rat nodose neurons expressed $P2X_{1/3}$ and $P2X_{2/3}$ heteromultimers. Sensory neurons from nodose ganglia express, in addition to $P2X_3$ receptor mRNA, significant levels of $P2X_1$, $P2X_2$ and $P2X_4$ receptor mRNAs, and some of these mRNAs are present in the same cell.

$P2Y_1$ receptors have been demonstrated immunohistochemically in rat and human nodose ganglia. Coexistence of functional P2Y receptors (acting via the inositol 1,4,5-trisphosphate pathway) and ryanodine receptors and their activation by ATP have been demonstrated in vagal sensory neurons from the rabbit nodose ganglion. Reverse transcription PCR (RT-PCR) has shown $P2Y_1$, $P2Y_2$, $P2Y_4$ and $P2Y_6$ receptor mRNA in rat nodose ganglia (Ruan and Burnstock 2003). $P2Y_1$ receptor immunoreactivity was found in over 80% of the sensory neurons, particularly small-diameter (neurofilament-negative) neurons, while $P2Y_4$ receptors were expressed in more medium- and large-diameter neurons. About 80% of the $P2X_3$ receptor immunoreactive neurons also stained for $P2Y_1$ receptors, while about 30% of the neurons showed colocalization of $P2Y_4$ with $P2X_3$ receptors.

2.3 *Trigeminal Ganglia*

Most of the facial sensory innervation is provided by nerve fibres originating in the trigeminal ganglion, comprising neurons that transduce mechanical, thermal and chemical stimuli, probably including odorant molecules. In trigeminal ganglia, $P2X_3$ receptor immunoreactivity is found in the cell bodies of both small and large neurons. Lower levels of immunoreactivity to $P2X_1$, $P2X_2$, $P2X_4$ and $P2X_6$ receptors appear to be present in these neurons. Forty percent of $P2X_2$ and 64% of $P2X_3$ receptor expressing cells were IB_4-positive and 33% of $P2X_2$ and 31% of $P2X_3$ receptor expressing cells were NF200-positive (Staikopoulos et al. 2007). About 40% of cells expressing $P2X_2$ receptors also expressed $P2X_3$ receptors and vice versa. Chronically applied NGF upregulated the function of $P2X_3$ receptors in trigeminal neurons without changing transient receptor potential vanilloid 1 (TRPV1) activity. IB_4-positive neurons release ATP by faster exocytosis compared with IB_4-negative neurons which release neuropeptides by slower exocytosis (Matsuka et al. 2007). Whole-cell patch-clamp studies of trigeminal neurons showed ATP-activated (both fast and slow) desensitizing currents in the majority of cells examined, but outward or biphasic currents also occurred in a small number of cells (Gu et al. 2006). Different types of cells show different types of ATP-activated currents related to different P2X subunit assemblies (Luo et al. 2006).

$P2Y_1$ and $P2Y_4$ receptor mRNA and protein are also expressed in rat trigeminal ganglia, with many neurons showing colocalization with $P2X_3$ receptors (Ruan and Burnstock 2003). In particular, only a small percentage of IB_4-binding neurons express $P2X_3$ receptors in trigeminal ganglia, whereas many peptidergic neurons express $P2X_3$ receptors.

Satellite glial cells in mouse trigeminal ganglia express P2Y receptors (possibly the $P2Y_1$ subtype). Single-cell calcium imaging demonstrated that both $P2Y_1$ and, to a lesser extent, $P2Y_{2,4,6,12,13}$ receptors on satellite glial cells contribute to ATP-induced calcium-dependent signalling in mixed neuron-glia primary cultures from mouse trigeminal ganglia (Ceruti et al. 2006).

2.4 *Petrosal Ganglia*

The petrosal ganglion provides sensory innervation of the carotid sinus and carotid body through the carotid sinus nerve. Acetylcholine (ACh) and ATP act as excitatory transmitters between cat glomus cells and petrosal ganglion neurons (Alcayaga et al. 2007), but independently of each other. ATP activates rat, cat and rabbit petrosal ganglia neurons in vitro via P2X receptors and evokes ventilatory reflexes in situ, which are abolished after bilateral chemosensory denervation. Dopamine inhibits ATP-induced responses of neurons of the cat petrosal ganglia.

2.5 *Retinal Ganglia*

Retinal ganglion cells on the eye receive information from both rods and cones and early papers about purinergic transmission in the retina have been reviewed (Pintor 2000). $P2X_2$ receptors have been identified in retinal ganglion cells, particularly within cone pathways (Puthussery and Fletcher 2006), while $P2X_3$ receptors are associated with both rod and cone bipolar cell axon terminals in the inner plexiform layer (Puthussery and Fletcher 2007). Functional studies have also identified $P2X_{2/3}$ heteromultimeric receptors in cultured rat retinal ganglion cells. $P2X_2$ receptors are also expressed on cholinergic amacrine cells of mouse retina and also GABAergic amacrine cells.

It was proposed that ATP, coreleased with ACh from retinal neurons, modulates light-evoked release of ACh by stimulating a glycinergic inhibitory feedback loop (Neal and Cunningham 1994). RT-PCR at the single-cell level revealed expression of $P2X_2$, $P2X_3$, $P2X_4$ and $P2X_5$ receptor mRNA in approximately one third of the bipolar cells (Wheeler-Schilling et al. 2001), $P2X_7$ receptors were identified on both inner and outer retinal ganglion cell layers of the primate and rat, and electron microscope analysis suggested that these receptors were localized in synapses. Stimulation of $P2X_7$ receptors elevated Ca^{2+} levels and killed retinal ganglion cells (Zhang et al. 2005) and may be involved in retinal cholinergic neuron density regulation.

$P2X_3$ receptors are present on Müller cells. Müller cells release ATP during Ca^{2+} wave propagation. While the potent $P2X_7$ agonist 3′-O-(4-benzoyl)benzoyl ATP killed retinal ganglion cells, this was prevented by the breakdown product, adenosine, via A_3 receptors (Zhang et al. 2006). Evidence has been presented for the involvement of $P2X_7$ receptors in outer retinal processing: $P2X_7$ receptors are expressed postsynaptically on horizontal cell processes as well as presynaptically on photoreceptor synaptic terminals in both rat and marmoset retinas (Puthussery et al. 2006).

2.6 *Intramural Enteric Sensory Neurons*

Most of the data about enteric sensory transmission are based on studies of the guinea pig ileum (Furness et al. 1998). The after hyperpolarization (AH) defined neurons appear to be the enteric sensory neurons, which represent about 30% of the neurons in the myenteric plexus. About 90% of Dogiel type II neurons in the guinea pig ileum exhibit slow AHs and many express the calcium-binding protein calbindin. These neurons are distinct from Dogiel type I, S neurons, which are motor neurons or interneurons. The functional properties of Dogiel type II (AH) sensory neurons have been reviewed recently (Blackshaw et al. 2007).

Several laboratories have studied purinergic signalling in the guinea pig myenteric and submucous neurons (Burnstock 2007). Exogenous and endogenous ATP, released during increase in intraluminal pressure, inhibits intestinal peristalsis in guinea pig. Exogenous ATP depresses peristalsis mostly via suramin- and PPADS-insensitive $P2X_4$ receptors, whereas endogenous purines probably act via $P2X_2$ and/or $P2X_3$ and/or $P2X_{2/3}$ receptors sensitive to both suramin and PPADS initiate peristalsis (Bian et al. 2003). ATP plays a major role in excitatory neuroneuronal transmission in both ascending and descending reflex pathways to the longitudinal and circular muscles of the guinea pig ileum triggered by mucosal stimulation. Experiments with $P2X_2$ and $P2X_3$ receptor knockout mice showed that peristalsis is impaired in the small intestine. $P2X_3$ receptors are dominant on neurons in the submucosal plexus of the rat ileum and distal colon and up to 70% of the neurons express calbindin, a marker for enteric sensory neurons (Xiang and Burnstock 2004a). $P2X_3$ receptor immunoreactivity has also been shown on sensory neurons in the *human* myenteric plexus.

Intracellular recordings from myenteric and submucosal neurons in guinea pig small intestine showed that ATP induced a transient depolarization of most AH-type neurons (Bertrand and Bornstein 2002; Monro et al. 2004) (Fig. 2a, c, d). Fast and slow depolarizations and Ca^{2+} responses of cultured guinea pig ileal submucosal neurons to ATP were mediated by P2X and P2Y receptors respectively. Slow excitatory postsynaptic potentials were mediated by $P2Y_1$ receptors in neurons in the submucosal plexus of guinea pig small intestine. ATP plays a major excitatory role, probably largely via $P2X_2$ receptors, in rat myenteric neurons, whether sensory neurons, motor neurons or interneurons. A $P2Y_1$ receptor has been cloned and characterized from guinea pig submucosa (Gao et al. 2006). About 40–60% of $P2X_3$ receptor immunoreactive neurons were immunoreactive for $P2Y_2$ receptors in the myenteric plexus and all $P2X_3$ receptor immunoreactive neurons expressed $P2Y_2$ receptors in the submucosal plexus (Xiang and Burnstock 2006). About 28–35% of $P2Y_6$ receptor immunoreactive neurons coexist with nitric oxide synthase (NOS), but not with calbindin, while all $P2Y_{12}$ receptor immunoreactive neurons were immunopositive for calbindin and appear to be AH intrinsic primary afferent neurons.

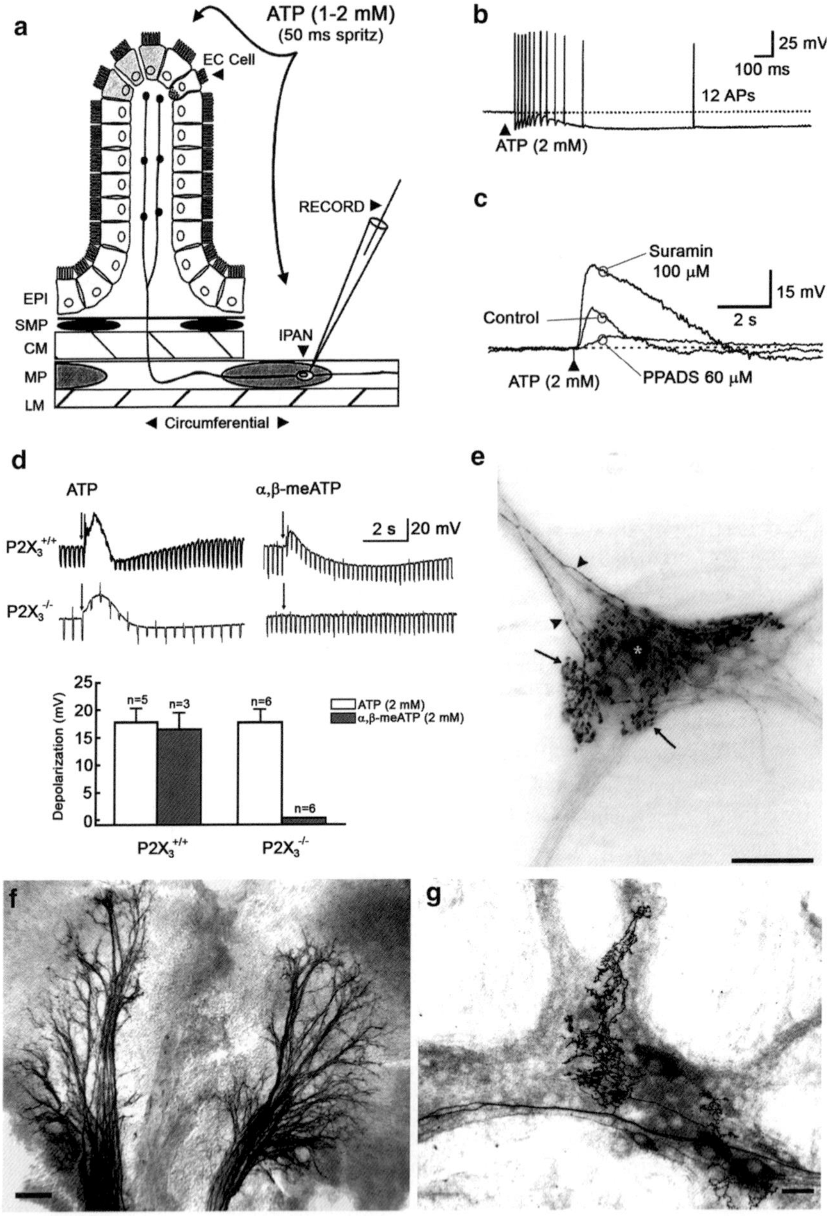

Fig. 2 Enteric sensory neurons. (**a**) Illustration of the experimental arrangement and the relation of the epithelium and the after hyperpolarization (Dogiel type II) sensory nerve terminals. *LM* longitudinal muscle, *MP* myenteric plexus, *CM* circular muscle, *SMP* submucosal plexus, *EPI* epithelium. Note that the intracellular recording electrode (*RECORD*) is impaling myenteric AH neurons [intrinsic primary afferent neurons (*IPAN*) at the *open circle*]. ATP and other agonists were applied to the mucosa and to the cell body of AH neurons via short-duration pressure ejection. Enterochromaffin cells (*EC Cell*) are present in about 1% of the total population

3 Peripheral Sensory Nerve Terminals

Sensory nerve terminals express purinoceptors and respond to ATP in many situations (Burnstock 2000, 2007). However, it has been shown that ATP sensitivity is not necessarily restricted to the terminals; increased axonal excitability to ATP and/or adenosine of unmyelinated fibres in rat vagus, sural and dorsal root nerves as well as human sural nerve has been described. During purinergic mechanosensory transduction, the ATP released from local epithelial cells acts on $P2X_3$, $P2X_{2/3}$ and $P2Y_1$ receptors on sensory nerve endings (see Sect. 5). In addition, released ATP is rapidly broken down by ectoenzymes to ADP (to act on $P2Y_1$, $P2Y_{12}$ and $P2Y_{13}$ receptors) or adenosine (to act on P1 receptors).

Since the seminal studies of Lewis in the 1920s, it has been well established that transmitters released following the passage of antidromic impulses down sensory nerve collaterals during "axon reflex" activity produce vasodilatation of skin vessels. The early work of Holton (1959) showing ATP release during antidromic stimulation of sensory collaterals, taken together with the evidence for glutamate in primary afferent sensory neurons, suggests that ATP and glutamate may be cotransmitters in these nerves. We know now that "axon reflex" activity is widespread in autonomic effector systems and forms an important physiological component of autonomic control (Maggi and Meli 1988; Rubino and Burnstock 1996). Calcitonin gene related peptide (CGRP) and substance P (SP) are well established as coexisting in sensory-motor nerves and, in some subpopulations, ATP is also likely to be a

---

Fig. 2 (continued) of epithelial cells. (**b**) Representative voltage trace from AH neurons during application of ATP to the mucosa; *dotted lines* in **b** and **c** indicate resting membrane potential. A brief application (100 ms; at the *filled triangle*) of ATP (2 mM) elicited a train of 12 action potentials that showed a slowing in frequency during the 1.1-s duration of the discharge. (**c**) Representative voltage recording from an intrinsic sensory neuron in the myenteric plexus. ATP was applied to the cell body and evoked a short latency depolarization – tetrodotoxin was present to block sodium-dependent action potentials. During superfusion with pyridoxal phosphate-6-azopheyl-2′,4′-disulphonic acid (60 μM), the ATP-evoked depolarization was blocked, whereas in the presence of suramin (100 μM), it was potentiated. (**d**) Effect of ATP and α,β-meATP in AH neurons from $P2X_3^{+/+}$ and $P2X_3^{-/-}$ mice. *Top panels*: Representative responses caused by ATP and α,β-meATP. ATP depolarized AH neurons from both types of mice. α,β-meATP caused depolarization of AH neurons in tissues from $P2X_3^{+/+}$ but not $P2X_3^{-/-}$ mice. *Bottom panel*: Pooled data from experiments illustrated in the *top panels*. (**e**) Morphology of intraganglionic laminar endings (IGLEs) revealed by $P2X_2$ receptor immunoreactivity in a group of three to four IGLEs at the surface of a myenteric ganglion in the duodenum. The axons that lead to the IGLEs also have $P2X_2$ receptor immunoreactivity (*arrowheads*). The IGLEs consist of clumps of axon dilatations, varying from small swellings (*arrows*) to large lamellae, one of which is indicated by an *asterisk*. *Scale bar* 50 μm. (**f**) $P2X_3$ receptor immunoreactivity in extrinsic vagal nerve fibres in the developing rat stomach with short branches at the ends at embryonic day 12. *Scale bar* 250 μm. (**g**) $P2X_3$ receptor immunoreactive neurons and IGLEs in myenteric plexus of rat stomach at postnatal day 60. *Scale bar* 30 μm. (**a**, **b** Reproduced from Bertrand and Bornstein 2002, with permission from the Society of Neuroscience; **c** reproduced from Bertrand 2003, with permission from Sage Publications; **d** reproduced from Bian et al. 2003, with permission from Blackwell Publishing; **e** reproduced from Castelucci et al. 2003, with kind permission from Springer Science and Business Media; **f**, **g** reproduced from Xiang and Burnstock 2004b, with kind permission from Springer Science and Business Media) cotransmitter (Burnstock 1993). Concurrent release of ATP and SP from guinea pig trigeminal ganglionic neurons in vivo has been described (Matsuka et al. 2001).

3.1 Carotid Body

The ventilatory response to decreased oxygen tension in the arterial blood is initiated by excitation of specialized oxygen-sensitive chemoreceptor cells in the carotid body that release neurotransmitter to activate endings of the sinus nerve afferent fibres. ATP and adenosine were shown early on to excite nerve endings in the carotid bifurcation (Lahiri et al. 2007).

Large amounts of adenine nucleotides are localized in glomus cells, stored within specific granules together with catecholamines and proteins, and there is evidence of ATP release from carotid chemoreceptor cells. Corelease of ATP and ACh from type I glomus chemoreceptor cells is a likely mechanism for chemosensory signalling in the carotid body in vivo (Nurse 2005; Zapata 2007). The ATP released during hypoxic and mechanical stimulation was shown to act on $P2X_{2/3}$ receptors on nerve fibres arising from the petrosal ganglion (Reyes et al. 2007). Immunoreactivity for $P2X_2$ and $P2X_3$ receptor subunits has been localized on rat carotid body afferent terminals surrounding clusters of glomus cells. $P2X_2$ and $P2X_{2/3}$ receptor deficiency resulted in a dramatic reduction in the responses of the carotid sinus nerve to hypoxia in an in vitro mouse carotid body-sinus nerve preparation (Rong et al. 2003) (Fig. 3). ATP mimicked the afferent discharge and PPADS blocked the hypoxia-induced discharge. ATP induces a rise in intracellular Ca^{2+} concentration in rat carotid body cultured glomus cells. Evidence that this mechanism is involved in hypercapnia as well as in hypoxia came from CO_2/pH chemosensory signalling in co-cultures of rat carotid body and petrosal neurons (Zhang and Nurse 2004). In fresh tissue slices of rat carotid body, low glucose stimulated ATP secretion (Zhang et al. 2007a). ATP, acting on $P2X_2$ receptors, contributed to modified chemoreceptor activity after *chronic* hypoxia, indicating a role for purinergic mechanisms in the adaptation of the carotid body in a chronic low-O_2 environment (He et al. 2006).

3.2 Lung

Pulmonary neuroepithelial bodies (NEBs) and more recently subepithelial receptor-like endings associated with smooth muscle (SMARs) have been shown to serve as sensory organs in the lung (Brouns et al. 2006). $P2X_3$ and $P2X_{2/3}$ receptors are expressed on a subpopulation of vagal sensory fibres that supply NEBs and SMARs which have their origin in the nodose ganglia (Fig. 4a). Sensory afferent fibres within the respiratory tract, which are sensitive to ATP, probably largely via $P2X_{2/3}$ receptors, have been implicated in vagal reflex activity (Taylor-Clark and

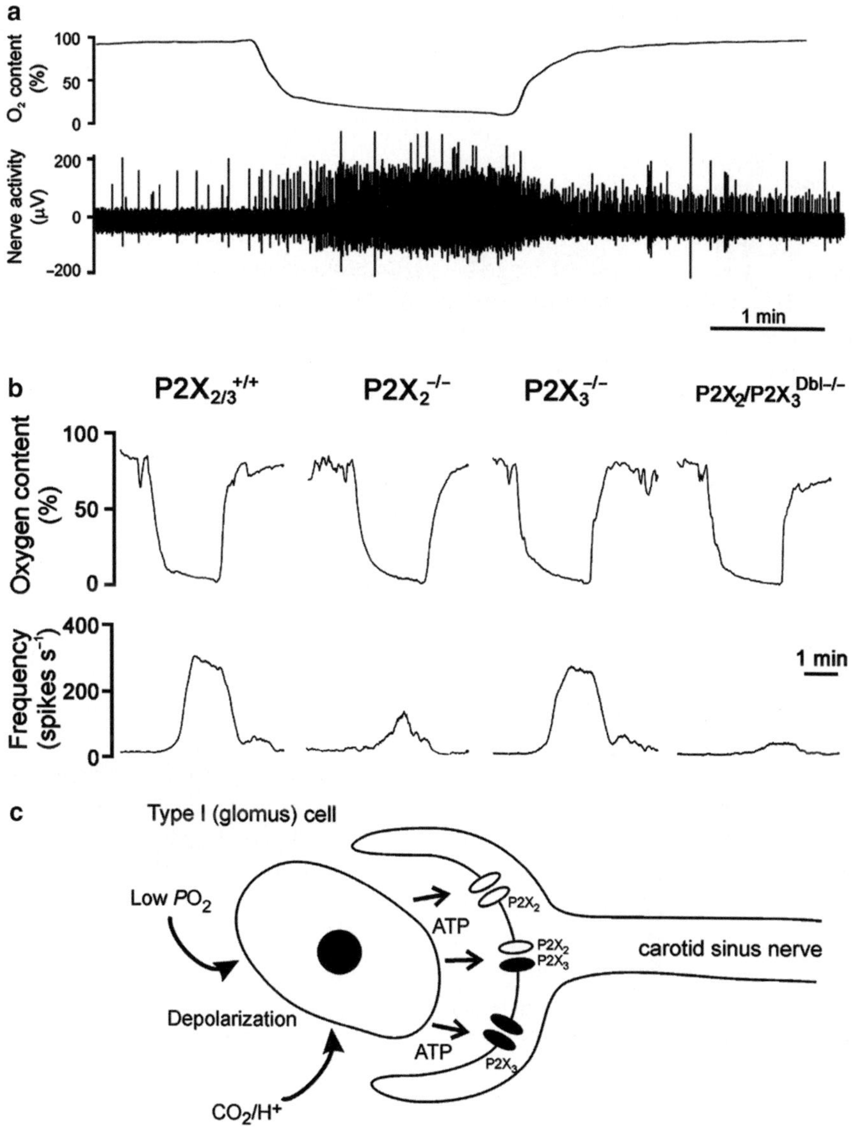

Fig. 3 Carotid body. (**a**) Representative recording of the afferent nerve responses to hypoxia in the isolated carotid body sinus nerve preparation taken from a wild-type mouse. Typical traces of changes in PO_2 and raw nerve activity. (**b**) Effects of ATP on carotid sinus nerve activity in wild-type mice and in $P2X_2$ ($P2X_2^{-/-}$)-, $P2X_3$ ($P2X_3^{-/-}$)- and $P2X_2$ and $P2X_3$ ($P2X_2/P2X_3^{Db-\,-/-}$)-deficient mice. (**c**) Hypothetical model of ATP involvement in the carotid body. P2X receptors containing the $P2X_2$ subunit play a pivotal role in transmitting information about arterial PO_2 and PCO_2 levels. A decrease in PO_2 or an increase in PCO_2/H^+ activates glomus cells, which release ATP as the main transmitter to stimulate afferent terminals of the sinus nerve via interaction with P2X receptors that contain the $P2X_2$ subunit, with or without the $P2X_3$ subunit. (**a** Reproduced and modified from Rong et al. 2003, with permission from the Society of Neuroscience; **b** courtesy of Weifang Rong; **c** reproduced from Spyer et al. 2004, with permission from Blackwell Publishing)

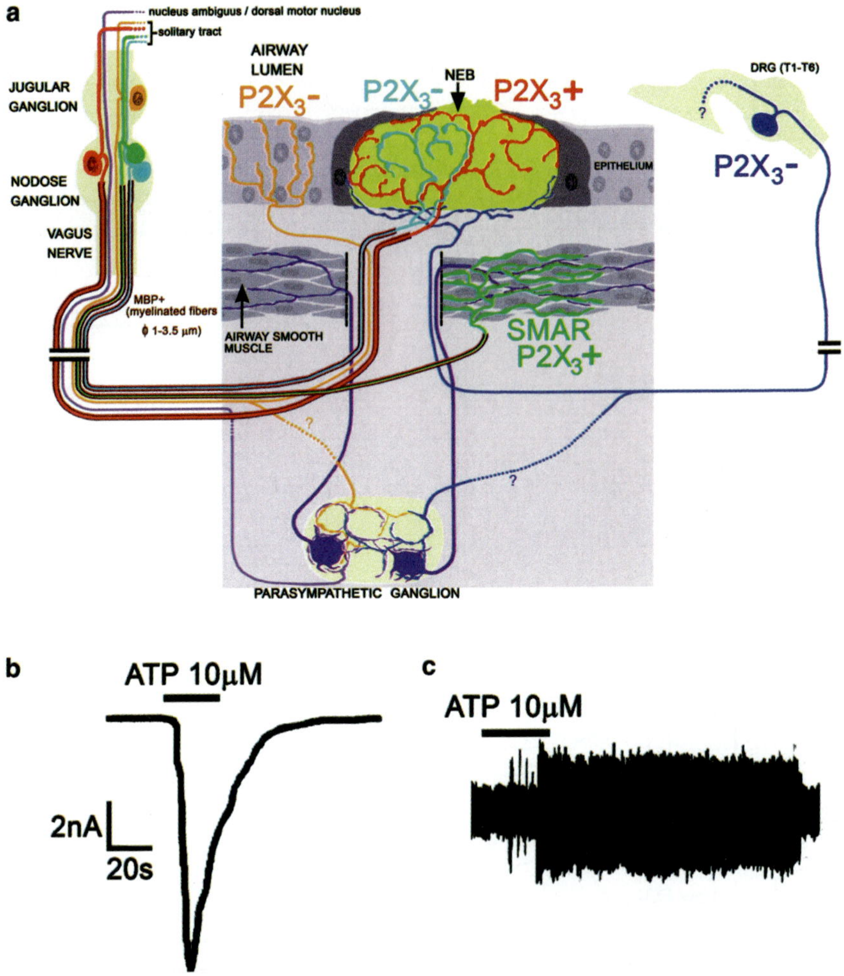

Fig. 4 Lung. (**a**) The main innervation of airway smooth muscle and of the sensory innervation of complex neuroendothelial body (NEB) receptors in rat airways. Nerve fibre populations are colour-coded. The *central* part of the scheme shows airway smooth muscle that receives laminar nerve terminals (SMAR; *green*) immunopositive for $P2X_3$ receptors that intercalate between the smooth muscle cells and nerve terminals from postganglionic parasympathetic neurons located in an airway ganglion (*bottom*; cholinergic neurons *purple*). The *top centre* part of the scheme represents a pulmonary NEB (*yellow*) and its extensive interactions with sensory nerve terminals. The *top left* part shows the myelinated vagal nodose afferent fibres immunopositive for $P2X_3$ receptors (*red*) and sensory fibres (*light blue*) that innervate the NEB but do not express $P2X_3$ receptors; C-fibre afferents that originate from the vagal jugular ganglion (*orange*) innervate the non-endocrine epithelium of large-diameter airways. The *top right* part represents dorsal root C-fibre afferents (*dark blue*) that innervate NEB but do not express $P2X_3$ receptors. ϕ diameter. (**b**) Representative inward ionic currents obtained with whole-cell patch recordings of nodose neurons retrogradely labelled from the lung. All neurons responded to ATP with a rapid inward current. (**c**) Representative extracellular recording of action potential discharge from

Undem 2006) (Fig. 4b, c), as well as in the cough and bradypneic reflexes (see Sect. 6.7). Quinacrine staining of NEBs indicates the presence of high concentrations of ATP in their secretory vesicles and it has been suggested that ATP is released in response to both mechanical stimulation during high-pressure ventilation and during hypoxia (Rich et al. 2003). NEBs are oxygen sensors especially in early development, before the carotid system has matured (Brouns et al. 2003).

Vagal C-fibres innervating the pulmonary system are derived from cell bodies situated in two distinct vagal sensory ganglia: the jugular (superior) ganglion neurons project fibres to the extrapulmonary airways (larynx, trachea, bronchus) and the lung parenchymal tissue, while the nodose (inferior) neurons innervate primarily structures within the lungs. Nerve terminals in the lungs from both jugular and nodose ganglia responded to capsaicin and bradykinin, but only the nodose C-fibres responded to α,β-meATP. In a study of bronchopulmonary afferent nerve activity of a mouse isolated perfused nerve-lung preparation it was found that C-fibres could be subdivided into two groups: fibres that conduct action potentials at less than 0.7 ms^{-1} and are responsive to capsaicin, bradykinin and ATP; and fibres that conduct action potentials on an average of 0.9 ms^{-1} and respond vigorously to ATP, but not to capsaicin or bradykinin (Kollarik et al. 2003). Both the TRPV1 receptor and P2X receptors mediate the sensory transduction of pulmonary reactive oxygen species, especially H_2O_2 and OH, by capsaicin-sensitive vagal lung afferent fibres.

The visceral pleura of the airways is often considered to be insensitive to painful stimuli and to lack sensory innervation. However, a recent paper has identified $P2X_3$ receptors on sensory fibres supplying the pleura, which appear to be myelinated and have a spinal origin (Pintelon et al. 2007).

3.3 Gut

ATP and α,β-meATP activate submucosal terminals of intrinsic sensory neurons in the guinea pig intestine (Bertrand and Bornstein 2002), supporting the hypothesis of Burnstock (2001a) that ATP released from mucosal epithelial cells has a dual action on $P2X_3$ and/or $P2X_{2/3}$ receptors in the subepithelial sensory nerve fibres. ATP acts on the terminals of low-threshold intrinsic enteric sensory neurons to initiate or modulate intestinal reflexes and acts on the terminals of high-threshold extrinsic sensory fibres to initiate pain (see Sects. 5.3, 6.1). Thirty-two percent of retrogradely labelled cells in the mouse DRG at levels T8–L1 and L6–S1, supplying sensory nerve fibres to the mouse distal colon, were immunoreactive for $P2X_3$ receptors (Robinson

Fig. 4 (continued) a nodose C-fibre ending with a receptive field within the right lung caused by tracheal infusion of ATP (10 μM). (**a** Modified from Adriaensen et al. 2006, and reproduced with permission from The American Physiological Society; **b** Reproduced from Undem et al. 2004, with permission from Blackwell Publishing; **c** reproduced from Taylor-Clark and Undem 2006, with permission from The American Physiological Society) et al. 2004). Extrinsic and possibly intrinsic sensory nerves associated with mucosal epithelial cells appear to be sensitive to pH, probably via $P2X_2$ and $P2X_{2/3}$ receptors (Holzer 2007).

Intraganglionic laminar nerve endings (IGLEs) are specialized mechanosensory endings of vagal afferent nerves in the rat stomach, arising from the nodose ganglion; they express $P2X_2$ and $P2X_3$ receptors and are probably involved in physiological reflex activity, especially in early postnatal development (Castelucci et al. 2003; Xiang and Burnstock 2004b) (Fig. 2e–g). α,β-meATP caused concentration-dependent excitation of IGLEs of vagal tension receptors in the guinea pig oesophagus, but evidence was presented against chemical transmission being involved in the mechanotransduction mechanism (Zagorodnyuk et al. 2003). A subpopulation of nodose vagal afferent nociceptive nerves sensitive to $P2X_3$ receptor agonists was later identified and shown to be different from the non-nociceptive vagal nerve mechanoreceptors (Yu et al. 2005).

3.4 *Urinary Bladder*

In the absence of $P2X_3$ receptors in mouse knockouts, the bladder is hyperactive (Cockayne et al. 2000; Vlaskovska et al. 2001). It has been claimed that suburothelial myofibroblast cells isolated from human and guinea pig bladder that are distinct from epithelial cells provide an intermediate regulatory step between urothelial ATP release and afferent excitation involved in the sensation of bladder fullness (Wu et al. 2004). The majority of lumbosacral neurons (93%) supplying the bladder were sensitive to α,β-meATP, compared with 50% of thoracolumbar neurons (Dang et al. 2004). Almost all sensory neurons in lumbosacral DRG innervating the bladder coexpress P2X, ASIC, and TRPV1 receptors, but not those in the thoracolumbar DRG neurons supplying the bladder, indicating that pelvic and hypogastric afferent pathways to the bladder are structurally and functionally distinct.

3.5 *Inner Ear*

The inner ear encompasses three organs: the cochlea, responsible for hearing; the vestibule, sensitive to gravity and acceleration; and the endolymphatic sac, devoid of sensory function. A role for ATP as a cotransmitter generating intracellular Ca^{2+} currents in cochlea inner hair cells was first proposed in 1990 (Housley et al. 2006). Later, various P2X and P2Y receptor subtypes were shown to be expressed in other cell types in the cochlea, including outer hair cells, Henson cells and Deiters cells in the organ of Corti. Physiological studies suggested that ATP acts as a neurotransmitter, but probably not as part of the efferent system as previously supposed, but rather as a cotransmitter with glutamate in auditory afferent nerves activated by glutamate released from hair cells and acting postsynaptically on the spiral ganglion neuron afferent dendrites (Housley et al. 2006). There are about 50,000 primary afferent neurons in the human cochlear and about half express $P2X_2$ (or $P2X_2$ variants) and probably $P2X_3$ receptors. ATP is released from K^+-depolarized organ of Corti in a Ca^{2+}-dependent manner and an increase in ATP levels in the endolymph has been demonstrated during sound exposure. The P2 receptor antagonist PPADS attenuated the effects of a moderately intense sound on cochlea mechanics. Nitric oxide enhances the ATP-induced intracellular Ca^{2+} increase in outer hair cells (Shen et al. 2006). $P2Y_2$ and/or $P2Y_4$ receptors mediate intercellular calcium wave propagation in supporting and epithelial cells in the organ of Corti (Piazza et al. 2007). Spiral ganglion neurons, located in the cochlear, convey to the brain stem the acoustic information arising from the mechanoelectrical transduction of the inner hair cells, express P2X receptors and are responsive to ATP (Dulon et al. 2006). P2X receptor signalling inhibits brain derived neurotrophic factor (BDNF)-mediated spiral ganglion neuron development in the neonatal rat cochlea, when synaptic reorganization is occurring in the cochlea (Greenwood et al. 2007).

3.6 *Eye*

Amacrine cells and the pigment epithelial cells themselves have been shown to release ATP as well as retinal astrocytes and inner retinal amacrine-like neurons (Burnstock 2007). ATP is also released from antidromically stimulated sensory nerve endings in the ciliary body (Maul and Sears 1979).

3.7 *Nasal Organ*

There are three types of epithelial cells in the nasal mucosa: non-keratinized, stratified squamous epithelium, respiratory epithelium and olfactory epithelium. Primary olfactory neurons lie in the olfactory epithelium and function to detect odiferous substances, sending information to the olfactory cortex. $P2X_2$ receptors are localized on different subpopulations of primary olfactory neurons located both in the olfactory epithelium and in vomeronasal organs, and on sensory fibres arising from the trigeminal ganglion (Gayle and Burnstock 2005).

Odorant recognition is mediated by olfactory receptors predominantly situated on the microvilli of olfactory receptor neurons in the nasal organ. Nucleotides act via purinoceptors on olfactory neurons as well as sustentacular supporting cells (Hegg et al. 2003). ATP released from olfactory epithelium modulates odour sensitivity and nociception. The majority of nasal trigeminal neurons lacked $P2X_3$ receptor-mediated currents, but showed $P2X_2$-mediated responses when stimulated by ATP (Damann et al. 2006).

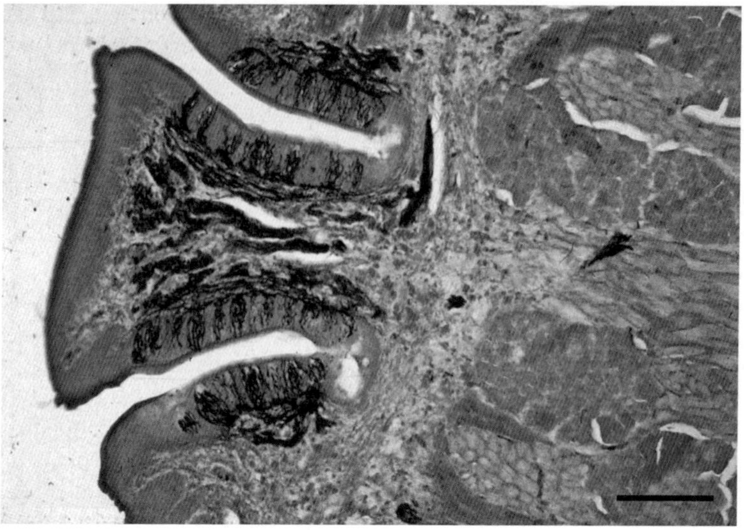

Fig. 5 Tongue. Distribution of $P2X_3$ receptor immunoreactivity in circumvallate papillae in rat tongue. *Scale bar* 200 μm. (Courtesy of Atossa Alavi)

3.8 Taste Buds

Taste bud cells and associated sensory nerve fibres express P2 receptors, including $P2X_2$ and $P2X_3$ receptor subunits (Bo et al. 1999) (Fig. 5) and $P2Y_1$ receptors (Kataoka et al. 2004). ATP is the key transmitter acting via $P2X_2$ and $P2X_3$ receptors on taste receptor cells detecting chemicals in the oral cavity (Finger et al. 2005). These authors showed that genetic elimination of $P2X_2$ and $P2X_3$ receptors abolished responses of the taste nerves, although the nerves remained responsive to touching, temperature and menthol and reduced responses to sweeteners, glutamate and bitter substances. They also showed that a bitter mixture containing denatonium and quinine stimulated release of ATP from the taste epithelium. Type A (but not type B and C) taste cells, defined electrophysiologically, which appear to be identical to type II cells, defined morphologically, have been shown to release ATP via connexin or pannexin hemichannels to activate $P2X_3$ receptors on sensory nerve endings (Huang et al. 2007; Romanov et al. 2007). Dystonin disruption, produced in mutant mice, resulted in a decrease in the number of vagal and glossopharyngeal sensory neurons, and in the number of taste buds as well as in the number of $P2X_3$ receptor labelled neurons and their peripheral endings in taste bud epithelium (Ichikawa et al. 2006). Other papers present data that suggest that $P2Y_2$ and $P2Y_4$ receptors also play a role in mediating taste cell responses to ATP and UTP (Bystrova et al. 2006). NTPDase2 has been shown to have a dominant presence on type 1 cells in mouse taste papillae (Bartel et al. 2006).

3.9 Skin, Muscle and Joints

It has been suggested that ATP receptors on keratinocytes might play a role in a variety of skin sensations (Denda et al. 2007). Ca^{2+} waves in human epidermal keratinocytes mediated by extracellular ATP, produce intracellular Ca^{2+} concentration elevation in DRG neurons, suggesting a dynamic cross talk between skin and sensory neurons mediated by extracellular ATP (Koizumi et al. 2004). ATP inhibits the heat response of the C-fibre polymodal receptor on a rat skin-nerve preparation at low concentrations, but facilitates it at high concentrations (Yajima et al. 2005).

P2 receptors on the endings of thin fibre muscle afferents play a role in evoking both the metabolic and the mechanoreceptor components of the exercise pressor reflex. PPADS attenuated the pressor response to contraction of the triceps muscle. ATP has been shown to be an effective stimulant of group IV receptors in mechanically sensitive muscle afferents (Kindig et al. 2007). Arterial injection of α,β-meATP in the blood supply of the triceps surae muscle evoked a pressor response that was a reflex localized to the cat hind limb and was reduced by P2X receptor blockade.

Sensory nerve fibres arising from the trigeminal ganglion supplying the temporomandibular joint have abundant receptors that respond to capsaicin, protons, heat and ATP; retrograde tracing revealed 25, 41 and 52% of neurons supplying this joint exhibited TRPV1 and $P2X_3$ receptors, respectively (Ichikawa et al. 2004).

3.10 Heart

An ATP-triggered vagal reflex has been described leading to suppression of sinus mode automaticity and atrioventricular nodal conduction (Pelleg and Hurt 1990). This is probably mediated by $P2X_{2/3}$ receptors located on vagal sensory nerve terminals in the left ventricle and lung (McQueen et al. 1998). This supports the hypothesis that ATP released from ischaemic myocytes is a mediator of atropine-sensitive bradyarrhythmias associated with left ventricular myocardial infarction (Xu et al. 2005).

4 Central Sensory Nerves

While the main areas of the central nervous system (CNS) concerned with control of autonomic function involving sensory nerves are the spinal cord, brain stem and hypothalamus (Burnstock 2007), the prefrontal cortex is implicated in the integration of sensory, limbic and autonomic information (Groenewegen and Uylings 2000). It seems likely that P1, P2X and P2Y receptors are involved in neurotransmission and neuromodulation of sensory pathways in the somatic, visual, olfactory, auditory and gustatory cortex (North and Verkhratsky 2006).

4.1 Spinal Cord

Spinal circuits, spinal afferent influx as well as descending influences from brain stem and hypothalamus work together in the integrative activities of the preganglionic sympathetic neurons, which regulate the activity on many organs. There was early identification of dense areas of acid phosphatase and 5′-nucleotidase activity in the substantia gelatinosa of the spinal cords of rats and mice and the possible implication for purinergic transmission was raised (Burnstock 2007).

P2X receptors mediate sensory synaptic transmission between primary afferent fibres and spinal dorsal horn neurons (Li et al. 1998). ATP-evoked increases in intracellular calcium were demonstrated in both neurons and glia of the dorsal spinal cord. ATP was shown to inhibit slow depolarization via P2Y receptors in substantia gelatinosa neurons. A recent study has identified $P2Y_1$ and $P2Y_4$ receptor mRNA in subpopulations of dorsal horn neurons (Kobayashi et al. 2006). $P2X_3$ immunoreactivity is present on the axon terminals of DRG neurons that extend across the entire mediolateral extent of inner lamina II of the dorsal horn. The immunolabelled nerve profiles in lamina II for $P2X_3$ receptors are located largely on terminals with ultrastructural characteristics of sensory afferent terminals (Llewellyn-Smith and Burnstock 1998). In contrast, although $P2X_2$ immunoreactivity is most prominent in lamina II, it is also seen in deeper layers, and only rarely overlaps with $P2X_3$ immunoreactivity. A TNP-ATP-resistant P2X ionic current has been reported on the central terminals of capsaicin-insensitive Aδ-afferent fibres that play a role modulating sensory transmission to lamina V nerves. At central terminals of primary afferent neurons, ATP has been shown to act both presynaptically facilitating glutamate release (Nakatsuka and Gu 2006) and postsynaptically (Fyffe and Perl 1984). P2X receptors are also expressed on glycinergic presynaptic nerve terminals.

ATP has been shown to be released from dorsal spinal cord synaptosomes. Morphine and capsaicin release purines from capsaicin-sensitive primary afferent nerve terminals in the spinal cord. In addition to acting as a fast excitatory synaptic transmitter, ATP facilitates excitatory transmission by increasing glutamate release and enhancing inhibitory neurotransmission mediated by both GABA and glycine. A different P2X receptor subtype (perhaps $P2X_{1/5}$ or $P2X_{4/6}$) was involved in long-lasting modulation in lamina V (Nakatsuka et al. 2003). The authors concluded that differential modulation of sensory inputs into different sensory regions by P2X receptor subtypes represents an important mechanism of sensory processing in the spinal cord dorsal horn. Blockade of P2X receptors in the dorsal horn with PPADS attenuates the cardiovascular "exercise pressor reflex" to activation of muscle afferents, while stimulation of P2X receptors enhances the reflex response (Gao et al. 2005).

4.2 *Nucleus Tractus Solitarius*

The nucleus tractus solitarius (NTS) (particularly neurons in the caudal NTS) is a central relay station for relaying viscerosensory information to respiratory, cardiovascular and digestive neuronal networks. Extracellular purines have been claimed to be the primary mediators signalling emergency changes in the internal environment in the CNS. Stimulation of P2X receptors in the NTS evokes hypotension with decreases in both cardiac output and total peripheral resistance (Kitchen et al. 2001). Injection of adenosine into the NTS produced dose-related decreases in heart rate and systolic and diastolic blood pressures. NTS A_{2A} receptor activation elicits hind limb vasodilatation. ATP and β,γ-methylene-ATP (β,γ-meATP) produced dose-related potent vasodepressor and bradycardic effects, suggesting that P2 as well as P1 receptors were involved. Hindquarter vasodilatation during defence reactions is mediated by P2X receptors in the NTS (Korim et al. 2007). Patch-clamp studies of neurons dissociated from rat NTS revealed P2 receptor-mediated responses and microinjection of P2 receptor agonists into the subpostremal NTS in anaesthetized rats produced reduction of arterial blood pressure probably via a $P2X_1$ or a $P2X_3$ receptor subtype, since α,β-meATP was particularly potent. The actions of ATP and adenosine in the NTS may be functionally linked to selectively coordinate the regulation of regional vasomotor tone.

Microinjections into the caudal NTS of anaesthetized spontaneously breathing cats showed that α,β-meATP elicited a distinct pattern of cardiorespiratory response, namely dose-related decrease in tidal volume and respiratory minute volume; at higher doses a pronounced apnoea was produced. This suggested that a P2X receptor was present, perhaps involved in the processing of sensation from pulmonary receptors related to the Breuer–Hering and pulmonary C-fibre reflexes. Impaired arterial baroreflex regulation of heart rate after blockade of P2 receptors in the NTS has been reported. Microinjection of ATP into caudal NTS of awake rats produces respiratory responses (Antunes et al. 2005) and purinergic mechanisms are probably involved in the sympathoexcitatory component of the chemoreflex (Braga et al. 2007). It has been suggested that there is a sensory afferent selective role of P2 receptors in the NTS for mediating the cardiac component of the peripheral chemoreceptor reflex (Paton et al. 2002). Activation of NTS A_1 receptors differentially inhibits baroreflex pathways controlling regional sympathetic outputs (Scislo et al. 2007).

The immunohistochemical distribution of P2X receptor subtypes in the NTS of the rat and colocalization of $P2X_2$ and $P2X_3$ immunoreactivity has been described in the NTS. At the electron microscope level, $P2X_3$ receptor positive boutons have been shown to synapse on dendrites and cell bodies and have complex synaptic relationships with other axon terminals and dendrites (Llewellyn-Smith and Burnstock 1998). $P2X_2$ receptors have been localized presynaptically in vagal afferent fibres in rat NTS. A whole-cell patch-clamp study of neurons in the caudal NTS led to the conclusion that ATP activates presynaptic $P1(A_1)$ receptors after breakdown to adenosine, reducing evoked release of glutamate from the primary afferent nerve terminals. Purinergic and vanilloid receptor activation releases glutamate from separate cranial afferent terminals in the NTS corresponding to myelinated and unmyelinated pathways in the NTS.

4.3 Ventrolateral Medulla

The ventrolateral medulla (VLM) contains a network of respiratory neurons that are responsible for the generation and shaping of respiratory rhythm; it also functions as a chemoreceptive area mediating the ventilating response to hypercapnia. Evidence has been presented that ATP acting on $P2X_2$ receptors expressed in VLM neurons influences these functions (Gourine et al. 2003). Recent studies suggest that P2X receptors on neurons in the raphe nucleus are also involved in respiratory regulation (Cao and Song 2007). It has also been shown in neonatal rats that respiratory rhythm generating networks in the pre-Bötzinger complex are very sensitive to $P2Y_1$ receptor activation and suggest a role for $P2Y_1$ receptors in respiratory motor control, particularly in the excitation of rhythm that occurs during hypoxia (Lorier et al. 2007).

Evidence has been presented to suggest that CO_2-evoked changes in respiration are mediated, at least in part, by P2X receptors in the retrofacial area of the VLM (Gourine 2005). CO_2–P2X-mediated actions were observed only in inspiratory neurons that have purinoceptors with pH sensitivity (characteristic of the $P2X_2$ receptor subtype) that could account for the actions of CO_2 in modifying ventilatory activity. During hypoxia, release of ATP in the VLM plays an important role in the hypoxic ventilatory response in rats. Adenosine acts as a neuromodulator of a variety of cardiorespiratory reflexes.

Intrathecal application of P2X receptor agonists and antagonists indicates that $P2X_3$ or $P2X_{2/3}$ receptors on the trigeminal primary afferent terminals in the medullary dorsal horn (trigeminal subnucleus caudalis) enhance trigeminal sensory transmission (Jennings et al. 2006).

4.4 Sensory Nuclei

$P1(A_1)$ adenosine receptor agonists presynaptically inhibit both GABAergic and glutamatergic synaptic transmission in periaqueductal grey neurons and adenosine suppresses excitatory glutamatergic inputs to rat hypoglossal motoneurons (Burnstock 2007). This is evidence for multiple P2X and P2Y subtypes in the rat medial vestibular nucleus.

P2X receptors are expressed in the medial nucleus of the trapezoid body of the auditory brain stem, where they act to facilitate transmitter release in the superior olivary complex (Watano et al. 2004). Although ATP potentiates release at both excitatory and inhibitory synapses, it does so via different P2X receptor subtypes expressed at different locations: $P2X_3$ receptors on cell bodies or axons of excitatory pathways and $P2X_1$ receptors on the presynaptic terminals of inhibitory pathways. A_1 rather than P2X receptors have been implicated during high-frequency glutamatergic synaptic transmission in the calyx of Held (Wong et al. 2006). P2 receptors modulate excitability, but do not mediate pH sensitivity of respiratory chemoreceptors in the retrotrapezoid nucleus on the ventral surface of the brain stem (Mulkey et al. 2006).

4.5 Trigeminal Mesencephalic Nucleus

Although the trigeminal mesencephalic nucleus (MNV) is located in the CNS, it contains cell bodies of primary afferent neurons that relay proprioceptive information exclusively. The MNV is known to contain mRNA for $P2X_2$, $P2X_4$, $P2X_5$ and $P2X_6$ subtypes. With in situ hybridization studies, higher levels of mRNA for $P2X_5$ were found in this nucleus than in any other brain area. ATP-gated ion channels (P2X receptors) were described in rat trigeminal MNV proprioceptive neurons from whole-cell and outside-out patch-clamp recording, possibly mediated by $P2X_5$ receptor homomultimers and $P2X_{2/5}$ heteromultimers (Patel et al. 2001).

4.6 Locus Coeruleus

There were early reports of modulation of neuronal activities in the locus coeruleus (LC) by adenosine. The first report of the action (depolarization) of ATP on P2 receptors on neurons in LC was by Harms et al. (1992). α,β-Methylene ADP was later shown to increase the firing rate of rat LC neurons. P2Y receptors are also present on LC neurons (Frohlich et al. 1996). Intracellular recordings from slices of rat LC led to the suggestion that ATP may be released either as the sole transmitter from purinergic neurons terminating in the LC or as a cotransmitter with noradrenaline (NA) from recurrent axon collaterals or dendrites of the LC neurons themselves (Poelchen et al. 2001). Microinjection of ATP or α,β-meATP into LC (and periaqueductal grey matter) led to changes in bladder function and arterial blood pressure (Rocha et al. 2001).

4.7 Area Postrema

Injection of adenosine into the area postrema (AP) produced decreased heart rate and systolic and diastolic blood pressure. Dense areas of $P2X_2$ receptor immunoreactivity were demonstrated in the rat AP and excitatory effects of ATP in rat AP neurons have been demonstrated (Sorimachi et al. 2006).

4.8 Hypothalamus

ATP and α,β-meATP excite neurosecretory vasopressin cells in the supraoptic nucleus (SON), an effect blocked by suramin. Suramin also blocked excitation produced by vagus nerve stimulation. There is evidence for cotransmitter release of ATP with NA at synapses in the hypothalamus stimulating vasopressin and oxytocin release (Song and Sladek 2006). ATP and the α_1-adrenoceptor agonist phenylephrine evoke synergistic stimulation of vasopressin and oxytocin release from the hypothalamoneurohypophyseal systems and the authors speculate that this allows for a sustained elevation of vasopressin release in response to extended stimuli such as severe haemorrhage, chronic hypotension or congestive heart failure. Excitatory effects of ATP via P2X receptors in acutely dissociated ventromedial hypothalamic neurons have been described. A role for adenosine A_1 receptors in mediating cardiovascular changes evoked during stimulation of the hypothalamic defence area has been postulated.

Purinergic regulation of stimulus-secretion coupling in the neurohypophysis has been reported. Ultrastructural localization of both $P2X_2$ and $P2X_6$ receptor immunoreactivity at both pre- and postsynaptic sites in the rat hypothalamoneurohypophyseal system has been described (Loesch and Burnstock 2001). From a study of the expression of P2X receptor subtypes in the SON using RT-PCR, in situ hybridization, Ca^{2+} imaging and whole-cell patch-clamp techniques, it was concluded that $P2X_3$ and $P2X_4$ receptors were predominant, but that $P2X_7$ receptors were also present. A study has shown that $P2X_5$ receptors are expressed on neurons containing vasopressin and NOS in the rat hypothalamus (Xiang et al. 2006). P2Y as well as P2X receptors mediate increases in intracellular calcium in supraoptic neurons produced by ATP (Song et al. 2007).

It has been suggested that ATP, cosecreted with vasopressin and oxytocin, may play a key role in the regulation of stimulus-secretion coupling in the neurohypophysis by acting through $P2X_2$ receptors increasing AVP release, and after breakdown to adenosine, acting via $P1(A_1)$ receptors (inhibiting N-type Ca^{2+} channels) to decrease neuropeptide release. Evidence for the involvement of purinergic signalling in hypothalamus and brain stem nuclei in body temperature regulation has been presented (Gourine et al. 2002). Early studies of the roles of adenosine in the hypothalamus have been reviewed (Burnstock 2003). Adenosine deaminase containing neurons in the posterior hypothalamus innervate mesencephalic primary sensory neurons, perhaps indicating purinergic control of jaw movements.

ATP injected into the paraventricular nucleus stimulates release of AVP, resulting in antidiuretic action through renal AVP (V_2) receptors, and ATP (but not ADP, AMP or adenosine) injected into the SON also decreased urine outflow (Mori et al. 1994). Stimulation of the hypothalamic defence area produces autonomic responses that include papillary dilatation, piloerection, tachypnoea, tachycardia and a marked pressor response. Luteinizing hormone releasing hormone (LHRH) is released from the hypothalamus in pulses at hourly intervals, which is essential for the maintenance of normal reproductive function. Studies of an in vivo culture preparation of

LHRH neurons show that ATP stimulates LHRH release, probably via $P2X_2$ and $P2X_4$ receptor subtypes, and may be involved in synchronization of the Ca^{2+} oscillations that appear to underlie the pulsatile release of LHRH (Terasawa et al. 2005). The authors also speculate that glial cells expressing $P2Y_1$ and $P2Y_2$ receptors may also participate in this process. $P2X_{1-6}$ receptor subunits are present on paraventricular nucleus neurons projecting to the rostral ventrolateral medulla in the rat, suggesting a role for ATP on the paraventricular nucleus in the regulation of sympathetic nerve activity.

5 Purinergic Mechanosensory Transduction

A hypothesis was proposed that purinergic mechanosensory transduction occurred in visceral tubes and sacs, including ureter, bladder and gut, where ATP released from epithelial cells during distension acted on $P2X_3$ homomeric and $P2X_{2/3}$ heteromeric receptors on subepithelial sensory nerves initiating impulses in both local sensory pathways and pathways to pain centres in the CNS (Burnstock 1999) (Fig. 6b). Subsequent studies of bladder, ureter and gut have produced evidence in support of this hypothesis as presented in the following sections.

5.1 Urinary Bladder

Mice lacking the $P2X_3$ receptor exhibited reduced inflammatory pain and marked urinary bladder hyporeflexia with reduced voiding frequency and increased voiding volume, suggesting that $P2X_3$ receptors are involved in mechanosensory transduction underlying both physiological voiding reflexes and inflammatory pain (Cockayne et al. 2000). A later study from this group, using $P2X_2$ knockout mice and $P2X_2$/$P2X_3$ double knockout mice, revealed a role for the $P2X_2$ subtype too in mediating the sensory effect of ATP (Cockayne et al. 2005). In a systematic study of purinergic mechanosensory transduction in the mouse urinary bladder, ATP was shown to be released from urothelial cells during distension and discharge initiated in pelvic sensory nerves, was mimicked by ATP and α,β-meATP and was attenuated by $P2X_3$ antagonists as well as in $P2X_3$ knockout mice (Fig. 6a); $P2X_3$ receptors were localized on suburothelial sensory nerve fibres (Vlaskovska et al. 2001). Single-unit analysis of sensory fibres in the mouse urinary bladder revealed both low- and high-threshold fibres sensitive to ATP contributing to physiological (non-nociceptive) and nociceptive mechanosensory transduction, respectively. The amilorode-sensitive mechanosensitive channels, including epithelial Na^+ channels, expressed in the rat bladder epithelium might be involved in the mechanosensory transduction mechanisms by controlling stretch-evoked ATP release (Du et al. 2007). TRPV1 receptors participate in normal bladder function and are essential for normal mechanically evoked purinergic signalling by ATP released from the urothelium. Purinergic agonists increase the excitability of afferent fibres to distension.

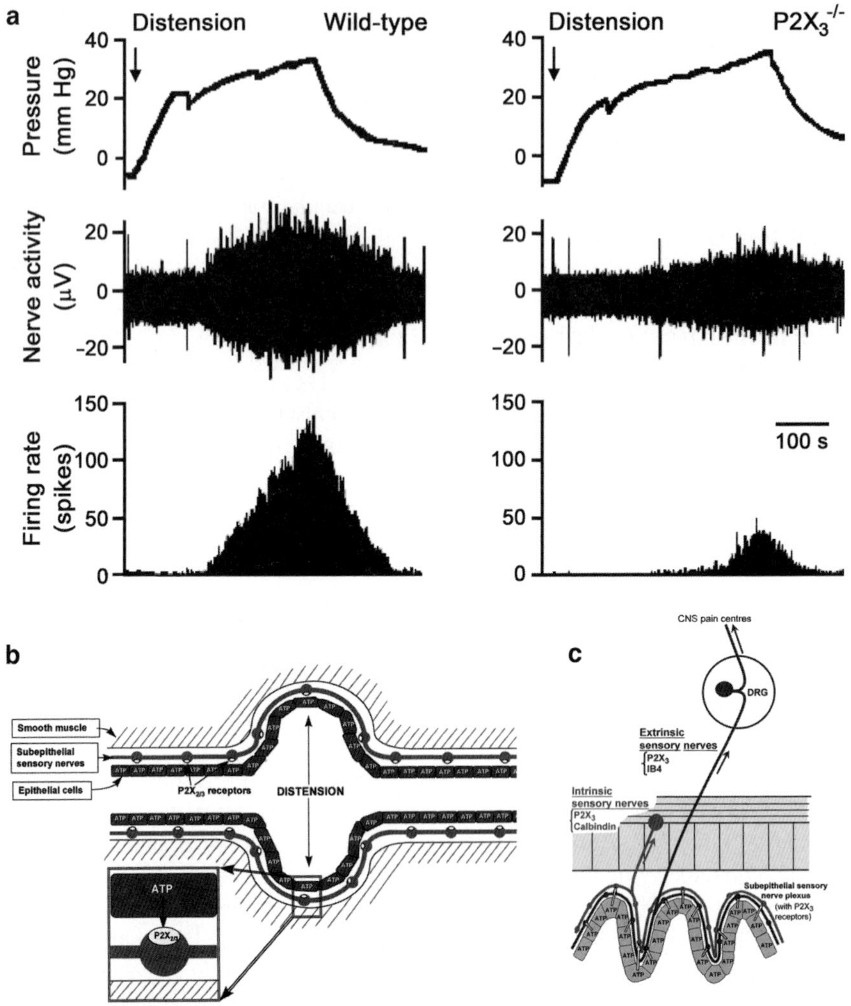

Fig. 6 Urinary bladder. (**a**) Comparison of the firing rate in sensory nerves during distension of the bladder in wild-type mice (*left*) and $P2X_3$ receptor deficient mice ($P2X_3^{-/-}$) (*right*). (**b**) Hypothesis for purinergic mechanosensory transduction in tubes (e.g. ureter, vagina, salivary and bile ducts, and gut) and sacs (e.g. urinary and gall bladders and lung). It is proposed that distension leads to release of ATP from epithelium lining the tube or sac, which then acts on $P2X_3$ and $P2X_{2/3}$ receptors on subepithelial sensory nerves to convey sensory/nociceptive information to the CNS. (**c**) Purinergic mechanosensory transduction in the gut. It is proposed that ATP released from mucosal epithelial cells during moderate distension acts preferentially on $P2X_3$ and/or $P2X_{2/3}$ receptors on low-threshold subepithelial intrinsic sensory nerve fibres (labelled with calbindin) to modulate peristaltic reflexes. ATP released during extreme (colic) distension also acts on $P2X_3$ and/or $P2X_{2/3}$ receptors on high-threshold extrinsic sensory nerve fibres (labelled with isolectin B4) that send messages via the DRG to pain centres in the CNS. (**a** Courtesy of Weifang Rong; **b** Reproduced from Burnstock 1999, with permission from Blackwell Publishing; **c** reproduced from Burnstock 2001a, with permission from John Wiley and Sons, Inc.)

Bladder sensory DRG neurons, projecting via pelvic nerves, express predominantly $P2X_{2/3}$ heteromultimer receptors. Stretch induces release of both ACh and ATP from urothelial cells of the human bladder.

ATP given intravesically stimulates the micturition reflex in awake, freely moving rats, probably by stimulating suburothelial C-fibres (Pandita and Andersson 2002). The findings of studies of resiniferatoxin desensitization of capsaicin-sensitive afferents on detrusor overactivity induced by intravesical ATP in conscious rats support the view that ATP has a role in mechanosensory transduction and that ATP-induced facilitation of the micturition reflex is mediated, at least partly, by nerves other than capsaicin-sensitive afferents (Brady et al. 2004). ATP has also been shown to induce a dose-dependent hypereflexia in conscious and anaesthetized mice, largely via capsaicin-sensitive C-fibres; these effects were dose-dependently inhibited by PPADS and TNP-ATP (Hu et al. 2004). $P2X_1$ and $P2X_3$ receptors play a fundamental role in the micturition reflex in female urethane-anaesthetized rats; $P2X_3$ receptor blockade by phenol red raised the pressure and volume thresholds for the reflex, while $P2X_1$ receptor blockade diminished motor activity associated with voiding (King et al. 2004).

It has been claimed that suburothelial myofibroblast cells isolated from human and guinea pig bladder that are distinct from epithelial cells provide an intermediate regulatory step between urothelial ATP release and afferent excitation involved in the sensation of bladder fullness (Wu et al. 2004). The roles of ATP released from urothelial cells and suburothelial myofibroblasts on various bladder functions have been considered at length in several reviews (e.g. Birder 2006) and evidence has been presented that urothelial-released ATP may alter afferent nerve excitability (de Groat 2006).

5.2 Ureter

The ureteric colic induced by the passage of a kidney stone causes severe pain. Distension of the ureter resulted in substantial ATP release from the urothelium in a pressure-dependent manner (Knight et al. 2002). Cell damage was shown not to occur during distension with scanning electron microscopy, and after removal of the urothelium there was no ATP release during distension. Evidence was presented that the release of ATP from urothelial cells was vesicular. Immunostaining of $P2X_3$ receptors in sensory nerves in the subepithelial region was reported. Multi-fibre recordings from ureter afferent nerves were made using a guinea pig preparation perfused in vitro (Rong and Burnstock 2004). Distension of the ureter resulted in a rapid, followed by maintained, increase in afferent nerve discharge. The rapid increase was mimicked by intraluminal application of ATP or α,β-meATP, and TNP-ATP attenuated these nerve responses to distension; the maintained increase was partly due to adenosine.

5.3 *Gut*

A hypothesis was proposed suggesting that purinergic mechanosensory transduction in the gut initiated both physiological reflex modulation of peristalsis via intrinsic sensory fibres and nociception via extrinsic sensory fibres (Burnstock 2001a) (Fig. 6c). Evidence in support of this hypothesis was obtained from a rat pelvic sensory nerve colorectal preparation (Wynn et al. 2003). Distension of the colorectum led to pressure-dependent increase in release of ATP from mucosal epithelial cells and also evoked pelvic nerve excitation. This excitation was mimicked by application of ATP and α,β-meATP and was attenuated by the selective $P2X_3$ and $P2X_{2/3}$ antagonist TNP-ATP and by PPADS. The sensory discharge was potentiated by ARL-67156, an ATPase inhibitor. Single-fibre analysis showed that high-threshold fibres were particularly affected by α,β-meATP. Lumbar splanchnic and sacral pelvic nerves convey different mechanosensory information from the colon to the spinal cord. Forty percent of lumbar splanchnic nerve afferents responded to α,β-meATP compared with only 7% of pelvic nerve afferents (Brierley et al. 2005). The $P2X_3$ receptor subtype predominates in AH-type neurons and probably participates in mechanosensory transduction (Raybould et al. 2004).

Purinergic mechanosensory transduction has also been implicated in reflex control of secretion, whereby ATP released from mucosal epithelial cells acts on $P2Y_1$ receptors on enterochromaffin cells to release 5-hydroxytryptamine, which leads to regulation of secretion either directly or via intrinsic reflex activity (Cooke et al. 2003; Xue et al. 2007).

5.4 *Uterus*

It has been hypothesized that tissue stress or damage in the uterine cervix during late pregnancy and parturition leads to ATP release and sensory signalling via P2X receptors (Papka et al. 2005). In support of this proposal, these authors have shown $P2X_3$ receptor immunoreactivity in axons in the cervix, in small and medium-sized neurons in L6-S1 DRG and in lamina II of the L6–S1 spinal cord segments and increases in $P2X_3$ receptor expression between pregnancy day 10 and parturition (day 22/23) in the rat cervix, although not in DRG or spinal cord.

5.5 *Tooth Pulp*

$P2X_3$ and $P2X_{2/3}$ receptors on sensory afferents in tooth pulp appear to mediate nociception (Alavi et al. 2001; Renton et al. 2003), perhaps from ATP released by mechanical distension or inflammation of odontoblasts. Mustard oil application to the tooth pulp in anaesthetized rats produced long-lasting central sensitization, reflected by increases in neuronal mechanoreceptive field size; TNP-ATP reversibly attenuated the mustard oil sensitization for more than 15 min (Hu et al. 2002). $P2X_3$ receptor expression is transiently upregulated and anterogradely transported in trigeminal sensory neurons after orthodontic tooth movement (Cao et al. 2006).

5.6 Tongue

$P2X_3$ receptors are abundantly present on sensory nerve terminals in the tongue (see Sect. 3.8), and ATP and α,β-meATP have been shown to excite trigeminal lingual nerve terminals in an in vitro preparation of intra-arterially perfused rat tongue mimicking nociceptive responses to noxious mechanical stimulation and high temperature (Rong et al. 2000). A purinergic mechanosensory transduction mechanism for the initiation of pain has been considered.

5.7 Skin and Joints

Skin cell damage causes action-potential firing and inward currents in sensory nerve fibres, which was eliminated by enzymatic degradation of ATP or blockade of P2X receptors, indicating release of cytosolic ATP (Cook and McCleskey 2002).

ATP has been shown to be a stimulant of articular nociceptors in the knee joint via $P2X_3$ receptors (Dowd et al. 1998) and also to some extent in lumbar intervertebral disc, but not as prominently as in the skin (Aoki et al. 2003). $P2Y_2$ receptor mRNA is expressed in both cultured normal and osteoarthritic chondrocytes taken from human knee joints and ATP was shown to be released by mechanical stimulation (Millward-Sadler et al. 2004).

6 Purinergic Sensory Pathology

6.1 Pain

There is much current interest in the involvement of purinergic signalling in pain and recent reviews are available (Burnstock 2006, 2007; McGaraughty and Jarvis 2006; Shieh et al. 2006; Inoue 2007).

There were early hints that ATP might be involved in pain, including the demonstration of pain produced by injection of ATP into human skin blisters and ATP participation in pain pathways in the spinal cord (see Sect. 1). $P2X_3$ ionotropic receptors were cloned in 1995 and shown to be localized predominantly on small nociceptive sensory neurons in DRG together with $P2X_{2/3}$ heteromultimer receptors.

Later, Burnstock (1996b) put forward a unifying purinergic hypothesis for the initiation of pain by ATP on nociceptive afferent nerves. It was suggested that ATP released as a cotransmitter with NA and neuropeptide Y from sympathetic nerve terminal varicosities might be involved in causalgia and reflex sympathetic dystrophy (see also Ren et al. 2006); that ATP released from vascular endothelial cells of microvessels during reactive hyperaemia is associated with pain in migraine, angina and ischaemia; and that ATP released from tumour cells (which contain very high levels), damaged during abrasive activity, reaches $P2X_3$ receptors on nociceptive sensory nerves. This was followed by an increasing number of papers expanding on this concept. Immunohistochemical studies have shown that the nociceptive fibres expressing $P2X_3$ receptors arose largely from the population of small neurons that were labelled with the lectin IB_4. IB_4-positive fibres expressing $P2X_3$ and $P2X_{2/3}$ receptors are C-fibres, but the smaller population of CGRP-positive fibres expressing $P2X_3$ and $P2X_{2/3}$ receptors appear to be Aδ-fibres. The central projections of these neurons were shown to be in inner lamina II of the dorsal horn and peripheral projections were demonstrated to skin, tooth pulp, tongue and subepithelial regions of visceral organs. A schematic illustrating the initiation of nociception on primary afferent fibres in the periphery and purinergic relay pathways in the spinal cord was presented by Burnstock and Wood (1996) (Fig. 7). The decreased sensitivity to noxious stimuli associated with the loss of IB_4-binding neurons expressing $P2X_3$ receptors indicates that these sensory neurons are essential for the signalling of acute pain. However, persistent pain during inflammation may also involve sensitization and/or spread of $P2X_3$ or $P2X_{2/3}$ receptors. In a study of the behavioural effects of intraplantar injections of ATP in freely moving rats, evidence was presented that ATP was more effective in exciting nociceptors in inflamed compared with normal skin (Hamilton et al. 2001). Cannabinoids appear to inhibit nociceptive responses produced by P2X receptors (Krishtal et al. 2006). Locally released ATP can sensitize large mechanosensitive afferent endings via P2 receptors, leading to increased nociceptive responses to pressure or touch; it has been suggested that such a mechanism, together with central changes in the dorsal horn, may contribute to touch-evoked pain. Enhanced expression of glial cell line derived neurotrophic factor (GDNF) in the skin can change the mechanical sensitivity of IB_4-positive nociceptive afferents expressing $P2X_3$ and $P2X_{2/3}$ receptors. Treatment with oxidized ATP, a selective inhibitor of $P2X_7$ receptors, reduced the hyperalgesia produced by complete Freund's adjuvant and carrageenan-induced inflammation in rats. Data have been presented to support a pathogenic role for keratinocyte-derived ATP in irritant dermatitis. Pain related to the musculoskeletal system (myofascial pain) is very common and ATP has been claimed to excite or sensitize myofascial nociceptors (Makowska et al. 2006).

The search is on for selective $P2X_3$ and $P2X_{2/3}$ receptor antagonists that are orally bioavailable and do not degrade in vivo for the treatment of pain (Burnstock 2006; Gever et al. 2006). Suramin, PPADS and reactive blue 2 have been used as non-selective antagonists at $P2X_3$ and $P2X_{2/3}$ receptors on nociceptive sensory nerve endings. PPADS has the advantage that it associates and dissociates approximately 100–10,000 times more slowly than other known antagonists. The

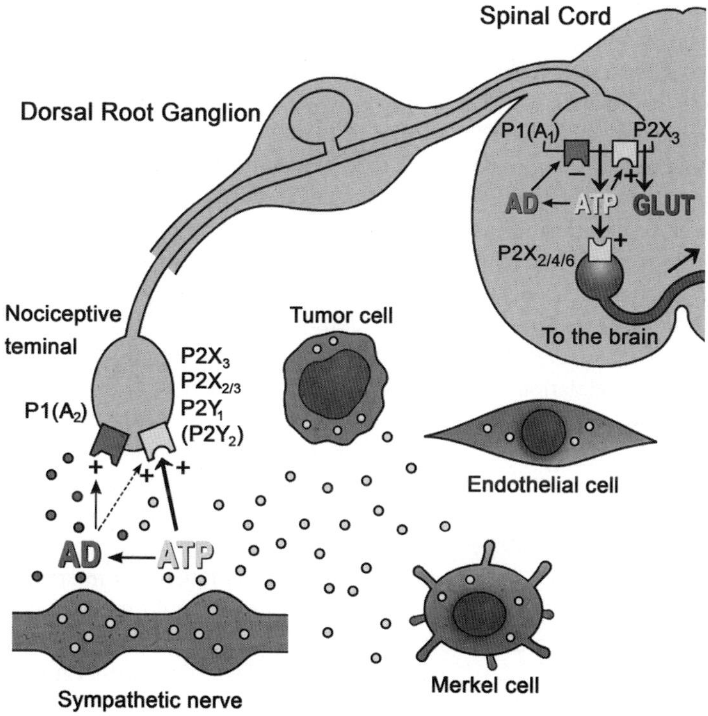

Fig. 7 Hypothetical schematic of the roles of purine nucleotides and nucleosides in pain pathways. At sensory nerve terminals in the periphery, $P2X_3$ and $P2X_{2/3}$ receptors have been identified as the principal P2X purinoceptors present, although recent studies have also shown expression of $P2Y_1$ and possibly $P2Y_2$ receptors on a subpopulation of $P2X_3$ receptor immunopositive fibres. Other known P2X purinoceptor subtypes (1–7) are also expressed at low levels in dorsal root ganglia. Although less potent than ATP, adenosine also appears to act on sensory terminals, probably directly via $P1(A_2)$ purinoceptors; however, it also acts synergistically (*broken black line*) to potentiate $P2X_{2/3}$ receptor activation, which also may be true for 5-hydroxytryptamine, capsaicin and protons. At synapses in sensory pathways in the CNS, ATP appears to act postsynaptically via $P2X_2$, $P2X_4$ and/or $P2X_6$ purinoceptor subtypes, perhaps as heteromultimers, and after breakdown to adenosine it acts as a prejunctional inhibitor of transmission via $P1(A_2)$ purinoceptors. $P2X_3$ receptors on the central projections of primary afferent neurons in lamina II of the dorsal horn mediate facilitation of glutamate and probably also ATP release. Sources of ATP acting on $P2X_3$ and $P2X_{2/3}$ receptors on sensory terminals include sympathetic nerves as well as endothelial, Merkel and tumour cells. (Modified from Burnstock and Wood 1996, and reproduced with permission from the American Physiological Society)

TNP-substituted nucleotide TNP-ATP is a very potent antagonist at both $P2X_3$ and $P2X_{2/3}$ receptors. A-317491 (synthesized by Abbott Laboratories) and compound RO3 (synthesized by Roche Palo Alto) are both effective $P2X_3$ and $P2X_{2/3}$ antagonists, the latter being orally bioavailable and stable in vivo. Antagonism of $P2X_1$

and $P2X_3$ receptors by phenol red has been reported and tetramethylpyrazine, a traditional Chinese medicine, used as an analgesic for dysmenorrhoea, was claimed to block $P2X_3$ receptor signalling. Antisense oligonucleotides have been used to downregulate the $P2X_3$ receptor, and in models of neuropathic (partial sciatic nerve ligation) and inflammatory (complete Freund's adjuvant) pain, inhibition of the development of mechanical hyperalgesia as well as significant reversal of established hyperalgesia were observed within 2 days of treatment (Stone and Vulchanova 2003). Combined antisense and RNA interference mediated treatment for specific inhibition of the recombinant rat $P2X_3$ receptor appears to be promising for pain therapy (Hemmings-Mieszczak et al. 2003). $P2X_3$ double-stranded short interfering RNA (siRNA) relieves chronic neuropathic pain and opens up new avenues for therapeutic pain strategies in man (Dorn et al. 2004).

P2Y receptors are also present on nociceptive sensory nerves and these are involved in modulation of pain transmission (Gerevich et al. 2007). With use of a mouse skin-sensory nerve preparation, evidence was presented that $P2Y_2$ receptors in the terminals of capsaicin-sensitive cutaneous sensory neurons mediate nociceptive transmission and further that P2Y signalling may contribute to mechanotransduction in low-threshold Aβ-fibres (Stucky et al. 2004). P2Y receptors appear to potentiate pain induced by chemical or physical stimuli via capsaicin-sensitive TRPV1 channels and it has been proposed that the functional interaction between $P2Y_2$ receptors and TRPV1 channels in nociceptors could underlie ATP-induced inflammatory pain (Ma and Quirion 2007). ATP-induced hyperalgesia was abolished in mice lacking TRPV1 receptors. A hypothesis that purinergic mechanosensory transduction occurs in visceral organs initiating nociception was discussed in Sect. 5.

Changes in central purinergic pathways that occur in chronic neuropathic pain have attracted considerable attention in recent years and have been well reviewed. There is purinoceptor involvement in nociceptive pathways in the spinal cord. For example, intrathecally administered P2 receptor antagonists, suramin and PPADS, produced antinociceptive effects in rats. ATP-activated P2X receptors in lamina II of the rat spinal cord play a role in transmitting or modulating nociceptive information. α,β-meATP-induced thermal hyperalgesia may be mediated by spinal $P2X_3$ receptors, perhaps by evoking glutamate release. Spinal endogenous ATP may play a role in capsaicin-induced neurogenic pain via $P2X_3$ or $P2X_{2/3}$ receptors and formalin-induced inflammatory pain via different P2X and/or P2Y receptors. Of the six lamina regions in the dorsal horn of the spinal cord, inner lamina II and lamina I are the major sensory regions involved in nociceptive transmission, as well as lamina V. Central terminals of nociceptive afferents coexpress ionotropic glutamate and $P2X_3$ receptors. Glial cells contribute to the α,β-meATP-induced long-term potentiation in the dorsal horn, which might be part of a cellular mechanism for the induction of persistent pain (Ikeda et al. 2007). An inhibitory role of supraspinal $P2X_{2/3}$ receptors on nociception in rats has been described (Fukui et al. 2006).

There are three potential sources of ATP release during sensory transmission in the spinal cord. ATP may be released from the central terminals of primary afferent neurons. ATP may be also released from astrocytes and/or postsynaptic dorsal horn neurons. The presence of $P2X_3$ mRNA-labelled neurons in the DRG increased 3 days after peripheral injury. $P2X_3$ receptors on DRG neurons increase their activity after inflammation and contribute to the hypersensitivity to mechanical stimulation. Evidence has been presented for increased release of ATP from DRG neurons on the side of the injury after induction of painful peripheral neuropathy by sciatic nerve entrapment; however, sensitization of $P2X_3$ receptors rather than a change in ATP release appears to be responsible for the neuropathic pain behaviour. For neuropathic pain, the tactile allodynia that follows peripheral nerve injury is reduced by A-134974, a novel adenosine kinase inhibitor acting at spinal sites. PPADS, TNP-ATP and apyrase attenuate central sensitization in nociceptive neurons in medullary dorsal horn, which suggests that release of ATP plays a key role in the central sensitization induced by injury or inflammation of peripheral tissues. Upregulated homomeric $P2X_3$ and heteromeric $P2X_{2/3}$ receptors augmented thermal hyperalgesia and mechanical allodynia, respectively, at the spinal level in the acute stage of chronic constriction injury; at the chronic stage (after 40 days), thermal hyperalgesia disappeared, but mechanical allodynia persisted. A-317491, a potent and selective antagonist of $P2X_3$ and $P2X_{2/3}$ receptors, reduces chronic inflammatory and neuropathic pain in the rat, but not acute, inflammatory or visceral pain. When A-317491 and also Compound A (US patent reference 2005/0209260A1) were administered spinally to animals after chronic nerve constriction injury, there was a reduction in sensory fibre responses, unmasking a central role for these P2X receptors and suggesting a potential role of their antagonists in the modulation of neuropathic pain (Sharp et al. 2006). Endogenous ATP acting on P2X receptors appears to be necessary for the induction of the postoperative pain characterized by mechanical allodynia. Suramin inhibits spinal cord microglia activation and long-term hyperalgesia induced by inflammation produced by formalin injection. Endogenous opioid mechanisms partially mediate spinal $P2X_3$/$P2X_{2/3}$ receptor-related antinociception in rat models of inflammatory and chemogenic pain, but not neuropathic pain (Chen et al. 2006).

Analgesic effects with intrathecal administration of P2Y receptor agonists UTP and UDP in a normal and neuropathic pain rat model have been reported, suggesting that $P2Y_2$ (and/or $P2Y_4$) and $P2Y_6$ receptors produce inhibitory effects in spinal pain transmission. It has been suggested that, while $P2X_3$ receptor activation leads to increased firing of DRG neurons and subsequently to increased release of sensory transmitter from their central processes, $P2Y_1$ receptor activation may decrease the release of sensory transmitter onto spinal cord neurons and may thereby partly counterbalance the algogenic effect of ATP. $P2Y_1$ receptor expression is upregulated in rat DRG neurons following transection of sciatic nerves and has been implicated in the mechanisms underlying neuropathic pain.

$P2X_7$ receptor activation of cultured astrocytes from rat brain increases the release of cysteinyl leukotrienes, which are potent lipid mediators of inflammation, further supporting a role for extracellular ATP as an integral component of the inflammatory brain pain response.

The roles of $P2X_4$ and $P2X_7$ receptors on microglia (immune cells) in neuropathic and inflammatory pain has attracted strong interest in the past few years

(Färber and Kettenmann 2006; Trang et al. 2006; Hughes et al. 2007). $P2X_4$ and $P2X_7$ knockout mice share a common pain-reduced phenotype, but apparently via different mechanisms (Chessell et al. 2006). Recently developed selective $P2X_7$ receptor antagonists, compound 15d (Nelson et al. 2006), A-740003 (Honore et al. 2006) and A-438079 (McGaraughty et al. 2007), reduce chronic inflammatory and neuropathic pain. After spinal cord injury, an increased number of lumbar microglia expressing the $P2X_4$ receptor in the spinal cord of rats with allodynia and hyperalgesia have been reported. Pharmacological blockade of $P2X_4$ receptors or intraspinal administration of $P2X_4$ antisense oligodeoxynucleotide reversed tactile allodynia caused by peripheral nerve injury without affecting acute pain behaviours in naïve animals (Tsuda et al. 2003).

Purinergic mechanisms are beginning to be explored in relation to cancer pain. It was suggested that the unusually high levels of ATP contained in tumour cells may be released by mechanical rupture to activate $P2X_3$ receptors on nearby nociceptive sensory nerve fibres. There is increased expression of $P2X_3$ receptors on CGRP immunoreactive epidermal sensory nerve fibres in a bone cancer pain model (Gilchrist et al. 2005) and in other cancers that involve mechanically sensitive tumours. For example, in bone tumours, destruction reduces the mechanical strength of the bone and antagonists that block the mechanically gated channels and/or ATP receptors in the richly innervated periosteum might reduce movement-associated pain. The hyperalgesia associated with tumours appears to be linked to increase in expression of $P2X_3$ receptors in nociceptive sensory neurons expressing CGRP by analogy with that described for increased $P2X_3$ receptor expression in a model of inflammatory colitis. Increased expression of $P2X_3$ receptors was also reported associated with thermal and mechanical hyperalgesia in a rat model of squamous cell carcinoma of the lower gingival (Nagamine et al. 2006).

6.2 Migraine

ATP has been implicated in the pathogenesis of pain during migraine via stimulation of primary afferent nerve terminals located in the cerebral microvasculature (Burnstock 1981, 1989; Fumagalli et al. 2006). $P2X_3$ receptors are expressed on primary afferent nerve terminals supplying cerebral vessels arising from trigeminal, nodose and spinal ganglia. Thus, $P2X_3$ receptor antagonists may be candidates for antimigraine drug development (Waeber and Moskowitz 2003). CGRP is expressed in human trigeminal neurons and is released during migraine attacks; a recent study shows that the algogenic action of CGRP is linked to sensitization of trigeminal $P2X_3$ nociceptive receptors, suggesting that trigeminal $P2X_3$ receptors may be a potential target for the early phase of migraine attack. There is also evidence that migraine is a chronic sympathetic nervous system disorder, with which there is an increase in release of sympathetic cotransmitters, including ATP, which may contribute to the initial vasospasm. ATP may contribute to pain in migraine by sensitizing nociceptors against acidosis via $P2Y_2$ receptor supported release of endogenous prostaglandin (Zimmermann et al. 2002). It has been suggested that there is an interaction of P2Y receptors on trigeminal sensory terminals with $P2X_3$ receptors after sensitization of trigeminal neurons with algogenic stimuli (e.g. NGF, BDNF or bradykinin) and that this may help identify new targets for the development of novel antimigraine drugs. It was shown recently that the majority of trigeminal primary afferent neurons innervating the dura mater express $P2X_2$ and/or $P2X_3$ receptors, suggesting that purines may be involved in nociceptive processing in migraine (Goadsby 2005).

6.3 *Diseases of Special Senses*

6.3.1 Eye

Purinergic signalling is widespread in the eye and novel therapeutic strategies are being developed for glaucoma, dry eye and retinal detachment. ATP, acting via both P2X and P2Y receptors, modulates retinal neurotransmission, affecting retinal blood flow and intraocular pressure. The ATP analogue β,γ-meATP is more effective in reducing intraocular pressure (40%) than are muscarinic agonists such as pilocarpine (25%) and β-adrenoceptor blockers (30%), raising the potential for the use of purinergic agents in glaucoma (Pintor et al. 2003). It was shown that rapid elevation of intraocular pressure leads to release of ATP that results in retinal ganglion cell injury and consequent visual defects (Resta et al. 2007).

6.3.2 Ear

ATP may regulate hearing sensitivity and thus may be useful in the treatment of Ménière's disease, tinnitus and sensorineural deafness (Housley et al. 2006). Sustained loud noise alters the response of outer hair cells in the inner ear to ATP and produces an upregulation of $P2X_2$ receptors, particularly at the site of outer hair cell sound transduction (Chen et al. 1995a), although with a longer time course of noise exposure up to 24 days, downregulation of P2X and P2Y receptor subtypes has been reported (Szücs et al. 2006). $P2X_2$ expression is also increased in spiral ganglion neurons, indicating that extracellular ATP acts as a modulator of auditory neurotransmission that is adaptive and dependent on the noise level (Wang et al. 2003). Excessive noise can irreversibly damage hair cell stereocilia, leading to deafness. Data have been presented showing that release of ATP from damaged hair cells is required for Ca^{2+} wave propagation through the support cells of the organ of Corti, involving P2Y receptors, and this may constitute the fundamental mechanism to signal the occurrence of hair cell damage (Gale et al. 2004). Noise-induced upregulation of NTPDase3 in the rat cochlear has been reported and its potential neuroprotective effect discussed (Vlajkovic et al. 2006).

6.3.3 Nasal Organs

Purinergic receptors have been described in the nasal mucosa, including the expression of $P2X_3$ receptors on olfactory neurons. Enhanced sensitivity to odours in the presence of P2 receptor antagonists suggests that low-level endogenous ATP normally reduces odour responsiveness. It appears that the induction of heat-shock proteins by noxious odour damage can be prevented by the in vivo administration of P2 receptor antagonists (Hegg and Lucero 2006). The predominantly suppressive effect of ATP in odour responses could play a role in the reduced odour sensitivity that occurs during acute exposure to noxious fumes and may be a novel neuroprotective mechanism. Purinergic receptors appear to play an integral role in signalling acute damage in the olfactory epithelium by airborne pollutants. Damaged cells release ATP, thereby activating purinergic receptors on neighbouring sustentacular cells, olfactory receptor neurons and basal cells.

6.4 Bladder Diseases

Purinergic signalling plays a role in afferent sensation from the bladder (see Sect. 3). Purinergic agonists acting on $P2X_3$ receptors in the bladder can sensitize bladder afferent nerves and these effects mimic the sensitizing effect of cystitis induced by cyclophosphamide (Nazif et al. 2007). Thus, $P2X_3$ receptors are a potential target for pharmacological manipulation in the treatment of both pain and detrusor instability. Subsensitivity of $P2X_3$ and $P2X_{2/3}$ receptors, but not vanilloid receptors, has been shown in L6–S1 DRG in the rat model of cyclophosphamide cystitis (Borvendeg et al. 2003). Release of ATP from urothelial cells with hypoosmotic mechanical stimulation was increased by over 600% in inflamed bladder from cyclophosphamide-treated animals; botulinum toxin inhibited this release (Smith et al. 2005). Botulinum neurotoxin type A is effective in the treatment of intractable detrusor overactivity; decreased levels of sensory receptors $P2X_3$ and/or TRPVI may contribute to its clinical effect (Apostolidis et al. 2005; Atiemo et al. 2005).

It is believed that the predominant sensory afferents involved in detecting bladder volume changes are the Aδ pelvic nerve afferents which convey information about the state of bladder fullness to spinal and supraspinal centres coordinating the micturition reflex (Andersson and Wein 2004). In contrast, the normally silent pelvic afferent C-fibres are thought to assume a prominent role under pathophysiological conditions, where they become hyperexcitable and convey information about noxious, inflammatory or painful stimuli, and evoke reflex contractions mainly through a localized spinal reflex. In the absence of $P2X_3$ receptors in mice knockouts, the bladder exhibits hyporeflexia, characterized by decreased voiding frequency and increased bladder capacity, but normal bladder pressures (Cockayne et al. 2000). The recently developed $P2X_3$ and $P2X_{2/3}$ antagonist RO3, which is orally bioavailable and metabolically stable, is being explored as a therapeutic agent for urinary tract dysfunction (Ford et al. 2006). The $P2X_3$ receptor is largely expressed in the IB_4 small nociceptive capsaicin-sensitive nerves in the DRG, so it is interesting that IB_4-conjugated saporin, a cytotoxin that destroys neurons binding IB_4, when administered intrathecally at the level of L6–S1 spinal cord, reduced bladder overactivity induced by ATP infusion. Voiding dysfunction involves $P2X_3$ receptors in conscious chronic spinal cord injured rats, which raises the possibility that $P2X_3$ receptor antagonists might be useful for the treatment of neurogenic bladder dysfunction. Chronic spinal cord injury results in a dramatic increase in muscarinic receptor-evoked release of ATP from primary afferents in the lumbosacral spinal cord and from the bladder (Salas et al. 2007).

Stretch-activated ATP release from bladder epithelial cells from patients with interstitial cystitis is significantly greater than from healthy cells and also in animal models of interstitial cystitis (Birder et al. 2004). The $P2X_3$ receptor subunit was upregulated during stretch of cultured urothelial cells from patients with interstitial cystitis. $P2X_2$ and $P2X_3$ receptor expression has been demonstrated on human bladder urothelial cells (as well as on afferent nerve terminals); the expression was greater in cells from interstitial cystitis bladder (Tempest et al. 2004).

Reduction of $P2X_3$ and $P2X_5$ receptors in human detrusor from adults with urge incontinence has been claimed (Moore et al. 2001). Overdistension of the bladder is caused by urinary retention, but it has also been used as a method for treating unstable bladder or interstitial cystitis, possibly damaging sensory nerve fibres. However, micturition problems often reoccur after overdistension treatment.

Recent reviews of management of detrusor dysfunction highlight the growing potential of therapeutic strategies related to purinergic sensory signalling (Ford et al. 2006; Ruggieri 2006).

6.5 Gut Disorders

The excitability of visceral afferent nerves is enhanced following injury, ischaemia and during inflammation, for example in irritable bowel syndrome (IBS). Under these conditions, substances are released from various sources that often act synergistically to cause sensitization of afferent nerves to mechanical or chemical stimuli. Receptors to these substances (including ATP) represent potential targets for drug treatment aimed at attenuating the inappropriate visceral sensation and subsequent reflex activities that underlie abnormal bowel function and visceral pain (Holzer 2004). α,β-meATP was shown to stimulate mechanosensitive mucosal and tension receptors in mouse stomach and oesophagus, leading to activity in vagal afferent nerves. The sensitizing effects of $P2X_3$ receptor agonists on mechanosensory function are induced in oesophagitis. $P2X_3$ purinergic signalling enhancement in an animal model of colonic inflammation has been described, owing, at least in part, to the appearance of $P2X_3$ receptor expression in a greater number of CGRP-labelled small nociceptive neurons in the DRG (Wynn et al. 2004). $P2X_3$ receptor expression is increased in the enteric plexuses in human IBS, suggesting a potential role in dysmotility and pain and the possibility that P2X receptors are potential targets for the drug treatment of IBS has been raised (Galligan 2004). It has also been suggested that agonists acting on P2X receptors on intrinsic enteric neurons may enhance gastrointestinal propulsion and secretion and that these drugs might be useful for treating constipation-predominant IBS, while P2X antagonists might be useful for treating diarrhoea-predominant IBS. The peripheral sensitization of $P2X_3$ receptors on vagal and spinal afferents in the stomach may contribute to dyspeptic symptoms and the development of visceral hyperalgesia (Dang et al. 2005). Enhanced activity in purinergic pathways occurs in postoperative ileus, but is reversed by orphanin FQ.

6.6 *Arthritis*

It was recognized early that the nervous system may contribute to the functional changes associated with rheumatoid arthritis. A role for purinergic signalling in rheumatic diseases has been considered (Green et al. 1991; Dowd et al. 1998; Seino et al. 2006). Quinacrine (Atabrine), a drug that binds strongly to ATP, has been used for the treatment of rheumatoid arthritis patients for many years. One of its mechanisms of action is to decrease levels of prostaglandin E_2 and cyclooxygenase-2, which are known to be produced following occupation of P2Y receptors by ATP. The articular fluid removed from arthritic joints contains high levels of ATP. Purinergic regulation of bradykinin-induced plasma extravasation and adjuvant-induced arthritis has been reported. ATP and UTP activate calcium-mobilizing $P2Y_2$ or $P2Y_4$ receptors and act synergistically with interleukin-1 to stimulate prostaglandin E_2 release from human rheumatoid synovial cells (Loredo and Benton 1998). Spinal P1 receptor activation has been claimed to inhibit inflammation and joint destruction in rat adjuvant-induced arthritis (Chan et al. 2007). When monoarthritis was induced by injection of complete Freund's adjuvant into the unilateral temporomandibular joint of the rat, the pain produced was associated with an increase in $P2X_3$ receptor positive small neurons in the trigeminal ganglion (Shinoda et al. 2005). Activation of P2X receptors in the rat temporomandibular joint induces nociception and blockage by PPADS decreases carrageenan-induced inflammatory hyperalgesia (Oliveira et al. 2005).

Evidence is accumulating to suggest that blockers of $P2X_7$ receptors may have a future as anti-inflammatory drugs (Ferrari et al. 2006). Oxidized ATP inhibits inflammatory pain in arthritic rats by inhibition of the $P2X_7$ receptor for ATP localized in nerve terminals (Dell'Antonio et al. 2002). The $P2X_7$ receptor antagonist AZD9056 has been reported to be in phase II clinical trials for rheumatoid arthritis (Okuse 2007).

6.7 Respiratory Diseases

Vagal afferent purinergic signalling may be involved in the hyperactivity associated with asthma and chronic obstructive pulmonary disease (Adriaensen and Timmermans 2004). The need to support the failing lung (acute respiratory distress syndrome) with mechanical ventilation is potentially life-saving but, unfortunately, alveolar overdistension and pulmonary shear stress may cause lung injury (ventilator-induced lung injury), increasing bronchoalveolar lavage leading to lung oedema. It has been suggested that ventilator-induced lung injury may involve stretch-associated release of ATP from neuroepithelial cell bodies and activation of sensory nerves and reflex responses (Rich et al. 2003). P2X receptors are involved in the reactive oxygen species evoked bradypneic reflex in anaesthetized rats (Ruan et al. 2006). Acid-sensitive vagal sensory pathways involved in the cough reflex may involve $P2X_2$ receptors (Kamei et al. 2005; Kollarik et al. 2007). P2X and $GABA_A$ receptors play an important role in CO_2 chemoreception and are involved in mediation of the ventilatory response to hypercapnia (Gourine 2005).

6.8 Central Disorders

Purinergic signalling appears to play a significant role in the regulation of body temperature during fever by central hypothalamic and brain stem nuclei (Gourine et al. 2004). Mice lacking the $P2X_3$ receptor subunit exhibit enhanced avoidance of both hot and cold thermal extremes (Shimizu et al. 2005). Evaluation of the roles of purinergic signalling in processing of the sympathoexcitatory component of the chemoreflex at the NTS level may illuminate the mechanisms underlying the sympathetic overactivity observed in pathophysiological conditions such as hypertension, obstructive sleep apnoea, and heart failure.

Although ethanol is probably the oldest and most widely used psychoactive drug, the cellular mechanisms by which it affects the nervous system have been poorly understood, although some insights in relation to purinergic P2 receptor signalling have emerged in recent years. Ethanol inhibits P2X receptor mediated responses of DRG neurons by an allosteric mechanism (Li et al. 1998). Ethanol differentially affects ATP-gated $P2X_3$ and $P2X_4$ receptor subtypes expressed in *Xenopus* oocytes (Davies et al. 2005).

7 Development of Purinergic Sensory Signalling

There are a limited number of studies of the roles of purinergic sensory signalling in both embryonic and postnatal development and in regeneration (Burnstock 2001b, 2007; Zimmermann 2006). An immunohistochemical study revealed intense labelling of $P2X_3$ receptors in the embryonic and postnatal (postnatal days 7 and 14; Fig. 8a), but not adult, rat brain. The staining was restricted to the hindbrain at embryonic day 16, in particular the mesencephalic trigeminal nucleus, the superior and inferior olive, the intermediate reticular zone, the spinal trigeminal tract and the prepositus hypoglossal nucleus. $P2X_3$ receptors first appeared in the hindbrain neural tube and sensory ganglia in embryonic day 11–11.5 embryos; at embryonic day 14.5 they appeared in the optic tract, NTS mesencephalic trigeminal nucleus, but $P2X_3$ immunoreactivity was downregulated in early postnatal brain stem. The $P2X_3$ receptor was coexpressed with the $P2X_2$ receptor in neurons in NTS and sensory ganglia (Cheung and Burnstock 2002). α,β-meATP is ineffective on glycinergic presynaptic nerve terminals projecting to rat substantia gelatinosa neurons at postnatal days 10–12, and is strongly active at postnatal days 28–30, perhaps contributing to the fine control of the pain signal in spinal cord dorsal horn neurons. In rat superficial dorsal horn, excitatory synapses mediated by both glutamate and ATP are functional from the first postnatal days. Distinct subtypes of P2X receptors have been shown to be functionally expressed at pre- and postsynaptic sites in lamina V neurons in rat dorsal spinal cord and it was suggested that purinergic signalling in deep dorsal horn neurons is more important during postnatal development (Shiokawa et al. 2006).

$P2X_3$ receptors are expressed in the trigeminal ganglia of zebrafish from a very early stage of development, most likely in neural crest-derived trigeminal cells rather than in placode-derived cells (Norton et al. 2000) (Fig. 8c). $P2X_3$ receptors were also expressed in the spinal sensory Rohan–Beard cells and in the putative lateral line ganglion in the early development of zebrafish. ATP-gated currents activated via $P2X_2$ and $P2X_3$ receptors in cultured embryonic rat DRG neurons show heterogeneity of time courses comparable to that seen in different adult subpopulations of dissociated adult DRG neurons (Labrakakis et al. 2000). Activation of P2X receptors on cultured embryonic DRG neurons results in the release of SP. Immunostaining of $P2X_3$ receptors was found in most neurons in embryonic mouse trigeminal ganglia and DRG, in contrast to adult ganglia, which express $P2X_3$ receptors only on small-diameter neurons (Ruan et al. 2004) (Fig. 8b). Nearly all sensory neurons in mouse DRG, trigeminal and nodose ganglia expressed $P2X_3$ receptors at embryonic day 14, but after birth there was a gradual decline to about 50% of neurons showing positive staining. IB_4-positive neurons in sensory ganglia did not appear until birth; the numbers increased to about 50% by postnatal day 14, when they were mostly colocalized with $P2X_3$ receptors. Responses to ATP have been described in ciliary neurons acutely dissociated from embryonic chick ciliary ganglia taken at day 14. ATP augments peptide release from neurons in embryonic DRG through activation of P2Y receptors. IB_4-binding DRG neurons (that express $P2X_3$ receptors) switch from NGF to GDNF dependence in early postnatal life.

While there are many studies of purinergic signalling in the retina of adult mammals, there are only a few reports about embryonic retina (Burnstock 2001b, 2007). Spontaneous waves of excitation in the developing mammalian retina are believed to play an important role in activity-dependent visual development of retinogeniculate connectivity. The earliest age at which spontaneous waves were

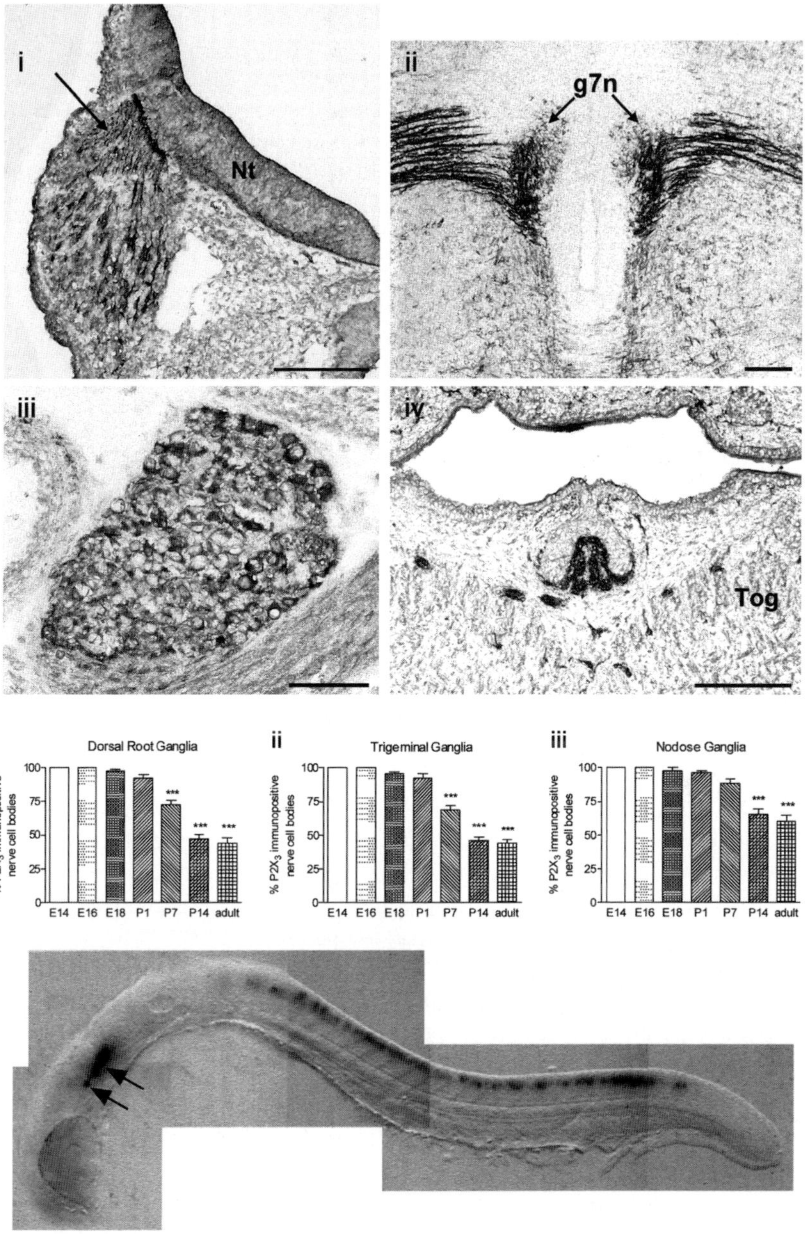

Fig. 8 Development of sensory nerves. (**a**) $P2X_3$ immunoreactivity in embryonic rat embryos. *i* $P2X_3$ immunoreactivity in an embryonic day 12.5 rat embryo. Transverse sections at the first branchial arch levels showing $P2X_3$ immunoreactivity (*arrow*) in the trigeminal ganglion. Note the expression of $P2X_3$ in the primitive spinal trigeminal tract between the trigeminal ganglion and the neural tube (*Nt*). *ii* $P2X_3$ immunoreactivity in an embryonic day 14.5 rat embryo. Coronal section at the pontine level showing the genu of the facial nerve (*g7n*) stained strongly with $P2X_3$ receptor

detected in rabbit retina was embryonic day 22 and the involvement of purinergic receptor activation in these waves was suggested. Suramin blocked the wave. Adenosine has also been implicated in chick retinal development; A_1 receptors may have different functions in the embryonic retina as compared with mature chick retina. Studies of embryonic chick neural retina have shown that the ATP-induced rise in intracellular Ca^{2+} is mediated by $P2Y_2$ or $P2Y_4$ receptors and that there is a dramatic decline of the ATP-induced rise in intracellular Ca^{2+} just before synaptogenesis. Suramin and reactive blue 2 almost completely block these responses. Injection of reactive blue 2 into early embryonic chicks produced severe effects in embryogenesis. ATP increased [^{3}H]thymidine incorporation in retinal cultures from embryonic day 3 and suramin and PPADS inhibited these activities. It was suggested that the change in Ca^{2+} signalling mediated by $P2Y_2$ or $P2Y_4$ receptors during development may underlie the differentiation of neuroepithelial cells or undifferentiated progenitor cells into neurons. ATP acting on P2 receptors is involved in the regulation of retinal progenitor cell proliferation at early embryonic stages, perhaps in collaboration with growth factors. ATP, probably via $P2Y_1$ receptors, stimulates proliferation of both bipolar and Müller cells in early developing chick retina at embryonic days 6–8. RT-PCR studies of $P2X_7$ mRNA in postnatal rats (postnatal days 23–210) showed positive identification in the retina. Changes in $P2Y_4$ receptor expression during development of rat cochlea outer sulcus cells have been described recently (Lee et al. 2007).

The perinatal development of nerves expressing $P2X_3$ receptors in the myenteric plexus of the rat stomach has been examined (Xiang and Burnstock 2004b). $P2X_3$ receptor immunoreactive nerves in the embryonic rat stomach are of both extrinsic and intrinsic origin. The extrinsic sensory nerve fibres first express $P2X_3$ receptors as early as embryonic day 12 and extend rapidly on to the whole stomach by embryonic day 14. In contrast, the intrinsic enteric neuron cell bodies showing $P2X_3$ immunoreactivity did not appear until birth (postnatal day 1), reached peak numbers by postnatal day 14, then decreased in maturing animals. IGLEs and intramuscular arrays expressing $P2X_3$ receptors were first seen postnatally at postnatal day 1 and postnatal day 7, respectively (Xiang and Burnstock 2004b). $P2X_3$ receptor immunoreactive neurons in the gastric myenteric plexus expressed calbindin only in the early postnatal days, while 14–21% of neurons from postnatal

Fig. 8 (continued) antibody. *iii* $P2X_3$ immunoreactivity in a neural-crest-derived nodose ganglion of an embryonic day 18.5 rat embryo. *iv* $P2X_3$ immunoreactivity in an embryonic day 18.5 rat embryo. Transverse section showing strong $P2X_3$ receptor staining in the taste bud of the tongue (*Tog*). *Scale bar* in *i* 200 μm, in *ii–iv* 100 μm. (**b**) Percentage of $P2X_3$-immunoreactive nerve cell bodies in sensory ganglia of mouse in embryonic and postnatal development. Note statistical significance indicated by *asterisks* relates to postnatal ages 7 days, 14 days and adult as compared with embryonic days 14, 16 and 18. $^{***}p < 0.001$. **c** Early expression of $P2X_3$ receptors in putative central and peripheral neural cells in a 24-h zebrafish embryo in which expression in the putative trigeminal ganglia cells has condensed to two spots (*arrows*) and in which expression in dorsal Rohon–Beard neurons is prominent. (**a** Reproduced from Cheung and Burnstock 2002, with permission from Wiley–Liss; **b** reproduced from Ruan et al. (2004), with kind permission from Springer Science and Business Media **c** reproduced from Norton et al. 2000, with permission from Elsevier) day 1 to postnatal day 60 increasingly expressed calretinin. About 20% of $P2X_3$ positive neurons coexpressed NOS throughout perinatal development.

Vagal sensory nerve terminals in rat lung express $P2X_3$ receptors from the first moment that they make contact with NEBs a few days before birth (Brouns et al. 2003). This is consistent with the important function of NEBs as oxygen sensors perinatally before the carotid body O_2-sensory system is fully developed at about 2 weeks after birth.

During embryonic development of the rat inner ear, $P2X_2$ receptor mRNA expression was present in the precursors of the cells bordering the cochlear endolymphatic compartment at embryonic day 12, as well as in spinal and vestibular ganglia (Housley et al. 2006). Both inner and outer hair cells did not exhibit $P2X_2$ receptor mRNA until after postnatal day 10 through postnatal day 12, concomitant with the onset of hearing. These data are consistent with roles for the $P2X_2$ receptor both in the process of labyrinthine development and in the regulation of auditory and vestibular sensory transduction. $P2X_1$ receptors provide the signal transduction pathway for development of afferent and efferent innervation of the sensory hair cells and purinergic influence on cochlea morphogenesis. $P2X_3$ receptor expression has been characterized in the mouse cochlea from embryonic day 16 using confocal immunofluorescence. From embryonic day 18 to postnatal day 6, spiral ganglion neuron cell bodies and peripheral neurites projecting to the inner and outer hair cells were labelled for $P2X_3$ receptor protein, but diminished around postnatal day 6, and were no longer detected at the onset of hearing (around postnatal day 11). These data suggest a role for $P2X_3$ receptor-mediated purinergic signalling in cochlea synaptic reorganization and establishment of neurotransmission that occurs just prior to the onset of hearing function (Huang et al. 2006).

Merkel cells appear in the epidermis of the planum nasale of rat fetuses from the 16th day of intrauterine development and sensory nerve fibres form close association with them by day 20. This is of interest since it is known that Merkel cells contain high levels of peptide-bound ATP and are in close association with sensory fibres expressing $P2X_3$ receptors (Burnstock and Wood 1996).

Studies of purinergic signalling in stem cells are beginning; the preliminary reports are encouraging and hopefully this will develop into a major new area of purinergic research (see, e.g., Mishra et al. 2006; Lin et al. 2007).

8 Evolution of Purinergic Sensory Mechanisms

Nucleosides and nucleotides are part of a primitive signalling system with potent actions in both invertebrates and lower vertebrates (Burnstock 1996a, 2007). For example, in the leech, ATP and ADP potently activated "noxious" and touch neurons. AMP was found to be the most potent chemoattractant of octopus, initiating a locomotor response; the suckers in the arms carry sensory organs with chemoreceptors that direct the arms towards a meal. There is considerable information about the effects of ATP and adenosine in crustaceans in the early literature, particularly by Carr and colleagues, which has been reviewed. The olfactory organs of the spiny lobsters *Panulirus argus* and *Panulirus interruptus* have different populations of purinergic chemoreceptors that are excited by AMP, ADP or ATP (Fig. 9a), via receptors that show similarities to P2 receptors described in vertebrates. These receptors reside on chemosensitive neurons that are contained within aesthetasc sensilla on the lateral filaments of the antennules. 5′-AMP odorant receptor sites have been localized ultrastructurally, utilizing 5′-AMP-biotin, along the entire dendritic region, including the transitional zone between inner and outer dendritic segments, the region that also contains 5′-ectonuclotidase and phosphatase. Since these receptors are more sensitive to the slowly degradable analogues of ATP, α,β-meATP and β,γ-meATP, they appear to be comparable to mammalian $P2X_1$ and $P2X_3$ receptors. Ectonucleotidases dephosphorylate adenine nucleotides to yield a nucleoside, which is internalized by an uptake system. Activation of olfactory and gustatory P2 receptors in lobsters induces a feeding behavioural response. ATP is an ideal stimulus for such animals that feed on wounded or recently killed animals, since ATP occurs at high concentrations in fresh animal flesh but decays rapidly as cells die. Since predators such as lobsters often inhabit crevices and only emerge to feed at night, foraging is directed principally by chemical stimuli, rather than visual or mechanical stimuli. ATP is detected in prey organisms, such as mussels and oysters, which contain high concentrations of nucleotides that are released when the animal dies. Olfactory purinoceptors have also been identified in the shrimp and blue crab. In lobsters and other decapod crustaceans, the sites of olfaction and gustation are anatomically distinct, the former in the antennules, the latter on the walking legs, maxillipeds and mouthparts. The sensilla on the walking legs of the spiny lobster have also been shown to possess ATP- and AMP-sensitive cells as well as enzymes that dephosphorylate purine nucleotides.

ATP released from mammalian erythrocytes stimulates the gorging responses in a variety of blood-feeding insects such as mosquitoes, black fly, horsefly, stable fly, tsetse fly and haematophagous ticks. Electrophysiological methods have been used to demonstrate that the apical sensilla of the labrum of mosquito express the ATP receptors involved in blood feeding (Fig. 9b). Novobiocin, which blocks ATP access to its binding site, inhibits the gorging response. The ED_{50} of ATP for tsetse fly females is 13 nM, while for males it is 140 nM; this level of sensitivity for detecting ATP is the highest recorded for an insect. Other chemosensory P2 receptors have been identified that are involved in the recognition of a blood meal in haematophagous insects. These represent a heterogeneous group. Many blood-feeding insects recognize ATP and related compounds as phagostimulants. In mosquitoes and tsetse flies, ATP is found to be more potent than ADP at stimulating feeding, while AMP is a very poor phagostimulant, indicating an ATP-selective P2 receptor. A similar ATP-selective receptor mediates the phagostimulatory response of insect larvae, suggesting that this response is not limited to the adult form. α,β-meATP and β,γ-meATP are less potent than ATP as phagostimulants in the tsetse fly, raising the possibility that a P2Y receptor maybe involved. A similar order of potency was found for the bug *Rhodnius*, while the potency order

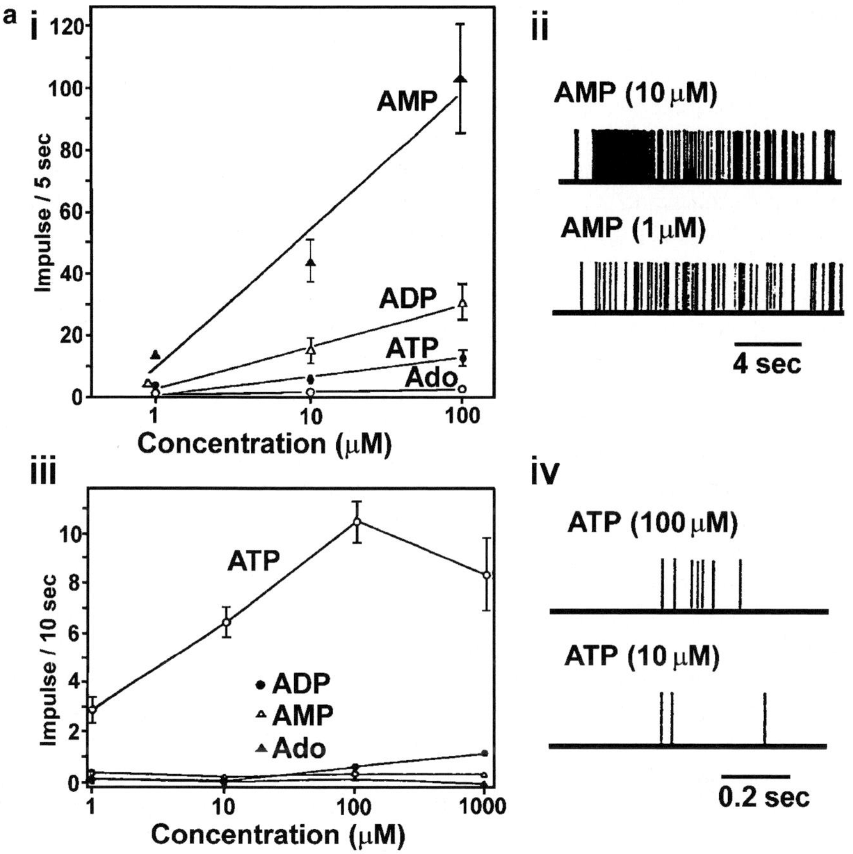

b

Nucleotide	ED_{50} [x] μmol/I	Phagostimulant index=(ED_{50}ATPx100)/ED_{50}test nucleotide)
Control	No feeding	__
Adenosine	No feeding	__
AMP	463.0	3
ADP	96.5	13
ATP	12.2	100
UTP	No feeding	__
2d ADP	248.5	5
2d ATP	24.9	49
2'3'dd ATP	1.2	1017

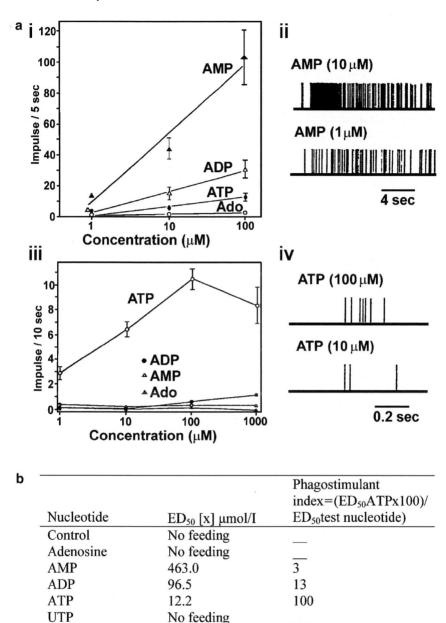

Fig. 9 Invertebrate sensory mechanisms. (**a**) Comparisons of response characteristics of AMP-sensitive and ATP-sensitive sensory nerves in the antennule of the spiny lobster. *i* response of AMP-best cells to the compounds indicated. *ii* series of action potentials produced by an AMP-best

was ADP > ATP > β,γ-meATP > AMP for the mosquito. ADP was also found to be the most potent phagostimulant of the horsefly. ADP-selective receptors, namely, $P2Y_1$, $P2Y_{12}$ and $P2Y_{13}$, have been identified in mammals. It is fascinating that apyrase (ATP diphosphohydrolase) has been reported to have exceptionally high activity in the salivary glands or saliva of blood-sucking insects, including the bug *Rhodnius*, tsetse fly, mosquito and sandfly. In all cases, since ADP induces platelet aggregation, breakdown of ADP by apyrase leads to enhanced haemorrhage and more effective blood sucking.

Taste chemosensilla sensitive to nucleotides have been identified in some non-haematophagous insects. ATP was first reported to be a feeding stimulant in a flea and tick. In the omnivorous common blowfly, ATP does not have a direct stimulatory action, but rather modulates the responses of the labilla sensilla; it reduces the responses to NaCl and fructose, but enhances responses to sucrose and glucose. Adenosine stimulates feeding in the African army worm; this larva of an owlmoth exclusively feeds on grasses. There are multiple nucleotide receptor sites in the labellar taste receptor cells of the flesh fly: ATP, ADP and AMP stimulate the sugar receptor cells, while the salt receptor cells only responded to GDP and to a lesser extent IDP and UDP. ATP receptors cloned in the platyhelminth *Schistosoma mansoni* and the protozoan *Dictyostelium* show surprisingly close similarity to mammalian P2X receptors (Agboh et al. 2004; Ludlow and Ennion 2006; Fountain et al. 2007).

9 Concluding Comments

This review has covered a wide spectrum of information about the roles of purinergic signalling in the physiological and pathophysiological processes of sensory nerves and mechanosensory transduction.

The last 10 years has been a period of rapid progress in identifying the numerous types of purinergic receptors and in understanding their relationships, pharmacological properties and intracellular transduction mechanisms. This progress has facilitated new appreciation of the wide spectrum of neural activities involving purinergic signalling, including the roles of ATP, ADP and adenosine in sensory signalling in both the peripheral nervous system and the CNS.

Fig. 9 (continued) cell to the concentration of AMP indicated. *iii* response of ATP-best cells to the compounds indicated. *iv* series of action potentials produced by an ATP-best cell to the concentrations of ATP indicated. Note the differences in time scale in *ii* and *iv*. (**b**) Values for the phagostimulant (gorging) response of the mosquito *Aedes aegypti* produced by different nucleotides dissolved in the control (150 mmol l^{-1} NaCl with 10 mmol l^{-1} $NaHCO_3$). There were also no feeding responses to GTP and ITP. *2d ADP* 2′-deoxy ADP, *2d ATP* 2′-deoxy ATP, *2′3′dd ATP* 2′3′-dideoxy ATP. (**a** Reproduced from Trapido-Rosenthal et al. 1989, with permission from Taylor and Francis; **b** reproduced from Werner-Reiss et al. 1999, with permission from Elsevier)

The chemistry of ATP in the extracellular environment is dynamic and complex, and more must be learned about the extracellular biochemistry and enzymes that regulate the synthesis and degradation of ATP outside the cell. The activity of ectonucleotidases in subcellular domains and how these enzymes change during development, disease and physiological state are still to be resolved. The development of selective inhibitors for the different subtypes of ectonucleotidases would be a valuable step forward.

While it is now clear that many different cell types release ATP, often acting on P2 receptors on sensory nerve terminals, we still await a clear understanding of the mechanisms that underlie ATP transport. Until recently, it was usually assumed that the source of extracellular ATP acting on purinoceptors was damaged or dying cells, but it is now recognized that the ATP release from healthy cells by mechanical distortion, hypoxia and various agents is a physiological mechanism (Bodin and Burnstock 2001; Lazarowski et al. 2003; Schwiebert et al. 2003). There is an active debate, however, about the precise transport mechanism(s) involved. There is compelling evidence for exocytotic vesicular release of ATP from nerves, but for ATP release from non-neuronal cells, various transport mechanisms have been proposed, including ATP binding cassette transporters, connexin or pannexin hemichannels or possibly plasmalemmal voltage-dependent anion channels, as well as vesicular release. Perhaps surprisingly, evidence was presented that the release of ATP from urothelial cells during purinergic mechanosensory transduction in the bladder and ureter (as well as from endothelial cells) is vesicular, since monensin and brefeldin A, which interfere with vesicular formation and trafficking, inhibited distension-evoked ATP release, but gadolinium, a stretch-activated channel inhibitor, and glibenclamide, an inhibitor of two members of the ATP binding cassette protein family, did not (Knight et al. 2002). Hopefully, when the ATP transport mechanisms become clearer, agents will be developed that will be able to enhance or inhibit ATP release, another useful way forward as a therapeutic strategy.

There are an increasing number of explorations of the therapeutic potential of purinergic signalling in various diseases of the nervous system and hopefully this will expand even further. Advances still depend on the serious endeavours of medicinal chemists to produce receptor subtype selective, small, orally bioavailable agonists and antagonists that survive degradation in vivo. However, other approaches are promising, including the development of agents that control the expression of receptors that inhibit ATP breakdown by selective inhibition of the known ectonucleotidases and agents that can be used to regulate ATP transport.

Knockout mice are available for a number of P1, P2X and P2Y receptor subtypes, but there are gaps that need to be filled and transgenic models that overexpress receptors, as well as antisense oligonucleotides, are also needed. The siRNA technique is only just beginning to be explored for purinergic signalling.

To conclude, while studies of purinergic sensory neurosignalling are moving forward rapidly and we are clearly on the steep slope of the growth curve, the field is still in its infancy and much new knowledge will hopefully emerge in the coming years.

References

Abbracchio MP, Burnstock G, Boeynaems J-M, Barnard EA, Boyer JL, Kennedy C, Knight GE, Fumagalli M, Gachet C, Jacobson KA, Weisman GA (2006) International Union of Pharmacology. Update and subclassification of the P2Y G protein-coupled nucleotide receptors: from molecular mechanisms and pathophysiology to therapy. Pharmacol Rev 58:281–341

Adriaensen D, Timmermans JP (2004) Purinergic signalling in the lung: important in asthma and COPD? Curr Opin Pharmacol 4:207–214

Adriaensen D, Brouns I, Pintelon I, De Proost I, Timmermans JP (2006) Evidence for a role of neuroepithelial bodies as complex airway sensors: comparison with smooth muscle-associated airway receptors. J Appl Physiol 101:960–970

Agboh KC, Webb TE, Evans RJ, Ennion SJ (2004) Functional characterization of a P2X receptor from *Schistosoma mansoni*. J Biol Chem 279:41650–41657

Alavi AM, Dubyak GR, Burnstock G (2001) Immunohistochemical evidence for ATP receptors in human dental pulp. J Dental Res 80:476–483

Alcayaga C, Varas R, Valdes V, Cerpa V, Arroyo J, Iturriaga R, Alcayaga J (2007) ATP- and ACh-induced responses in isolated cat petrosal ganglion neurons. Brain Res 1131:60–67

Andersson KE, Wein AJ (2004) Pharmacology of the lower urinary tract: basis for current and future treatments of urinary incontinence. Pharmacol Rev 56:581–631

Antunes VR, Bonagamba LG, Machado BH (2005) Hemodynamic and respiratory responses to microinjection of ATP into the intermediate and caudal NTS of awake rats. Brain Res 1032:85–93

Aoki Y, Ohtori S, Takahashi K, Ino H, Ozawa T, Douya H, Chiba T, Moriya H (2003) $P2X_3$-immunoreactive primary sensory neurons innervating lumbar intervertebral disc in rats. Brain Res 989:214–220

Apostolidis A, Popat R, Yiangou Y, Cockayne D, Ford AP, Davis JB, Dasgupta P, Fowler CJ, Anand P (2005) Decreased sensory receptors $P2X_3$ and TRPV1 in suburothelial nerve fibers following intradetrusor injections of botulinum toxin for human detrusor overactivity. J Urol 174:977–982

Arthur DB, Akassoglou K, Insel PA (2005) $P2Y_2$ receptor activates nerve growth factor/TrkA signaling to enhance neuronal differentiation. Proc Natl Acad Sci USA 102:19138–19143

Atiemo H, Wynes J, Chuo J, Nipkow L, Sklar GN, Chai TC (2005) Effect of botulinum toxin on detrusor overactivity induced by intravesical adenosine triphosphate and capsaicin in a rat model. Urology 65:622–626

Bartel DL, Sullivan SL, Lavoie EG, Sévigny J, Finger TE (2006) Nucleoside triphosphate diphosphohydrolase-2 is the ecto-ATPase of type I cells in taste buds. J Comp Neurol 497:1–12

Bertrand PP (2003) ATP and sensory transduction in the enteric nervous system. Neuroscientist 9:243–260

Bertrand PP, Bornstein JC (2002) ATP as a putative sensory mediator: activation of intrinsic sensory neurons of the myenteric plexus via P2X receptors. J Neurosci 22:4767–4775

Bian X, Ren J, DeVries M, Schnegelsberg B, Cockayne DA, Ford AP, Galligan JJ (2003) Peristalsis is impaired in the small intestine of mice lacking the $P2X_3$ subunit. J Physiol 551:309–322

Birder LA (2006) Urinary bladder urothelium: molecular sensors of chemical/thermal/mechanical stimuli. Vasc Pharmacol 45:221–226

Birder LA, Ruan HZ, Chopra B, Xiang Z, Barrick S, Buffington CA, Roppolo JR, Ford AP, de Groat WC, Burnstock G (2004) Alterations in P2X and P2Y purinergic receptor expression in urinary bladder from normal cats and cats with interstitial cystitis. Am J Physiol Renal Physiol 287:F1084–F1091

Blackshaw LA, Brookes SJ, Grundy D, Schemann M (2007) Sensory transmission in the gastrointestinal tract. Neurogastroenterol Motil 19:1–19

Bleehen T, Keele CA (1977) Observations on the algogenic actions of adenosine compounds on human blister base preparation. Pain 3:367–377
Bo X, Alavi A, Xiang Z, Oglesby I, Ford A, Burnstock G (1999) Localization of ATP-gated $P2X_2$ and $P2X_3$ receptor immunoreactive nerves in rat taste buds. Neuroreport 10:1107–1111
Bodin P, Burnstock G (2001) Purinergic signalling: ATP release. Neurochem Res 26:959–969
Borvendeg SJ, Al Khrasani M, Rubini P, Fischer W, Allgaier C, Wirkner K, Himmel HM, Gillen C, Illes P (2003) Subsensitivity of P2X but not vanilloid 1 receptors in dorsal root ganglia of rats caused by cyclophosphamide cystitis. Eur J Pharmacol 474:71–75
Bradbury EJ, Burnstock G, McMahon SB (1998) The expression of $P2X_3$ purinoceptors in sensory neurons: effects of axotomy and glial-derived neurotrophic factor. Mol Cell Neurosci 12:256–268
Brady CM, Apostolidis A, Yiangou Y, Baecker PA, Ford AP, Freeman A, Jacques TS, Fowler CJ, Anand P (2004) $P2X_3$-immunoreactive nerve fibres in neurogenic detrusor overactivity and the effect of intravesical resiniferatoxin. Eur Urol 46:247–253
Braga VA, Soriano RN, Braccialli AL, de Paula PM, Bonagamba LG, Paton JF, Machado BH (2007) Involvement of L-glutamate and ATP in the neurotransmission of the sympathoexcitatory component of the chemoreflex in the commissural nucleus tractus solitarii of awake rats and in the working heart-brainstem preparation. J Physiol 581:1129–1145
Brierley SM, Carter R, Jones W III, Xu L, Robinson DR, Hicks GA, Gebhart GF, Blackshaw LA (2005) Differential chemosensory function and receptor expression of splanchnic and pelvic colonic afferents in mice. J Physiol 567:267–281
Brouns I, Van Genechten J, Burnstock G, Timmermans J-P, Adriaensen D (2003) Ontogenesis of $P2X_3$ receptor-expressing nerve fibres in the rat lung, with special reference to neuroepithelial bodies. Biomed Res 14:80–86
Brouns I, Pintelon I, De Proost I, Alewaters R, Timmermans JP, Adriaensen D (2006) Neurochemical characterisation of sensory receptors in airway smooth muscle: comparison with pulmonary neuroepithelial bodies. Histochem Cell Biol 125:351–367
Burnstock G (1981) Pathophysiology of migraine: a new hypothesis. Lancet 317:1397–1399
Burnstock G (1989) The role of adenosine triphosphate in migraine. Biomed Pharmacother 43:727–736
Burnstock G (1993) Introduction: changing face of autonomic and sensory nerves in the circulation. In: Edvinsson L, Uddman R (eds) Vascular innervation and receptor mechanisms: new perspectives. Academic, San Diego, pp 1–22
Burnstock G (1996a) Purinoceptors: ontogeny and phylogeny. Drug Dev Res 39:204–242
Burnstock G (1996b) A unifying purinergic hypothesis for the initiation of pain. Lancet 347:1604–1605
Burnstock G (1999) Release of vasoactive substances from endothelial cells by shear stress and purinergic mechanosensory transduction. J Anat 194:335–342
Burnstock G (2000) P2X receptors in sensory neurones. Br J Anaesth 84:476–488
Burnstock G (2001a) Purine-mediated signalling in pain and visceral perception. Trends Pharmacol Sci 22:182–188
Burnstock G (2001b) Purinergic signalling in development. In: Abbracchio MP, Williams M (eds) Purinergic and pyrimidinergic signalling I – molecular, nervous and urinogenitary system function. Handbook of experimental pharmacology, vol 151/I. Springer, Berlin, pp 89–127
Burnstock G (2003) Purinergic receptors in the nervous system. In: Schwiebert EM (ed) Purinergic receptors and signalling. Current topics in membranes, vol 54. Academic, San Diego, pp 307–368
Burnstock G (2006) Purinergic P2 receptors as targets for novel analgesics. Pharmacol Therap 110:433–454
Burnstock G (2007) Physiology and pathophysiology of purinergic neurotransmission. Physiol Rev 87:659–797
Burnstock G, Knight GE (2004) Cellular distribution and functions of P2 receptor subtypes in different systems. Int Rev Cytol 240:31–304

Burnstock G, Wood JN (1996) Purinergic receptors: their role in nociception and primary afferent neurotransmission. Curr Opin Neurobiol 6:526–532
Bystrova MF, Yatzenko YE, Fedorov IV, Rogachevskaja OA, Kolesnikov SS (2006) P2Y isoforms operative in mouse taste cells. Cell Tissue Res 323:377–382
Cao Y, Song G (2007) Purinergic modulation of respiration via medullary raphe nuclei in rats. Respir Physiol Neurobiol 155:114–120
Cao Y, Lai W-L, Chen Y-X (2006) Differential regulation of $P2X_3$ protein expression in the rat trigeminal ganglion after experimental tooth movement. West China J Stomatol 24:389–392
Castelucci P, Robbins HL, Furness JB (2003) $P2X_2$ purine receptor immunoreactivity of intraganglionic laminar endings in the mouse gastrointestinal tract. Cell Tissue Res 312:167–174
Ceruti C, Fumagalli M, Verderio C, Abbracchio MP (2006) Nucleotides as neurotransmitters of pain in migraine: a role for P2Y receptors in primary cultures from mouse trigeminal ganglia. In: Proceedings of the American Society for Neuroscience, Atlanta, GA, 14-18 October 2006
Chan ESL, Fernandez P, Cronstein BN (2007) Adenosine in inflammatory joint diseases. Purinergic Signal 3:145–152
Chen C, Nenov A, Bobbin RP (1995a) Noise exposure alters the response of outer hair cells to ATP. Hear Res 88:215–221
Chen CC, Akopian AN, Sivilotti L, Colquhoun D, Burnstock G, Wood JN (1995b) A P2X purinoceptor expressed by a subset of sensory neurons. Nature 377:428–431
Chen CL, Broom DC, Liu Y, de Nooij JC, Li Z, Cen C, Samad OA, Jessell TM, Woolf CJ, Ma Q (2006) Runx1 determines nociceptive sensory neuron phenotype and is required for thermal and neuropathic pain. Neuron 49:365–377
Chessell IP, Hatcher JP, Hughes JP, Ulmann L, Green P, Mander PK, Reeve AJ, Rassendren F (2006) The role of $P2X_7$ and $P2X_4$ in pain processing; common or divergent pathways? Purinergic Signal 2:46–47
Cheung K-K, Burnstock G (2002) Localisation of $P2X_3$ and co-expression with $P2X_2$ receptors during rat embryonic neurogenesis. J Comp Neurol 443:368–382
Cockayne DA, Hamilton SG, Zhu Q-M, Dunn PM, Zhong Y, Novakovic S, Malmberg AB, Cain G, Berson A, Kassotakis L, Hedley L, Lachnit WG, Burnstock G, McMahon SB, Ford APDW (2000) Urinary bladder hyporeflexia and reduced pain-related behaviour in $P2X_3$-deficient mice. Nature 407:1011–1015
Cockayne DA, Dunn PM, Zhong Y, Hamilton SG, Cain GR, Knight GE, Ruan H-Z, Ping Y, Nunn P, Bei M, McMahon SB, Burnstock G, Ford APDW (2005) $P2X_2$ knockout mice and $P2X_2$/$P2X_3$ double knockout mice reveal a role for the $P2X_2$ receptor subunit in mediating multiple sensory effects of ATP. J Physiol 567:621–639
Collier HO, James GWL, Schneider C (1966) Antagonism by aspirin and fenamates of bronchoconstriction and nociception induced by adenosine-5′-triphosphate. Nature 212:411–412
Cook SP, McCleskey EW (2002) Cell damage excites nociceptors through release of cytosolic ATP. Pain 95:41–47
Cooke HJ, Wunderlich J, Christofi FL (2003) "The force be with you": ATP in gut mechanosensory transduction. News Physiol Sci 18:43–49
Damann N, Rothermel M, Klupp BG, Mettenleiter TC, Hatt H, Wetzel CH (2006) Chemosensory properties of murine nasal and cutaneous trigeminal neurons identified by viral tracing. BMC Neurosci 7:46
Dang K, Bielefeldt K, Gebhart GF (2004) Distinct P2X receptors on thoracolumbar and lumbosacral dorsal root ganglion neurons innervating the rat urinary bladder. Abstract viewer/itinerary planner. Program no. 2856.1 2004. Society for Neuroscience, Washington
Dang K, Bielfeldt K, Lamb K, Gebhart GF (2005) Gastric ulcers evoke hyperexcitability and enhance P2X receptor function in rat gastric sensory neurons. J Neurophysiol 93:3112–3119
Davies DL, Kochegarov AA, Kuo ST, Kulkarni AA, Woodward JJ, King BF, Alkana RL (2005) Ethanol differentially affects ATP-gated $P2X_3$ and $P2X_4$ receptor subtypes expressed in Xenopus oocytes. Neuropharmacology 49:243–253

de Groat WC (2006) Integrative control of the lower urinary tract: preclinical perspective. Br J Pharmacol 147:S25–S40

Dell'Antonio G, Quattrini A, Cin ED, Fulgenzi A, Ferrero ME (2002) Relief of inflammatory pain in rats by local use of the selective $P2X_7$ ATP receptor inhibitor, oxidized ATP. Arthritis Rheumatism 46:3378–3385

Denda M, Nakatani M, Ikeyama K, Tsutsumi M, Denda S (2007) Epidermal keratinocytes as the forefront of the sensory system. Exp Dermatol 16:157–161

Dorn G, Patel S, Wotherspoon G, Hemmings-Mieszczak M, Barclay J, Natt FJ, Martin P, Bevan S, Fox A, Ganju P, Wishart W, Hall J (2004) siRNA relieves chronic neuropathic pain. Nucleic Acids Res 32:e49

Dowd E, McQueen DS, Chessell IP, Humphrey PPA (1998) P2X receptor-mediated excitation of nociceptive afferents in the normal and arthritic rat knee joint. Br J Pharmacol 125:341–346

Du S, Araki I, Mikami Y, Zakoji H, Beppu M, Yoshiyama M, Takeda M (2007) Amiloride-sensitive ion channels in urinary bladder epithelium involved in mechanosensory transduction by modulating stretch-evoked adenosine triphosphate release. Urology 69:590–595

Dulon D, Jagger DJ, Lin X, Davis RL (2006) Neuromodulation in the spiral ganglion: shaping signals from the organ of corti to the CNS. J Membr Biol 209:167–175

Dunn PM, Zhong Y, Burnstock G (2001) P2X receptors in peripheral neurones. Prog Neurobiol 65:107–134

Färber K, Kettenmann H (2006) Purinergic signaling and microglia. Pflugers Arch Eur J Physiol 452:615–621

Ferrari D, Pizzirani C, Adinolfi E, Lemoli RM, Curti A, Idzko M, Panther E, Di Virgilio F (2006) The $P2X_7$ receptor: a key player in IL-1 processing and release. J Immunol 176:3877–3883

Finger TE, Danilova V, Barrows J, Bartel DL, Vigers AJ, Stone L, Hellekant G, Kinnamon SC (2005) ATP signaling is crucial for communication from taste buds to gustatory nerves. Science 310:1495–1499

Ford AP, Gever JR, Nunn PA, Zhong Y, Cefalu JS, Dillon MP, Cockayne DA (2006) Purinoceptors as therapeutic targets for lower urinary tract dysfunction. Br J Pharmacol 147:S132–S143

Fountain SJ, Parkinson K, Young MT, Cao L, Thompson CR, North RA (2007) An intracellular P2X receptor required for osmoregulation in *Dictyostelium discoideum*. Nature 448:200–203

Frohlich R, Boehm S, Illes P (1996) Pharmacological characterization of P_2 purinoceptor types in rat locus coeruleus neurons. Eur J Pharmacol 315:255–261

Fukui M, Nakagawa T, Minami M, Satoh M, Kaneko S (2006) Inhibitory role of supraspinal $P2X_3$/$P2X_{2/3}$ subtypes on nociception in rats. Mol Pain 2:19–25

Fumagalli M, Ceruti S, Verderio C, Abbracchio MP (2006) ATP as a neurotransmitter of pain in migraine: a functional role for P2Y receptors in primary cultures from mouse trigeminal sensory ganglia. Purinergic Signal 2:120–121

Furness JB, Kunze WA, Bertrand PP, Clerc N, Bornstein JC (1998) Intrinsic primary afferent neurons of the intestine. Prog Neurobiol 54:1–18

Fyffe REW, Perl ER (1984) Is ATP a central synaptic mediator for certain primary afferent fibres from mammalian skin? Proc Natl Acad Sci USA 81:6890–6893

Gale JE, Piazza V, Ciubotaru CD, Mammano F (2004) A mechanism for sensing noise damage in the inner ear. Curr Biol 14:526–529

Galligan JJ (2004) Enteric P2X receptors as potential targets for drug treatment of the irritable bowel syndrome. Br J Pharmacol 141:1294–1302

Gao Z, Kehoe V, Sinoway LI, Li J (2005) Spinal P2X receptor modulates reflex pressor response to activation of muscle afferents. Am J Physiol Heart Circ Physiol 288:H2238–H2243

Gao N, Hu HZ, Zhu MX, Fang X, Liu S, Gao C, Wood JD (2006) The $P2Y_1$ purinergic receptor expressed by enteric neurones in guinea-pig intestine. Neurogastroenterol Motil 18:316–323

Gayle S, Burnstock G (2005) Immunolocalisation of P2X and P2Y nucleotide receptors in the rat nasal mucosa. Cell Tissue Res 319:27–36

Gerevich Z, Zadori Z, Müller C, Wirkner K, Schröder W, Rubini P, Illes P (2007) Metabotropic P2Y receptors inhibit P2X3 receptor-channels via G protein-dependent facilitation of their desensitization. Br J Pharmacol 151:226–236

Gever J, Cockayne DA, Dillon MP, Burnstock G, Ford APDW (2006) Pharmacology of P2X channels. Pflugers Arch Eur J Physiol 452:513–537

Gilchrist LS, Cain DM, Harding-Rose C, Kov AN, Wendelschafer-Crabb G, Kennedy WR, Simone DA (2005) Re-organization of $P2X_3$ receptor localization on epidermal nerve fibers in a murine model of cancer pain. Brain Res 1044:197–205

Goadsby PJ (2005) Migraine, allodynia, sensitisation and all of that. Eur Neurol 53:10–16

Gourine AV (2005) On the peripheral and central chemoreception and control of breathing: an emerging role of ATP. J Physiol 568:715–724

Gourine AV, Melenchuk EV, Poputnikov DM, Gourine VN, Spyer KM (2002) Involvement of purinergic signalling in central mechanisms of body temperature regulation in rats. Br J Pharmacol 135:2047–2055

Gourine AV, Atkinson L, Deuchars J, Spyer KM (2003) Purinergic signalling in the medullary mechanisms of respiratory control in the rat: respiratory neurones express the $P2X_2$ receptor subunit. J Physiol 552:197–211

Gourine AV, Dale N, Gourine VN, Spyer KM (2004) Fever in systemic inflammation: roles of purines. Front Biosci 9:1011–1022

Green PG, Basbaum AI, Helms C, Levine JD (1991) Purinergic regulation of bradykinin-induced plasma extravasation and adjuvant-induced arthritis in the rat. Proc Natl Acad Sci USA 88:4162–4165

Greenwood D, Jagger DJ, Huang LC, Hoya N, Thorne PR, Wildman SS, King BF, Pak K, Ryan AF, Housley GD (2007) P2X receptor signaling inhibits BDNF-mediated spiral ganglion neuron development in the neonatal rat cochlea. Development 134:1407–1417

Groenewegen HJ, Uylings HB (2000) The prefrontal cortex and the integration of sensory, limbic and autonomic information. Prog Brain Res 126:3–28

Gu YZ, Yin GF, Guan BC, Li ZW (2006) Characteristics of P2X purinoceptors in the membrane of rat trigeminal ganglion neurons. Sheng Li Xue Bao 58:164–170

Hamilton SG, McMahon SB, Lewin GR (2001) Selective activation of nociceptors by P2X receptor agonists in normal and inflamed rat skin. J Physiol 534:437–445

Harms L, Finta EP, Tschöpl M, Illes P (1992) Depolarization of rat locus coeruleus neurons by adenosine 5′-triphosphate. Neuroscience 48:941–952

He L, Chen J, Dinger B, Stensaas L, Fidone S (2006) Effect of chronic hypoxia on purinergic synaptic transmission in rat carotid body. J Appl Physiol 100:157–162

Hegg CC, Lucero MT (2006) Purinergic receptor antagonists inhibit odorant-induced heat shock protein 25 induction in mouse olfactory epithelium. Glia 53:182–190

Hegg CC, Greenwood D, Huang W, Han P, Lucero MT (2003) Activation of purinergic receptor subtypes modulates odor sensitivity. J Neurosci 23:8291–8301

Hemmings-Mieszczak M, Dorn G, Natt FJ, Hall J, Wishart WL (2003) Independent combinatorial effect of antisense oligonucleotides and RNAi-mediated specific inhibition of the recombinant rat $P2X_3$ receptor. Nucleic Acids Res 31:2117–2126

Holton P (1959) The liberation of adenosine triphosphate on antidromic stimulation of sensory nerves. J Physiol (Lond) 145:494–504

Holzer P (2004) Gastrointestinal pain in functional bowel disorders: sensory neurons as novel drug targets. Expert Opin Ther Targets 8:107–123

Holzer P (2007) Taste receptors in the gastrointestinal tract. V. Acid sensing in the gastrointestinal tract. Am J Physiol Gastrointest Liver Physiol 292:G699–G705

Honore P, Donnelly-Roberts D, Namovic MT, Hsieh G, Zhu CZ, Mikusa JP, Hernandez G, Zhong C, Gauvin DM, Chandran P, Harris R, Medrano AP, Carroll W, Marsh K, Sullivan JP, Faltynek CR, Jarvis MF (2006) A-740003 [*N*-(1-{[(cyanoimino)(5-quinolinylamino) methyl]amino}-2, 2-dimethylpropyl)-2-(3,4-dimethoxyphenyl)acetamide], a novel and selective $P2X_7$ receptor antagonist, dose-dependently reduces neuropathic pain in the rat. J Pharmacol Exp Ther 319:1376–1385

Housley GD, Marcotti W, Navaratnam D, Yamoah EN (2006) Hair cells – beyond the transducer. J Membr Biol 209:89–118

Hu B, Chiang CY, Hu JW, Dostrovsky JO, Sessle BJ (2002) P2X receptors in trigeminal subnucleus caudalis modulate central sensitization in trigeminal subnucleus oralis. J Neurophysiol 88:1614–1624

Hu ST, Gever J, Nunn PA, Ford AP, Zhu Q-M (2004) Cystometric studies with ATP, PPADS and TNP-ATP in conscious and anaesthetised C57BL/6 mice. J Urol 171:461–462

Huang LC, Ryan AF, Cockayne DA, Housley GD (2006) Developmentally regulated expression of the $P2X_3$ receptor in the mouse cochlea. Histochem Cell Biol 125:681–692

Huang YJ, Maruyama Y, Dvoryanchikov G, Pereira E, Chaudhari N, Roper SD (2007) The role of pannexin 1 hemichannels in ATP release and cell-cell communication in mouse taste buds. Proc Natl Acad Sci USA 104:6436–6441

Hughes JP, Hatcher JP, Chessell IP (2007) The role of $P2X_7$ in pain and inflammation. Purinergic Signal 3:163–169

Ichikawa H, Fukunaga T, Jin HW, Fujita M, Takano-Yamamoto T, Sugimoto T (2004) VR1-, VRL-1- and $P2X_3$ receptor-immunoreactive innervation of the rat temporomandibular joint. Brain Res 1008:131–136

Ichikawa H, De Repentigny Y, Kothary R, Sugimoto T (2006) The survival of vagal and glossopharyngeal sensory neurons is dependent upon dystonin. Neuroscience 137:531–536

Ikeda H, Tsuda M, Inoue K, Murase K (2007) Long-term potentiation of neuronal excitation by neuron-glia interactions in the rat spinal dorsal horn. Eur J Neurosci 25:1297–1306

Inoue K (2007) P2 receptors and chronic pain. Purinergic Signal 3:135–144

Jahr CE, Jessell TM (1983) ATP excites a subpopulation of rat dorsal horn neurones. Nature 304:730–733

Jennings EA, Christie MJ, Sessle BJ (2006) ATP potentiates neurotransmission in the rat trigeminal subnucleus caudalis. Neuroreport 17:1507–1510

Kamei J, Takahashi Y, Yoshikawa Y, Saitoh A (2005) Involvement of P2X receptor subtypes in ATP-induced enhancement of the cough reflex sensitivity. Eur J Pharmacol 528:158–161

Kataoka S, Toyono T, Seta Y, Ogura T, Toyoshima K (2004) Expression of $P2Y_1$ receptors in rat taste buds. Histochem Cell Biol 121:419–426

Kindig AE, Hayes SG, Kaufman MP (2007) Purinergic 2 receptor blockade prevents the responses of group IV afferents to post-contraction circulatory occlusion. J Physiol 578:301–308

King BF, Knowles I, Burnstock G, Ramage A (2004) Investigation of the effects of P2 purinoceptor ligands on the micturition reflex in female urethane-anaesthetised rats. Br J Pharmacol 142:519–530

Kitchen AM, Collins HL, DiCarlo SE, Scislo TJ, O'Leary DS (2001) Mechanisms mediating NTS P2x receptor-evoked hypotension: cardiac output vs. total peripheral resistance. Am J Physiol Heart Circ Physiol 281:H2198–H2203

Knight GE, Bodin P, de Groat WC, Burnstock G (2002) ATP is released from guinea pig ureter epithelium on distension. Am J Physiol Renal Physiol 282:F281–F288

Kobayashi K, Fukuoka T, Yamanaka H, Dai Y, Obata K, Tokunaga A, Noguchi K (2006) Neurons and glial cells differentially express P2Y receptor mRNAs in the rat dorsal root ganglion and spinal cord. J Comp Neurol 498:443–454

Koizumi S, Fujishita K, Inoue K, Shigemoto-Mogami Y, Tsuda M, Inoue K (2004) Ca^{2+} waves in keratinocytes are transmitted to sensory neurons: the involvement of extracellular ATP and $P2Y_2$ receptor activation. Biochem J 380:329–338

Kollarik M, Dinh QT, Fischer A, Undem BJ (2003) Capsaicin-sensitive and -insensitive vagal bronchopulmonary C-fibres in the mouse. J Physiol 551:869–879

Kollarik M, Ru F, Undem BJ (2007) Acid-sensitive vagal sensory pathways and cough. Pulm Pharmacol Ther 20:402–411

Korim WS, Ferreira-Neto ML, Cravo SLD (2007) Role of NTS P2x receptors in cardiovascular adjustments during alerting defense reactions. FASEB J 21:5750.16

Krishtal OA, Marchenko SM, Pidoplichko VI (1983) Receptor for ATP in the membrane of mammalian sensory neurones. Neurosci Lett 35:41–45

Krishtal O, Lozovaya N, Fedorenko A, Savelyev I, Chizhmakov I (2006) The agonists for nociceptors are ubiquitous, but the modulators are specific: P2X receptors in the sensory neurons are modulated by cannabinoids. Pflugers Arch Eur J Physiol 453:353–360

Labrakakis C, Gerstner E, MacDermott AB (2000) Adenosine triphosphate-evoked currents in cultured dorsal root ganglion neurons obtained from rat embryos: desensitization kinetics and modulation of glutamate release. Neuroscience 101:1117–1126

Lahiri S, Mitchell CH, Reigada D, Roy A, Cherniack NS (2007) Purines, the carotid body and respiration. Respir Physiol Neurobiol 157:123–129

Lazarowski ER, Boucher RC, Harden TK (2003) Mechanisms of release of nucleotides and integration of their action as P2X- and P2Y-receptor activating molecules. Mol Pharmacol 64:785–795

Lee JH, Heo JH, Kim CH, Chang SO, Kim CS, Oh SH (2007) Changes in $P2Y_4$ receptor expression in rat cochlear outer sulcus cells during development. Hear Res 228:201–211

Lewis C, Neidhart S, Holy C, North RA, Buell G, Surprenant A (1995) Coexpression of $P2X_2$ and $P2X_3$ receptor subunits can account for ATP-gated currents in sensory neurons. Nature 377:432–435

Li P, Calejesan AA, Zhou M (1998) ATP P_{2X} receptors and sensory synaptic transmission between primary afferent fibers and spinal dorsal horn neurons in rats. J Neurophysiol 80:3356–3360

Lin JH, Takano T, Arcuino G, Wang X, Hu F, Darzynkiewicz Z, Nunes M, Goldman SA, Nedergaard M (2007) Purinergic signaling regulates neural progenitor cell expansion and neurogenesis. Dev Biol 302:356–366

Llewellyn-Smith IJ, Burnstock G (1998) Ultrastructural localization of $P2X_3$ receptors in rat sensory neurons. Neuroreport 9:2245–2250

Loesch A, Burnstock G (2001) Immunoreactivity to $P2X_6$ receptors in the rat hypothalamo-neurohypophysial system: an ultrastructural study with ExtrAvidin and colloidal gold-silver immunolabelling. Neuroscience 106:621–631

Loredo GA, Benton HP (1998) ATP and UTP activate calcium-mobilizing P2U-like receptors and act synergistically with interleukin-1 to stimulate prostaglandin E_2 release from human rheumatoid synovial cells. Arthritis Rheumatism 41:246–255

Lorier AR, Huxtable AG, Robinson DM, Lipski J, Housley GD, Funk GD (2007) $P2Y_1$ receptor modulation of the pre-Bötzinger complex inspiratory rhythm generating network in vitro. J Neurosci 27:993–1005

Ludlow M, Ennion S (2006) A putative *Dictyostelium discoideum* P2X receptor. Purinergic Signal 2:81–82

Luo J, Yin GF, Gu YZ, Liu Y, Dai JP, Li C, Li ZW (2006) Characterization of three types of ATP-activated current in relation to P2X subunits in rat trigeminal ganglion neurons. Brain Res 1115:9–15

Ma W, Quirion R (2007) Inflammatory mediators modulating the transient receptor potential vanilloid 1 receptor: therapeutic targets to treat inflammatory and neuropathic pain. Expert Opin Ther Targets 11:307–320

Maggi CA, Meli A (1988) The sensory-efferent function of capsaicin-sensitive sensory neurons. Gen Pharmacol 19:1–43

Makowska A, Panfil C, Ellrich J (2006) ATP induces sustained facilitation of craniofacial nociception through P2X receptors on neck muscle nociceptors in mice. Cephalalgia 26:697–706

Matsuka Y, Neubert JK, Maidment NT, Spigelman I (2001) Concurrent release of ATP and substance P within guinea pig trigeminal ganglia in vivo. Brain Res 915:248–255

Matsuka Y, Edmonds B, Mitrirattanakul S, Schweizer FE, Spigelman I (2007) Two types of neurotransmitter release patterns in isolectin B4-positive and negative trigeminal ganglion neurons. Neuroscience 144:665–674

Maul E, Sears M (1979) ATP is released into the rabbit eye by antidromic stimulation of the trigeminal nerve. Invest Ophthalmol Vis Sci 18:256–262

McGaraughty S, Jarvis MF (2006) Purinergic control of neuropathic pain. Drug Dev Res 67:376–388

McGaraughty S, Chu KL, Namovic MT, Donnelly-Roberts DL, Harris RR, Zhang XF, Shieh CC, Wismer CT, Zhu CZ, Gauvin DM, Fabiyi AC, Honore P, Gregg RJ, Kort ME, Nelson DW, Carroll WA, Marsh K, Faltynek CR, Jarvis MF (2007) $P2X_7$-related modulation of pathological nociception in rats. Neuroscience 146:1817–1828

McQueen DS, Bond SM, Moores C, Chessell I, Humphrey PP, Dowd E (1998) Activation of P2X receptors for adenosine triphosphate evokes cardiorespiratory reflexes in anaesthetized rats. J Physiol 507:843–855

Millward-Sadler SJ, Wright MO, Flatman PW, Salter DM (2004) ATP in the mechanotransduction pathway of normal human chondrocytes. Biorheology 41:567–575

Mishra SK, Braun N, Shukla V, Füllgrabe M, Schomerus C, Korf HW, Gachet C, Ikehara Y, Sévigny J, Robson SC, Zimmermann H (2006) Extracellular nucleotide signaling in adult neural stem cells: synergism with growth factor-mediated cellular proliferation. Development 133:675–684

Monro RL, Bertrand PP, Bornstein JC (2004) ATP participates in three excitatory postsynaptic potentials in the submucous plexus of the guinea pig ileum. J Physiol 556:51–584

Moore KH, Ray FR, Barden JA (2001) Loss of purinergic $P2X_3$ and $P2X_5$ receptor innervation in human detrusor from adults with urge incontinence. J Neurosci 21:C166:1–6

Mori M, Tsushima H Matsuda T (1994) Antidiuretic effects of ATP induced by microinjection into the hypothalamic supraoptic nucleus in water-loaded and ethanol-anesthetized rats. Jpn J Pharmacol 66:445–450

Mulkey DK, Mistry AM, Guyenet PG, Bayliss DA (2006) Purinergic P2 receptors modulate excitability but do not mediate *p*H sensitivity of RTN respiratory chemoreceptors. J Neurosci 26:7230–7233

Nagamine K, Ozaki N, Shinoda M, Asai H, Nishiguchi H, Mitsudo K, Tohnai I, Ueda M, Sugiura Y (2006) Mechanical allodynia and thermal hyperalgesia induced by experimental squamous cell carcinoma of the lower gingiva in rats. J Pain 7:659–670

Nakatsuka T, Gu JG (2006) P2X purinoceptors and sensory transmission. Pflugers Arch Eur J Physiol 452:598–607

Nakatsuka T, Tsuzuki K, Ling JX, Sonobe H, Gu JG (2003) Distinct roles of P2X receptors in modulating glutamate release at different primary sensory synapses in rat spinal cord. J Neurophysiol 89:3243–3252

Nazif O, Teichman JM, Gebhart GF (2007) Neural upregulation in interstitial cystitis. Urology 69:24–33

Neal M, Cunningham J (1994) Modulation by endogenous ATP of the light-evoked release of ACh from retinal cholinergic neurones. Br J Pharmacol 113:1085–1087

Nelson DW, Gregg RJ, Kort ME, Perez-Medrano A, Voight EA, Wang Y, Grayson G, Namovic MT, Donnelly-Roberts DL, Niforatos W, Honore P, Jarvis MF, Faltynek CR, Carroll WA (2006) Structure-activity relationship studies on a series of novel, substituted 1-benzyl-5-phenyltetrazole $P2X_7$ antagonists. J Med Chem 49:3659–3666

North RA (2002) Molecular physiology of P2X receptors. Physiol Rev 82:1013–1067

North RA, Verkhratsky A (2006) Purinergic transmission in the central nervous system. Pflugers Arch Eur J Physiol 452:479–485

Norton WHJ, Rohr KB, Burnstock G (2000) Embryonic expression of a $P2X_3$ receptor encoding gene in zebrafish. Mech Dev 99:149–152

Nurse CA (2005) Neurotransmission and neuromodulation in the chemosensory carotid body. Auton Neurosci 120:1–9

Okuse K (2007) Pain signalling pathways: from cytokines to ion channels. Int J Biochem Cell Biol 39:490–496

Oliveira MC, Parada CA, Veiga MC, Rodrigues LR, Barros SP, Tambeli CH (2005) Evidence for the involvement of endogenous ATP and P2X receptors in TMJ pain. Eur J Pain 9:87–93

Pandita RK, Andersson KE (2002) Intravesical adenosine triphosphate stimulates the micturition reflex in awake, freely moving rats. J Urol 168:1230–1234

Papka RE, Hafemeister J, Storey-Workley M (2005) P2X receptors in the rat uterine cervix, lumbosacral dorsal root ganglia, and spinal cord during pregnancy. Cell Tissue Res 321:35–44

Patel MK, Khakh BS, Henderson G (2001) Properties of native P2X receptors in rat trigeminal mesencephalic nucleus neurones: lack of correlation with known, heterologously expressed P2X receptors. Neuropharmacology 40:96–105

Paton JF, De Paula PM, Spyer KM, Machado BH, Boscan P (2002) Sensory afferent selective role of P2 receptors in the nucleus tractus solitarii for mediating the cardiac component of the peripheral chemoreceptor reflex in rats. J Physiol 543:995–1005

Pelleg A, Hurt CM (1990) Evidence for ATP-triggered vagal reflex in the canine heart in vivo. Ann N Y Acad Sci 603:441–442

Piazza V, Ciubotaru CD, Gale JE, Mammano F (2007) Purinergic signalling and intercellular Ca^{2+} wave propagation in the organ of Corti. Cell Calcium 41:77–86

Pintelon I, Brouns I, De Proost I, Van Meir F, Timmermans JP, Adriaensen D (2007) Sensory receptors in the visceral pleura: neurochemical coding and live staining in whole mounts. Am J Respir Cell Mol Biol 36:541–551

Pintor J (2000) Purinergic signalling in the eye. In: Burnstock G, Sillito AM (eds) Nervous control of the eye. Harwood, Amsterdam, pp 171–210

Pintor J, Peral A, Pelaez T, Martin S, Hoyle CH (2003) Presence of diadenosine polyphosphates in the aqueous humor: their effect on intraocular pressure. J Pharmacol Exp Therap 304:342–348

Poelchen W, Sieler D, Wirkner K, Illes P (2001) Co-transmitter function of ATP in central catecholaminergic neurons of the rat. Neuroscience 102:593–602

Puthussery T, Fletcher EL (2006) $P2X_2$ receptors on ganglion and amacrine cells in cone pathways of the rat retina. J Comp Neurol 496:595–609

Puthussery T, Fletcher EL (2007) Neuronal expression of $P2X_3$ purinoceptors in the rat retina. Neuroscience 146:403–414

Puthussery T, Yee P, Vingrys AJ, Fletcher EL (2006) Evidence for the involvement of purinergic $P2X_7$ receptors in outer retinal processing. Eur J Neurosci 24:7–19

Raybould HE, Cooke HJ, Christofi FL (2004) Sensory mechanisms: transmitters, modulators and reflexes. Neurogastroenterol Motil 16:60–63

Ren Y, Zou X, Fang L, Lin Q (2006) Involvement of peripheral purinoceptors in sympathetic modulation of capsaicin-induced sensitization of primary afferent fibers. J Neurophysiol 96:2207–2216

Renton T, Yiangou Y, Baecker PA, Ford AP, Anand P (2003) Capsaicin receptor VR1 and ATP purinoceptor $P2X_3$ in painful and nonpainful human tooth pulp. J Orofac Pain 17:245–250

Resta V, Novelli E, Vozzi G, Scarpa C, Caleo M, Ahluwalia A, Solini A, Santini E, Parisi V, Di Virgilio F, Galli-Resta L (2007) Acute retinal ganglion cell injury caused by intraocular pressure spikes is mediated by endogenous extracellular ATP. Eur J Neurosci 25:2741–2754

Reyes EP, Fernández R, Larraín C, Zapata P (2007) Effects of combined cholinergic-purinergic block upon cat carotid body chemoreceptors in vitro. Respir Physiol Neurobiol 156:17–22

Rich PB, Douillet CD, Mahler SA, Husain SA, Boucher RC (2003) Adenosine triphosphate is released during injurious mechanical ventilation and contributes to lung edema. J Trauma 55:290–297

Robinson DR, McNaughton PA, Evans ML, Hicks GA (2004) Characterization of the primary spinal afferent innervation of the mouse colon using retrograde labelling. Neurogastroenterol Motil 16:113–124

Rocha I, Burnstock G, Spyer KM (2001) Effect on urinary bladder function and arterial blood pressure of the activation of putative purine receptors in brainstem areas. Auton Neurosci 88:6–15

Romanov RA, Rogachevskaja OA, Bystrova MF, Jiang P, Margolskee RF, Kolesnikov SS (2007) Afferent neurotransmission mediated by hemichannels in mammalian taste cells. EMBO J 26:657–667

Rong W, Burnstock G (2004) Activation of ureter nociceptors by exogenous and endogenous ATP in guinea pig. Neuropharmacology 47:1093–1101

Rong W, Burnstock G, Spyer KM (2000) P2X purinoceptor-mediated excitation of trigeminal lingual nerve terminals in an in vitro intra-arterially perfused rat tongue preparation. J Physiol 524:891–902

Rong W, Gourine A, Cockayne DA, Xiang Z, Ford APDW, Spyer KM, Burnstock G (2003) Pivotal role of nucleotide $P2X_2$ receptor subunit mediating ventilatory responses to hypoxia: knockout mouse studies. J Neurosci 23:11315–11321

Ruan H-Z, Burnstock G (2003) Localisation of $P2Y_1$ and $P2Y_4$ receptors in dorsal root, nodose and trigeminal ganglia of the rat. Histochem Cell Biol 120:415–426

Ruan H-Z, Moules E, Burnstock G (2004) Changes in P2X purinoceptors in sensory ganglia of the mouse during embryonic and postnatal development. Histochem Cell Biol 122:539–551

Ruan H-Z, Birder LA, de Groat WC, Tai C, Roppolo J, Buffington A, Burnstock G (2005) Localization of P2X and P2Y receptors in dorsal root ganglia of the cat. J Histochem Cytochem 53:1273–1282

Ruan T, Lin YS, Lin KS, Kou YR (2006) Mediator mechanisms involved in TRPV1 and P2X receptor-mediated, ROS-evoked bradypneic reflex in anesthetized rats. J Appl Physiol 101:644–654

Rubino A, Burnstock G (1996) Capsaicin-sensitive sensory-motor neurotransmission in the peripheral control of cardiovascular function. Cardiovasc Res 31:467–479

Ruggieri MR Sr (2006) Mechanisms of disease: role of purinergic signaling in the pathophysiology of bladder dysfunction. Nat Clin Pract Urol 3:206–215

Salas NA, Somogyi GT, Gangitano DA, Boone TB, Smith CP (2007) Receptor activated bladder and spinal ATP release in neurally intact and chronic spinal cord injured rats. Neurochem Int 50:45–350

Salter MW, Henry JL (1985) Effects of adenosine 5′-monophosphate and adenosine 5′-triphosphate on functionally identified units in the cat spinal dorsal horn. Evidence for a differential effect of adenosine 5′-triphosphate on nociceptive vs non-nociceptive units. Neuroscience 15:15–825

Schwiebert EM, Zsembery A, Geibel JP (2003) Cellular mechanisms and physiology of nucleotide and nucleoside release from cells: current knowledge, novel assays to detect purinergic agonists, and future directions. Curr Top Membr 54:31–58

Scislo TJ, Ichinose T, O'Leary DS (2007) Activation of NTS A_1 adenosine receptors differentially resets baroreflex control of adrenal (ASNA) and renal (RSNA) sympathetic nerve activity. FASEB J 21:582.15

Seino D, Tokunaga A, Tachibana T, Yoshiya S, Dai Y, Obata K, Yamanaka H, Kobayashi K, Noguchi K (2006) The role of ERK signaling and the P2X receptor on mechanical pain evoked by movement of inflamed knee joint. Pain 123:193–203

Sharp CJ, Reeve AJ, Collins SD, Martindale JC, Summerfield SG, Sargent BS, Bate ST, Chessell IP (2006) Investigation into the role of $P2X_3$/$P2X_{2/3}$ receptors in neuropathic pain following chronic constriction injury in the rat: an electrophysiological study. Br J Pharmacol 148:845–852

Shen J, Harada N, Nakazawa H, Kaneko T, Izumikawa M, Yamashita T (2006) Role of nitric oxide on ATP-induced Ca^{2+} signaling in outer hair cells of the guinea pig cochlea. Brain Res 1081:101–112

Shieh C-C, Jarvis MF, Lee C-H, Perner RJ (2006) P2X receptor ligands and pain. Expert Opin Ther Patents 16:1113–1127

Shimizu I, Iida T, Guan Y, Zhao C, Raja SN, Jarvis MF, Cockayne DA, Caterina MJ (2005) Enhanced thermal avoidance in mice lacking the ATP receptor $P2X_3$. Pain 116:96–108

Shinoda M, Ozaki N, Asai H, Nagamine K, Sugiura Y (2005) Changes in $P2X_3$ receptor expression in the trigeminal ganglion following monoarthritis of the temporomandibular joint in rats. Pain 116:42–51

Shiokawa H, Nakatsuka T, Furue H, Tsuda M, Katafuchi T, Inoue K, Yoshimura M (2006) Direct excitation of deep dorsal horn neurones in the rat spinal cord by the activation of postsynaptic P2X receptors. J Physiol 573:753–763

Smith CP, Vemulakonda VM, Kiss S, Boone TB, Somogyi GT (2005) Enhanced ATP release from rat bladder urothelium during chronic bladder inflammation: effect of botulinum toxin A. Neurochem Int 47:291–297

Song Z, Sladek CD (2006) Site of ATP and phenylephrine synergistic stimulation of vasopressin release from the hypothalamo-neurohypophyseal system. J Neuroendocrinol 18:266–272

Song Z, Vijayaraghavan S, Sladek CD (2007) ATP increases intracellular calcium in supraoptic neurons by activation of both P2X and P2Y purinergic receptors. Am J Physiol Regul Integr Comp Physiol 292:R423–R431

Sorimachi M, Wakamoria M, Akaikeb N (2006) Excitatory effect of ATP on rat area postrema neurons. Purinergic Signal 2:545–557

Spyer KM, Dale N, Gourine AV (2004) ATP is a key mediator of central and peripheral chemosensory transduction. Exp Physiol 89:53–59

Staikopoulos V, Sessle BJ, Furness JB, Jennings EA (2007) Localization of $P2X_2$ and $P2X_3$ receptors in rat trigeminal ganglion neurons. Neuroscience 144:208–216

Stone LS, Vulchanova L (2003) The pain of antisense: in vivo application of antisense oligonucleotides for functional genomics in pain and analgesia. Adv Drug Deliv Rev 55:1081–1112

Stucky CL, Medler KA, Molliver DC (2004) The P2Y agonist UTP activates cutaneous afferent fibers. Pain 109:36–44

Szücs A, Szappanos H, Batta TJ, Tóth A, Szigeti GP, Panyi G, Csernoch L, Sziklai I (2006) Changes in purinoceptor distribution and intracellular calcium levels following noise exposure in the outer hair cells of the guinea pig. J Membr Biol 213:135–141

Taylor-Clark T, Undem BJ (2006) Transduction mechanisms in airway sensory nerves. J Appl Physiol 101:950–959

Tempest HV, Dixon AK, Turner WH, Elneil S, Sellers LA, Ferguson DR (2004) P2X and P2X receptor expression in human bladder urothelium and changes in interstitial cystitis. BJU Int 93:1344–1348

Terasawa E, Keen KL, Grendell RL, Golos TG (2005) Possible role of 5′-adenosine triphosphate in synchronization of Ca^{2+} oscillations in primate luteinizing hormone-releasing hormone neurons. Mol Endocrinol 19:2736–2747

Trang T, Beggs S, Salter MW (2006) Purinoceptors in microglia and neuropathic pain. Pflugers Arch Eur J Physiol 452:645–652

Trapido-Rosenthal HG, Carr WE, Gleeson RA (1989) Biochemistry of purinergic olfaction. The importance of nucleotide dephosphorylation. In: Brand JG, Teeter H, Cagan RH, Kare MR (eds) Receptor events and transduction in taste and olfaction. Chemical senses, vol 1. Dekker, New York, pp 243–262

Tsuda M, Inoue K (2006) P2X receptors in sensory neurons. Curr Top Membr 57:277–310

Tsuda M, Shigemoto-Mogami Y, Koizumi S, Mizokoshi A, Kohsaka S, Salter MW, Inoue K (2003) $P2X_4$ receptors induced in spinal microglia gate tactile allodynia after nerve injury. Nature 424:778–783

Undem BJ, Chuaychoo B, Lee MG, Weinreich D, Myers AC, Kollarik M (2004) Subtypes of vagal afferent C-fibres in guinea-pig lungs. J Physiol 556:905–917

US 2005/0209260 A1 (Hoffmann-La Roche Pharmaceuticals) Broka CA, Carter DS, Dillon MP, Hawley RC, Jahangir A, Lin CJJ, Parish DW (Sep 22, 2005). Diaminopyrimidines as $P2X_3$ and $P2X_{2/3}$ antagonists.

Vlajkovic SM, Vinayagamoorthy A, Thorne PR, Robson SC, Wang CJ, Housley GD (2006) Noise-induced up-regulation of NTPDase3 expression in the rat cochlea: implications for auditory transmission and cochlear protection. Brain Res 1104:55–63

Vlaskovska M, Kasakov L, Rong W, Bodin P, Bardini M, Cockayne DA, Ford APDW, Burnstock G (2001) $P2X_3$ knockout mice reveal a major sensory role for urothelially released ATP. J Neurosci 21:5670–5677

Waeber C, Moskowitz MA (2003) Therapeutic implications of central and peripheral neurologic mechanisms in migraine. Neurology 61:S9–S20

Wang JC, Raybould NP, Luo L, Ryan AF, Cannell MB, Thorne PR, Housley GD (2003) Noise induces up-regulation of $P2X_2$ receptor subunit of ATP-gated ion channels in the rat cochlea. Neuroreport 14:817–823

Wang LC, Xiong W, Zheng J, Zhou Y, Zheng H, Zhang C, Zheng LH, Zhu XL, Xiong ZQ, Wang LY, Cheng HP, Zhou Z (2006) The timing of endocytosis after activation of a G-protein-coupled receptor in a sensory neuron. Biophys J 90:3590–3598

Watano T, Calvert JA, Vial C, Forsythe ID, Evans RJ (2004) P2X receptor subtype-specific modulation of excitatory and inhibitory synaptic inputs in the rat brainstem. J Physiol 558:745–757

Werner-Reiss U, Galun R, Crnjar R, Liscia A (1999) Sensitivity of the mosquito *Aedes aegypti* (Culicidae) labral apical chemoreceptors to phagostimulants. J Insect Physiol 45:629–636

Wheeler-Schilling TH, Marquordt K, Kohler K, Guenther E, Jabs R (2001) Identification of purinergic receptors in retinal ganglion cells. Brain Res Mol Brain Res 92:177–180

Wong AY, Billups B, Johnston J, Evans RJ, Forsythe ID (2006) Endogenous activation of adenosine A1 receptors, but not P2X receptors, during high-frequency synaptic transmission at the calyx of Held. J Neurophysiol 95:3336–3342

Wu C, Sui GP, Fry CH (2004) Purinergic regulation of guinea pig suburothelial myofibroblasts. J Physiol 559:231–243

Wynn G, Rong W, Xiang Z, Burnstock G (2003) Purinergic mechanisms contribute to mechanosensory transduction in the rat colorectum. Gastroenterology 125:1398–1409

Wynn G, Bei M, Ruan H-Z, Burnstock G (2004) Purinergic component of mechanosensory transduction is increased in a rat model of colitis. Am J Physiol Gastrointest Liver Physiol 287:G647–G657

Xiang Z, Burnstock G (2004a) $P2X_2$ and $P2X_3$ purinoceptors in the rat enteric nervous system. Histochem Cell Biol 121:169–179

Xiang Z, Burnstock G (2004b) Development of nerves expressing $P2X_3$ receptors in the myenteric plexus of rat stomach. Histochem Cell Biol 122:111–119

Xiang Z, Burnstock G (2006) Distribution of $P2Y_6$ and $P2Y_{12}$ receptors: their colocalisation with calbindin, calretinin and nitric oxide synthase in the guinea pig enteric nervous system. Histochem Cell Biol 125:327–336

Xiang Z, He C, Burnstock G (2006) $P2X_5$ receptors are expressed on neurons containing arginine vasopressin and neuronal nitric oxide synthase in the rat hypothalamus. Brain Res 1099:56–63

Xu J, Kussmaul W, Kurnik PB, Al-Ahdav M, Pelleg A (2005) Electrophysiological-anatomic correlates of ATP-triggered vagal reflex in the dog. V. Role of purinergic receptors. Am J Physiol Regul Integr Comp Physiol 288:R651–R655

Xue J, Askwith C, Javed NH, Cooke HJ (2007) Autonomic nervous system and secretion across the intestinal mucosal surface. Auton Neurosci 133:55–63

Yajima H, Sato J, Giron R, Nakamura R, Mizumura K (2005) Inhibitory, facilitatory, and excitatory effects of ATP and purinergic receptor agonists on the activity of rat cutaneous nociceptors in vitro. Neurosci Res 51:405–416

Yu S, Undem BJ, Kollarik M (2005) Vagal afferent nerves with nociceptive properties in guinea-pig oesophagus. J Physiol 563:831–842

Zagorodnyuk VP, Chen BN, Costa M, Brookes SJ (2003) Mechanotransduction by intraganglionic laminar endings of vagal tension receptors in the guinea-pig oesophagus. J Physiol 553:575–587

Zapata P (2007) Is ATP a suitable co-transmitter in carotid body arterial chemoreceptors? Respir Physiol Neurobiol 157:106–115

Zarei MM, Toro B, McCleskey EW (2004) Purinergic synapses formed between rat sensory neurons in primary culture. Neuroscience 126:195–201

Zhang M, Nurse CA (2004) CO_2/*p*H chemosensory signaling in co-cultures of rat carotid body receptors and petrosal neurons: role of ATP and ACh. J Neurophysiol 92:3433–3445

Zhang X, Zhang M, Laties AM, Mitchell CH (2005) Stimulation of $P2X_7$ receptors elevates Ca^{2+} and kills retinal ganglion cells. Invest Ophthalmol Vis Sci 46:2183–2191

Zhang X, Zhang M, Laties AM, Mitchell CH (2006) Balance of purines may determine life or death of retinal ganglion cells as A_3 adenosine receptors prevent loss following $P2X_7$ receptor stimulation. J Neurochem 98:566–575

Zhang M, Buttigieg J, Nurse CA (2007a) Neurotransmitter mechanisms mediating low-glucose signalling in cocultures and fresh tissue slices of rat carotid body. J Physiol 578:735–750

Zhang X, Chen Y, Wang C, Huang LY (2007b) Neuronal somatic ATP release triggers neuron-satellite glial cell communication in dorsal root ganglia. Proc Natl Acad Sci USA 104:9864–9869

Zimmermann H (2006) Nucleotide signaling in nervous system development. Pflugers Arch Eur J Physiol 452:573–588

Zimmermann K, Reeh PW, Averbeck B (2002) ATP can enhance the proton-induced CGRP release through P2Y receptors and secondary PGE_2 release in isolated rat dura mater. Pain 97:259–265

Sensory-Nerve-Derived Neuropeptides: Possible Therapeutic Targets

Elizabeth S. Fernandes, Sabine M. Schmidhuber, and Susan D. Brain

Contents

Abstract This review examines our developing understanding of the families and activities of some of the best known sensory-nerve-derived inflammatory neuropeptides, namely substance P, calcitonin gene-related peptide and galanin. Evidence to date shows involvement of these transmitters in a wide range of systems that includes roles as inflammatory modulators. There is an increasing understanding of the mechanisms involved in the release of the peptides from sensory nerves and these are key in understanding the potential of neuropeptides in modulating inflammatory responses and may also provide novel targets for anti-inflammatory therapy. The neuropeptides released act via specific G protein coupled receptors, most of which have now been cloned. There is knowledge of selective agonists and antagonists for many subtypes within these families. The study

S.D. Brain (✉)
Cardiovascular Division, King's College London, Franklin-Wilkins Building, Waterloo Campus, London SE1 9NH, UK
sue.brain@kcl.ac.uk

B.J. Canning and D. Spina (eds.), *Sensory Nerves*,
Handbook of Experimental Pharmacology 194, DOI: 10.1007/978-3-540-79090-7_11,

of neuropeptides in animal models has additionally revealed pathophysiological roles that in turn have led to the development of new drugs, based on selective receptor antagonism.

Keywords Neuropeptides, Substance P, CGRP, Galanin

Abbreviations

AM	Adrenomedullin
AM_1	Adrenomedullin receptor type 1
AM_2	Adrenomedullin receptor type 2
CGRP	Calcitonin gene-related peptide
CL	Calcitonin receptor-like receptor
DRG	Dorsal root ganglia
GAL	Galanin
GALP	Galanin-like peptide
GMAP	Galanin-message-associated peptide
mRNA	Messenger RNA
NKA	Neurokinin A
NKB	Neurokinin B
RAMP	Receptor activity modifying protein
SP	Substance P
TRPV1	Transient receptor potential vanilloid 1

1 Introduction

A diverse range of chemically distinct neuropeptides are contained in and released from a range of sensory nerves. They exhibit selective patterns of localization within the peripheral and central nervous system and they possess the ability to stimulate a range of diverse biological activities. One of the earliest to be intensively researched was the opioid family. This was soon followed by a sustained focus on substance P (SP), the later interest that developed in calcitonin gene-related peptide (CGRP) and the more recent interest in galanin (GAL). Interest in and research into these and other neuropeptides remains high, despite a lack of evidence of a primary pathological role for these peptides in many cases. This lack of research information is often due to difficulties in obtaining ligands for use as experimental tools that are specific enough to act in a selective manner to either enhance or block activity or synthesis. Furthermore, it is now becoming more common to discover that a structurally related peptide or peptides can be released from non-neuronal tissues, which can act via the same receptors as the neuronal sources. This adds another level of interest as well as complexity to unravelling their importance in biological systems.

In this chapter we will discuss the activities of three neuropeptide families that are associated with pain and inflammation pathways and which we have studied in skin. The first of these is SP. This was the first neuropeptide to be discovered more than 70 years ago by Von Euler and Gaddum (1931), and remains under substantial investigation. We will also evaluate evidence that the CGRP and GAL families could play pivotal roles in diseases that involve vascular inflammation.

2 Sensory-Nerve-Derived Neuropeptides

The sensory nerves that contain and release neuroptides are of mixed type composed of unmyelinated sensory C-fibres that are most abundant, with also myelinated Aδ-fibres. They innervate most organs, with a particular dense perivascular network of nerves around blood vessels, where nerve endings often terminate in close association with endothelial cells. Their classic neurogenic inflammatory roles will be considered first and this will be followed by a discussion of their role in disease. Evidence indicating the neuronal participation and nerve-derived transmitters in vascular events were revealed more than one century ago. In 1876, it was proposed by Stricker that sensory afferent nerves might be involved in the inflammatory process. Indeed, the antidromic stimulation of peripheral sensory nerves leads to cutaneous vasodilatation (Bayliss 1901). This is a component of the well-studied "triple response" to injury that is easily observed in Caucasian human skin (Lewis 1927) in response to insect bites and other punctate injuries. The response has three major components. One is a wheal, or swelling, due to oedema formation, that is secondary to increased microvascular permeability. The second is local reddening that is due to increased blood flow at the site of injury. The third is a flare that can be observed for up to several centimetres around the injury. The flare is a consequence of a sensory-nerve-mediated axon reflex where antidromic stimulation of sensory nerves that are linked via a collateral system leads to the release from perivascular nerve endings of neuropeptides. Since then, much evidence has accumulated showing that activation of sensory nerves by a range of stimuli such as local depolarization, axonal or dorsal root reflexes leads to the release of biologically active molecules (Richardson and Vasko 2002). It is now understood that axon reflexes involving sensory nerves occur in most tissues of the body and are central to the response of skin to injury. Whilst these acute vasoactive responses are easily observed in this experimental model, there is now evidence to suggest that neuropeptides also have roles in modulating more chronic aspects of inflammatory responses in a range of tissues. However, a direct pivotal role of neuropeptides in skin disease has yet to be proven.

The pungent agent from chilli peppers, capsaicin, is an important pharmacological tool and was shown to activate sensory nerves some time ago (Jancsó et al. 1967, 1977). Capsaicin at first activates and then desensitizes sensory nerves and evidence using capsaicin to deplete or block sensory nerves has established the concept that sensory nerves are involved in pain and inflammatory syndromes.

More recently, the transient receptor potential vanilloid 1 (TRPV1) has been established as the ion channel receptor that is activated by capsaicin and related vanilloids (Caterina et al. 1997). The first antagonist to be described was capsazepine (Bevan et al. 1992). Today a range of TRPV1 ligands exist and are being examined for their efficacy in both preclinical and clinical models of pain and inflammation. Endogenous stimuli that mediate sensory nerve activation are discussed elsewhere in this book. However, a range of related ion channels and mediators may also play important roles (Chahl 2004; Brain and Cox 2006).

3 Substance P and the Tachykinin Family

The tachykinin family is formed by peptides that include SP, neurokinin A (NKA) and neurokinin B (NKB). These peptides are widely distributed in both the central and the peripheral nervous system and they exert their actions by activating three different seven transmembrane domain G protein coupled receptors known as NK_1, NK_2 and NK_3 (Buck 1988; Maggi 1995; Brain and Cox 2006). It is now established that SP exhibits higher affinity for the NK_1 receptor, while NKA and NKB preferentially bind to NK_2 and NK_3 receptors, respectively (Mussap et al. 1993; Regoli et al. 1994). Figure 1 shows the biosynthesis of SP, NKA (NPK and NPγ) as well as their respective preferred receptors. The efforts in studying and identifying selective and competitive antagonists for NK_1, NK_2 and NK_3 receptors allowed considerable and important progress in understanding the pathophysiological role of this family of peptides (Regoli et al. 1994; Khawaja and Rogers 1996). Neurokinins are implicated in distinct biological events, many of which are associated with the inflammatory process (Fig. 2). They include plasma extravasation, vasodilatation (Germonpré et al. 1995; Holzer 1998) and other cardiovascular responses (Regoli et al. 1994; Walsh and McWilliams 2006; Dzurik et al. 2007), smooth-muscle contraction and relaxation, salivary secretion (Holzer-Petsche 1995), airway contraction (Joos et al. 1995) and immune responses (Koon and Pothoulakis 2006; Ikeda et al. 2007).

SP and other neurokinins are released to exert effects synergistically with other neuropeptides such as CGRP and vasoactive intestinal peptide (Brain and Williams 1985; Maggi 1997; Holzer 1998; Richardson and Vasko 2002; Brain and Cox 2006). These substances, when released, act on target cells in the periphery such as mast cells, immune cells and vascular smooth muscle, leading to inflammation which is characterized by redness and warmth, swelling and hypersensitivity (Richardson and Vasko 2002).

SP is a undecapeptide widely distributed in the central, peripheral and enteric nervous system (Diz et al. 2002) and is considered a potent mediator of neurogenic inflammation, acting as a cotransmitter in primary afferent nerve fibres. There is also a large body of evidence implicating a role for SP as a "pain-transmitter" mediator (Weber et al. 2001; Vachon et al. 2004; Gradl et al. 2007). SP is a vasodilator, especially in large blood vessels, but is better known for its ability to

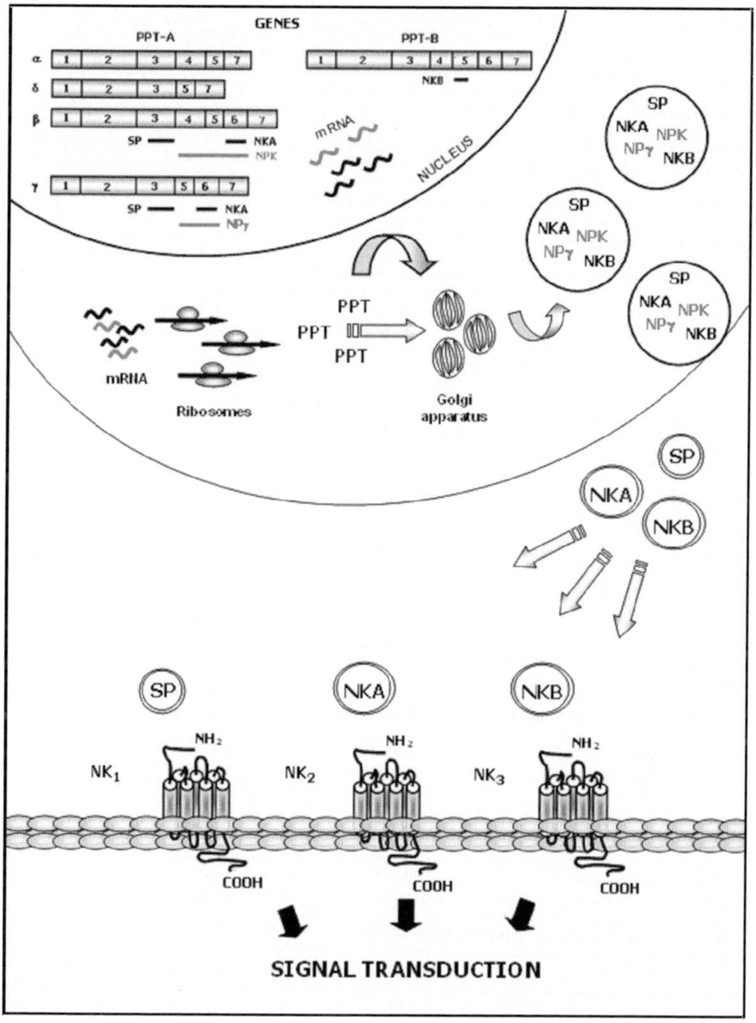

Fig. 1 Two genes are involved in substance P (SP), neurokinin A (NKA) and neurokinin B (NKB) expression. The *PPT-A* gene is represented by four distinct subtypes (α, δ, β and γ). SP can be generated from exon 3 via all *PPT-A* gene variants, while NKA and its elongated forms (NPK and NPγ) can only be generated via β and γ variants. The *PPT-B* gene can only decode NKB. Following both *PPT-A* and *PPT-B* transcription, a prepropeptide (*PPT*) is formed inside the ribosomes and cleaved in the Golgi apparatus, producing SP, NKA (NPK and NPγ) and NKB that remain in intracellular vesicles until there are further stimuli. Once stimulated, neuronal and non-neuronal cells release tachykinins, allowing them to bind to their receptors and activate their intracellular pathways. Tachykinin receptors NK_1, NK_2 and NK_3 are G protein coupled receptors. SP bind with higher affinity to the NK_1 receptor, while NKA and NKB preferentially bind to NK_2 and NK_3 receptors, respectively

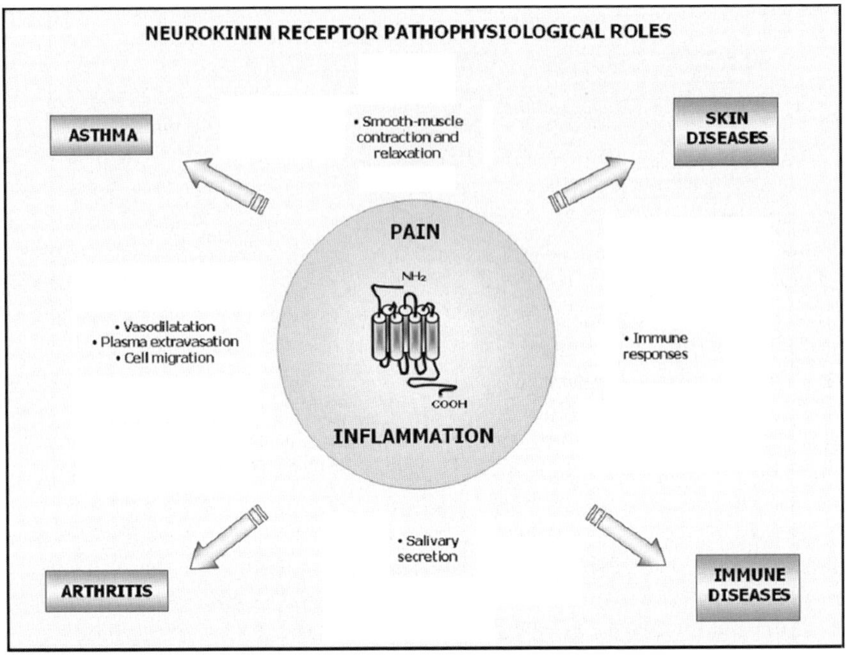

Fig. 2 Tachykinins, acting via their receptors, exert both physiological and pathological effects throughout different systems. They can regulate vascular permeability and vasodilatation, leading to increased plasma leakage. They can drive cell migration into an inflammatory site, control salivary secretion, stimulate smooth-muscle contraction and relaxation and activate immune cells controlling immune responses. All these ubiquitous effects are normally well regulated, but in some situations, the effects of tachykinins can become deleterious and participate in a negative manner in the disease process

increase microvascular permeability leading to oedema formation (Holzer 1998; Fig. 4). SP affects vascular permeability by two main pathways: (1) activation of endothelial NK_1 receptors to increase plasma leakage and (2) mast cell degranulation to release oedema-induced amines (Foreman et al. 1983). SP and its receptor NK_1 are proposed to be involved in a range of inflammatory diseases such as arthritis, inflammatory bowel disease, airway disease, dermatitis and psoriasis (Eysselein and Nast 1991; Keeble and Brain 2004; Peters et al. 2006; Saraceno et al. 2006; Pavlovic et al. 2008; Gross and Pothoulakis 2007).

SP also has a role in immune responses (Koon and Pothoulakis 2006; Zhang et al. 2007). In fact, SP can drive cellular infiltration indirectly by inducing cytokine release (Peters et al. 2006). The role of SP will be explored in a range of diseases.

3.1 An Inflammatory Role for Substance P in Arthritis

There is compelling evidence supporting the role of neurokinins in joint disease. SP is widely distributed in nerves localized in joints (Iwasaki et al. 1995). SP-positive cells are also found surrounding blood vessels in the joint and also SP-containing neurons are located in bone marrow, some of which communicate with the synovium (Iwasaki et al. 1995). This SP expression suggests that this peptide could be released in the joint causing the hyperaemia and increased vascular permeability observed in the diseased joint (Campos and Calixto 2000). On the other hand, a reduction in SP-containing nerves in the synovium, mainly in tissues with higher cell influx, has been reported; thus, it could be suggested that SP expression can be upregulated and downregulated depending on the stage of the disease (Konttinen et al. 1992; Keeble and Brain 2004). Changes in SP expression also occur in the dorsal horn (Garrett et al. 1995). This can vary according to the animal model being studied (Sluka and Westlund 1993; Bulling et al. 2001). NK_1 receptor expression can be altered in arthritis (Kar et al. 1994). Other studies have reported an increased concentration of SP and also CGRP in both ankle joints and dorsal root ganglia (DRG) in a rat adjuvant arthritis model (Ahmed et al. 1995). Exogenous SP administration into the joint causes plasma extravasation and vasodilatation in normal animals (Lam and Ferrell 1993; Lam and Wong 1996; Ferrell et al. 1997). Non-peptide orally administrable neurokinin antagonists have been used to establish the potential mechanisms and importance of neurokinins in arthritis; however, controversial data have been collected. Intra-articular injection of the NK_1 receptor antagonist L-703606 before but not after joint inflammation induction had beneficial effects on inflammatory pain in the rat knee (Hong et al. 2002). Another NK_1 antagonist, CP99994, was capable of preventing both pain and inflammation induced by kaolin and carrageenan when given directly into the knee joint (Sluka et al. 1997). Thus, direct intraknee administration of NK_1 antagonists could represent a very useful therapy for arthritis.

3.2 Substance P in Skin Diseases

There are substantial reports suggesting a role for neuropeptides in skin diseases. SP mediates pain and itch sensation via small-diameter C fibres integrated into the dorsal horn of the spinal cord (Saraceno et al. 2006). Peripheral release of SP may initiate secondary release of inflammatory mediators in diseased skin (Peters et al. 2006). In fact, findings relate neuropeptide release to several skin diseases. Psoriatic plaques express higher number of intraepidermal SP-positive nerve fibres when compared with normal skin in immunohistochemistry and immunofluorescence studies (Al'Abadie et al. 1995; Chan et al. 1997; Jiang et al. 1998). Controversially, Pincelli et al. (1992) showed lower levels of SP using a radioimmunoassay technique. These discrepant data could be related to different methods used to study SP involvement. SP can act via a receptor-independent effect on skin resident mast cells. However, receptor-mediated effects via other skin resident cells such as keratinocytes and fibroblasts also need to be considered. Human and murine keratinocytes express functional NK_1 receptors with high affinity for SP (Steinhoff et al. 2003; Peters et al. 2006). Also, SP induces proliferation of murine and human dermal keratinocytes and fibroblasts (Nilsson et al. 1985; Tanaka et al. 1988; Scholzen et al. 1998). In addition, SP promotes fibroblast migration in an NK_1-independent way (Khaler et al. 1993). In various experimental models of cutaneous inflammation, SP has been shown to exacerbate inflammation via a wide variety of proinflammatory and immunoregulatory effects (Goetzl et al. 1985; Shepherd et al. 2005). In addition to the release of neuropeptides in a skin disease, their actions over the immune system are being speculated upon. SP is capable of causing tumour necrosis factor α release from mast cells independent of NK_1 receptor activation (Ansel et al. 1993), while keratinocyte-derived interleukin-1 can activate cutaneous and infiltrating cells, triggering the additional axonal transport and release of neuropeptides from sensory nerves (Jeanjean et al. 1995; Viac et al. 1996). Neuropeptide-induced hyperaemia can contribute to cell influx by increasing vascular permeability and SP increases cell adhesion by upregulating vascular and intercellular cell adhesion molecule 1 (Lindsey et al. 2000; Peters et al. 2006). SP can also stimulate natural killer cells, lymphocyte and eosinophil activation (Lindsey et al. 2000; Foster and Cunningham 2003; Feistritzer et al. 2003; Peters et al. 2006; Ikeda et al. 2007).

3.3 Substance P and Sepsis

Various studies in both human and animals have investigated a link between SP release and immune responses. Evidence is accumulating from studies involving gastrointestinal inflammatory conditions and sepsis. Elevated systemic levels of SP are detected in patients with postoperative sepsis and they are related to the lethal outcome of sepsis (Beer et al. 2002). Previous studies showed increased levels of SP in both plasma and lung in septic mice and that lung inflammation and damage are attenuated by the genetic ablation of SP, suggesting a crucial role for SP in sepsis (Puneet et al. 2006). Also, H_2S upregulates SP generation, which drives the inflammatory response in the sepsis induced by cecal ligation puncture by activating NK_1 receptors (Zhang et al. 2007). On the other hand, NK_1, NK_2 and NK_3 receptors do not appear to be related to the acute production of nitric oxide detected in the peritoneal cavity of animals with severe sepsis induced by lipopolysaccharide (Clark et al. 2007). These differences could be related to the target site (lung and peritoneal cavity) as well as to the animal model evaluated.

3.4 Substance P and the Gut

Accumulating evidence indicates that the NK_1 receptor and SP are involved in the immunoregulatory circuit in several pathophysiological gut responses (Koon and Pothoulakis 2006). It was previous demonstrated that treatment with the NK_1 receptor CP-96345 inhibited all secretory and inflammatory responses associated with the production of toxin A released from *Clostridium difficile* in the rat gut (Pothoulakis et al. 1994). Also, it was demonstrated that toxin A causes an increase of SP in the DRG followed by an increase of SP in the intestinal mucosa (Castagliuolo et al. 1994). In addition, the NK_1 receptor is found to be upregulated in the Peyer's patches and mesenteric lymph nodes of mice treated with *Salmonella* (Kincy-Cain and Bost 1996). Administration of the NK_1 receptor antagonist spantide II resulted in early onset of *Salmonella* infection, increased mortality and reduction of interleukin-12 and interferon-γ messenger RNA (mRNA) levels in the intestinal mucosal (Kincy-Cain and Bost 1996). A potential role for SP in parasitic infections such as *Trichinella spiralis*, *Nippostrongylus brasiliensis* and *Schistossoma mansoni* is also being investigated (Woodbury et al. 1984; Bienenstock et al. 1987; Stead et al. 1987; Neil et al. 1991; Blum et al. 1993, 1999; Khan and Collins 2004).

3.5 Clinical Trials with the Tachykinin Receptor Antagonists

During the 1980s and 1990s a number of non-peptide receptor antagonists for the major vasoactive receptor for SP (the tachykinin NK_1 receptor) were developed. However, published results from clinical trials in this area are disappointing and it is now generally understood that NK_1 antagonists do not have a beneficial effect in the treatment of human inflammatory conditions. The mixed peptide NK_1 and NK_2 receptor antagonist FK224 and the non-peptide selective NK_1 receptor antagonist CP99994 were tested in clinical trials and both had negative effects. This was a disappointing finding as NK_1 receptors had been shown to be involved in bronchoconstriction, mucus secretion, microvascular leakage and vasodilatation (Joos et al. 1995). NK_1 antagonists were also tested as an analgesic in osteoarthritis pain (Goldstein et al. 2000). Lanepitant is a selective NK_1 receptor antagonist that blocks neurogenic inflammation and pain transmission, but clinical trials showed it to be not effective in the osteoarthritis condition. It has been suggested that this lack of effect of FK244, CP99994 and lanepitant could be related to either insufficient doses tested or the pharmacokinetic or pharmacodynamic properties of the compounds (Joos et al. 1995; Goldstein et al. 2000). Importantly, independently of the immune system, two NK_1 antagonists had significant beneficial effects in placebo-controlled clinical trials of patients with moderate and severe depression (e.g. Kramer et al. 2004). However, this effect was not supported in later trials and NK_1 antagonists are not used clinically as antidepressants. The incidence of side effects was low. Furthermore, a clinical use for NK_1 antagonists has been found in the treatment of emesis, associated with cancer therapies. The addition of an NK_1 receptor antagonist to standard therapy improved the incidence of emesis side effects in the acute and especially in the delayed phase by approximately 20% (Chawla et al. 2003). The possibility that NK_2 and NK_3 receptor antagonists may also have therapeutic roles, especially in gut inflammation, has also been debated (Lecci et al. 2004; Sanger 2004).

4 Calcitonin Gene-Related Peptide

The 37 amino acid CGRP is synthesized following the tissue-specific expression of CGRP mRNA in nerves by the calcitonin gene (Brain and Grant 2004) (Fig. 3, Table1). The most common form of CGRP is αCGRP (otherwise known as CGRPI), and the second form of CGRP (αCGRP or CGRPII) has more than 90% structural similarity to αCGRP. It is formed from a distinct gene and is found in some tissues, such as the gut. A family of CGRP-like peptides exists that includes adrenomedullin (AM), produced in vascular tissues in disease, and amylin, which is primarily localized to pancreatic tissue. All members of the family share structural homology, although this is quite low (25–40%), and some biological activities, such as vasodilation, where the potency ranking is CGRP $>$ AM $>$ amylin. CGRP is widely distributed in both the central and the peripheral nervous system, where it is found commonly colocalized with SP, as well as with other neuropeptides in sensory nerves.

The vasodilator activity of CGRP is well established, and it has been suggested to be one of the most potent microvascular vasodilators known (Brain et al. 1985). CGRP does not appear to play a primary role in the physiological regulation of blood pressure, although evidence is increasing to suggest a role at the specific level of individual tissues or organs. In particular, it would appear that CGRP may have important roles in mediating Raynaud's disease and migraine. The injection of femtomolar amounts of CGRP into skin leads to increased cutaneous blood flow, due to its potent effects in the microcirculation, in a range of species, including humans, with higher doses inducing responses that have longer durations of action (Brain et al. 1985). Furthermore, CGRP, in common with other known vasodilators, can act to potentiate inflammatory oedema formation induced by mediators of increased permeability such as SP (Brain and Williams 1985) (Fig. 4).

CGRP and its related peptides act via a family of unique receptors. Originally in studies of antagonist potency they were classified as CGRP1 and CGRP2, where the peptide CGRP antagonist $CGRP_{8-37}$ antagonized the CGRP1 receptor, but not the CGRP2 receptor (Brain and Grant 2004). It is now realized that CGRP1 is the primary vascular receptor for CGRP. The importance of the CGRP2 receptor is still unclear. However, more is now known about the other members of this family of receptors. The CGRP family is composed of a seven transmembrane G protein coupled calcitonin receptor-like receptor (CL) that links with a single membrane

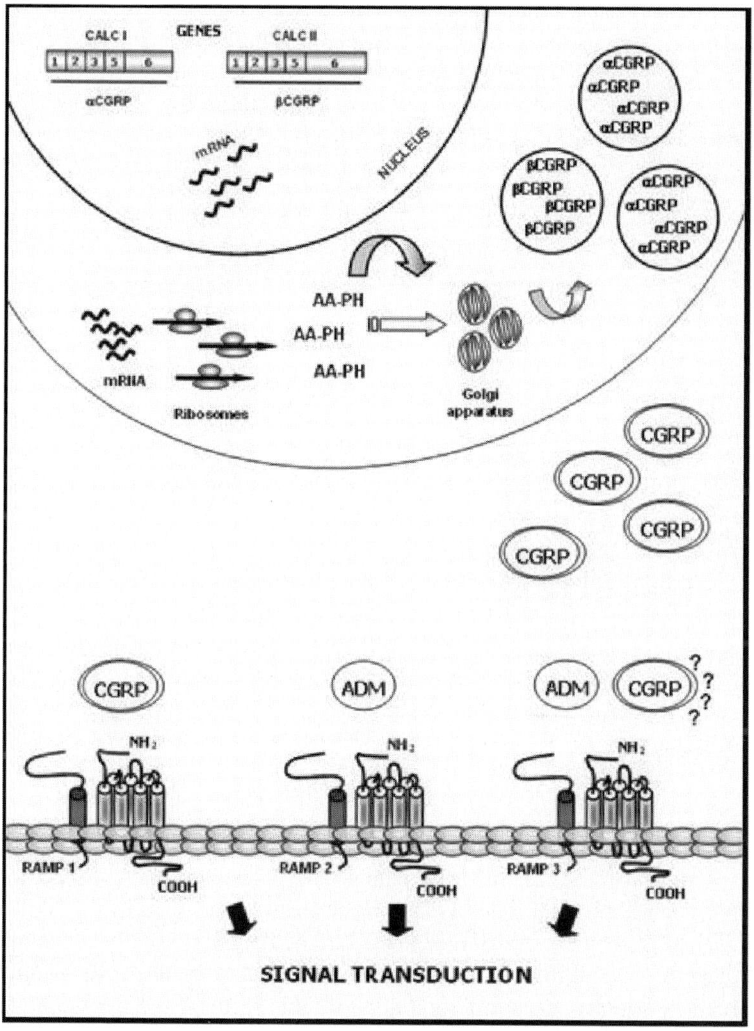

Fig. 3 Two distinct genes carry the information that encodes calcitonin gene-related peptide (CGRP). The *CALC I* gene is linked to αCGRP expression, while *CALC II* is linked to βCGRP expression. Following transcription, an amino acid preprohormone (*AA-PH*) is formed inside the ribosomes and then cleaved in the Golgi apparatus to give αCGRP and βCGRP, which remains in neuronal intracellular vesicles until there are further stimuli. CGRP is released from stimulated cells and after that binds to its receptor, leading to activation of specific intracellular pathways. A family of CGRP-like peptides exists that includes adrenomedullin (ADM) and amylin, both of which are released from non-neuronal sources

spanning receptor activity modifying protein (RAMP; McLatchie et al. 1998). CL is important for ligand binding, whereas the RAMP component is important for the phenotype of the receptor and its location at the cell surface. There are three RAMPs: RAMP1, RAMP2 and RAMP3. CL when linked to RAMP1 acts as a

Table 1 The human amino acid sequences of selected neuropeptides

Substance P – 11 amino acids	Arg-Pro-Lys-Pro-Gln-Gln-Phe-Phe-Gly-Leu-Met-NH_2
Calcitonin gene-related peptide – 37 amino acids	H-Ala-Cys-Asp-Thr-Ala-Thr-Cys-Val-Thr-His-Arg-Leu-Ala-Gly-Leu-Leu-Ser-Arg-Ser-Gly-Gly-Val-Val-Lys-Asn-Asn-Phe-Val-Pro-Thr-Asn-Val-Gly-Ser-Lys-Ala-Phe-NH_2
Galanin – 30 amino acids	Gly-Trp-Thr-Leu-Asn-Ser-Ala-Gly-Tyr-Leu-Leu-Gly-Pro-His-Ala-Val-Gly-Asn-His-Arg-Ser-Phe-Ser-Asp-Lys-Asn-Gly-Leu-Thr-Ser

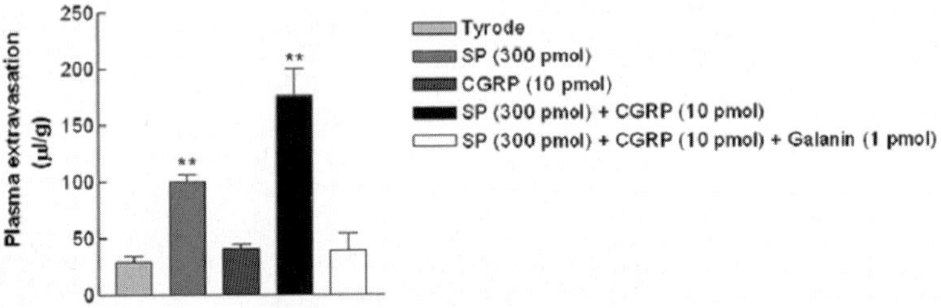

Fig. 4 Effect of the SP, CGRP and galanin on plasma extravasation in dorsal murine skin. Plasma extravasation was induced by intradermal injection of SP and CGRP and the effect of coinjected galanin is shown. Results are expressed as plasma extravasation ($\mu l\ g^{-1}$) (mean $\pm$ standard error of the mean) measured over 30 min, by the ^{125}I-bovine serum albumin method. Responses that are significantly different from the corresponding sites treated with Tyrode solution are shown. $^{**}p < 0.01$

CGRP receptor, which can also bind AM. CL when with RAMP2 is an AM receptor type 1 (AM_1) receptor, whereas CL with RAMP3 leads to an AM receptor type 2 (AM_2), about which the least is known. The increased blood flow induced by CGRP is mediated by the CGRP receptor (CL/RAMP1). It is usually considered that CGRP acts via smooth muscle receptors associated with a cyclic AMP accumulation mechanism. Certainly in the microcirculation, this seems to be the major mechanism. However, vascular relaxation can also occur via a nitric oxide dependent endothelium-dependent mechanism. Potent small-molecule CGRP antagonists are now becoming available. BIBN4096BS is a potent competitive antagonist of primate CGRP1 receptors (Doods et al. 2000) with a 200-fold greater affinity in human compared with rodent tissues; however, it lacks oral availability. The non-peptide antagonist MK-0974 developed by Merck is orally active (Salvatore et al. 2008).

CGRP is distributed widely in the trigeminal vascular system. BIBN4096BS and MK-0974 have both been shown to be effective in lessening the common headache pain associated with migraine. Initially both compounds were found to block neurogenic vasodilatation in animal models that mimicked the trigeminal activation that occurs in migraine (Doods et al. 2000; Salvatore et al. 2008). It is hypothesized that intracranial extracerebral blood vessels (e.g. middle meningeal artery and its dural arterioles) that feed into the dura mater vasodilate and that this process is involved in initiating pain due to the activation of perivascular sensory nociceptive nerve fibres. In addition, there is probably a more direct neuronal involvement (Storer et al. 2004). The intravenous administration of BIBN4096BS has been shown to be successful in phase II clinical trials (Olesen et al. 2004). The orally active MK-0974 has also been shown to be active in relieving migraine and further clinical trials are in progress (see Doods et al. 2007 for a review). Thus, CGRP antagonists may be an important treatment for migraine. To date triptans have been widely used, but their use is contraindicated in patients with coronary disease owing to an increased risk of coronary vasospasm. The CGRP antagonists do not appear to share this adverse effect.

5 Galanin and Related Peptides

The 29 amino acid peptide GAL, originally isolated from porcine intestine (Tatemoto 1983), is localized in primary sensory neurons and has a widespread distribution in the central nervous system (Bartfai et al. 1993). The N-terminal 1-15 amino acids are highly conserved, although human GAL is unique in having 30 amino acids with no amidation of the N-terminus (Evans and Shine 1991). GAL-related peptides include GAL-message-associated peptide (GMAP), which derives from the same peptide precursor gene product as GAL, GAL-like peptide (GALP), which is encoded by a different gene, and the recently discovered peptide alarin, which is encoded by a splice variant of the *GALP* gene (Lang et al. 2007) (Fig. 5).

The effects of GAL are mediated by three G protein coupled receptor subtypes, referred to as GalR1, GalR2 and GalR3, which are uniquely distributed throughout the central nervous system and periphery (Burgevin et al. 1995; Fathi et al. 1998; Kolakowski et al. 1998). Since all three subtypes have substantial differences in functional coupling and subsequent signalling activity, a variety of ligands have been developed to elucidate the specific role for each receptor in mediating the broad spectrum of physiological effects of the GALP family (Lang et al. 2007).

GAL is involved in multiple functions in the central and peripheral nervous system of many mammalian species (Bartfai et al. 1993), and these include control of food intake and gonadotropic axis (Crawley 1999; Landry et al. 2000; Gundlach 2002; Rossmanith et al. 1996) learning and memory (Kinney et al. 2002), mood regulation as well as pathophysiological processes such as neurodegeneration/ neuroregeneration (Kerr et al. 2000, 2001) as well as seizure activity and pain (Liu and Hokfelt 2002). By comparison, much less is known about GMAP, although the distributions of the two gene products overlap in most of the regions identified so far. GMAP has been suggested to be involved in modifying nociception (Hao et al. 1999). GALP mRNA and protein distribution in the central nervous

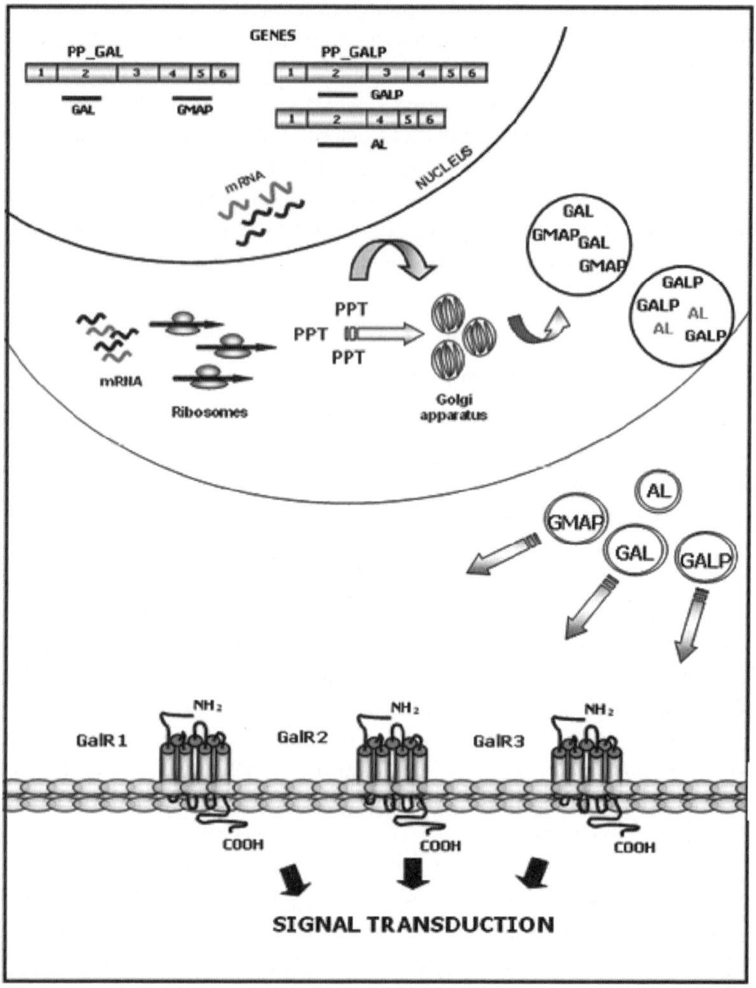

Fig. 5 Preprogalanin (*PP-GAL*) is encoded by a single-copy gene organized into six small exons. Galanin is proteolytically processed from this precursor propeptide along with galanin-message-associated peptide (*GMAP*). Preprogalanin-like peptide (*PP-GALP*) comprises six exons with a structural organization similar to that of galanin. Posttranscriptional splicing leads to exclusion of exon 3, resulting in a frame shift and a novel precursor protein. This protein harbours the signal sequence of PP-GALP and the first five amino acids of the mature galanin-like peptide followed by another 20 amino acids and proteolytic cleavage leads to alarin (*AL*). Galanin-related peptides are released from stimulated cells and bind to galanin receptors 1–3 (GalR1, GalR2, GalR3), leading to activation of specific intracellular pathways. To date, there is no information about the putative alarin receptor(s) and their activation pathways

system is limited when compared with that of GAL, being detected only in the hypothalamic arcuate nucleus, the median eminence and the posterior pituitary (Jureus et al. 2001; Cunningham et al. 2004; Larm et al. 2000; Takatsu et al. 2001). GALP has been implicated in both the homeostatic regulation of feeding and body weight, as well as the control of the hypothalamic–pituitary–gonadal axis (Krasnow et al. 2003; Gottsch et al. 2004). Intracerebroventricular injections of GALP alter food intake and body weight in a time-dependent manner in rats and mice (Matsumot et al. 2002). Furthermore, GALP stimulates the secretion of both gonadotropin-releasing hormone and luteinizing hormone in female rats and induces sexual behaviour in males (Fraley et al. 2004). Alarin, which originates from a splice variant of the GALP mRNA, was first described in human neuroblastic tumours (Santic et al. 2006). Interestingly GALP and alarin possess vasoactive properties and this will be discussed in the following.

5.1 *Galanin and Pain Processing*

GAL and its three receptors are expressed in DRG neurons and in the spinal cord (Landry et al. 2005), which indicates a role in nociception. The role of GAL in the regulation of pain processing have led to controversial results. Work into GAL demonstrates biphasic, dose dependent effects in neuropathic pain and inflammation (Liu et al. 2001; Xu et al. 2000). High doses of exogenous GAL delivered by intrathecal infusion ease neuropathic pain behaviour following peripheral nerve injury (Hao et al. 1999; Liu et al. 2001), while low doses of GAL or GalR1/GalR2 agonists increase pain sensitivity to thermal and mechanical pain (Flatters et al. 2002; Liu et al. 2001). Extensive research over many years has examined the role of GAL in neurodegeneration/neuroregeneration in neuropathic models, focusing mainly on expression of GAL in DRG neurons (Hokfelt et al. 1987). Normally only a few DRG neurons show detectable GAL levels, but after various types of peripheral nerve injury the peptide is dramatically upregulated with an increased release of GAL in the spinal dorsal horn (Hokfelt et al. 1987). Furthermore, GAL has trophic actions on DRG neurons, promoting neurite outgrowth, and plays a role in neuronal development (Holmes et al. 2000; Elliott-Hunt et al. 2004; Mahoney et al. 2003). Data suggest that GalR2 is the primary receptor involved in these regenerative functions this is supported by finding that neuritis outgrowth is induced in GAL-knockout animals using a selective GalR2 agonist (Mahoney et al. 2003). GAL has also been implicated in the control of neurogenesis in normal and injured brain (Shen et al. 2003; Elliott-Hunt et al. 2004; Mazarati et al. 2004) and also its level is elevated in some pathological conditions, including Alzheimer's disease (Chan-Palay 1988; Mufson et al. 1993).

5.2 *Galanin and the Gastrointestinal Tract*

The GALP family has also been implicated in functional regulation of the peripheral nervous system (Liu and Hokfelt 2002; Holmes et al. 2005) and various peripheral organs, such as the pancreas, the heart and the gastrointestinal tract

(Ahren and Lindskog 1992; Ahrens et al. 2006; Potter and Smith-White 2005; Sarnelli et al. 2004). GAL is also found in nerves and other cells in bone and joint tissues (Mc Donald et al. 2003). GAL was originally isolated from porcine small intestine (Tatemoto et al. 1983), and the gastrointestinal tract has been a primary target for uncovering possible physiological functions. It has been demonstrated that GAL inhibits gastric acid secretion (Schepp et al. 1990; Mungan et al. 1992; Kisfalvi et al. 2000) and inhibits the release of numerous pancreatic peptides (Bauer et al. 1989; Flowe et al. 1992; Herzig et al. 1993; Brodish et al. 1994). GAL is also able to modulate gastrointestinal motility, either via direct action on intestinal smooth muscle cells (Delvaux et al. 1991; Botella et al. 1992; Umer et al. 2005) or by indirect neuromodulatory mechanisms (Yau et al. 1986; Brown et al. 1990; Mulholland et al. 1992; Sarnelli et al. 2004). Importantly, it has recently been shown that GAL is involved in inflammatory processes affecting the gastrointestinal tract. In an experimental model of acute and chronic colitis: a single intraperitoneal injection of GAL reduced the formation of gastric ulcers and diminished the production of inflammatory response modifiers such as tumour necrosis factor α (Talero et al. 2006, 2007).

5.3 Vascular Effects of Galanin in the Cutaneous Microvasculature

Recently, a vasomodulatory/inflammatory role of the GALP family in murine skin was described, where GAL, GALP and alarin inhibit inflammatory oedema formation and reduce dorsal skin microvascular blood flow, with a potency ranking of GAL > GALP > alarin (Schmidhuber et al. 2007). This was the first demonstration of a biological activity of alarin. Accordingly, GAL inhibits plasma extravasation induced either chemically or by antidromic C-fibre stimulation (Xu et al. 1991; Green et al. 1992) and SP- and histamine-induced plasma extravasation was inhibited by GAL in the rat hindpaw (Xu et al. 1991) and in pigeon skin (Jancsó et al. 2000). Furthermore, a selective regional vasoconstriction potential of GAL in possums and cats was demonstrated by Courtice et al. (1994) and later confirmed in the hamster cheek pouch, measured by the change of arteriolar diameter (Dagar et al. 2003). The combined evidence suggests that GAL is a potent microvascular constrictor agent.

A first hint of a role for GAL in the plasticity in the cutaneous system was provided by Ji et al. (1995), who demonstrated that upregulation of GAL and its binding sites occurs in rat skin upon inflammation. Reverse-transcription PCR analysis revealed GalR2 and GalR3 mRNA expression but no GalR1 in dorsal murine skin, implying that the vasomodulatory action of GAL is mediated primarily by GalR2 or GalR3 in the murine model (Schmidhuber et al. 2007). Importantly, the vascular function of GAL might not be limited to the cutaneous microvasculature and should therefore prompt further studies to evaluate possible roles in different vascular systems.

In summary, the potent biological activities of GAL suggest that it may be an important physiological mediator. In addition, it plays a role in pathological situations and the search for its precise activities requires more attention. GAL receptors are potential therapeutic targets, especially in inflammatory processes affecting the gastrointestinal tract and inflammatory skin disorders.

6 Conclusions

Studies in the neuropeptide field have produced a range of peptides with diverse biological activities. Surprisingly, there have been few therapeutic successes that have involved neuropeptide blockage. Certainly, the lack of analgesic and anti-inflammatory activity of the NK_1 antagonists in humans has puzzled many. However, NK_1 antagonists do attenuate emesis associated with chemotherapy in the clinic. The findings that CGRP antagonists are beneficial in clinical trials involving migraine are promising and this may yield an important new class of drugs for the treatment of migraine. On the other hand, the therapeutic potential of GAL has not been fully investigated to our knowledge.

Acknowledgement E.S.F. is funded by the Arthritis Research Campaign and by a postdoctoral grant from Conselho de Desenvolvimento Cientifico e Tecnologico (CNPq, Brazil).

References

Ahmed M, Bjurholm A, Srinivasan GR, Lundeberg T, Theodorsson E, Schultzberg M, Kreicbergs A (1995) Capsaicin effects on substance P and CGRP in rat adjuvant arthritis. Regul Pept 55:85–102

Ahren B, Wierup N, Sundler F (2006) Neuropeptides and the regulation of islet function. Diabetes 55(Suppl 2):S98–S107

Ahrens B, Lindskog S (1992) Galanin and the regulation of islet hormone secretion. Int J Pancreatol 1:147–160

Al'Abadie MS, Senior HJ, Bleehen SS, Gawkrodger DJ (1995) Neuropeptides and general neuronal marker in psoriasis – an immunohistochemical study. Clin Exp Dermatol 20:384–389

Ansel JC, Brown JR, Payan DG, Brown MA (1993) Substance P selectively activates *TNF*-α gene expression in murine mast cells. J Immunol 150:4478–4485

Bartfai T, Hokfelt T, Langel U (1993) Galanin – a neuroendocrine peptide. Crit Rev Neurobiol 7:229–274

Bauer FE, Zintel A, Kenny MJ, Calder D, Ghatei MA, Bloom SR (1989) Inhibitory effect of galanin on postprandial gastrointestinal motility and gut hormone release in humans. Gastroenterology 97:260–264

Bayliss WM (1901) On the origin from the spinal cord of the vaso-dilator fibres of the hind-limb, and on the nature of these fibres. J Physiol 26:173–209

Beer S, Weighardt H, Emmanuilidis K, Harzenetter MD, Matevossian E, Heidecke CD, Bartels H, Siewert JR, Holzmann B (2002) Systemic neuropeptide levels as predictive indicators for lethal outcome in patients with postoperative sepsis. Crit Care Med 30:1794–1798

Bevan S, Hothi S, Hughes G, James IF, Rang HP, Shah K, Walpole CS, Yeats JC (1992) Capsazepine: a competitive antagonist of the sensory neurone excitant capsaicin. Br J Pharmacol 107:544–552

Bienenstock J, Tomioka M, Matsuda H, Stead RH, Quinonez G, Simon GT, Coughlin MD, Denburg JA (1987) The role of mast cells in inflammatory processes: evidence for nerve/mast cell interactions. Int Arch Allergy Appl Immunol 82:238–243

Blum AM, Metwali A, Cook G, Mathew RC, Elliott D, Weinstock JV (1993) Substance P modulates antigen-induced, IFN-gamma production in murine Schistosomiasis mansoni. J Immunol 151:225–233

Blum AM, Metwali A, Kim-Miller M, Li J, Qadir K, Elliott DE, Lu B, Fabry Z, Gerard N, Weinstock JV (1999) The substance P receptor is necessary for a normal granulomatous response in murine schistosomiasis mansoni. J Immunol 162:6080–6085

Botella A, Delvaux M, Bueno L, Frexinos J (1992) Intracellular pathways triggered by galanin to induce contraction of pig ileum smooth muscle cells. J Physiol 458:475–486

Brain SD, Cox HM (2006) Neuropeptides and their receptors: innovative science providing novel therapeutic targets. Br J Pharmacol 147(Suppl 1):S202–S211

Brain SD, Grant AD (2004) Vascular actions of calcitonin gene-related peptide and adrenomedullin. Physiol Rev 84:903–934

Brain SD, Williams TJ (1985) Inflammatory oedema induced by synergism between calcitonin gene-related peptide (CGRP) and mediators of increased vascular permeability. Br J Pharmacol 86:855–860

Brain SD, Williams TJ, Tippins JR, Morris HR, MacIntyre I (1985) Calcitonin gene-related peptide is a potent vasodilator. Nature 313:54–56

Brodish RJ, Kuvshinoff BW, Fink AS, McFadden DW (1994) Inhibition of pancreatic exocrine secretion by galanin. Pancreas 9:297–303

Brown DR, Hildebrand KR, Parsons AM, Soldani G (1990) Effects of galanin on smooth muscle and mucosa of porcine jejunum. Peptides 11:497–500

Buck SH (1988) Multiple receptors for the tachykinin peptides. Proc West Pharmacol Soc 31: 45–47

Bulling DG, Kelly D, Bond S, McQueen DS, Seckl JR (2001) Adjuvant-induced joint inflammation causes very rapid transcription of beta-preprotachykinin and *alpha-CGRP* genes in innervating sensory ganglia. J Neurochem 77:372–382

Burgevin MC, Loquet I, Quarteronet D, Habert-Ortoli E (1995) Cloning, pharmacological characterization, and anatomical distribution of a rat cDNA encoding for a galanin receptor. J Mol Neurosci 6:33–41

Campos MM, Calixto JB (2000) Neurokinin mediation of edema and inflammation. Neuropeptides 34:314–322

Castagliuolo I, LaMont JT, Letourneau R, Kelly C, O'Keane JC, Jaffer A, Theoharides TC, Pothoulakis C (1994) Neuronal involvement in the intestinal effects of *Clostridium difficile* toxin A and *Vibrio cholerae* enterotoxin in rat ileum. Gastroenterology 107:657–665

Caterina MJ, Schumacher MA, Tominaga M, Rosen TA, Levine JD, Julius D (1997) The capsaicin receptor: a heat-activated ion channel in the pain pathway. Nature 389:816–824

Chahl LA (2004) Hydrogen sulphide: an endogenous stimulant of capsaicin-sensitive primary afferent neurons? Br J Pharmacol 142:1–2

Chan J, Smoller BR, Raychauduri SP, Jiang WY, Farber EM (1997) Intraepidermal nerve fiber expression of calcitonin gene-related peptide, vasoactive intestinal peptide and substance P in psoriasis. Arch Dermatol Res 289:611–616

Chan-Palay V (1988) Galanin hyperinnervates surviving neurons of the human basal nucleus of Meynert in dementias of Alzheimer's and Parkinson's disease: a hypothesis for the role of galanin in accentuating cholinergic dysfunction in dementia. J Comp Neurol 273:543–557

Chawla SP, Grunberg SM, Gralla RJ et al (2003) Establishing the dose of the oral NK1 antagonist aprepitant for the prevention of chemotherapy-induced nausea and vomiting. Cancer 97: 2290–2300

Clark N, Keeble J, Fernandes ES, Starr A, Liang L, Sugden D, de Winter P, Brain SD (2007) The transient receptor potential vanilloid 1 (TRPV1) receptor protects against the onset of sepsis after endotoxin. FASEB J 21:3747–3755

Courtice GP, Hales JR, Potter EK (1994) Selective regional vasoconstriction underlying pressor effects of galanin in anaesthetized possums compared with cats. J Physiol 481:439–45

Crawley JN (1999) The role of galanin in feeding behavior. Neuropeptides 33:369–375

Cunningham MJ (2004) Galanin-like peptide as a link between metabolism and reproduction. J Neuroendocrinol 16:717–723

Dagar S, Onyüksel H, Akhter S, Krishnadas A, Rubinstein I (2003) Human galanin expresses amphipathic properties that modulate its vasoreactivity in vivo. Peptides 24:1373–1380

Delvaux M, Botella A, Fioramonti J, Frexinos J, Bueno L (1991) Galanin induces contraction of isolated cells from circular muscle layer of pig ileum. Regul Pept 32:369–374

Diz DI, Jessup JA, Westwood BM, Bosch SM, Vinsant S, Gallagher PE, Averill DB (2002) Angiotensin peptides as neurotransmitters/neuromodulators in the dorsomedial medulla. Clin Exp Pharmacol Physiol 29:473–482

Doods H, Hallermayer G, Wu D, Entzeroth M, Rudolf K, Engel W, Eberlein W (2000) Pharmacological profile of BIBN4096BS, the first selective small molecule CGRP antagonist. Br J Pharmacol 129:420–423

Doods H, Arndt K, Rudolf K (2007) CGRP antagonists: unravelling the role of CGRP in migraine. Trends Pharmacol Sci 28:580–587

Dzurik MV, Diedrich A, Black B, Paranjape SY, Raj SR, Byrne DW, Robertson D (2007) Endogenous substance P modulates human cardiovascular regulation at rest and during orthostatic load. J Appl Physiol 102:2092–2097

Elliott-Hunt CR, Marsh B, Bacon A, Pope R, Vanderplank P, Wynick D (2004) Galanin acts as a neuroprotective factor to the hippocampus. Proc Natl Acad Sci USA 101:5105–5110

Evans HF, Shine J (1991) Human galanin: Molecular cloning reveals a unique structur. Endocrinology 129:1682–1684

Eysselein VE, Nast CC (1991) Neuropeptides and inflammatory bowel disease. Z Gastroenterol Verh 26:253–257

Fathi Z, Battaglino PM, Iben LG et al (1998) Molecular characterization, pharmacological properties and chromosomal localization of the human GALR2 galanin receptor. Brain Res Mol Brain Res 58:156–169

Feistritzer C, Clausen J, Sturn DH, Djanani A, Gunsilius E, Wiedermann CJ, Kähler CM (2003) Natural killer cell functions mediated by the neuropeptide substance P. Regul Pept 116:119–126

Ferrell WR, Lockhart JC, Karimian SM (1997) Tachykinin regulation of basal synovial blood flow. Br J Pharmacol 121:29–34

Flatters SJ, Fox AJ, Dickenson A (2002) Nerve injury induces plasticity that results in spinal inhibitory effects of galanin. Pain 98:249–258

Flowe KM, Lally KM, Mulholland MW (1992) Galanin inhibits rat pancreatic amylase release via cholinergic suppression. Peptides 13:487–492

Foreman JC, Jordan CC, Piotrowski W (1983) Interaction of neurotensin with the substance P receptor mediating histamine release from rat mast cells and the flare in human skin. 77:531–539

Foster AP, Cunningham FM (2003) Substance P induces activation, adherence and migration of equine eosinophils. J Vet Pharmacol Ther 26:131–138

Fraley GS, Thomas-Smith SE, Acohido BV, Steiner RA, Clifton DK (2004) Stimulation of sexual behavior in the male rat by galanin-like peptide. Horm Behav 46:551–557

Garrett NE, Kidd BL, Cruwys SC, Tomlinson DR (1995) Changes in preprotachykinin mRNA expression and substance P levels in dorsal root ganglia of monoarthritic rats: comparison with changes in synovial substance P levels. Brain Res 675:203–207

Germonpré PR, Joos GF, Pauwels RA (1995) Characterization of the neurogenic plasma extravasation in the airways. Arch Int Pharmacodyn Ther 329:185–203

Goetzl EJ, Chernov T, Renold F, Payan DG (1985) Neuropeptide regulation of the expression of immediate hypersensitivity. J Immunol 135:802s–805s

Goldstein DJ, Wang O, Todd LE, Gitter BD, DeBrota DJ, Iyengar S (2000) Study of the analgesic effect of lanepitant in patients with osteoarthritis pain. Clin Pharmacol Ther 67:419–426

Gottsch ML, Clifton DK, Steiner RA (2004) Galanin-like peptide as a link in the integration of metabolism and reproduction. Trends Endocrinol Metab 15:215–221

Gradl G, Finke B, Schattner S, Gierer P, Mittlmeier T, Vollmar B (2007) Continuous intra-arterial application of substance P induces signs and symptoms of experimental complex regional pain syndrome (CRPS) such as edema, inflammation and mechanical pain but no thermal pain. Neuroscience 148:757–765

Green PG, Basbaum AI, Levine JD (1992) Sensory neuropeptide interactions in the production of plasma extravasation in the rat. Neuroscience 50:745–749

Gross KJ, Pothoulakis C (2007) Role of neuropeptides in inflammatory bowel disease. Inflamm Bowel Dis 13:918–932

Gundlach AL (2002) Galanin/GALP and galanin receptors: Role in central control of feeding, body weight/obesity and reproduction? Eur J Pharmaol 440:255–268

Hao JX, Shi TJ, Xu IS, Kaupilla T, Xu XJ, Hökfelt T, Bartfai T, Wiesenfeld-Hallin Z (1999) Intrathecal galanin alleviates allodynia-like behaviour in rats after partial peripheral nerve injury. Eur J Neurosci 11:427–432

Herzig KH, Brunke G, Schön I, Schäffer M, Fölsch UR (1993) Mechanism of galanin's inhibitory action on pancreatic enzyme secretion: Modulation of cholinergic transmission-studies in vivo and in vitro. Gut 34:1616–1621

Hökfelt T, Wiesenfeld-Hallin Z, Villar M, Melander T (1987) Increase of galanin-like immunoreactivity in rat dorsal root ganglion cells after peripheral axotomy. Neurosci Lett 83:217–220

Holmes FE, Mahoney S, King VR, Bacon A, Kerr NC, Pachnis V, Curtis R, Priestley JV, Wynick D (2000) Targeted disruption of the galanin gene reduces the number of sensory neurons and their regenerative capacity. Proc Natl Acad Sci USA 97:1563–11568

Holmes FE, Mahoney SA, Wynick D (2005) Use of genetically engineered transgenic mice to investigate the role of galanin in the peripheral nervous system after injury. Neuropeptides 39:191–199

Holzer P (1998) Neurogenic vasodilatation and plasma leakage in the skin. Gen Pharmacol 30:5–11

Holzer-Petsche U (1995) Tachykinin receptors in gastrointestinal motility. Regul Pept 57:19–42

Hong SK, Han JS, Min SS, Hwang JM, Kim YI, Na HS, Yoon YW, Han HC (2002) Local neurokinin-1 receptor in the knee joint contributes to the induction, but not maintenance, of arthritic pain in the rat. Neurosci Lett 322:21–24

Ikeda Y, Takei H, Matsumoto C, Mase A, Yamamoto M, Takeda S, Ishige A, Watanabe K (2007) Administration of substance P during a primary immune response amplifies the secondary immune response via a long-lasting effect on CD8+ T lymphocytes. Arch Dermatol Res 299:345–351

Iwasaki A, Inoue K, Hukuda S (1995) Distribution of neuropeptide-containing nerve fibers in the synovium and adjacent bone of the rat knee joint. Clin Exp Rheumatol 13:173–178

Jancsó N, Jancsó-Gabor A, Szolcsanyi J (1967) Direct evidence for neurogenic inflammation and its prevention by denervation and by pretreatment with capsaicin. Br J Pharmacol Chemother 31:138–151

Jancsó G, Kiraly E, Jancsó-Gabor A (1977) Pharmacologically induced selective degeneration of chemosensitive primary sensory neurones. Nature 270:741–743

Jancsó G, Sántha P, Horváth V, Pierau F (2000) Inhibitory neurogenic modulation of histamine-induced cutaneous plasma extravasation in the pigeon. Regul Pept 95:75–80

Jeanjean AP, Moussaoui SM, Maloteaux JM, Laduron PM (1995) Interleukin-1β induces long-term increase of axonally transported opiate receptors and substance P. Neuroscience 68:151–157
Ji RR, Zhang X, Zhang Q, Dagerlind A, Nilsson S, Wiesenfeld-Hallin Z, Hökfelt T (1995) Central and peripheral expression of galanin in response to inflammation. Neuroscience 68:563–576
Jiang WY, Raychaudhuri SP, Farber EM (1998) Double-labeled immunofluorescence study of cutaneous nerves in psoriasis. Int J Dermatol 37:572–574
Joos GF, Kips JC, Peleman RA, Pauwels RA (1995) Tachykinin antagonists and the airways. Arch Int Pharmacodyn Ther 329:205–219
Juréus A, Cunningham MJ, Li D, Johnson LL, Krasnow SM, Teklemichael DN, Clifton DK, Steiner RA (2001) Distribution and regulation of galanin-like peptide (GALP) in the hypothalamus of the mouse. Endocrinology 142:5140–5144
Kähler CM, Sitte BA, Reinisch N, Wiedermann CJ (1993) Stimulation of the chemotactic migration of human fibroblasts by substance P. Eur J Pharmacol 249:281–286
Kar S, Rees RG, Quirion R (1994) Altered calcitonin gene-related peptide, substance P and enkephalin immunoreactivities and receptor binding sites in the dorsal spinal cord of the polyarthritic rat. Eur J Neurosci 6:345–354
Keeble JE, Brain SD (2004) A role for substance P in arthritis? Neurosci Lett 361:176–179
Kerr BJ, Cafferty WB, Gupta YK, Bacon A, Wynick D, McMahon SB, Thompson SW (2000) Galanin knockout mice reveal nociceptive deficits following peripheral nerve injury. Eur J Neurosci 12:793–802
Kerr BJ, Gupta Y, Pope R, Thompson SW, Wynick D, McMahon SB (2001) Endogenous galanin potentiates spinal nociceptive processing following inflammation. Pain 93:267–277
Khan WI, Collins SM (2004) Immune-mediated alteration in gut physiology and its role in host defence in nematode infection. Parasite Immunol 26:319–326
Khawaja AM, Rogers DF (1996) Tachykinins: receptor to effector. Int J Biochem Cell Biol 28:721–738
Kincy-Cain T, Bost KL (1996) Increased susceptibility of mice to Salmonella infection following in vivo treatment with the substance P antagonist, spantide II. J Immunol 157:255–264
Kinney JW, Starosta G, Holmes A, Wrenn CC, Yang RJ, Harris AP, Long KC, Crawley JN (2002) Deficits in trace cued fear conditioning in galanin-treated rats and galanin-overexpressing transgenic mice. Learn Mem 9:178–190
Kisfalvi I Jr, Burghardt B, Bálint A, Zelles T, Vizi ES, Varga G (2000) Antisecretory effects of galanin and its putative antagonists M15, M35 and C7 in the rat stomach. J Physiol Paris 94:37–42
Kolakowski LF, O'Neill GP, Howard AD et al (1998) Molecular characterization and expression of cloned human galanin receptors GALR2 and GALR3. J Neurochem 71:2239–2251
Konttinen YT, Hukkanen M, Segerberg M, Rees R, Kemppinen P, Sorsa T, Saari H, Polak JM, Santavirta S (1992) Relationship between neuropeptide immunoreactive nerves and inflammatory cells in adjuvant arthritic rats. Scand J Rheumatol 21:55–59
Koon HW, Pothoulakis C (2006) Immunomodulatory properties of substance P: the gastrointestinal system as a model. Ann N Y Acad Sci 1088:23–40
Kramer MS, Winokur A, Kelsey J et al (2004) Demonstration of the efficacy and safety of a novel substance P (NK1) receptor antagonist in major depression. Neuropsychopharmacology 29:385–392
Krasnow SM, Fraley GS, Schuh SM, Baumgartner JW, Clifton DK, Steiner RA (2003) A role of galanin-like peptide in the integration of feeding, body weight regulation, and reproduction in the mouse. Endocrinology 144:813–822
Lam FY, Wong MC (1996) Characterization of tachykinin receptors mediating plasma extravasation and vasodilatation in normal and acutely inflamed knee joints of the rat. Br J Pharmacol 118:2107–2114
Lam FY, Ferrell WR, Scott DT (1993) Substance P-induced inflammation in the rat knee joint is mediated by neurokinin 1 (NK1) receptors. Regul Pept 46:198–201

Landry M, Roche D, Vila-Porcile E, Calas A (2000) Effects of centrally administered galanin (1–16) on galanin expression in the rat hypothalamus. Peptides 21:1725–1733

Landry M, Liu HX, Shi TJ, Brumovsky P, Nagy F, Hökfelt T (2005) Galaninergic mechanisms at the spinal level: focus on histochemical phenotyping. Neuropeptides 39:223–231

Lang R, Gundlach AL, Kofler B (2007) The galanin peptide family: receptor pharmacology, pleiotropic biological actions, and implications in health and disease. Pharmacol Ther 115:177–207

Larm JA, Gundlach AL (2000) Galanin-like peptide (GALP) mRNA expression is restricted to arcuate nucleus of hypothalamus in adult male rat brain. Neuroendocrinology 72:67–71

Lecci A, Capriati A, Maggi CA (2004) Tachykinin NK2 receptor antagonists for the treatment of irritable bowel syndrome. Br J Pharmacol 141:1249–1263

Lewis T, Zotterman Y (1927) Vascular reactions of the skin to injury: part VIII. The resistance of the human skin to constant currents, in relation to injury and vascular response. J Physiol 62:280–288

Lindsey KQ, Caughman SW, Olerud JE, Bunnett NW, Armstrong CA, Ansel JC (2000) Neural regulation of endothelial cell-mediated inflammation. J Investig Dermatol Symp Proc 5:74–78

Liu H, Hockfelt T (2002) The participation of galanin in pain processing at the spinal level. Trends Pharmacol Sci 23:468–474

Liu HX, Brumovsky P, Schmidt R, Brown W, Payza K, Hodzic L, Pou C, Godbout C, Hökfelt T (2001) Receptor subtype-specific pronociceptive and analgesic actions of galanin in the spinal cord: Selective actions via GalR1 and GalR2 receptors. Proc Natl Acad Sci USA 98:9960–9964

Maggi CA (1995) The mammalian tachykinin receptors. Gen Pharmacol 26:911–944

Maggi CA (1997) Tachykinins as peripheral modulators of primary afferent nerves and visceral sensitivity. Pharmacol Res 36:153–169

Mahoney SA, Hosking R, Farrant S, Holmes FE, Jacoby AS, Shine J, Iismaa TP, Scott MK, Schmidt R, Wynick D (2003) The second galanin receptor GalR2 plays a key role in neurite outgrowth from adult sensory neurons. J Neurosci 23:416–421

Matsumoto Y, Watanabe T, Adachi Y, Itoh T, Ohtaki T, Onda H, Kurokawa T, Nishimura O, Fujino M (2002) Galanin-like peptide stimulates food intake in the rat. Neurosci Lett 322:67–69

Mazarati A, Lu X, Kilk K, Langel U, Wasterlain C, Bartfai T (2004) Galanin type 2 receptors regulate neuronal survival, susceptibility to seizures and seizure-induced neurogenesis in the dentate gyrus. Eur J Neurosci 19:3235–3244

McDonald AC, Schuijers JA, Shen PJ, Gundlach AL, Grills BL (2003) Expression of galanin and galanin receptor-1 in normal bone and during fracture repair in the rat. Bone 33:788–797

McLatchie LM, Fraser NJ, Main MJ, Wise A, Brown J, Thompson N, Solari R, Lee MG, Foord SM (1998) RAMPs regulate the transport and ligand specificity of the calcitonin-receptor-like receptor. Nature 393:333–339

Mufson EJ, Cochran E, Benzing W, Kordower JH (1993) Galaninergic innervation of the cholinergic vertical limb of the diagonal band (Ch2) and bed nucleus of the stria terminalis in aging. Alzheimer's disease and Down's syndrome. Dementia 4:237–250

Mulholland MW, Schoeneich S, Flowe K (1992) Galanin inhibition of enteric cholinergic neurotransmission: Guanosine triphosphate-binding protein interactions with adenylate cyclase. Surgery 112:195–201

Mungan Z, Ozmen V, Ertan A, Coy DH, Baylor LM, Rice JC, Rossowski WJ (1992) Structural requirements for galanin inhibition of pentagastrin-stimulated gastric acid secretion in conscious rats. Eur J Pharmacol 214:53–57

Mussap CJ, Geraghty DP, Burcher E (1993) Tachykinin receptors: a radioligand binding perspective. J Neurochem 60:1987–2009

Neil GA, Blum A, Weinstock JV (1991) Substance P but not vasoactive intestinal peptide modulates immunoglobulin secretion in murine schistosomiasis. Cell Immunol 135:394–401

Nilsson J, von Euler AM, Dalsgaard CJ (1985) Stimulation of connective tissue cell growth by substance P and substance K. Nature 315:61–63

Olesen J, Diener HC, Husstedt IW, Goadsby PJ, Hall D, Meier U, Pollentier S, Lesko LM (2004) Calcitonin gene-related peptide receptor antagonist BIBN 4096 BS for the acute treatment of migraine. N Engl J Med 350:1104–1110

Pavlovic S, Daniltchenko M, Tobin DJ, Hagen E, Hunt SP, Klapp BF, Arck PC, Peters EM (2008) Further exploring the brain-skin connection: stress worsens dermatitis via substance P-dependent neurogenic inflammation in mice. J Invest Dermatol 128:434–446

Peters EM, Ericson ME, Hosoi J, Seiffert K, Hordinsky MK, Ansel JC, Paus R, Scholzen TE (2006) Neuropeptide control mechanisms in cutaneous biology: physiological and clinical significance. J Invest Dermatol 126:1937–1947

Pincelli C, Fantini F, Romualdi P, Sevignani C, Lesa G, Benassi L, Giannetti A (1992) Substance P is diminished and vasoactive intestinal peptide is augmented in psoriatic lesions and these peptides exert disparate effects on the proliferation of cultured human keratinocytes. J Invest Dermatol 98:421–427

Pothoulakis C, Castagliuolo I, LaMont JT, Jaffer A, O'Keane JC, Snider RM, Leeman SE (1994) CP-96,345, a substance P antagonist, inhibits rat intestinal responses to *Clostridium difficile* toxin A but not cholera toxin. Proc Natl Acad Sci USA 91:947–951

Potter EK, Smith-White MA (2005) Galanin modulates cholinergic neurotransmission in the heart. Neuropeptides 39:345–348

Puneet P, Hegde A, Ng SW, Lau HY, Lu J, Moochhala SM, Bhatia M (2006) Preprotachykinin-A gene products are key mediators of lung injury in polymicrobial sepsis. J Immunol 176:3813–3820

Regoli D, Boudon A, Fauchere JL (1994) Receptors and antagonists for substance P and related peptides. Pharmacol Rev 46:551–599

Richardson JD, Vasko MR (2002) Cellular mechanisms of neurogenic inflammation. J Pharmacol Exp Ther 302:839–845

Rossmanith WG, Clifton DK, Steiner RA (1996) Galanin gene expression in hypothalamic GnRH-containing neurons in the rat: a model for autocrine regulation. Horm Metab 28:257–266

Salvatore C, Hershey J, Corcoran H et al (2008) Pharmacological characterization of MK-0974 [*N*-[(3*R*,6*S*)-6-(2,3-difluorophenyl)-2-oxo-1-(2,2,2-trifluoroethyl)azepan-3-yl]-4-(2-oxo-2,3-dihydro-1*H*-imidazo[4,5-b]pyridin-1-yl)piperidine-1-carboxamide], a potent and orally active calcitonin gene-related peptide receptor antagonist for the treatment of migraine. J Pharmacol Exp Ther 324:416–421

Sanger GJ (2004) Neurokinin NK1 and NK3 receptors as targets for drugs to treat gastrointestinal motility disorders and pain. Br J Pharmacol 141:1303–1312

Santic R, Fenninger K, Graf K et al (2006) Gangliocytes in neuroblastic tumors express alarin, a novel peptide derived by differential splicing of the galanin-like peptide gene. J Mol Neurosci 29:145–152

Saraceno R, Kleyn CE, Terenghi G, Griffiths CE (2006) The role of neuropeptides in psoriasis. Br J Dermatol 155:876–882

Sarnelli G, Vanden Berghe P, Raeymaekers P, Janssens J, Tack J (2004) Inhibitory effects of galanin on evoked $[Ca^{2+}]$i responses in cultured myenteric neurons. Am J Physiol Gastrointest Liver Physiol 286:G1009–G1014

Schepp W, Prinz C, Tatge C, Håkanson R, Schusdziarra V, Classen M (1990) Galanin inhibits gastrin release from isolated rat gastric G-cells. Am J Physiol 258:G596–G602

Schmidhuber SM, Santic R, Tam CW, Bauer JW, Kofler B, Brain SD (2007) Galanin-like peptides exert potent vasoactive functions in vivo. J Invest Dermatol 127:716–721

Scholzen T, Armstrong CA, Bunnett NW, Luger TA, Olerud JE, Ansel JC (1998) Neuropeptides in the skin: interactions between the neuroendocrine and the skin immune systems. Exp Dermatol 7:81–96

Shen PJ, Larm JA, Gundlach AL (2003) Expression and plasticity of galanin systems in cortical neurons, oligodendrocyte progenitors and proliferative zones in normal brain and after spreading depression. Eur J Neurosci 18:1362–1376
Shepherd AJ, Beresford LJ, Bell EB, Miyan JA (2005) Mobilisation of specific T cells from lymph nodes in contact sensitivity requires substance P. J Neuroimmunol 164:115–123
Sluka KA, Westlund KN (1993) Behavioral and immunohistochemical changes in an experimental arthritis model in rats. Pain 55:367–377
Sluka KA, Milton MA, Willis WD, Westlund KN (1997) Differential roles of neurokinin 1 and neurokinin 2 receptors in the development and maintenance of heat hyperalgesia induced by acute inflammation. Br J Pharmacol 120:1263–1273
Stead RH, Tomioka M, Quinonez G, Simon GT, Felten SY, Bienenstock J (1987) Intestinal mucosal mast cells in normal and nematode-infected rat intestines are in intimate contact with peptidergic nerves. Proc Natl Acad Sci USA 84:2975–2979
Steinhoff M, Ständer S, Seeliger S, Ansel JC, Schmelz M, Luger T (2003) Modern aspects of cutaneous neurogenic inflammation. Arch Dermatol 139:1479–1488
Storer RJ, Akerman S, Goadsby PJ (2004) Calcitonin gene-related peptide (CGRP) modulates nociceptive trigeminovascular transmission in the cat. Br J Pharmacol 142:1171–1181
Takatsu Y, Matsumoto H, Ohtaki T, Kumano S, Kitada C, Onda H, Nishimura O, Fujino M (2001) Distribution of galanin-like peptide in the rat brain. Endocrinology 142:1626–1634
Talero E, Sánchez-Fidalgo S, Ramón Calvo J, Motilva V (2006) Galanin in the trinitrobenzene sulfonic acid rat model of experimental colitis. Int Immunopharmacol 6:1404–1412
Talero E, Sánchez-Fidalgo S, Calvo JR, Motilva V (2007) Chronic administration of galanin attenuates the TNBS-induced colitis in rats. Regul Pept 141:96–104
Tanaka T, Danno K, Ikai K, Imamura S (1988) Effects of substance P and substance K on the growth of cultured keratinocytes. J Invest Dermatol 90:399–401
Tatemoto K, Rökaeus A, Jörnvall H, McDonald TJ, Mutt V (1983) Galanin – a novel biologically active peptide from porcine intestine. FEBS Lett 164:124–128
Umer A, Ługowska H, Sein-Anand J, Rekowski P, Ruczyński J, Petrusewicz J, Korolkiewicz RP (2005) The contractile effects of several substituted short analogues of porcine galanin in isolated rat jejunal and colonic smooth muscle strips. Pharmacol Res 52:283–289
Vachon P, Masse R, Gibbs BF (2004) Substance P and neurotensin are up-regulated in the lumbar spinal cord of animals with neuropathic pain. Can J Vet Res 68:86–92
Viac J, Gueniche A, Doutremepuich JD, Reichert U, Claudy A, Schmitt D (1996) Substance P and keratinocyte activation markers: an in vitro approach. Arch Dermatol Res 288:85–90
Von Euler US, Gaddum JH (1931) An unidentified depressor substance in certain tissue extracts. J Physiol 72:74–87
Walsh DA, McWilliams F (2006) Tachykinins and the cardiovascular system. Curr Drug Targets 7:1031–1042
Weber M, Birklein F, Neundörfer B, Schmelz M (2001) Facilitated neurogenic inflammation in complex regional pain syndrome. Pain 91:251–257
Woodbury RG, Miller HR, Huntley JF, Newlands GF, Palliser AC, Wakelin D (1984) Mucosal mast cells are functionally active during spontaneous expulsion of intestinal nematode infections in rat. Nature 312:450–452
Xu XJ, Hao JX, Wiesenfeld-Hallin Z, Håkanson R, Folkers K, Hökfelt T (1991) Spantide II, a novel tachykinin antagonist, and galanin inhibit plasma extravasation induced by antidromic C-fiber stimulation in rat hindpaw. Neuroscience 42:731–737
Xu XJ, Hökfelt T, Bartfai T, Wiesenfeld-Hallin Z (2000) Galanin and spinal nociceptive mechanisms: Recent advances and therapeutic implications. Neuropeptides 34:137–147
Yau WM, Dorsett JA, Youther ML (1986) Evidence for galanin as an inhibitory neuropeptide on myenteric cholinergic neurons in the guinea pig small intestine. Neurosci Lett 72:305–308
Zhang H, Hegde A, Ng SW, Adhikari S, Moochhala SM, Bhatia M (2007) Hydrogen sulfide up-regulates substance P in polymicrobial sepsis-associated lung injury. J Immunol 179:4153–4160

Cytokine and Chemokine Regulation of Sensory Neuron Function

Richard J. Miller, Hosung Jung, Sonia K. Bhangoo, and Fletcher A. White

Contents

Abstract Pain normally subserves a vital role in the survival of the organism, prompting the avoidance of situations associated with tissue damage. However, the sensation of pain can become dissociated from its normal physiological role. In conditions of neuropathic pain, spontaneous or hypersensitive pain behavior occurs in the absence of the appropriate stimuli. Our incomplete understanding of the mechanisms underlying chronic pain hypersensitivity accounts for the general ineffectiveness of currently available options for the treatment of chronic pain syndromes. Despite its complex pathophysiological nature, it is clear that neuropathic pain is associated with short- and long-term changes in the excitability of sensory neurons in the dorsal root ganglia (DRG) as well as their central connections. Recent evidence suggests that the upregulated expression of inflammatory cytokines in association with tissue damage or infection triggers the observed hyperexcitability of pain sensory neurons. The actions of inflammatory cytokines synthesized by DRG neurons and associated glial cells, as well as by astrocytes and microglia in the spinal cord, can produce changes in the excitability of nociceptive sensory neurons. These changes include rapid alterations in the properties of ion

R.J. Miller (✉)
Molecular Pharmacology and Structural Biochemistry, Northwestern University, Chicago, IL, USA
r-miller10@northwestern.edu

B.J. Canning and D. Spina (eds.), *Sensory Nerves*,
Handbook of Experimental Pharmacology 194, DOI: 10.1007/978-3-540-79090-7_12,

channels expressed by these neurons, as well as longer-term changes resulting from new gene transcription. In this chapter we review the diverse changes produced by inflammatory cytokines in the behavior of sensory neurons in the context of chronic pain syndromes.

Keywords Cytokine, Chemokine, DRG, Pain, Inflammation

1 Introduction

Primary afferent sensory neurons are responsible for processing important sensory information, including temperature, touch, proprioception, and pain. The cell bodies of these pseudounipolar neurons are found in the dorsal root ganglia (DRG), which are situated outside the central nervous system. DRG neurons exhibit a wide range of sizes and degrees of myelination. Neurons that transmit afferent information about potentially damaging stimuli that lead to the perception of pain are known as "nociceptors" (*noci-* is derived from the Latin for "hurt"). These nociceptive sensory neurons are subdivided into two groups on the basis of nerve fiber types: (1) fast conducting myelinated Aδ-fibers, which convey the initial stimulus of nociception (mechanosensitive or mechanothermal), and (2) slowly conducting, unmyelinated C-fibers, which transmit a less intense nociceptive sensation. Nociceptors have both a peripheral connection innervating potentially diseased or traumatized nerves, muscles, tendons, organs, and epithelia, and a centrally projecting axon that enters the central nervous system. This central axon conveys "nociceptive" information to second-order neurons in the dorsal horn of the spinal cord. Neural connections from the dorsal horn to the thalamus and from there to the cortex relay this noxious information to higher centers of conscious and emotional experience. The central axons of primary afferent nociceptive neurons also provide information to polysynaptic spinal cord interneurons, which are essential for the initiation of the nociceptive withdrawal reflex. These neurons trigger motor reflexes that are important for the avoidance of potentially harmful painful stimuli. Descending pathways originating in the cortex and/or midbrain provide modulatory feedback signals at the level of the spinal cord that also regulate the nociceptive experience, thereby providing a closed loop feedback control of this behavior. Additionally, impulses can travel back along the peripheral axon of the nociceptive sensory neuron toward the distal nerve endings, resulting in the local release of neuropeptides in the injury environment. This neuropeptide release produces vasodilatation, venule permeability, plasma extravasation, edema, and leukocyte influx – a process termed "neurogenic inflammation" (Fig. 1).

Although pain clearly plays an important survival role in safeguarding the individual from potential sources of tissue destruction, the perception of pain can also be the result of a dysfunctional nervous system. Typically, the local response to various types of injury or infection involves the release of peripheral chemical

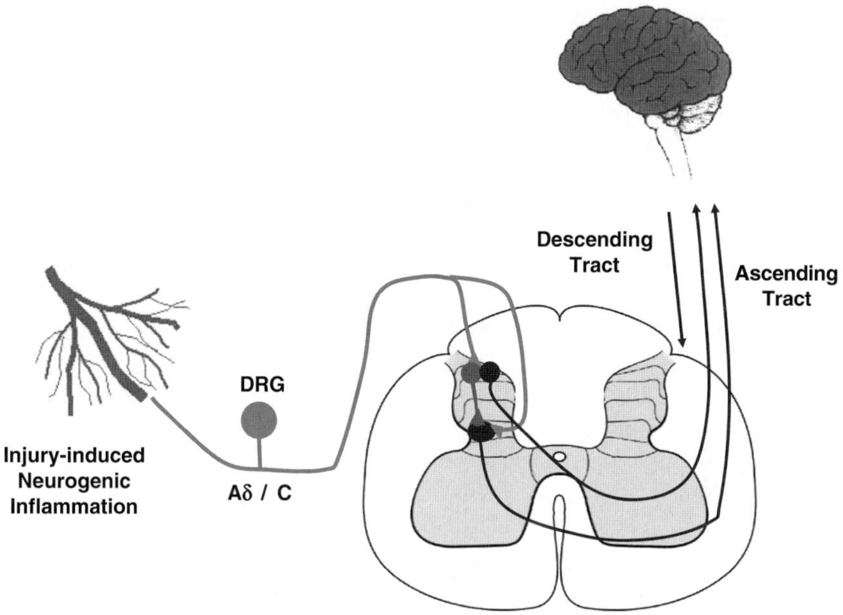

Fig. 1 Nociceptive pathways in the dorsal root ganglia (DRG) and central nervous system. Axons of nociceptors transmit information from the periphery to second-order neurons in the dorsal horn of the spinal cord. Neural connections from the dorsal horn to the thalamus and from there to the cortex relay this noxious information to higher centers of the central nervous system. The central axons of primary afferent nociceptive neurons also provide information to polysynaptic spinal cord interneurons, which are essential for the withdrawal reflex. Descending pathways originating in the cortex and/or midbrain provide modulatory feedback signals at the level of the spinal cord. Impulses can also travel back along the peripheral axon toward the distal nerve endings, resulting in neurogenic inflammation

mediators. These injury-associated factors produce two effects. One role is to attract leukocytes to the point of injury as part of the inflammatory response (Charo and Ransohoff 2006), and the other is to sensitize nociceptors, enhancing their responses to painful stimuli (Zimmermann 2001). The increased excitatory activity of nociceptors produces increased transmitter release in the spinal cord, enhancing neuronal activity in pain pathways in the central nervous system, a phenomenon known as spinal sensitization (Woolf 1983). Under some circumstances, nociceptor-driven electrical activity in the spinal cord becomes divorced from normal physiological function and pathological condition, so pain is produced in the absence of any appropriate stimulus (Campbell et al. 1988; Torebjork et al. 1992). This is now known as pathological, or "neuropathic," pain.

Neuropathic pain is experienced in association with many types of injury to the nervous system or as a consequence of diabetes, cancer, infectious agents (e.g., HIV-1), or the toxic side effects of diverse drug regimens. From the behavioral point of view, neuropathic pain is associated with different types of painful responses to a mechanical stimulus, including *allodynia* (pain evoked by a normally innocuous stimulus) and *hyperalgesia* (enhanced pain evoked by a noxious stimulus).

From the therapeutic point of view, neuropathic pain is an extremely intractable problem. Once established, pain of this type is not readily susceptible to treatment with nonsteroidal anti-inflammatory drugs. Moreover, although opiates may be employed acutely or for chronic pain states (e.g., terminal cancer), alleviation of neuropathic pain is more problematic as high doses are often required, narrowing the therapeutic index (Hempenstall et al. 2005). The remaining available drugs used to treat these syndromes (tricyclic antidepressants, antiepileptics) are not particularly effective and are also associated with a number of negative side effects (Watson 2000). Hence, a complete understanding of the cellular and molecular processes involved in the development of neuropathic pain is essential for the development of novel therapies.

In general, neuropathic pain is the result of abnormal activity of nociceptive neurons. This activity is thought to initially result from the increased neuronal expression and activation of ion channels and receptors that mediate the abnormal generation of action potentials and synaptic transmission in primary afferent nociceptive neurons and/or other parts of the pain pathway. But what causes these changes to occur? It is presumed that some peripheral event provokes primary afferent nociceptive neurons to express different sets of genes, resulting in a new and abnormal chronically hyperexcitable "pain" phenotype.

It has been shown that peripheral nerve injury (trauma-, disease-, or drug-induced) can trigger a wide variety of cellular changes in sensory neurons and, as we have discussed, neuropathic pain following peripheral nerve injury is a consequence of enhanced excitability associated with the chronic sensitization of nociceptive neurons in the peripheral and central nervous systems. Interestingly, following a peripheral nerve injury, not only a subset of injured (Wall and Devor 1983; Kajander et al. 1992; Kim et al. 1993; Amir et al. 1999), but also neighboring noninjured peripheral sensory neurons exhibit spontaneous, ectopic discharges (Tal and Devor 1992; Sheth et al. 2002; Ma et al. 2003; Obata et al. 2003; Liu and Eisenach 2005; Xie et al. 2005). Abnormal excitability of pain neurons may even extend to the spinal cord dorsal horn contralateral to the nerve injury (Sluka et al. 2001, 2007; Raghavendra et al. 2004; Tanaka et al. 2004; Twining et al. 2004; Romero-Sandoval et al. 2005; Bhangoo et al. 2007a; Jung et al. 2007). Although it is clear that molecular changes in the sensory ganglia and spinal cord dorsal horn are responsible for chronic pain, it remains a mystery as to what event(s) are critical for its development and maintenance.

2 Peripheral Nerve Injury and Inflammation

One important development in our understanding of the cellular and molecular processes that produce neuropathic pain concerns the role of the immune system. Immunity can be dissociated into two different phases – innate and acquired.

Acquired immunity involves the phenomenon of immunological memory and includes the antibody and lymphocyte responses to specific antigens. The forerunner to acquired immunity is the innate immune response. This more basic type of immunity involves a generalized immune cell response to a variety of toxic or pathological intrusions into physiological homeostasis. Molecules such as Toll-like receptors (TLRs), Nod-like receptors, and RIG-like receptors expressed by numerous types of cells, including leukocytes, Schwann cells, neurons, astrocytes, and microglia, can recognize shared molecular patterns expressed by infectious agents, cell debris, or other cellular detritus initiating a cascade of cytokine synthesis that orchestrates a general cellular response to these potential problems (Tanga et al. 2005; Creagh and O'Neill 2006; Kim et al. 2007; Tawfik et al. 2007; Watkins et al. 2007b). As noted before, this response is inflammatory in nature and involves the recruitment of leukocytes to areas of tissue damage. The activation of innate immune inflammatory responses is also frequently linked to the development of disease. In the present context, it is believed that the innate immune response to injury plays a prominent role in the establishment of chronic pain states, extending beyond its role in promoting the influx and activation of leukocytes. Although inflammatory and neuropathic pain syndromes are often considered distinct entities, emerging evidence suggests that proinflammatory cytokines produced in association with the innate immune response are clearly implicated in the actual development and maintenance of neuropathic pain, and are a necessary prelude to its development. As such, both neuroinflammatory and associated immune responses following nerve damage may contribute as much to the development and maintenance of neuropathic pain as the initial nerve damage itself.

The traditional view of the post-nerve-trauma environment has been that the influx of leukocytes associated with inflammation was responsible for secreting the chemical mediators that produced pain. However, as we shall discuss, current evidence suggests that the role of the inflammatory response in the generation of pain is not limited to effects produced by the influx of leukocytes per se. Thus, it is currently believed that the proinflammatory cytokines that drive chronic pain behavior may be derived from the cellular elements of the nervous system itself, and that these molecules can act directly on receptors expressed by neurons and other cells of the nervous system (White et al. 2005a). The effects produced by these factors may lead to chronic hyperexcitability and alterations in gene expression by nociceptors, abnormal processing of pain signals, and enhanced pain states. In this way, signaling pathways designed to facilitate a protective response to tissue injury become sources of chronic pathological pain. Generally speaking, the development of chronic pain behavior seems to require the participation of cells in both the peripheral nerve and the dorsal horn of the spinal cord. For example, at various points in time following the initial nerve injury, cytokine synthesis is upregulated in the peripheral nerve, including by DRG satellite cells and nerve-associated Schwann cells, as well as in central elements in the dorsal horn, including microglia and astrocytes (McMahon et al. 2005). Leukocyte influx may also be a participating event. It is clear that complex interactive signaling occurs between various cell types that ultimately results in long-term changes in the excitability of neurons in the pain pathway. Thus, activated sensory neurons can signal to microglia, microglia can signal to neurons, Schwann cells and satellite glial cells can signal to DRG neurons, and vice versa. Ultimately, nociceptive neurons become hyperexcitable and their communication with neurons in the dorsal horn becomes "sensitized." The molecular signatures of this increased nerve activity involve changes in the complement of receptors and ion channels expressed by neurons as well as the neurotransmitters they use. The molecules that orchestrate these changes are inflammatory cytokines.

The question therefore arises as to exactly which inflammatory cytokines are concerned with the development and maintenance of pain states across time and what molecular signaling processes underlie the development of pain hypersensitivity? Furthermore, which cellular elements in the peripheral nerve or dorsal horn of the spinal cord are responsible for the elaboration of cytokine synthesis and subsequently how do these molecules produce their effects? The innate immune response is associated with the development of a complex cascade of cytokine expression in which many inflammatory mediators are synthesized in a mutually dependent manner. What is the precise order and cellular localization of the molecules involved in such cascades? It is likely that several important cytokines are concerned in the establishment of the phenotype that characterizes neuropathic pain. As we shall now discuss, considerable progress has been made on the identification and mechanism of action of proalgesic cytokines. It is now clear that in response to injury or infection, cytokines can be produced by both neurons and glia and this can occur both peripherally and centrally. Cytokines can also be produced by immune cells that participate in the response to injury, infection, or toxicity. Once synthesized by these different types of cells, cytokines produce both short-term and long-term effects on the excitability of sensory neurons. Some of these effects are produced by the cytokines themselves and some by the upregulated synthesis and release of downstream mediators under their control. Thus, the cytokine response is a complex interlocking series of events that ultimately results in long-term changes in nociceptor behavior.

3 Early Events in Sensory Nerve Cytokine Signaling

As we have discussed, it is clear that many of the events that ultimately give rise to chronic pain hypersensitivity initiate a "cascade" of cytokine production, which in turn produces the observed alterations in sensory neuron behavior. These cytokine cascades appear to start with the production of certain key multifunctional cytokines that initiate and orchestrate the subsequent production of further downstream cytokines and numerous other proalgesic mediators. The first cytokines linked to inflammatory hypernociception have frequently been shown to be interleukin-1β (IL-1β) (Ferreira et al. 1988) and tumor necrosis factor α (TNF-α) (Cunha et al. 1992). These cytokines may produce direct effects on sensory neurons and may give rise to further downstream mediators, including other cytokines, chemokines, prostanoids, neurotrophins, NO, kinins, lipids, ATP, and members of the complement pathway (Park and Vasko 2005; Ma and Quirion 2006; Pezet and McMahon 2006; Levin et al. 2008; White et al. 2007b; Donnelly-Roberts et al. 2008; Ting et al. 2008). Upregulation of IL-1β and TNF-α represents one of the earliest events observed in sensory nerves in response to trauma or infection. For example, after chronic constriction injury to the sciatic nerve, levels of both TNF-α and IL-1β in the injured nerve increased over tenfold within 1 h (Uceyler et al. 2007). Both of these cytokines are capable of upregulating the synthesis of numerous downstream mediators and can produce pain hypersensitivity behaviors when administered locally to the skin, systemically, or into the spinal cord (Opree and Kress 2000; Schafers et al. 2003a, b; McMahon et al. 2005). Indeed, elaboration of local cytokine synthesis appears to be sufficient to produce all of the subsequent molecular changes that underlie chronic pain (White et al. 2007a). On the other hand, inhibition of TNF-α or IL-1β action, using neutralizing antibodies or similar strategies, inhibits the development of chronic pain behavior in a variety of models (Schafers and Sommer 2007). For example, TNF-α antibodies attenuate the development of thermal hyperalgesia and mechanical allodynia in several models of neuropathic pain (Cunha et al. 2007; Sasaki et al. 2007; Zanella et al. 2008). Results such as these have encouraged the view that manipulation of cytokine synthesis at an early point in the development of chronic pain behavior with reagents of this type may have a therapeutic role to play in the treatment of chronic pain syndromes.

Despite an enormous amount of work on inflammatory stimulus-induced cytokine cascades and the development of pain hypersensitivity, very few groups have investigated the mechanisms of maintenance of chronic pain. One recent investigation has provided evidence that there are two distinct mechanisms contributing to the development of chronic pain states. The early mechanistic state is dependent on calcium as the use of a calpain inhibitor can diminish both IL-1β and TNF-α levels 1 h after injury, whereas inhibitors of excitatory synaptic transmission (e.g., with the NMDA receptor blocker MK801) did not affect the cytokine levels. In sharp contrast, MK801 successfully diminished IL-1β and TNF-α levels at 3 days, while calpain inhibitors had no effect (Uceyler et al. 2007). Thus, it is possible that one element of chronic pain maintenance is dependent on the activity of the sensory neurons.

Elucidating the exact sequence of cellular and molecular events that leads to the initiation of pain-related cytokine cascades is clearly an important task. It is reasonable to ask what kinds of molecular mechanisms are directly proximal to the original insult and serve as the initiators of all of these subsequent events. Although the answer to this question in not completely clear, there is good evidence that the earliest events are the same as those identified as upstream initiating signals that trigger the innate immune response. For example, the activation of TLRs is one possible entry point into the cytokine pathway that results in the upregulated synthesis of master pleiotropic cytokines such as TNF-α, IL-1β, and frequently also interleukin-6 (IL-6) (Fig. 2). This makes sense because as we discussed earlier, TLRs are initiators of the innate immune response in numerous other cases as well (Martin and Wesche 2002; Guo and Schluesener 2007). The ligands that activate TLRs are pathogen-associated

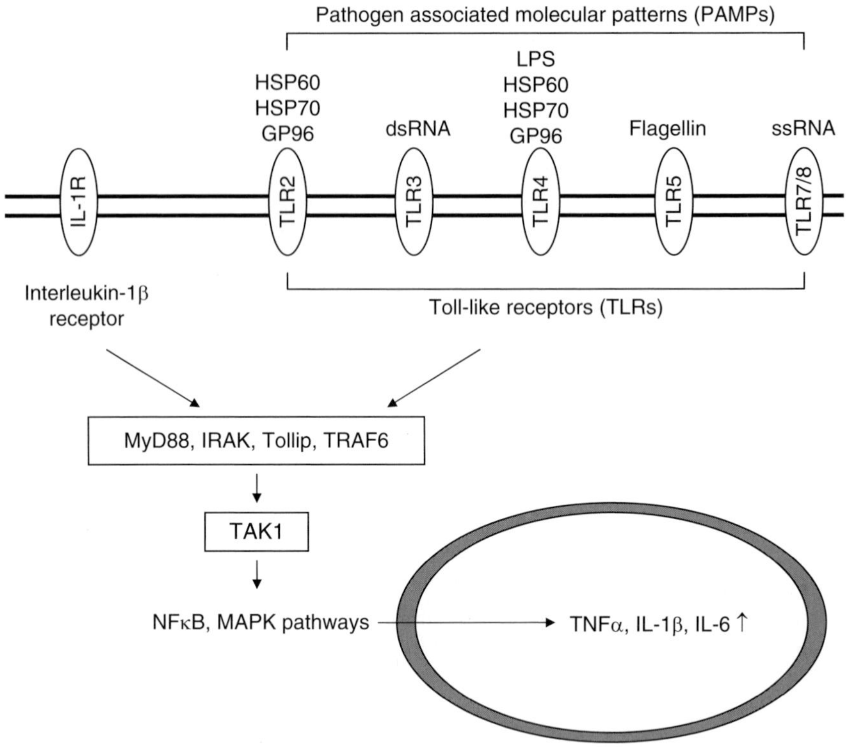

Fig. 2 The Toll-like receptor (TLR) pathway. TLR activation initiates the innate immune response, which is thought to lead to the detrimental cytokine cascade in chronic pain. Activation of TLR signaling proceeds via a family of adaptor proteins which includes the protein MyD88, the interleukin-1 receptor associated kinase, Toll interacting protein, and the adapter protein TRAF6. These proteins activate the kinase TAK1, which ultimately leads to the activation of signaling cascades including nuclear factor κB and mitogen activated protein kinase (MAPK) pathways. The activation of these pathways can then direct the synthesis of cytokines such as tumor necrosis factor α (TNF-α), interleukin-1β (IL-1β), and interleukin-6 (IL-6). Both TLRs and receptors for IL-1β have similar structures and share a cytoplasmic motif. Activation of both types of receptors recruits a scaffolding complex that leads to upregulation of the production of similar cytokines

epitopes, or "pathogen-associated molecular patterns." These elements include molecular components of viruses such as nucleic acids which can activate TLRs 7/8 (single-stranded RNA) or TLR3 (double-stranded RNA). Similarly, molecules from bacteria, including cell wall components such as lipopolysaccharide from Gram-negative bacteria, can activate TLR4. TLR5 mediates the immune response to bacterial flagellins. In addition, molecules released from cells undergoing stress or degradation following injury may also act as signals (Dalpke and Heeg 2002). These include toxicity- or injury-induced release of the heat shock proteins HSP60, HSP70 and/or GP96, which, in turn, activate TLR2 and TLR4 (Vabulas et al. 2002).

Thirteen functional TLRs are known to exist in mammals and several of these forms are expressed by different types of cells known to be important in generating chronic pain behavior (Martin and Wesche 2002; Guo and Schluesener 2007). These include DRG neurons, microglia, astrocytes, Schwann cells, different types of leukocytes, and different peripheral target tissues such as skin (keratinocytes). TLRs are single-pass transmembrane proteins that exist as preassembled homodimers or heterodimers depending on the situation. In some cases, further ancillary membrane proteins are also required for the binding of pathogen-associated molecular patterns and resulting TLR activation. This includes the requirement for the proteins MD-2 and CD14 in binding of lipopolysaccharide by TLR4. Activation of TLR signaling proceeds via a family of adaptor proteins that produce activation of protein kinases and ultimately of transcription factors such as nuclear factor κB. These transcription factors can then direct the synthesis of cytokines such as TNF-α at the gene transcriptional level. Interestingly, elements of TLR "signalosome" are shared with signaling intermediates produced by activation of the IL-1β receptor (IL-1R) (Boraschi and Tagliabue 2006). IL-1βR is also a dimer consisting of two chains, the IL-1R type 1 (IL-1R1) and the IL-1R accessory protein (IL-1RacP). Both TLRs and receptors for IL-1β have similar structures and share a cytoplasmic motif, the Toll/IL-r receptor (TIR) domain. Activation of both types of receptors recruits a scaffolding complex that includes the protein MyD88, the interleukin-1 receptor associated kinase (IRAK), the Toll interacting protein (Tollip) and the adapter protein TRAF6. Recruitment and activation of this signaling complex then leads to activation of the kinase TAK1 that produces phosphorylation and activation of regulatory kinases in different important downstream signaling pathways such as those involved in nuclear factor κB or mitogen activated protein kinase (MAPK) activity. Activation of such signaling pathways ultimately leads to upregulation of the production of cytokines such as TNF-α or IL-1β itself. The fact that TLRs and IL-1Rs share downstream signaling motifs means that activation of TLRs produces a great deal of amplification of their own signaling consequences. The involvement of TLR function in the generation of neuropathic pain is highlighted by recent observations demonstrating reduced pain behavior and inflammatory cytokine upregulation in the spinal cords of TLR2 and four knockout mice (Tanga et al. 2005; Kim et al. 2007). These data imply that damaged, infected, or poisoned neurons or glia release factors that activate TLRs, leading to the synthesis and release of TNF-α and other important cytokines. TLR2 and TLR4, which have been particularly implicated in these events, are expressed by microglia (Tanga et al. 2005; Kim et al. 2007). This interaction implies that cytokine production by these cells in particular may be very early events in the pathway leading from injury to aberrant pain behavior.

If the early production of cytokines is important in the generation of pain we must then ask exactly how such molecules produce the observed phenotypic changes in peripheral nerves and the central connections that underlie pain. It is clear that both sensory neurons and the peripheral and central glial cells associated with them are capable of both elaborating and responding to TNF-α, suggesting a complex network of interdependent signaling occurs between these various cellular elements of sensory nerves (Schafers et al. 2003a, b; Ohtori et al. 2004; Takeda et al. 2007). As we shall discuss further, cytokines such as TNF-α clearly produce changes in the behavior of sensory neurons at a variety of levels. Some of the long-term changes in behavior require alterations in gene transcription and protein expression. However, it is also clear that TNF-α and other upstream cytokines can produce very rapid changes in neuronal excitability which do not seem to require alterations in gene transcription. These changes in excitability probably arise from direct effects of cytokine signaling on the properties of important ion channels, including voltage-dependent sodium channels and transient receptor potential (TRP) channels expressed by sensory nerves (Fig. 3). Presumably, these kinds of effects are the earliest influences on nociceptor excitability produced by cytokines once they have been synthesized and released. For example, perfusion of DRG in vitro with TNF-α produces a rapid increase in A- and C-fiber discharge and also a rapid increase of calcitonin gene-related peptide (CGRP) release from the terminals of nociceptors in the spinal cord (Opree and Kress 2000). How might such

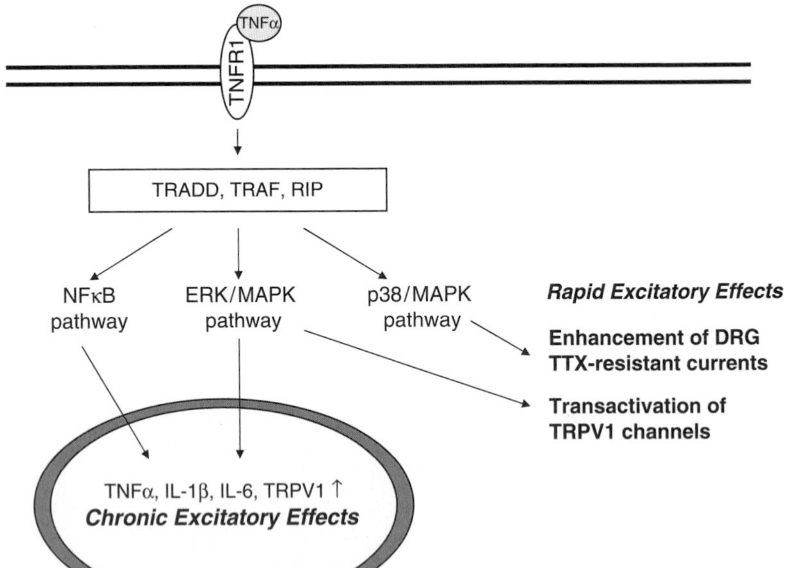

Fig. 3 Possible molecular mechanisms of TNF-α action. TNF-α produces changes in the behavior of sensory neurons at a variety of levels. While some long-term changes in behavior require alterations in gene transcription and protein expression, TNF-α and other upstream cytokines can produce very rapid changes in neuronal excitability as well. These changes in excitability probably arise from direct effects of cytokine signaling on the properties of important ion channels, including voltage-dependent sodium channels and transient receptor potential (TRP) channels expressed by sensory nerves. Activation of TNF-α receptors (TNFRs) produces a wide array of signaling options beginning with recruitment of TNFR-associated death domain protein, receptor-interacting protein, and TNFR-associated factor 2. These proteins go on to activate extracellular-signal-related kinase/MAPK, p38/MAPK, and NFκB pathways

rapid effects on neuronal excitability be produced? TNF-α produces its effects via the activation of two TNF-α receptor subtypes, TNFR1 and TNFR2 (MacEwan 2002). TNFR1 is expressed exclusively on neuronal cells and the TNFR2 is mostly expressed on macrophages and/or monocytes in the DRG under inflammatory conditions (Li et al. 2004). Actions via TNFR1 r appear to be the most relevant to the development of pain behavior because (1) mechanical hyperalgesia induced by exogenous TNF-α or by inflammation is reduced in TNFR1 but not in TNFR2 knockout mice and (2) TNFR1 but not TNFR2 neutralizing antibodies as well as antisense RNA against TNFR1 can reduce experimentally induced hyperalgesia (Sommer et al. 1998; Parada et al. 2003). How can the action of TNF-α on sensory neurons produce rapid changes in excitability? Interestingly, the ability of TNF-α to produce thermal, but not mechanical sensitization was reduced in TRP vanilloid 1 (TRPV1) knockout mice, suggesting that another conductance was the target underlying TNF-α induced mechanical pain hypersensitivity (Jin and Gereau 2006). Consistent with this idea, it was also observed that application of TNF-α to DRG neurons in culture produced a rapid (within 1 min) enhancement of the amplitude of the tetrodotoxin (TTX)-resistant sodium current in these cells (Jin and Gereau 2006). As with TLRs and IL-1R discussed above, activation of TNF-α receptors produces a wide array of signaling options, including activation of the MAPK pathway. In the present context, it was observed that inhibitors of the p38 MAPK could selectively abolish TNF-α induced mechanical pain hypersensitivity and enhancement of the DRG TTX-resistant sodium current. These data suggest a model in which the rapid effects of TNF-α might involve activation of TNFR1 expressed by nociceptors leading to enhanced mechanical hypersensitivity mediated by p38-induced phosphorylation of TTX-resistant sodium current subunits together with thermal hypersensitivity produced by actions on TRPV1 (Jin and Gereau 2006).

In keeping with this hypothesis, it is clear that treatment of DRG neurons with TNF-α also produces rapid upregulation of TRPV1 function and expression. While addition of TNF-α to cultured DRG neurons alone did not directly lead to the release of CGRP, the addition of a thermal stimulus enhanced the release of this neuropeptide, implying that rapid transactivation of TRPV1 by TNF-α can also occur (Jin and Gereau 2006; Hensellek et al. 2007). In addition, TNF-α was also able to produce subsequent upregulation of TRPV1 protein expression when applied to cultured DRG neurons employing a pathway involving extracellular-signal-related kinase rather than p38 signaling. However, this effect required chronic treatment of the cells (more than 8 h) (Jin and Gereau 2006; Hensellek et al. 2007). Hence, it is clear that TNF-α can produce both rapid and long-term excitatory effects on DRG neurons through a variety of molecular mechanisms. The observation that TNF-α expression in DRG neurons, as well as by microglia (Ohtori et al. 2004; Jin and Gereau 2006), is an early event following tissue injury suggests that rapid autocrine excitation of DRG nociceptors by TNF-α may be of importance in the initiation of the cytokine-mediated cascade that eventually results in pain hypersensitivity. The multiple cellular sources of TNF-α together with the multiple effects it can produce on DRG excitability over a broad time course illustrate the complex nature of the impact of inflammatory cytokines on the function of pain sensory neurons.

It is possible that other important upstream cytokines can also produce rapid excitatory signaling in DRG neurons. For example, it is known that DRG neurons can express IL-1β and IL-6 under some circumstances, as well as components of the IL-1R and IL-6 receptor complexes, suggesting that both of these cytokines may also produce direct effects on DRG neuron excitability (Gadient and Otten 1996; Inoue et al. 1999; Gardiner et al. 2002; Lee et al. 2004; Li et al. 2005; Nilsson et al. 2005) (Fig. 4). In the case of IL-6, DRG neurons have been shown to express the glycoprotein 130 (gp130) cytokine receptor subunit, a common feature of all cytokine receptors in the IL-6 family (Gadient and Otten 1996; Thompson et al. 1998; Gardiner et al. 2002; Summer et al. 2008). DRG neurons also express the gp130 binding subunit for the IL-6 related cytokine leukemia inhibitory factor, although the binding component for IL-6 itself (glycoprotein 80) has not been detected (Opree and Kress 2000; Gardiner et al. 2002). Addition of IL-6 to cultured DRG neurons was not effective by itself, but was able to rapidly (minutes) sensitize TRPV1 conductances to heat as well as to stimulate CGRP release, provided that the IL-6 was first primed with a soluble fragment of its receptor (Obreja et al. 2005).

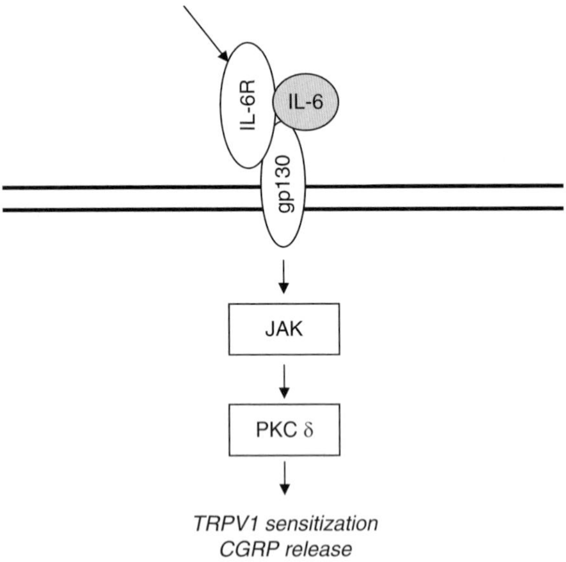

Fig. 4 Rapid effects of the IL-6 pathway. DRG neurons can express IL-6 under some circumstances, as well as components of the IL-6 receptor complexes, suggesting that it can also produce direct effects on DRG neuron excitability. DRG neurons have been shown to express the glycoprotein 130 cytokine receptor subunit, a common feature of all cytokine receptors in the IL-6 family. IL-6 is able to rapidly sensitize vanilloid 1 (TRPV1) conductances to heat as well as to stimulate calcitonin gene-related peptide release via Janus kinase and protein kinase Cδ pathways. It is likely that the binding portion of the IL-6 receptor can be provided *in trans*

Appropriately, for a gp130-linked receptor, Janus kinase and protein kinase C inhibitors inhibited the enhancement of TRPV1 sensitivity. The fact that IL-6 only functions when added together with a soluble form of its binding subunit suggests that it may be activated *in trans* by soluble IL-6 receptors secreted from other cell types in the vicinity.

IL-1β was also unable to increase DRG excitability by itself, but as with IL-6 and TNF-α, produced rapid increases in the sensitivity of TRPV1 and heat-activated CGRP release, implying that IL-1β can also transactivate TRPV1 expressed by DRG neurons (Obreja et al. 2002). It appears that DRG neurons express all the molecular components required for IL-1β signaling and these can be upregulated in inflammatory pain states (Inoue et al. 1999; Li et al. 2005). In the related trigeminal ganglia, it was observed that following the induction of inflammation with complete Freund's adjuvant, IL-1β was highly expressed by satellite glial cells, whereas IL-1R was expressed in the cell bodies of trigeminal neurons. Addition of IL-1β produced rapid excitation of these neurons. Moreover, an IL-1β antagonist reduced complete Freund's adjuvant induced neuronal hyperexcitability, again suggesting a role for cytokine signaling in the development of hyperexcitability of pain sensory neurons (Takeda et al. 2008). In summary, the major upstream cytokines that are rapidly induced in association with the innate immune response can excite DRG neurons by a variety of mechanisms. Some of these effects are too rapid to involve effects on gene transcription and are likely to involve kinase regulation of important conductances such as sodium currents and TRP channels. Molecules such as TNF-α, IL-1β, and IL-6 can be rapidly upregulated by microglia in the spinal cord and frequently by peripheral elements such as the sensory neurons themselves or their associated glial cells. Whatever the cellular source of the cytokines produced in response to injury, increases in sensory neuron excitability are likely to be one of the first cytokine-induced effects that lead to changes in neuronal phenotypes underlying chronic pain. Moreover, these same cytokines may also have rapid electrophysiological effects on second-order neurons in the dorsal horn, so effects on neuronal excitability induced by cytokines may be an early feature of the cytokine response in pain at numerous points in the neuraxis (Kawasaki et al. 2008).

4 Chemokines, Glia, and Chronic Pain

The previous discussion focused on the role of upstream cytokines and their receptors expressed by neurons in particular. It is clear that these molecules are expressed by other types of cells in the DRG and central nervous system, which may also participate in the development and maintenance of neuropathic pain. Some cytokine/receptor signaling events following peripheral injury or infection appear to be primarily mediated by molecular and/or morphological remodeling of glial cells that in turn become a source of inflammatory mediators. It has been proposed that such "activated" Schwann cells, DRG satellite cells, astrocytes, and microglia also play an essential role in the development of chronic pain hypersensitivity (Watkins and Maier 2003). Indeed, drugs that inhibit the activation of these cells have also been reported to interfere with the development of chronic pain behavior, presumably by suppressing the release of inflammatory mediators such as cytokines associated with their activation.

A real "paradigm shift" in pain research has been the recognition that reciprocal communication between neurons and microglia is important in regulating the quiescent and reactive states of glial cells. Glial receptors for inflammatory cytokines, ATP, neuropeptides, neurotransmitters, neurotrophic factors, and chemokines appear to contribute to these events. A clear example of signaling between DRG neurons and microglia in the spinal cord involves the chemokine fractalkine/CX3CL1 and its receptor CX3CR1(Verge et al. 2004; Zhuang et al. 2007). Fractalkine has an unusual structure for a chemokine in that it is tethered to the membrane by means of a transmembrane mucin-like stalk. Normally fractalkine is expressed by neurons and its receptor is particularly highly expressed by microglia (Verge et al. 2004). Fractalkine can signal to its receptor on target microglia in a "tethered" state or it can be released following proteolytic cleavage producing a soluble form of the chemokine that can act at a distance (Milligan et al. 2004). Injection of fractalkine into the spinal cord produces pain hypersensitivity. Moreover, production of soluble fractalkine has been observed in some chronic pain models (Milligan et al. 2004, 2005; Lindia et al. 2005; Zhuang et al. 2007). Recent studies have revealed how fractalkine may act in vivo. It has been demonstrated that the enzyme cathepsin S, which can cleave tethered membrane-bound fractalkine to its soluble form, can itself be released from activated microglia (Clark et al. 2007). The released fractalkine can then act upon microglia to upregulate the release of proallodynic inflammatory mediators such as those discussed above. Thus, fractalkine may act as a neuron to a microglia messenger that amplifies ongoing pain-producing mechanisms. This model also illustrates the fact that neurons and glia can interact in a variety of complex ways to elaborate ongoing pain stimuli producing the mediators that may then initiate transcriptional and other changes resulting in chronic neuronal hyperexcitability and pain. In addition to the example of fractalkine, activated spinal microglia also express C-C chemokine receptor 2 (CCR2) and C-X-C chemokine receptor 3 (CXCR3), making them potential targets for the chemokines monocyte chemotactic protein 1 (MCP-1) or interferon-γ inducing protein 10 (IP-10) upregulated and released from DRG neurons, (Abbadie et al. 2003; Flynn et al. 2003; Tanuma et al. 2006), as we shall now discuss.

5 Downstream Cytokine Signaling

A relatively novel family of cytokines that has now been linked to the induction and maintenance of chronic pain are the chemotactic cytokines (chemokines). Chemokines are small, secreted proteins that exert all of their known effects through the activation of G protein coupled receptors. Chemokines were originally identified as migrational effectors for the attraction of different classes of leukocytes in association with the development of inflammation (Charo and Ransohoff 2006). Several subfamilies of chemokines and their receptors are known to exist. Most chemokines are not constitutively expressed at high levels, their production and secretion being normally associated with activation of the inflammatory response. Thus, the synthesis of most chemokines is usually greatly stimulated through the action of one of the major upstream inflammatory cytokines discussed earlier. An exception to this rule is the chemokine stromal cell derived factor 1 (SDF-1/CXCL12). SDF-1 is the most evolutionarily ancient member of the chemokine family and existed phylogenetically prior to the development of an immune system, indicating that chemokine signaling originally played a role other than the regulation of leukocyte chemotaxis (Huising et al. 2003; Knaut et al. 2003). Still, chemotaxis appears to be one ancient function of this chemokine as well. In mammals, SDF-1 signaling through its major receptor, C-X-C chemokine receptor 4 (CXCR4), has been shown to be important for the development of the embryo where SDF-1 regulates the migration of the stem/progenitor cells that form numerous tissues (Tachibana et al. 1998; Lu et al. 2002). Postnatally, this signaling system is still used in this way to retain hematopoietic stem cells in the bone marrow (Wright et al. 2002).

Although chemokines clearly have a central role in orchestrating the normal inflammatory response, the pathogenesis of many chronic inflammatory conditions such as atherosclerosis, arthritis, and inflammatory bowel disease has been shown to be mediated in large part by the actions of chemokines (Charo and Ransohoff 2006). In addition, numerous neurological conditions which are accompanied by activation of the innate immune response during their onset or progression appear to involve the action of chemokines in their pathogenesis. These include autoimmune disorders (e.g., multiple sclerosis), neurodegenerative disorders (e.g., cerebral ischemic injury, Parkinson's, Huntington's, and Alzheimer's diseases) as well as virus-based diseases (e.g., HIV-1 and herpes simplex) (Streit et al. 2001; Cartier et al. 2005; Ubogu et al. 2006). This chemokine-mediated component is also likely to extend to the pathogenesis and maintenance of chronic pain in both disease-related conditions (e.g., multiple sclerosis, HIV-1, and herpes simplex) and following trauma, all of which are associated with innate immune responses and prolonged expression of chemokines and their receptors by the cellular elements of the nervous system (White et al. 2005a). This being the case, interference with chemokine function represents a promising approach for the development of both novel anti-inflammatory medication and the treatment of chronic pain conditions.

6 Chemokines and Their Receptors in Acute and Chronic Pain

There is now a large amount of data indicating that chemokines and their receptors can influence both the acute and chronic phases of pain. However, why is chemokine function of particular interest in this regard? It has become apparent that the cellular elements of the nervous system (e.g., neurons, glia, and microglia) are able to both synthesize and respond to chemokines, something that is quite independent of their traditional role in the regulation of leukocyte chemotaxis and function. Oh et al. (2001) first demonstrated that the simple injection of the chemokines SDF-1, regulated upon activation, normal T cell expressed, and secreted (RANTES/CCL5), or macrophage inflammatory protein 1α (MIP-1α/CCL3) into the adult rat hind paw produced dose-dependent tactile allodynia. These authors also demonstrated that cultured DRG neurons expressed numerous types of chemokine receptors, indicating that the observed pain behavior might result from a direct action of chemokines on these neurons. In support of this possibility, chemokines were found to strongly excite DRG neurons in culture (White et al. 2005b; Sun et al. 2006) and chemokine-induced excitation was associated with the release of pain related neurotransmitters such as substance P and CGRP (Qin et al. 2005; Jung et al. 2008). The cellular mechanism underlying chemokine-induced excitation of sensory neurons in culture has been shown to have at least two components. The first of these is the transactivation of TRP cation channels, such as TRPV1 and TRP ankyrin 1 (TRPA1), which are also expressed by populations of nociceptive neurons (Bandell et al. 2004; Ruparel et al. 2008; Jung et al. 2008), and the second of these is inhibition of K^+ conductances that normally regulate neuronal excitability. MIP-1α, for example, can enhance the thermal sensitivity of TRPV1 (Zhang et al. 2005). The receptor for MIP-1α, C-C chemokine receptor 1 (CCR1), is expressed by more than 85% of cultured DRG neurons which also express TRPV1 (Zhang et al. 2005). Activation of other chemokine receptors such as CCR2 expressed by cultured DRG neurons (see below) also produces excitation through transactivation of both TRPV1 and TRPA1 (Jung et al. 2008). In the former instance, the mechanism of activation appears to be due to phospholipase C induced removal of tonic phosphatidylinositol 4,5-bisphosphate mediated channel block (Chuang et al. 2001), whereas in the second instance the transactivation appears to involve a protein kinase C mediated event (Cesare and McNaughton 1996; Premkumar and Ahern 2000; Sugiura et al. 2002). Importantly, TRPA1 activation is central to acute pain, neuropeptide release, and neurogenic inflammation (McNamara et al. 2007; Trevisani et al. 2007). These data suggest that chemokine-induced excitation involving TRP channel activation may be of key importance to driving increased excitation observed in chronic pain states.

A significant question is whether such data, mostly obtained in cell culture studies, have relevance to the situation prevailing in chronic pain states in vivo. A key role for chemokines and their receptors in chronic pain has come from the results of experiments using several accepted models of neuropathic pain in rodents. These models include sciatic nerve transaction (Taskinen and Roytta 2000; Subang and Richardson 2001), partial ligation of the sciatic nerve (Abbadie et al. 2003; Tanaka et al. 2004; Lindia et al. 2005), chronic constriction injury of the sciatic nerve (Milligan et al. 2004; Kleinschnitz et al. 2005; Zhang and De Koninck 2006), chronic compression of the L_4L_5 DRG, a rodent model of spinal stenosis (White et al. 2005b; Sun et al. 2006), lysophosphatidylcholine-induced focal nerve demyelination (Bhangoo et al. 2007a; Jung et al. 2008), bone cancer pain (Vit et al.

2006; Khasabova et al. 2007), and zymosan-induced inflammatory pain (Milligan et al. 2004; Verge et al. 2004; Xie et al. 2006). Each of these models resulted in upregulation of one or more chemokine receptors by DRG neurons associated with, or in close proximity to, the injury. Moreover, in several instances it has also been demonstrated that sensory neurons will actually upregulate the synthesis of chemokines in addition to their cognate receptors (White et al. 2005b; Sun et al. 2006; Bhangoo et al. 2007a; Jung et al. 2007, 2008). Thus, in association with chronic pain the same DRG neuron may upregulate both a chemokine and its receptor, suggesting some form of cell autologous regulation of DRG excitability by these molecules may occur. For example, it might be imagined that under these circumstances DRG neurons could release chemokines that would then activate receptors expressed by the same neuron or by others in the vicinity. As chemokines can excite DRG neurons, this process might contribute to the neuronal hyperexcitability observed under these circumstances (White et al. 2005b; Sun et al. 2006). As chemokines are also of central importance in the recruitment of leukocytes, they would have a unique role in simultaneously coordinating inflammation and neuronal excitability.

One good example of the validity of this type of model concerns the potential role of the chemokine MCP-1 and its receptor CCR2 in the genesis of neuropathic pain. The role of MCP-1/CCR2 signaling in neuropathic pain states was suggested following peripheral nerve injury in genetically engineered mice lacking CCR2 receptors (Abbadie et al. 2003). These receptor knockout mice failed to display mechanical hyperalgesia following partial ligation of the sciatic nerve without a detectable change in acute pain behavior, while transgenic mice overexpressing glial MCP-1 production exhibited enhanced nociceptive responses (Menetski et al. 2007).

In keeping with these results, both CCR2 and its preferred ligand, MCP-1, are extensively upregulated in sensory neurons following chronic compression of the DRG (White et al. 2005b) and focal demyelination of the sciatic nerve (Bhangoo et al. 2007a). Functionally, many of these injured neurons respond to the exogenous administration of MCP-1 with membrane threshold depolarization, action potentials, and Ca^{2+} mobilization. Appropriately, these MCP-1-induced excitatory events were not observed in control animals and the use of a CCR2 receptor antagonist effectively reversed hypernociception (Bhangoo et al. 2007a). Subsequent investigations have revealed that two ionic mechanisms contribute to the excitatory effects of MCP-1; a non-voltage-dependent, depolarizing current with the properties of a nonselective cation conductance, quite possibly a TRP channel (Jung et al. 2008), and activation of another nonv-oltage-dependent depolarizing current with characteristics similar to those of a nonselective cation conductance (Sun et al. 2006).

Such chemokine-induced excitatory effects on sensory neurons may further facilitate the axonal transport and the release of excitatory neuropeptides, such as CGRP (Qin et al. 2005) and substance P from the terminals of DRG neurons in the spinal cord. Zhang and De Koninick (2006) recently demonstrated that MCP-1 is also present in central afferent fibers in the spinal cord. Thus, electrical activity due to peripheral nerve injury may also stimulate central afferent release of MCP-1 into the spinal cord dorsal horn, further activating CCR2-expressing microglial cells or central neurons (Abbadie et al. 2003; Bursztajn et al. 2004; Zhang and De Koninck 2006). Neurons from the dorsal horn express CCR2 receptors and MCP-1/CCR2 signaling reduces the inhibitory effects of GABA on these cells. Hence, release of MCP-1 may mediate excitatory effects at the level of both the DRG and the spinal cord.

Overall, these results suggest that injury-induced expression of MCP-1 may, in effect, function as a neurotransmitter in DRG neurons and may be central to the maintenance of chronic neuropathic pain states. Moreover, examination of the distribution of MCP-1 at a subcellular level following its synthesis in cultured DRG neurons has revealed that it is initially processed via the *trans*-Golgi network and packaged into the same synaptic vesicles as the peptide neurotransmitter CGRP (Jung et al. 2008). Vesicles that contain both proteins can be observed in the neuronal soma and following transport to nerve terminals. Depolarization of these neurons results in calcium-dependent release of MCP-1 either from the soma or from the nerve terminals (Jung et al. 2008). Presumably release of the chemokine from the cell soma within the DRG would have the effect of depolarizing neighboring CCR2-expressing neurons, eliciting excitation and promoting further MCP-1 release within the DRG or within the dorsal horn or the spinal cord, where it could interact with CCR2-expressing neurons and glia. In this way upregulation of MCP-1 and CCR2 might be an important component of DRG hyperexcitability and maintenance of chronic pain. It is interesting to note that in the brain the chemokine CCL21/exodus has also been shown to be upregulated by neurons following excitotoxic stimulation and to be packaged into secretory vesicles and released upon neuronal depolarization (de Jong et al. 2005). Thus, it appears that when chemokines are expressed in neurons under different circumstances they may generally play a novel role as neurotransmitters. MCP-1 and CCR2, as well as certain other chemokines and chemokine receptors, exhibit an exceptionally prolonged upregulation in the injury-associated DRG (White et al. 2005b; Zhang and De Koninck 2006; Bhangoo et al. 2007a, b), and the trigeminal ganglion following peripheral nerve injury (White et al. 2006) or herpes simplex virus infection (Theil et al. 2003; Cook et al. 2004; Wickham et al. 2005), supporting the possibility that this type of signaling could contribute to the chronic nature of neuropathic pain.

Overall, the evidence suggests that prolonged chemokine and chemokine receptor expression in sensory ganglia may well be a significant contributor to many injury-induced and virus-associated neuropathic pain syndromes (Fig. 5). This being the case, it is also of interest to define the signaling pathways in DRG neurons that result in the upregulation of chemokine and chemokine receptor expression as they may represent novel targets for intervention in the treatment of chronic pain. In the case of CCR2 receptors, some information on this issue has been obtained (Jung and Miller 2008). Analysis of the structure of the mouse and human CCR2 genes revealed several upstream regulatory elements that might potentially mediate the action of different transcription factors. Included in these is a conserved binding site for the transcription factor nuclear factor of activated T cells (NFAT) (Jung and Miller 2008). Members of the NFAT family of proteins are expressed by DRG neurons and expression of constitutively active NFAT derivatives produced upre-

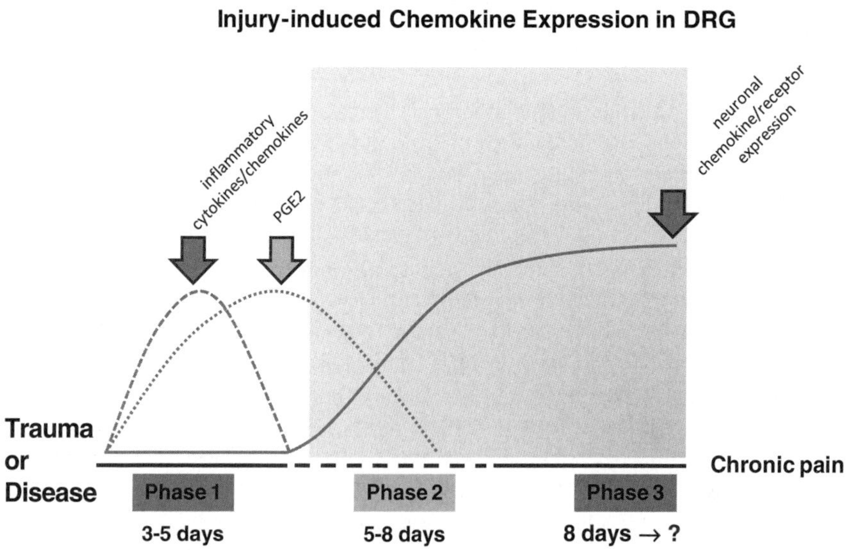

Fig. 5 Injury-induced chemokine expression in DRG. Evidence suggests that prolonged chemokine and chemokine receptor expression in sensory ganglia may be a significant contributor to neuropathic pain syndromes. It is likely that chemokines affect neuronal hyperexcitability by transactivating TRP channels. While proinflammatory cytokines such as TNF-α, IL-6 and prostaglandin E are expressed early on and contribute to the genesis of chronic pain, evidence suggests that chemokines are expressed at later time points and may act as the trigger to convert the acute pain to one that is chronic in nature

gulation of CCR2 receptors in these neurons (Jung and Miller 2008). NFAT is activated by being dephosphorylated by the calcium-dependent phophatase calcineurin. When the intracellular calcium concentration is increased in DRG neurons following depolarization via voltage-dependent calcium channels, calcineurin/NFAT activation effectively modulates increases in CCR2 expression (Jung and Miller 2008). This then provides a possible pathway for the induction of CCR2 in the context of neuropathic pain. Some upstream mediator is envisaged as initially depolarizing DRG neurons, leading to calcium influx and CCR2 upregulation. Once CCR2 has been upregulated, signaling via CCR2 could increase DRG excitation further and potentiate ongoing excitability. Interestingly, although MCP-1 is upregulated by DRG neurons together with CCR2 in chronic pain (White et al. 2005b), MCP-1 is not a target gene for NFAT regulation. On the other hand, we have observed that MCP-1 is upregulated in DRG neurons by the action of the cytokine TNF-α (Jung and Miller 2008). Indeed, as discussed earlier, TNF-α is known to increase the excitability of DRG neurons by a variety of mechanisms (Nicol et al. 1997; Sorkin and Doom 2000). In addition, TNF-α may also act as an upstream regulator of chemokine signaling in these cells and the chemokines produced may help to maintain the hyperexcitability of nociceptors. Such a possibility would also help to explain why increased DRG excitability extends to uninjured neurons that are both ipsilateral and contralateral to the nerve injury, observations that suggest an important role for diffusible mediators in triggering these events.

Although most of the data obtained on chemokine signaling in the DRG in the context of neuropathic pain concern the role of MCP-1/CCR2, it is clear that other types of chemokine signaling may also be dynamically regulated under similar conditions. Upregulated expression of the CXCR3, CXCR4, and C-C chemokine receptor 5 (CCR5) receptors as well as their chemokine ligands has also been observed in populations of DRG neurons in chronic pain models (Bhangoo et al. 2007a, b). As with CCR2, upregulation of some of these chemokine receptors appears to be NFAT-dependent (e.g., CCR5), whereas upregulation of others is not (e.g., CXCR4) (Jung and Miller 2008). The precise expression patterns and time course of upregulation of these diverse chemokine signaling systems differ in each case, and so the details of how they each participates in pain behavior may vary according to the circumstances and will require further clarification. Nevertheless, the fact that chemokines are packaged into neurotransmitter secretory vesicles in DRG neurons indicates that they may play a neuromodulatory role in chronic pain (de Jong et al. 2005; Jung and Miller 2008). It is interesting to note that in the case of SDF-1 and MCP-1 these vesicle populations are clearly different (unpublished observations), indicating that even when two chemokines are secreted by the same neuron they may subserve somewhat different functions.

As an example of the role of chemokine signaling in chronic pain one might consider peripheral nervous system and central nervous system inflammatory demyelinating diseases such as Guillain-Barre syndrome, Charcot-Marie-Tooth disease types 1 and 4, and multiple sclerosis, which are frequently accompanied by a neuropathic pain syndrome (Carter et al. 1998; Boukhris et al. 2007). Epidemiological studies suggest that chronic pain syndromes afflict 50–80% of patients with multiple sclerosis and 70–90% of individuals with Guillain-Barre syndrome (Moulin 1998). Disease-related components that may be central to this overall pattern of symptoms of neuropathic pain include axon and Wallerian degeneration (Bruck 2005), which may act as a trigger for the cytokine cascades that result in the upregulation and chronic expression of chemokines and their cognate receptors (Mahad et al. 2002; Charo and Ransohoff 2006).

Studies of several rodent models of demyelinating diseases known to elicit neuropathic pain behavior, including late-developing peripheral axon demyelination in *periaxin* knockout mice (Gillespie et al. 2000), lysophosphatidylcholine-induced transient focal demyelination of the sciatic nerve in mice and rats (Wallace et al. 2003; Bhangoo et al. 2007a; Jung et al. 2008) and the late, acute clinical phase of experimental autoimmune neuritis (Moalem-Taylor et al. 2007), have indicated a possible role for chemokine-mediated signaling in these models. Recent studies on rats and mice subjected to transient focal demyelination of the sciatic nerve revealed chronic upregulation of MCP-1, IP-10/CXCL10, and the chemokine receptors CCR2, CCR5, and CXCR4 in primary sensory neurons (Bhangoo et al. 2007a). Application of these same chemokines to neurons isolated from DRG of animals following demyelination produced an increase in excitation. Thus, upregulation of these chemokines and their receptors may effectively drive the chronic excitability and pain behavior in demyelinating diseases of this type. It is also of interest that administration of small-molecule CCR2 receptor antagonists to these animals afforded some relief from ongoing pain, further indicating the role of chemokine signaling and the potential therapeutic effectiveness of inhibiting these events (Bhangoo et al. 2007a).

As in the case of upstream inflammatory cytokines such as TNF-α, glia in the DRG and peripheral nerve may also represent a source of, and a target for, the action of chemokines. For example, in response to nerve injury MCP-1 is upregulated in Schwann cells (Toews et al. 1998; Taskinen and Roytta 2000; Orlikowski et al. 2003). Thus, these cells might also represent a source of chemokine release for the activation of CCR2 chemokine receptors upregulated in adjacent DRG neurons.

The key involvement of chemokine signaling between glia and DRG neurons appears to be likely in certain chronic pain states such as those experienced in association with HIV-1 infection. This has particular relevance for the present discussion, as the cellular receptors for glycoprotein 120 (gp120), the HIV-1 coat protein, are the CXCR4 and CCR5 chemokine receptors. One example of an HIV-1 associated pain syndrome is distal symmetrical polyneuropathy (DSP), which affects as many as one third of all HIV-1 infected individuals (Skopelitis et al. 2006). This painful sensory neuropathy frequently begins with paresthesias in the fingers and toes, progressing over weeks to months, followed by the development of pain, often of a burning and lancinating nature, which can make walking very difficult. Measurements of pain hypersensitivity have demonstrated allodynia and hyperalgesia in HIV-1 infected individuals. Interestingly, as is the case of HIV-1 associated effects on the central nervous system, there is no productive infection of peripheral neurons by the virus. Thus, indirect effects of HIV-1 must lead to the development of this pain state.

In addition to the effects of inflammatory mediators (including chemokines) released by virally infected leukocytes, there are at least two ways in which HIV-1 induced DSP may involve the direct effects of HIV-1 gp120 on chemokine receptors in the DRG: (1) viral protein shedding in the peripheral nervous system might enable gp120 to produce painful neuropathy via glial to neuronal signaling in the DRG and/or spinal cord (Milligan et al. 2000; Keswani et al. 2003) or (2) by the direct activation of CCR5/CXCR4-bearing sensory neurons by gp120 (Herzberg and Sagen 2001; Oh et al. 2001; Wallace et al. 2007). Indeed, Keswani et al. (2003, 2006) have presented a model in which gp120 can act in both these ways. In the first instance, these authors demonstrated that binding of gp120 to CXCR4 receptors expressed by DRG satellite glial cells upregulates the release of the chemokine RANTES, which can then activate CCR5 receptors expressed by DRG neurons. In the second instance, gp120 can directly bind to and activate CXCR4 receptors expressed by DRG neurons (Oh et al. 2001). Moreover, this initial excitation of DRG neurons by gp120 and/or glial mediators might produce Ca^{2+}-dependent upregulation of CCR2 expression by these neurons by the mechanisms discussed above (Jung and Miller 2008), leading to a second level of chemokine-mediated excitation. In support of such a model we have observed that treatment of the sciatic nerve with a T-tropic gp120 subsequently leads to MCP-1 and CCR2 upregulation (unpublished observations), which would also be expected to promote excitation of DRG neurons.

Complicating matters further, AIDS patients who are treated by highly active, antiretroviral therapeutical (HAART) agents can also develop a painful sensory neuropathy. Intriguingly, the symptoms of this syndrome are clinically indistinguishable from those of HIV-1 induced DSP, including a burning sensation in the hands and feet and hypersensitivity to pain (Snider et al. 1983; Pardo et al. 2001; Skopelitis et al. 2006). The fact that the two syndromes are usually seen in association with one another makes diagnosis more difficult.

Recent studies have shed new light on the mechanisms of HAART-induced DSP and the role of chemokine signaling in particular. It was observed that the drug 2′,3′-dideoxycytidine (zalcitabine, or ddC) produced neuropathic pain behavior together with upregulated expression of both SDF-1 and CXCR4 in DRG satellite glial cells and some neurons. This suggests that SDF-1 release from DRG glia might be involved in the autologous regulation of excitatory substances from these same cells and that released SDF-1 might directly excite DRG neurons. Significantly, zalcitabine-induced pain was completely blocked by the CXCR4 antagonist AMD3100, illustrating the key role of CXCR4 signaling in this behavior. (Bhangoo et al. 2007b). Hence, the proallodynic actions of both HIV-1 and zalcitabine are dependent on chemokine signaling between DRG glia and neurons.

7 Chemokine Interactions with Other Neurotransmitters

As we have discussed, chemokines and their receptors expressed by DRG neurons in chronic pain conditions may contribute to nociceptor hyperexcitability in many instances by directly exciting these neurons. However, other consequences of chemokine signaling may also indirectly contribute to pain behavior. One important example of this concerns chemokine interactions with the endogenous opioid system. Generally speaking, activation of μ-opioid receptors in the DRG and dorsal horn reduces neuronal excitability and synaptic transmission at synapses between nociceptors and first-order neurons in the spinal cord. This is believed to be one of the mechanisms by which opiates reduce pain behavior. However, it has been demonstrated that upregulation of chemokine signaling routinely modulates μ-opioid receptor function (Szabo et al. 2002; Zhang et al. 2005). One mechanism through which this may occur is by heterologous desensitization resulting from the effects of chemokine receptor activation on μ-receptor function (Grimm et al. 1998; Chen et al. 2007). In addition, fluorescence resonance energy transfer studies have demonstrated that some chemokine receptors can directly dimerize with μ-opioid receptors, raising the possibility that this interaction may also alter μ-receptor signaling (Toth et al. 2004). Interestingly, the opposite may also be true as the μ-opiate receptor agonist DAMGO can downregulate chemokine activation of chemokine receptors, something that may account for opiate-drug-induced immune suppression (Patel et al. 2006).

A particularly interesting interaction between cytokine/chemokine and opioid signaling seems to occur in the context of chronic opioid use. As has now been well documented, chronic opioid use or opioid withdrawal may result in significant hyperalgesia and this may present itself as a clinically significant problem (DeLeo et al. 2004; Watkins et al. 2007c). Although mechanisms such as those discussed above suggest that some chemokine/opioid interactions may be responsible for the downregulation of opioid effects in pain, they do not explain the development of pain hypersensitivity. However, several hypotheses do try to accommodate this phenomenon. According to one view, the normal opioid-induced analgesic effects that are observed are always concomitantly accompanied by opposing opioid-mediated hyperalgesic effects (Hutchinson et al. 2007). These latter effects are not mediated by the actions of opioids on neurons, but on glia (Watkins et al. 2007a). Thus, it is proposed that the activation of microglia by drugs such as morphine normally results in the upregulation of inflammatory cytokines by these cells as well as a reduction in the synthesis of anti-inflammatory cytokines such as interleukin-10 (Johnston et al. 2004; Milligan et al. 2006; Hutchinson et al. 2007; Ledeboer et al. 2007; Liang et al. 2008). The triggering of this cytokine cascade eventually results in pain hypersensitivity as described above. Viewed in this way, the proalgesic effects of chronic opioid use are another version of the "neuroinflammatory" response that is associated with pain hypersensitivity syndromes. This is even more the case given that it is also proposed that the opioid receptors that are expressed by microglia are none other than the TLR4 receptors (Hutchinson et al. 2007). It has been shown that unlike the effects of morphine on μ-receptors that are stereospecifically blocked by the opioid antagonist naloxone (only the – isomer being effective), the ability of morphine to activate TLR4 receptors is inhibited by both (+)-naloxone and (–)-naloxone. It is suggested that these proalgesic effects eventually overwhelm the antinociceptive effects of morphine to shift the balance to pain-producing rather than pain-preventing behavior. Recently, we have observed that chronic morphine treatment produces an upregulation of SDF-1 expression by DRG sensory neurons and that morphine-induced pain hypersensitivity is blocked by the CXCR4 antagonist AMD3100 (Wilson et al. 2008). As we have discussed, chemokines are often among the proteins synthesized downstream of cytokine cascades and can act directly on DRG neurons to enhance their excitability (White et al. 2005b; Sun et al. 2006). Hence, it is possible that this represents a further example of this phenomenon.

As we have discussed, chemokines expressed by DRG neurons may also be responsible for chemoattractant effects resulting in leukocyte influx into the ganglia. Some leukocytes can actively secrete opioid peptides, an action which is potentially analgesic (Labuz et al. 2006; Rittner et al. 2006). Thus, chemokines may be potentially proalgesic by directly exciting DRG neurons and downregulating opioid signaling as well as potentially analgesic owing to their effects on endorphin release from leukocytes. How these diverse effects play out in the context of chronic pain behavior is incompletely understood, and may have different degrees of importance depending on the precise type of pain syndrome under consideration. Clearly, numerous cellular mechanisms through which upregulated chemokine signaling might occur result in pain hypersensitivity or related phenomena.

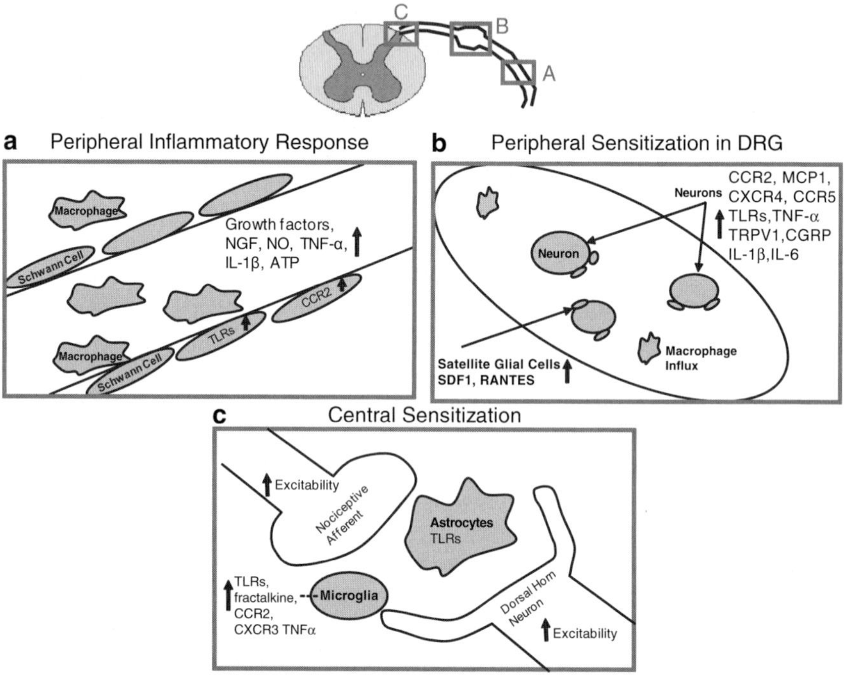

Fig. 6 Injury-induced changes in the nociceptive pathway. In neuropathic pain, nociceptive pathways are altered at all levels of the central and peripheral nervous systems. Inflammatory cytokines and chemokines may play a key role in coordinating injury-associated nociceptive events as they regulate the inflammatory response and can simultaneously act upon elements of the nervous system, including the peripheral nerve (**a**), the DRG (**b**), and the dorsal horn of the spinal cord (**c**). Rapid effects of these molecules can alter the excitability of neurons, and the sensitization of ion channels involved in the neuropathic pain mechanism. Slower effects of cytokines include altered gene expression, which could the result in the subsequent upregulation of other proinflammatory cytokines, and ion channel expression. These events, which occur in many different cell types, when taken together result in an altered state of excitability that contributes to the chronic pain state. *NGF* nerve growth factor, *NO* nitric oxide, *TNF-α* tumor necrosis factor α, *IL-1β* interleukin-1β, *TLR* Toll-like receptor, *ATP* adenosine triphosphate, *TRPV1* transient receptor potential vanilloid 1, *CGRP* calcitonin gene-related peptide, *IL-6* interleukin-6, *CCR2* C-C chemokine receptor 2, *CXCR3* C-X-C chemokine receptor 3, *CXCR4* C-X-C chemokine receptor 4, *MCP-1* monocyte chemotactic protein 1, *SDF-1* stromal cell derived factor 1, *RANTES* regulated upon activation, normal T cell expressed and secreted

8 Conclusions

Recent research has made it clear that inflammatory processes are critical for the development of states of chronic pain and for the changes in behavior of pain neurons that accompany these syndromes. The development of such behavior may involve reciprocal signaling interactions between the different cellular elements of the central and peripheral nervous systems. As we have discussed here, inflammatory cytokines and chemokines seem to be one set of molecules that play a key role in coordinating injury-associated nociceptive events as they serve to regulate inflammatory responses and can simultaneously act upon elements of the nervous system (Fig. 6). Importantly, chemokines in DRG neurons seem to act as upregulatable neurotransmitters that produce excitatory effects in the DRG and spinal cord through a variety of mechanisms. The ability of small-molecule antagonists of CCR2 and CXCR4 receptors to ameliorate ongoing pain hypersensitivity in animal models clearly indicates the importance of chemokine signaling in this behavior. Furthermore, antibodies to cytokines such as TNF-α also prevent the development of chronic pain. We therefore conclude that targeting inflammatory cytokine and chemokine signaling may provide a novel form of therapeutic intervention into states of chronic pain.

Acknowledgements F.A.W acknowledges NIH grants NS049136, National Multiple Sclerosis Society Pilot Award, and Illinois Excellence in Medicine, State of Illinois. R.J.M. acknowledges NIH grants NS043095, DA013141, and MH040165.

References

Abbadie C, Lindia JA, Cumiskey AM, Peterson LB, Mudgett JS, Bayne EK, DeMartino JA, MacIntyre DE, Forrest MJ (2003) Impaired neuropathic pain responses in mice lacking the chemokine receptor CCR2. Proc Natl Acad Sci USA 100:7947–7952

Amir R, Michaelis M, Devor M (1999) Membrane potential oscillations in dorsal root ganglion neurons: role in normal electrogenesis and neuropathic pain. J Neurosci 19:8589–8596

Bandell M, Story GM, Hwang SW, Viswanath V, Eid SR, Petrus MJ, Earley TJ, Patapoutian A (2004) Noxious cold ion channel TRPA1 is activated by pungent compounds and bradykinin. Neuron 41:849–857

Bhangoo S, Ren D, Miller RJ, Henry KJ, Lineswala J, Hamdouchi C, Li B, Monahan PE, Chan DM, Ripsch MS, White FA (2007a) Delayed functional expression of neuronal chemokine receptors following focal nerve demyelination in the rat: a mechanism for the development of chronic sensitization of peripheral nociceptors. Mol Pain 3:38

Bhangoo SK, Ren D, Miller RJ, Chan DM, Ripsch MS, Weiss C, McGinnis C, White FA (2007b) CXCR4 chemokine receptor signaling mediates pain hypersensitivity in association with antiretroviral toxic neuropathy. Brain Behav Immun 21:581–591

Boraschi D, Tagliabue A (2006) The interleukin-1 receptor family. Vitam Horm 74:229–254

Boukhris S, Magy L, Khalil M, Sindou P, Vallat JM (2007) Pain as the presenting symptom of chronic inflammatory demyelinating polyradiculoneuropathy (CIDP). J Neurol Sci 254:33–38

Bruck W (2005) The pathology of multiple sclerosis is the result of focal inflammatory demyelination with axonal damage. J Neurol 252(Suppl 5):v3–v9

Bursztajn S, Rutkowski MD, Deleo JA (2004) The role of the *N*-methyl-D-aspartate receptor NR1 subunit in peripheral nerve injury-induced mechanical allodynia, glial activation and chemokine expression in the mouse. Neuroscience 125:269–275

Campbell JN, Raja SN, Meyer RA, Mackinnon SE (1988) Myelinated afferents signal the hyperalgesia associated with nerve injury. Pain 32:89–94

Carter GT, Jensen MP, Galer BS, Kraft GH, Crabtree LD, Beardsley RM, Abresch RT, Bird TD (1998) Neuropathic pain in Charcot–Marie–Tooth disease. Arch Phys Med Rehabil 79: 1560–1564

Cartier L, Hartley O, Dubois-Dauphin M, Krause K-H (2005) Chemokine receptors in the central nervous system: role in brain inflammation and neurodegenerative diseases. Brain Res Rev 48:16–42

Cesare P, McNaughton P (1996) A novel heat-activated current in nociceptive neurons and its sensitization by bradykinin. Proc Natl Acad Sci USA 93:15435–15439

Charo IF, Ransohoff RM (2006) The many roles of chemokines and chemokine receptors in inflammation. N Engl J Med 354:610–621

Chen X, Geller EB, Rogers TJ, Adler MW (2007) Rapid heterologous desensitization of antinociceptive activity between mu or delta opioid receptors and chemokine receptors in rats. Drug Alcohol Depend 88:36–41

Chuang H-h, Prescott ED, Kong H, Shields S, Jordt S-E, Basbaum AI, Chao MV, Julius D (2001) Bradykinin and nerve growth factor release the capsaicin receptor from PtdIns(4,5)P2-mediated inhibition. Nature 411:957–962

Clark AK, Yip PK, Grist J, Gentry C, Staniland AA, Marchand F, Dehvari M, Wotherspoon G, Winter J, Ullah J, Bevan S, Malcangio M (2007) Inhibition of spinal microglial cathepsin S for the reversal of neuropathic pain. Proc Natl Acad Sci USA 104:10655–10660

Cook WJ, Kramer MF, Walker RM, Burwell TJ, Holman HA, Coen DM, Knipe DM (2004) Persistent expression of chemokine and chemokine receptor RNAs at primary and latent sites of herpes simplex virus 1 infection. Virol J 1:5

Creagh EM, O'Neill LA (2006) TLRs, NLRs and RLRs: a trinity of pathogen sensors that co-operate in innate immunity. Trends Immunol 27:352–357

Cunha FQ, Poole S, Lorenzetti BB, Ferreira SH (1992) The pivotal role of tumour necrosis factor alpha in the development of inflammatory hyperalgesia. Br J Pharmacol 107:660–664

Cunha TM, Verri WA Jr, Fukada SY, Guerrero AT, Santodomingo-Garzon T, Poole S, Parada CA, Ferreira SH, Cunha FQ (2007) TNF-alpha and IL-1beta mediate inflammatory hypernociception in mice triggered by B1 but not B2 kinin receptor. Eur J Pharmacol 573:221–229

Dalpke A, Heeg K (2002) Signal integration following Toll-like receptor triggering. Crit Rev Immunol 22:217–250

de Jong EK, Dijkstra IM, Hensens M, Brouwer N, van Amerongen M, Liem RS, Boddeke HW, Biber K (2005) Vesicle-mediated transport and release of CCL21 in endangered neurons: a possible explanation for microglia activation remote from a primary lesion. J Neurosci 25:7548–7557

DeLeo JA, Tanga FY, Tawfik VL (2004) Neuroimmune activation and neuroinflammation in chronic pain and opioid tolerance/hyperalgesia. Neuroscientist 10:40–52

Donnelly-Roberts D, McGaraughty S, Shieh CC, Honore P, Jarvis MF (2008) Painful purinergic receptors. J Pharmacol Exp Ther 324:409–415

Ferreira SH, Lorenzetti BB, Bristow AF, Poole S (1988) Interleukin-1 beta as a potent hyperalgesic agent antagonized by a tripeptide analogue. Nature 334:698–700

Flynn G, Maru S, Loughlin J, Romero IA, Male D (2003) Regulation of chemokine receptor expression in human microglia and astrocytes. J Neuroimmunol 136:84–93

Gadient RA, Otten U (1996) Postnatal expression of interleukin-6 (IL-6) and IL-6 receptor (IL-6R) mRNAs in rat sympathetic and sensory ganglia. Brain Res 724:41–46

Gardiner NJ, Cafferty WB, Slack SE, Thompson SW (2002) Expression of gp130 and leukaemia inhibitory factor receptor subunits in adult rat sensory neurones: regulation by nerve injury. J Neurochem 83:100–109

Gillespie CS, Sherman DL, Fleetwood-Walker SM, Cottrell DF, Tait S, Garry EM, Wallace VC, Ure J, Griffiths IR, Smith A, Brophy PJ (2000) Peripheral demyelination and neuropathic pain behavior in periaxin-deficient mice. Neuron 26:523–531

Grimm MC, Ben-Baruch A, Taub DD, Howard OM, Resau JH, Wang JM, Ali H, Richardson R, Snyderman R, Oppenheim JJ (1998) Opiates transdeactivate chemokine receptors: delta and mu opiate receptor-mediated heterologous desensitization. J Exp Med 188:317–325

Guo LH, Schluesener HJ (2007) The innate immunity of the central nervous system in chronic pain: the role of Toll-like receptors. Cell Mol Life Sci 64:1128–1136

Hempenstall K, Nurmikko TJ, Johnson RW, A'Hern RP, Rice AS (2005) Analgesic therapy in postherpetic neuralgia: a quantitative systematic review. PLoS Med 2:e164

Hensellek S, Brell P, Schaible HG, Brauer R, Segond von Banchet G (2007) The cytokine TNF-alpha increases the proportion of DRG neurones expressing the TRPV1 receptor via the TNFR1 receptor and ERK activation. Mol Cell Neurosci 36:381–391

Herzberg U, Sagen J (2001) Peripheral nerve exposure to HIV viral envelope protein gp120 induces neuropathic pain and spinal gliosis. J Neuroimmunol 116:29–39

Huising MO, Stet RJ, Kruiswijk CP, Savelkoul HF, Lidy Verburg-van Kemenade BM (2003) Molecular evolution of CXC chemokines: extant CXC chemokines originate from the CNS. Trends Immunol 24:307–313

Hutchinson MR, Bland ST, Johnson KW, Rice KC, Maier SF, Watkins LR (2007) Opioid-induced glial activation: mechanisms of activation and implications for opioid analgesia, dependence, and reward. Sci World J 7:98–111

Inoue A, Ikoma K, Morioka N, Kumagai K, Hashimoto T, Hide I, Nakata Y (1999) Interleukin-1beta induces substance P release from primary afferent neurons through the cyclooxygenase-2 system. J Neurochem 73:2206–2213

Jin X, Gereau RWt (2006) Acute p38-mediated modulation of tetrodotoxin-resistant sodium channels in mouse sensory neurons by tumor necrosis factor-alpha. J Neurosci 26:246–255

Johnston IN, Milligan ED, Wieseler-Frank J, Frank MG, Zapata V, Campisi J, Langer S, Martin D, Green P, Fleshner M, Leinwand L, Maier SF, Watkins LR (2004) A role for proinflammatory cytokines and fractalkine in analgesia, tolerance, and subsequent pain facilitation induced by chronic intrathecal morphine. J Neurosci 24:7353–7365

Jung H, Miller RJ (2008) Activation of the nuclear factor of activated T cells (NFAT) mediates upregulation of CCR2 chemokine receptors in dorsal root ganglion (DRG) neurons: A possible mechanism for activity-dependent transcription in DRG neurons in association with neuropathic pain. Mol Cell Neurosci 37:170–177

Jung J, Bhangoo SK, Fitzgerald MP, Miller RJ, White FA (2007) Expression of functional chemokine receptors in bladder-associated sensory neurons following focal demyelination of sciatic nerve. In: 2007 neuroscience meeting planner. Program no. 185.188. Society for Neuroscience, San Diego

Jung H, Toth PT, White FA, Miller RJ (2008) Monocyte chemoattractant protein-1 functions as a neuromodulator in dorsal root ganglia neurons. J Neurochem 104:254–263

Kajander KC, Wakisaka S, Bennett GJ (1992) Spontaneous discharge originates in the dorsal root ganglion at the onset of a painful peripheral neuropathy in the rat. Neurosci Lett 138: 225–228

Kawasaki Y, Zhang L, Cheng JK, Ji RR (2008) Cytokine mechanisms of central sensitization: distinct and overlapping role of interleukin-1beta, interleukin-6, and tumor necrosis factor-alpha in regulating synaptic and neuronal activity in the superficial spinal cord. J Neurosci 28:5189–5194

Keswani SC, Polley M, Pardo CA, Griffin JW, McArthur JC, Hoke A (2003) Schwann cell chemokine receptors mediate HIV-1 gp120 toxicity to sensory neurons. Ann Neurol 54:287–296

Keswani SC, Jack C, Zhou C, Hoke A (2006) Establishment of a rodent model of HIV-associated sensory neuropathy. J Neurosci 26:10299–10304

Khasabova IA, Stucky CL, Harding-Rose C, Eikmeier L, Beitz AJ, Coicou LG, Hanson AE, Simone DA, Seybold VS (2007) Chemical interactions between fibrosarcoma cancer cells and sensory neurons contribute to cancer pain. J Neurosci 27:10289–10298

Kim SH, Na HS, Sheen K, Chung JM (1993) Effects of sympathectomy on a rat model of peripheral neuropathy. Pain 55:85–92

Kim D, Kim MA, Cho IH, Kim MS, Lee S, Jo EK, Choi SY, Park K, Kim JS, Akira S, Na HS, Oh SB, Lee SJ (2007) A critical role of Toll-like receptor 2 in nerve injury-induced spinal cord glial cell activation and pain hypersensitivity. J Biol Chem 282:14975–14983

Kleinschnitz C, Brinkhoff J, Sommer C, Stoll G (2005) Contralateral cytokine gene induction after peripheral nerve lesions: dependence on the mode of injury and NMDA receptor signaling. Brain Res Mol Brain Res 136:23–28

Knaut H, Werz C, Geisler R, Nusslein-Volhard C (2003) A zebrafish homologue of the chemokine receptor Cxcr4 is a germ-cell guidance receptor. Nature 421:279–282

Labuz D, Berger S, Mousa SA, Zollner C, Rittner HL, Shaqura MA, Segovia-Silvestre T, Przewlocka B, Stein C, Machelska H (2006) Peripheral antinociceptive effects of exogenous and immune cell-derived endomorphins in prolonged inflammatory pain. J Neurosci 26:4350–4358

Ledeboer A, Jekich BM, Sloane EM, Mahoney JH, Langer SJ, Milligan ED, Martin D, Maier SF, Johnson KW, Leinwand LA, Chavez RA, Watkins LR (2007) Intrathecal interleukin-10 gene therapy attenuates paclitaxel-induced mechanical allodynia and proinflammatory cytokine expression in dorsal root ganglia in rats. Brain Behav Immun 21:686–698

Lee HL, Lee KM, Son SJ, Hwang SH, Cho HJ (2004) Temporal expression of cytokines and their receptors mRNAs in a neuropathic pain model. Neuroreport 15:2807–2811

Levin ME, Jin JG, Ji RR, Tong J, Pomonis JD, Lavery DJ, Miller SW, Chiang LW (2008) Complement activation in the peripheral nervous system following the spinal nerve ligation model of neuropathic pain. Pain 137(1):182–201

Li Y, Ji A, Weihe E, Schafer MK-H (2004) Cell-specific expression and lipopolysaccharide-induced regulation of tumor necrosis factor {alpha} (TNF{alpha}) and TNF receptors in rat dorsal root ganglion. J Neurosci 24:9623–9631

Li M, Shi J, Tang JR, Chen D, Ai B, Chen J, Wang LN, Cao FY, Li LL, Lin CY, Guan XM (2005) Effects of complete Freund's adjuvant on immunohistochemical distribution of IL-1 beta and IL-1R I in neurons and glia cells of dorsal root ganglion. Acta Pharmacol Sin 26:192–198

Liang DY, Shi X, Qiao Y, Angst MS, Yeomans DC, Clark JD (2008) Chronic morphine administration enhances nociceptive sensitivity and local cytokine production after incision. Mol Pain 4:7

Lindia JA, McGowan E, Jochnowitz N, Abbadie C (2005) Induction of CX3CL1 expression in astrocytes and CX3CR1 in microglia in the spinal cord of a rat model of neuropathic pain. J Pain 6:434–438

Liu B, Eisenach JC (2005) Hyperexcitability of axotomized and neighboring unaxotomized sensory neurons is reduced days after perineural clonidine at the site of injury. J Neurophysiol 94:3159–3167

Lu M, Grove EA, Miller RJ (2002) Abnormal development of the hippocampal dentate gyrus in mice lacking the CXCR4 chemokine receptor. Proc Natl Acad Sci USA 99:7090–7095

Ma C, Shu Y, Zheng Z, Chen Y, Yao H, Greenquist KW, White FA, LaMotte RH (2003) Similar electrophysiological changes in axotomized and neighboring intact dorsal root ganglion neurons. J Neurophysiol 89:1588–1602

Ma W, Quirion R (2006) Targeting invading macrophage-derived PGE2, IL-6 and calcitonin gene-related peptide in injured nerve to treat neuropathic pain. Expert Opin Ther Targets 10:533–546

MacEwan DJ (2002) TNF receptor subtype signalling: differences and cellular consequences. Cell Signal 14:477–492

Mahad DJ, Howell SJL, Woodroofe MN (2002) Expression of chemokines in the CSF and correlation with clinical disease activity in patients with multiple sclerosis. J Neurol Neurosurg Psychiatry 72:498–502

Martin MU, Wesche H (2002) Summary and comparison of the signaling mechanisms of the Toll/interleukin-1 receptor family. Biochim Biophys Acta 1592:265–280

McMahon SB, Cafferty WB, Marchand F (2005) Immune and glial cell factors as pain mediators and modulators. Exp Neurol 192:444–462

McNamara CR, Mandel-Brehm J, Bautista DM, Siemens J, Deranian KL, Zhao M, Hayward NJ, Chong JA, Julius D, Moran MM, Fanger CM (2007) TRPA1 mediates formalin-induced pain. Proc Natl Acad Sci USA 104(33):13525–13530

Menetski J, Mistry S, Lu M, Mudgett JS, Ransohoff RM, Demartino JA, Macintyre DE, Abbadie C (2007) Mice overexpressing chemokine ligand 2 (CCL2) in astrocytes display enhanced nociceptive responses. Neuroscience 149:706–714

Milligan ED, Mehmert KK, Hinde JL, Harvey LO Jr, Martin D, Tracey KJ, Maier SF, Watkins LR (2000) Thermal hyperalgesia and mechanical allodynia produced by intrathecal administration of the human immunodeficiency virus-1 (HIV-1) envelope glycoprotein, gp120. Brain Res Mol Brain Res 861:105–116

Milligan ED, Zapata V, Chacur M, Schoeniger D, Biedenkapp J, O'Connor KA, Verge GM, Chapman G, Green P, Foster AC, Naeve GS, Maier SF, Watkins LR (2004) Evidence that exogenous and endogenous fractalkine can induce spinal nociceptive facilitation in rats. Eur J Neurosci 20:2294–2302

Milligan E, Zapata V, Schoeniger D, Chacur M, Green P, Poole S, Martin D, Maier SF, Watkins LR (2005) An initial investigation of spinal mechanisms underlying pain enhancement induced by fractalkine, a neuronally released chemokine. Eur J Neurosci 22:2775–2782

Milligan ED, Soderquist RG, Malone SM, Mahoney JH, Hughes TS, Langer SJ, Sloane EM, Maier SF, Leinwand LA, Watkins LR, Mahoney MJ (2006) Intrathecal polymer-based interleukin-10 gene delivery for neuropathic pain. Neuron Glia Biol 2:293–308

Moalem-Taylor G, Allbutt HN, Iordanova MD, Tracey DJ (2007) Pain hypersensitivity in rats with experimental autoimmune neuritis, an animal model of human inflammatory demyelinating neuropathy. Brain Behav Immun 21:699–710

Moulin DE (1998) Pain in central and peripheral demyelinating disorders. Neurol Clin 16:889–898

Nicol GD, Lopshire JC, Pafford CM (1997) Tumor necrosis factor enhances the capsaicin sensitivity of rat sensory neurons. J Neurosci 17:975–982

Nilsson A, Moller K, Dahlin L, Lundborg G, Kanje M (2005) Early changes in gene expression in the dorsal root ganglia after transection of the sciatic nerve; effects of amphiregulin and PAI-1 on regeneration. Brain Res Mol Brain Res 136:65–74

Obata K, Yamanaka H, Fukuoka T, Yi D, Tokunaga A, Hashimoto N, Yoshikawa H, Noguchi K (2003) Contribution of injured and uninjured dorsal root ganglion neurons to pain behavior and the changes in gene expression following chronic constriction injury of the sciatic nerve in rats. Pain 101:65–77

Obreja O, Rathee PK, Lips KS, Distler C, Kress M (2002) IL-1 beta potentiates heat-activated currents in rat sensory neurons: involvement of IL-1RI, tyrosine kinase, and protein kinase C. FASEB J 16:1497–1503

Obreja O, Biasio W, Andratsch M, Lips KS, Rathee PK, Ludwig A, Rose-John S, Kress M (2005) Fast modulation of heat-activated ionic current by proinflammatory interleukin-6 in rat sensory neurons. Brain 128:1634–1641

Oh SB, Tran PB, Gillard SE, Hurley RW, Hammond DL, Miller RJ (2001) Chemokines and glycoprotein120 produce pain hypersensitivity by directly exciting primary nociceptive neurons. J Neurosci 21:5027–5035

Ohtori S, Takahashi K, Moriya H, Myers RR (2004) TNF-alpha and TNF-alpha receptor type 1 upregulation in glia and neurons after peripheral nerve injury: studies in murine DRG and spinal cord. Spine 29:1082–1088

Opree A, Kress M (2000) Involvement of the proinflammatory cytokines tumor necrosis factor-alpha, IL-1beta, and IL-6 but not IL-8 in the development of heat hyperalgesia: effects on heat-evoked calcitonin gene-related peptide release from rat skin. J Neurosci 20:6289–6293

Orlikowski D, Chazaud B, Plonquet A, Poron F, Sharshar T, Maison P, Raphael J-C, Gherardi RK, Creange A (2003) Monocyte chemoattractant protein 1 and chemokine receptor CCR2 productions in Guillain-Barre syndrome and experimental autoimmune neuritis. J Neuroimmunol 134:118–127

Parada CA, Yeh JJ, Joseph EK, Levine JD (2003) Tumor necrosis factor receptor type-1 in sensory neurons contributes to induction of chronic enhancement of inflammatory hyperalgesia in rat. Eur J Neurosci 17:1847–1852

Pardo CA, McArthur JC, Griffin JW (2001) HIV neuropathy: insights in the pathology of HIV peripheral nerve disease. J Peripher Nerv Syst 6:21–27

Park KA, Vasko MR (2005) Lipid mediators of sensitivity in sensory neurons. Trends Pharmacol Sci 26:571–577

Patel JP, Sengupta R, Bardi G, Khan MZ, Mullen-Przeworski A, Meucci O (2006) Modulation of neuronal CXCR4 by the micro-opioid agonist DAMGO. J Neurovirol 12:492–500

Pezet S, McMahon SB (2006) Neurotrophins: mediators and modulators of pain. Annu Rev Neurosci 29:507–538

Premkumar LS, Ahern GP (2000) Induction of vanilloid receptor channel activity by protein kinase C. Nature 408:985–990

Qin X, Wan Y, Wang X (2005) CCL2 and CXCL1 trigger calcitonin gene-related peptide release by exciting primary nociceptive neurons. J Neurosci Res. doi:10.1002/jnr.20612

Raghavendra V, Tanga FY, DeLeo JA (2004) Complete Freunds adjuvant-induced peripheral inflammation evokes glial activation and proinflammatory cytokine expression in the CNS. Eur J Neurosci 20:467–473

Rittner HL, Labuz D, Schaefer M, Mousa SA, Schulz S, Schafer M, Stein C, Brack A (2006) Pain control by CXCR2 ligands through Ca^{2+}-regulated release of opioid peptides from polymorphonuclear cells. FASEB J 20(14):2627–2629

Romero-Sandoval EA, McCall C, Eisenach JC (2005) Alpha2-adrenoceptor stimulation transforms immune responses in neuritis and blocks neuritis-induced pain. J Neurosci 25:8988–8994

Ruparel NB, Patwardhan AM, Akopian AN, Hargreaves KM (2008) Homologous and heterologous desensitization of capsaicin and mustard oil responses utilize different cellular pathways in nociceptors. Pain 135(3):271–279

Sasaki N, Kikuchi S, Konno S, Sekiguchi M, Watanabe K (2007) Anti-TNF-alpha antibody reduces pain-behavioral changes induced by epidural application of nucleus pulposus in a rat model depending on the timing of administration. Spine 32:413–416

Schafers M, Sommer C (2007) Anticytokine therapy in neuropathic pain management. Expert Rev Neurother 7:1613–1627

Schafers M, Svensson CI, Sommer C, Sorkin LS (2003a) Tumor necrosis factor-alpha induces mechanical allodynia after spinal nerve ligation by activation of p38 MAPK in primary sensory neurons. J Neurosci 23:2517–2521

Schafers M, Lee DH, Brors D, Yaksh TL, Sorkin LS (2003b) Increased sensitivity of injured and adjacent uninjured rat primary sensory neurons to exogenous tumor necrosis factor-alpha after spinal nerve ligation. J Neurosci 23:3028–3038

Sheth RN, Dorsi MJ, Li Y, Murinson BB, Belzberg AJ, Griffin JW, Meyer RA (2002) Mechanical hyperalgesia after an L5 ventral rhizotomy or an L5 ganglionectomy in the rat. Pain 96:63–72

Skopelitis EE, Kokotis PI, Kontos AN, Panayiotakopoulos GD, Konstantinou K, Kordossis T, Karandreas N (2006) Distal sensory polyneuropathy in HIV-positive patients in the HAART era: an entity underestimated by clinical examination. Int J STD AIDS 17:467–472

Sluka KA, Kalra A, Moore SA (2001) Unilateral intramuscular injections of acidic saline produce a bilateral, long-lasting hyperalgesia. Muscle Nerve 24:37–46

Sluka KA, Radhakrishnan R, Benson CJ, Eshcol JO, Price MP, Babinski K, Audette KM, Yeomans DC, Wilson SP (2007) ASIC3 in muscle mediates mechanical, but not heat, hyperalgesia associated with muscle inflammation. Pain 129:102–112

Snider WD, Simpson DM, Nielsen S, Gold JW, Metroka CE, Posner JB (1983) Neurological complications of acquired immune deficiency syndrome: analysis of 50 patients. Ann Neurol 14:403–418

Sommer C, Schmidt C, George A (1998) Hyperalgesia in experimental neuropathy is dependent on the TNF receptor 1. Exp Neurol 151:138–142

Sorkin LS, Doom CM (2000) Epineurial application of TNF elicits an acute mechanical hyperalgesia in the awake rat. J Peripher Nerv Syst 5:96–100

Streit WJ, Conde JR, Harrison JK (2001) Chemokines and alzheimer's disease. Neurobiol Aging 22:909–913

Subang MC, Richardson PM (2001) Influence of injury and cytokines on synthesis of monocyte chemoattractant protein-1 mRNA in peripheral nervous tissue. Eur J Neurosci 13:521–528

Sugiura T, Tominaga M, Katsuya H, Mizumura K (2002) Bradykinin lowers the threshold temperature for heat activation of vanilloid receptor 1. J Neurophysiol 88:544–548

Summer GJ, Romero-Sandoval EA, Bogen O, Dina OA, Khasar SG, Levine JD (2008) Proinflammatory cytokines mediating burn-injury pain. Pain 135:98–107

Sun JH, Yang B, Donnelly DF, Ma C, LaMotte RH (2006) MCP-1 enhances excitability of nociceptive neurons in chronically compressed dorsal root ganglia. J Neurophysiol 96:2189–2199

Szabo I, Chen XH, Xin L, Adler MW, Howard OM, Oppenheim JJ, Rogers TJ (2002) Heterologous desensitization of opioid receptors by chemokines inhibits chemotaxis and enhances the perception of pain. Proc Natl Acad Sci USA 99:10276–10281

Tachibana K, Hirota S, Iizasa H, Yoshida H, Kawabata K, Kataoka Y, Kitamura Y, Matsushima K, Yoshida N, Nishikawa S, Kishimoto T, Nagasawa T (1998) The chemokine receptor CXCR4 is essential for vascularization of the gastrointestinal tract. Nature 393:591–594

Takeda M, Tanimoto T, Kadoi J, Nasu M, Takahashi M, Kitagawa J, Matsumoto S (2007) Enhanced excitability of nociceptive trigeminal ganglion neurons by satellite glial cytokine following peripheral inflammation. Pain 129:155–166

Takeda M, Takahashi M, Matsumoto S (2008) Contribution of activated interleukin receptors in trigeminal ganglion neurons to hyperalgesia via satellite glial interleukin-1beta paracrine mechanism. Brain Behav Immun 22(7):1016–1023

Tal M, Devor M (1992) Ectopic discharge in injured nerves: comparison of trigeminal and somatic afferents. Brain Res 579:148–151

Tanaka T, Minami M, Nakagawa T, Satoh M (2004) Enhanced production of monocyte chemoattractant protein-1 in the dorsal root ganglia in a rat model of neuropathic pain: possible involvement in the development of neuropathic pain. Neurosci Res 48:463–469

Tanga FY, Nutile-McMenemy N, DeLeo JA (2005) The CNS role of Toll-like receptor 4 in innate neuroimmunity and painful neuropathy. Proc Natl Acad Sci USA 102:5856–5861

Tanuma N, Sakuma H, Sasaki A, Matsumoto Y (2006) Chemokine expression by astrocytes plays a role in microglia/macrophage activation and subsequent neurodegeneration in secondary progressive multiple sclerosis. Acta Neuropathol (Berl) 112:195–204

Taskinen HS, Roytta M (2000) Increased expression of chemokines (MCP-1, MIP-1alpha, RANTES) after peripheral nerve transection. J Peripher Nerv Syst 5:75–81

Tawfik VL, Nutile-McMenemy N, Lacroix-Fralish ML, Deleo JA (2007) Efficacy of propentofylline, a glial modulating agent, on existing mechanical allodynia following peripheral nerve injury. Brain Behav Immun 21:238–246

Theil D, Derfuss T, Paripovic I, Herberger S, Meinl E, Schueler O, Strupp M, Arbusow V, Brandt T (2003) Latent herpesvirus infection in human trigeminal ganglia causes chronic immune response. Am J Pathol 163:2179–2184

Thompson SW, Priestley JV, Southall A (1998) gp130 Cytokines, leukemia inhibitory factor and interleukin-6, induce neuropeptide expression in intact adult rat sensory neurons in vivo: time-course, specificity and comparison with sciatic nerve axotomy. Neuroscience 84:1247–1255

Ting E, Guerrero AT, Cunha TM, Verri WA Jr, Taylor SM, Woodruff TM, Cunha FQ, Ferreira SH (2008) Role of complement C5a in mechanical inflammatory hypernociception: potential use of C5a receptor antagonists to control inflammatory pain. Br J Pharmacol 153:1043–1053

Toews AD, Barrett C, Morell P (1998) Monocyte chemoattractant protein 1 is responsible for macrophage recruitment following injury to sciatic nerve. J Neurosci Res 53:260–267

Torebjork HE, Lundberg LE, LaMotte RH (1992) Central changes in processing of mechanoreceptive input in capsaicin-induced secondary hyperalgesia in humans. J Physiol 448: 765–780

Toth PT, Ren D, Miller RJ (2004) Regulation of CXCR4 receptor dimerization by the chemokine SDF-1alpha and the HIV-1 coat protein gp120: a fluorescence resonance energy transfer (FRET) study. J Pharmacol Exp Ther 310:8–17

Trevisani M, Siemens J, Materazzi S, Bautista DM, Nassini R, Campi B, Imamachi N, Andre E, Patacchini R, Cottrell GS, Gatti R, Basbaum AI, Bunnett NW, Julius D, Geppetti P (2007) 4-Hydroxynonenal, an endogenous aldehyde, causes pain and neurogenic inflammation through activation of the irritant receptor TRPA1. Proc Natl Acad Sci USA 104(33):13519–13524

Twining CM, Sloane EM, Milligan ED, Chacur M, Martin D, Poole S, Marsh H, Maier SF, Watkins LR (2004) Peri-sciatic proinflammatory cytokines, reactive oxygen species, and complement induce mirror-image neuropathic pain in rats. Pain 110:299–309

Ubogu EE, Cossoy MB, Ransohoff RM (2006) The expression and function of chemokines involved in CNS inflammation. Trends Pharmacol Sci 27:48–55

Uceyler N, Tscharke A, Sommer C (2007) Early cytokine expression in mouse sciatic nerve after chronic constriction nerve injury depends on calpain. Brain Behav Immun 21:553–560

Vabulas RM, Wagner H, Schild H (2002) Heat shock proteins as ligands of Toll-like receptors. Curr Top Microbiol Immunol 270:169–184

Verge GM, Milligan ED, Maier SF, Watkins LR, Naeve GS, Foster AC (2004) Fractalkine (CX3CL1) and fractalkine receptor (CX3CR1) distribution in spinal cord and dorsal root ganglia under basal and neuropathic pain conditions. Eur J Neurosci 20:1150–1160

Vit JP, Ohara PT, Tien DA, Fike JR, Eikmeier L, Beitz A, Wilcox GL, Jasmin L (2006) The analgesic effect of low dose focal irradiation in a mouse model of bone cancer is associated with spinal changes in neuro-mediators of nociception. Pain 120:188–201

Wall PD, Devor M (1983) Sensory afferent impulses originate from dorsal root ganglia as well as from the periphery in normal and nerve injured rats. Pain 17:321–339

Wallace VCJ, Cottrell DF, Brophy PJ, Fleetwood-Walker SM (2003) Focal lysolecithin-induced demyelination of peripheral afferents results in neuropathic pain behavior that is attenuated by cannabinoids. J Neurosci 23:3221–3233

Wallace VC, Blackbeard J, Segerdahl AR, Hasnie F, Pheby T, McMahon SB, Rice AS (2007) Characterization of rodent models of HIV-gp120 and anti-retroviral-associated neuropathic pain. Brain 130(10):2688–2702

Watkins LR, Maier SF (2003) Glia: a novel drug discovery target for clinical pain. Nat Rev Drug Discov 2:973–985

Watkins LR, Hutchinson MR, Milligan ED, Maier SF (2007a) "Listening" and "talking" to neurons: implications of immune activation for pain control and increasing the efficacy of opioids. Brain Res Rev 56:148–169

Watkins LR, Hutchinson MR, Ledeboer A, Wieseler-Frank J, Milligan ED, Maier SF (2007b) Glia as the "bad guys": Implications for improving clinical pain control and the clinical utility of opioids. Brain Behav Immun 21:131–146

Watkins LR, Hutchinson MR, Ledeboer A, Wieseler-Frank J, Milligan ED, Maier SF (2007c) Norman Cousins Lecture. Glia as the "bad guys": implications for improving clinical pain control and the clinical utility of opioids. Brain Behav Immun 21:131–146

Watson CP (2000) The treatment of neuropathic pain: antidepressants and opioids. Clin J Pain 16: S49–S55

White FA, Bhangoo SK, Miller RJ (2005a) Chemokines: integrators of pain and inflammation. Nat Rev Drug Discov 4:834–844

White FA, Sun J, Waters SM, Ma C, Ren D, Ripsch M, Steflik J, Cortright DN, Lamotte RH, Miller RJ (2005b) Excitatory monocyte chemoattractant protein-1 signaling is up-regulated in sensory neurons after chronic compression of the dorsal root ganglion. Proc Natl Acad Sci USA 102:14092–14097

White FA, Bauer WR, Jellish WS, Chan DM, LaMotte RH, Miller RJ (2006) MCP-1/CCL2 and CCR2 upregulation following partial ligation of the infraorbital nerve: possible involvement in the development and maintenance of trigeminal neuralgia. J Pain 7:628

White FA, Monahan P, LaMotte RH (2007a) Chemokines and their receptors in the nervous system: a link to neuropathic pain. In: Watkins LA, DeLeo JA, Sorkin L (eds) Immune and glial activation in pain. IASP, Seattle

White FA, Jung H, Miller RJ (2007b) Chemokines and the pathophysiology of neuropathic pain. Proc Natl Acad Sci USA 104:20151–20158

Wickham S, Lu B, Ash J, Carr DJ (2005) Chemokine receptor deficiency is associated with increased chemokine expression in the peripheral and central nervous systems and increased resistance to herpetic encephalitis. J Neuroimmunol 162:51–59

Wilson N, Ripsch MS, Miller RJ, White FA (2008) Morphine-induced hypernociception is reversed with the CXCR4 receptor antagonist, AMD3100. Society for Neuroscience annual meeting, Washington

Woolf CJ (1983) Evidence for a central component of post-injury pain hypersensitivity. Nature 306:686–688

Wright DE, Bowman EP, Wagers AJ, Butcher EC, Weissman IL (2002) Hematopoietic stem cells are uniquely selective in their migratory response to chemokines. J Exp Med 195:1145–1154

Xie W, Strong JA, Meij JT, Zhang JM, Yu L (2005) Neuropathic pain: early spontaneous afferent activity is the trigger. Pain 116:243–256

Xie WR, Deng H, Li H, Bowen TL, Strong JA, Zhang JM (2006) Robust increase of cutaneous sensitivity, cytokine production and sympathetic sprouting in rats with localized inflammatory irritation of the spinal ganglia. Neuroscience 142(3):809–822:809-822

Zanella JM, Burright EN, Hildebrand K, Hobot C, Cox M, Christoferson L, McKay WF (2008) Effect of etanercept, a tumor necrosis factor-alpha inhibitor, on neuropathic pain in the rat chronic constriction injury model. Spine 33:227–234

Zhang J, De Koninck Y (2006) Spatial and temporal relationship between monocyte chemoattractant protein-1 expression and spinal glial activation following peripheral nerve injury. J Neurochem 97:772–783

Zhang N, Inan S, Cowan A, Sun R, Wang JM, Rogers TJ, Caterina M, Oppenheim JJ (2005) A proinflammatory chemokine, CCL3, sensitizes the heat- and capsaicin-gated ion channel TRPV1. Proc Natl Acad Sci USA 102:4536–4541

Zhuang ZY, Kawasaki Y, Tan PH, Wen YR, Huang J, Ji RR (2007) Role of the CX3CR1/p38 MAPK pathway in spinal microglia for the development of neuropathic pain following nerve injury-induced cleavage of fractalkine. Brain Behav Immun 21:642–651

Zimmermann M (2001) Pathobiology of neuropathic pain. Eur J Pharmacol 429:23–37

The Role of Peptides in Central Sensitization

V.S. Seybold

Contents

Abstract Peptides released in the spinal cord from the central terminals of nociceptors contribute to the persistent hyperalgesia that defines the clinical experience of chronic pain. Using substance P (SP) and calcitonin gene-related peptide (CGRP) as examples, this review addresses the multiple mechanisms through which peptidergic neurotransmission contributes to the development and maintenance

V.S. Seybold
Department of Neuroscience, University of Minnesota, 6-145 Jackson Hall, 321 Church St., S.E., Minneapolis, MN 55455, USA
vseybold@umn.edu

B.J. Canning and D. Spina (eds.), *Sensory Nerves*,
Handbook of Experimental Pharmacology 194, DOI: 10.1007/978-3-540-79090-7_13,

of chronic pain. Activation of CGRP receptors on terminals of primary afferent neurons facilitates transmitter release and receptors on spinal neurons increases glutamate activation of AMPA receptors. Both effects are mediated by cAMP-dependent mechanisms. Substance P activates neurokinin receptors (3 subtypes) which couple to phospholipase C and the generation of the intracellular messengers whose downstream effects include depolarizing the membrane and facilitating the function of AMPA and NMDA receptors. Activation of neurokinin-1 receptors also increases the synthesis of prostaglandins whereas activation of neurokinin-3 receptors increases the synthesis of nitric oxide. Both products act as retrograde messengers across synapses and facilitate nociceptive signaling in the spinal cord. Whereas these cellular effects of CGRP and SP at the level of the spinal cord contribute to the development of increased synaptic strength between nociceptors and spinal neurons in the pathway for pain, the different intracellular signaling pathways also activate different transcription factors. The activated transcription factors initiate changes in the expression of genes that contribute to long-term changes in the excitability of spinal and maintain hyperalgesia.

Keywords Calcitonin gene-related peptide, Substance P, Neurokinin, Spinal cord, Hyperalgesia, NFAT, CREB, Receptor, Inflammation

Abbreviations

AMPA	α-Amino-3-hydroxy-5-methyl-4-isoxazolepropionate
cAMP	Cyclic AMP
CaMK	Ca^{2+}/calmodulin-dependent protein kinase
CGRP	Calcitonin gene-related peptide
COX	Cyclo-oxygenase
CRE	Cyclic AMP response element
CREB	Cyclic AMP response element binding protein
CRLR	Calcitonin receptor-like receptor
ERK	Extracellular-signal-regulated kinase
mRNA	Messenger RNA
NFAT	Nuclear factor of activated T cells
NK1	Neurokinin 1
NK2	Neurokinin 2
NK3	Neurokinin 3
NKA	Neurokinin A
NKB	Neurokinin B
NOS	Nitric oxide synthase
NSAID	Nonsteroidal anti-inflammatory drug
pCREB	Phosphorylated cyclic AMP response element binding protein
PGE2	Prostaglandin E_2
PPT-A	Preprotachykinin A
RAMP	Receptor activity modifying protein
RCP	Receptor component protein
SP	Substance P

1 Introduction

Peptides released in the spinal cord from the central terminals of nociceptors contribute to the persistent hyperalgesia that defines the clinical experience of chronic pain. At a cellular level, hyperalgesia is mediated by an increase in synaptic signaling among neurons in the pathway for sensation of pain, and this process is referred to as "central sensitization." Using substance P (SP) and calcitonin gene-related peptide (CGRP) as examples, this review will address the multiple mechanisms through which peptidergic neurotransmission contributes to the development and maintenance of chronic pain, especially pain associated with inflammation. Although the specific contribution of SP and CGRP to the maintenance of central sensitization following peripheral nerve injury has been questioned because their synthesis decreases in dorsal root ganglion neurons affected by the lesion of peripheral nerves (Villar et al. 1989; Zhang et al. 1996), recent evidence indicates that release of SP and CGRP in the spinal cord in a model of nerve injury does contribute to the maintenance of neuropathic pain (Lee and Kim 2007). Moreover, these two peptides are of specific interest because pharmaceutical companies have invested in the development of antagonists for neurokinin receptors activated by SP and the receptor activated by CGRP on the basis of compelling preclinical data described in this review. Whereas there is some success in treatment of migraine headaches with CGRP receptor antagonists (Durham 2004; Edvinsson 2005), the clinical impact of neurokinin 1 (NK1) receptor antagonists has been greatly disappointing (Hill 2000). There are varied opinions concerning the poor antihyperalgesic effect of NK1 receptor antagonists in humans, including whether appropriate animal species were used to test compounds in preclinical studies (Urban and Fox 2000) and the choice of assays for defining clinical efficacy (Hill 2000; Urban and Fox 2000; Laird 2001). These are noteworthy issues, and this review will pose one more: involvement of multiple neurokinin receptors. SP and its related tachykinins activate at least three subtypes of neurokinin receptors. These receptors have complementary physiological effects that converge on increasing the excitability of spinal neurons. Furthermore, emerging evidence indicates that the intracellular signaling pathways activated by SP and CGRP ultimately have long-term consequences in regulating the expression of genes for proteins that would maintain central sensitization and hyperalgesia. This long-term effect has implications for defining the duration of treatment that is needed to judge the clinical efficacy of a receptor antagonist.

1.1 Concept of Central Sensitization

Peripheral injury results in increased activation of sensory neurons in the pathway for the sensation of pain. As a consequence of the increase in neuronal activity, there is a leftward shift in the stimulus–response function for the perception of pain.

This shift is perceived as hyperalgesia (increased sensation to stimuli that would normally be perceived as moderately uncomfortable) and allodynia (perception of normally innocuous stimuli as painful). These changes are frequently accompanied by spontaneous pain. Hyperalgesia (and allodynia) are further subdivided into hyperalgesia at the site of injury (primary hyperalgesia) and hyperalgesia outside the area of injury (secondary hyperalgesia).

Hyperalgesia, allodynia, and spontaneous pain are encoded by increased efficacy of synapses of sensory neurons onto spinal neurons that project to rostral regions involved in pain sensation and modulation. The increased synaptic efficacy is reflected in increased spontaneous activity of spinal neurons as well as an increase in the size of their receptive fields and a decrease in the intensity of a peripheral stimulus that is sufficient to evoke synaptic potentials (Hylden et al. 1989, Neugebauer and Schaible 1990; Woolf and King 1990). Sensitization of nociceptors alone cannot account for the changes observed in the spinal neurons: the increased excitability of spinal neurons can be induced by electrical stimuli when the site of injury is anesthetized (Hylden et al. 1989), and even following electrical stimulation of C-fibers in the absence of injury (Cook et al. 1987).

Cellular changes both pre- and postsynaptically underlie the increase in synaptic efficacy that contributes to the increased excitability of spinal neurons following peripheral injury. Presynaptically, an increase in release of transmitter from terminals of nociceptive neurons results in activation of a greater number of neurotransmitter receptors and a higher frequency of receptor activation. Postsynaptically, an increase in synaptic current in response to the same amount of transmitter and a decrease in threshold for generation of an action potential further increase the probability of neuronal firing in response to synaptic input (see Ji et al. 2003 for a review). These changes constitute central sensitization and necessarily account for the expanded receptive fields of dorsal horn neurons and the secondary hyperalgesia that accompany peripheral injury.

1.2 Phases of Central Sensitization

In describing the biochemical events that contribute to central sensitization, it is useful to categorize the processes as contributing to either the induction of central sensitization (acute) or the maintenance of central sensitization (long term). Acutely (within seconds to hours), increased synaptic efficacy is mediated largely by posttranslational modifications of proteins by kinases in peripheral terminals of primary afferent neurons and at synapses in the pathway for nociception. For spinal neurons, this may be reflected in phosphorylation of glutamate receptors thereby increasing the conductance of their channels in response to neurotransmitter binding. In addition, phosphorylation of ion channels that contribute to the resting membrane potential or ion channels that contribute to the active membrane properties of central neurons promotes an increase in excitability. The net effect is an increase in synaptic strength and central sensitization. However, phosphorylation events are transient: protein phosphatases remove the phosphate group, returning receptors or ion channel proteins to their basal levels of function. Thus, posttranslational modifications of proteins can account for the induction of central sensitization, but these processes cannot account for the maintenance of central sensitization over days or longer. Changes in expression of receptors, enzymes, and voltage-dependent ion channels that participate in neurotransmission are necessary to maintain the change in excitability of spinal neurons that underlies persistent hyperalgesia. This review will focus on how two peptides released from sensory neurons contribute to central sensitization at the time of peripheral injury as well as how these peptides may evoke enduring increases in synaptic strength through changes in gene expression (i.e., neuroadaptation).

2 Contribution of Peptides to Central Sensitization

Whereas a large body of evidence indicates that glutamate is the small-molecule neurotransmitter responsible for rapid excitatory synaptic transmission between sensory neurons and dorsal horn neurons, an interesting aspect of central sensitization is that it requires the activation of C-fibers (Cook et al. 1987). C-fibers, which have unmyelinated axons, arise from small neurons within dorsal root and cranial nerve ganglia. These small neurons robustly express a variety of peptides. More specifically, peptides occur predominately in the small neurons that express TrkA receptors (see the chapter by Fernandes et al. in this volume).

The nature of peptidergic neurotransmission makes these neuromodulators ideal messengers of long-term neuroadaptation. First, peptides are sequestered in large dense core vesicles that reside farther from the synaptic density relative to the small secretory vesicles that contain glutamate, and the Ca^{2+} used to couple action potentials to transmitter release from vesicles enters through voltage-dependent Ca^{2+} channels within the synaptic density. Thus, higher firing frequencies are required for the intracellular Ca^{2+} concentration to reach the threshold for release of peptides compared with that for small-molecule neurotransmitters (Lundberg et al. 1989; Verhage et al. 1991). Consequently, peptide release increases with persistent stimuli. Second, peptides activate G protein coupled receptors which initiate cascades of enzyme activity culminating in the activation of kinases which phosphorylate proteins. Protein phosphorylation contributes to development of central sensitization, but it is also required for the activation of transcription factors that regulate gene expression for long-term neuroadaptation. Third, peptidergic neurotransmission is best described as volume transmission (reviewed by Agnati et al. 2006) as opposed to spatially discrete synaptic transmission mediated by small-molecule neurotransmitters such as amino acids. One factor that contributes to volume transmission is that the primary mechanism for termination of peptide responses is degradation of the peptide by extracellular peptidases. The capacity for degradation by peptidases can be overwhelmed by high concentrations of peptides in the extracellular space resulting in diffusion of peptides over relatively large distances. In addition, the affinity of peptide receptors for their ligands is generally very high, in the low nanomolar range. Thus, only a small amount of a peptide is necessary to activate its receptors, further increasing the effective distance from its release site. Through these mechanisms, therefore, a peptide released from one source may bind to its receptors expressed within a large volume of the spinal cord. These factors are complemented by the large volume within which neurons spread their dendrites. Consequently, spinal neurons that express a peptide receptor have the capacity to sample a large volume of synaptic space.

2.1 SP and CGRP as Prototypic Peptides in Central Sensitization

This review focuses on the role of two peptides: SP and CGRP. These two peptides are the most widely studied of those released by primary afferent neurons, which follows from observations that they are the most widely expressed by primary afferent neurons (McCarthy and Lawson 1989, 1990). SP and CGRP coexist to a large extent (70%) in terminals of primary afferent neurons in the dorsal horn of the spinal cord (Tuchscherer and Seybold 1989). Consequently, they are released in response to the same noxious stimuli (Yaksh et al. 1980; Duggan et al. 1988; Morton and Hutchison 1989), encoding moderate to intense stimuli (Duggan et al. 1995; Allen et al. 1997). Early evidence supporting a role for these peptides in central sensitization includes observations that SP and CGRP are expressed in more muscle afferents compared with cutaneous afferents (O'Brien et al. 1989; Perry and Lawson 1998). This differential distribution correlates with evidence that electrical stimulation of muscle afferents in naïve animals generates a more robust central sensitization of spinal neurons compared with stimulation of cutaneous nerves (Wall and Woolf 1984). Furthermore, the expression of SP and CGRP by primary afferent neurons is rapidly increased in response to peripheral inflammation (Donaldson et al. 1992) such that the releasable pool of peptide is maintained in the face of a 40% decrease in peptide content in the dorsal horn (Galeazza et al. 1995) and an increase in spontaneous as well as evoked release in the spinal cord (Schaible et al. 1990; Garry and Hargreaves 1992). Together these changes provide the context in which activation of SP and CGRP receptors in the spinal cord may contribute to both acute and long-term modulation of synaptic transmission underlying nociception. In addition, SP and CGRP receptors couple to different signal transduction mechanisms providing integration of diverse cellular mechanisms to support central sensitization.

3 CGRP Receptors

3.1 Endogenous Ligands

CGRP occurs as two isoforms (α and β) that exhibit high sequence homology even though they are derived from different genes. Rat α-CGRP differs from rat β-CGRP by one amino acid (a glutamate instead of a lysine at amino acid number 35; Amara et al. 1985), but their potency at rat CGRP receptors is the same (see Juaneda et al. 2000 for a review). Both α-CGRP and β-CGRP messenger RNAs (mRNAs) are expressed in small and medium-sized dorsal root ganglion neurons, sometimes within the same neurons (Noguchi et al. 1990): however, α-CGRP levels are threefold to sixfold higher than β-CGRP levels in rat dorsal root ganglion neurons (Mulderry et al. 1988). It is noteworthy that dorsal root ganglion neurons are the sole source of CGRP in the dorsal spinal cord (Tuchscherer and Seybold 1989).

3.2 Components of CGRP Receptors

The discovery of CGRP is credited to molecular biology (it was deduced from the structure of the gene for calcitonin; Amara et al. 1982; Rosenfeld et al. 1983), so it is somehow fitting that its receptors are progressive in design as well. Unlike most peptide receptors for which functional activity is contained in a single seven-transmembrane-domain protein, CGRP receptors are composed of at least three different proteins. CGRP receptors contain the seven-transmembrane-domain protein known as the calcitonin receptor-like receptor (CRLR) that is common to both CGRP and adrenomedullin receptors. The potency of CGRP in activating this receptor, however, is determined by the coexpression of a member of a family of smaller proteins called "receptor activity modifying proteins" (RAMPs) which have a single transmembrane domain. Within this family, RAMP1 confers high-affinity binding of CRLR for CGRP (McLatchie et al. 1998; Oliver et al. 2001). A third protein, which is a member of a family of receptor component proteins (RCPs), also contributes to a functional CGRP receptor (Evans et al. 2000). It is likely that different complexes formed by the CRLR protein with RAMPs and RCPs contribute to the high- and low-affinity binding sites of CGRP receptors in brain and peripheral tissues (Galeazza et al. 1991). In primary afferent neurons and spinal neurons, the receptor antagonist $CGRP_{8-37}$ inhibits the majority of responses mediated by CGRP. This antagonist specificity implicates the involvement of CGRP1 receptors (Poyner 1995).

3.3 Signal Transduction of CGRP Receptors

The primary signal transduction mechanism of CGRP receptors in the spinal cord is activation of adenylyl cyclase (Parsons and Seybold 1997; Seybold et al. 2003b). In primary cultures of rat spinal cord, CGRP induces formation of cyclic AMP (cAMP) over a broad range of concentrations that parallels occupancy of high- and low-affinity binding to spinal CGRP receptors. The occurrence of spare receptors is limited to high-affinity receptors. Whereas activation of guanylyl cyclase occurs at high concentrations of CGRP (micromolar range; Parsons and Seybold 1997), there is no direct evidence of CGRP receptors coupling to phospholipase C in spinal neurons. Observations that behavioral effects of intrathecal CGRP are blocked by treatment with a protein kinase C inhibitor (Sun et al. 2004) must be interpreted with caution. This observation is likely due to the activation of protein kinase C secondary to the release of other neurotransmitters (e.g., glutamate and SP). In primary cultures of neonatal rat spinal cord, functional low-affinity CGRP receptors are only associated with nonneuronal components of the cultures (e.g., glial cells, endothelial cells), and these receptors couple to the formation of both cyclic GMP and cAMP. Independent observations confirm that CGRP receptors on astrocytes (Lazar et al. 1991; Moreno et al. 2002) and endothelial cells (Moreno et al. 2002) generate cAMP with a potency comparable to the low-affinity receptor for CGRP in spinal cord cultures. The functional significance of the low-affinity receptors remains to be determined, but it is interesting to speculate that CGRP receptors on astrocytes may contribute to central sensitization by facilitating recycling of glutamate released from primary afferent nociceptors. It would also be interesting to explore whether the increase in cyclic GMP in response to CGRP is mediated by a nitric oxide dependent mechanism.

3.4 Distribution of CGRP Receptors within the Spinal Cord

When the distribution of CGRP receptors in the spinal cord was first described using radiohistochemistry (i.e., receptor autoradiography; Tschopp et al. 1985; Inagaki et al. 1986), a mismatch was noted between the distribution of CGRP-immunoreactive varicosities and high-affinity CGRP binding sites (Kruger et al. 1988). CGRP-immunoreactive varicosities are most numerous in the superficial laminae of the dorsal horn, where only a low level of high-affinity binding sites is detected. The low level of binding sites may reflect a low expression of CGRP receptor proteins. This concept is supported by in situ hybridization studies that have detected only low levels of RAMP1 and RCP mRNAs in the spinal cord of naïve rats (Oliver et al. 2001). Despite apparent differences in densities of CGRP-containing terminals and receptors, the level of functional receptors is sufficient to have significant physiological consequences (see below). In contrast to the disparities in the localization of CGRP-immunoreactive varicosities and binding sites or

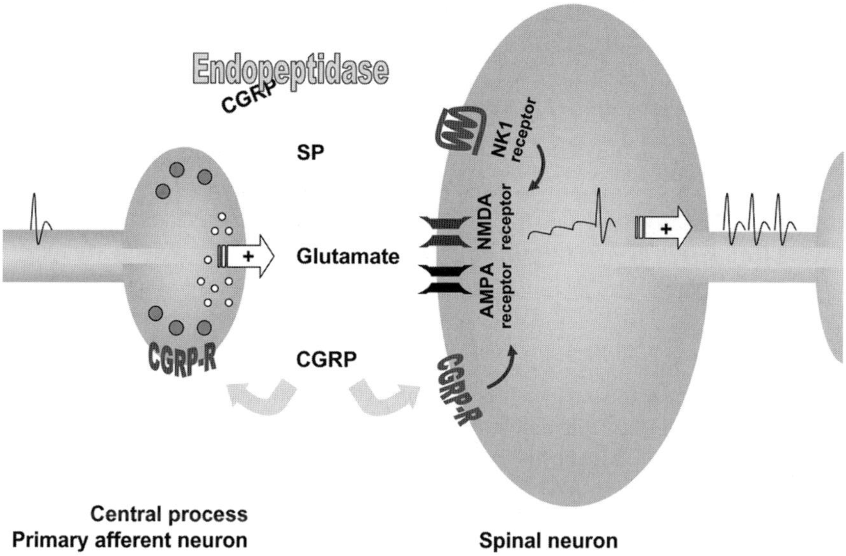

Fig. 1 Calcitonin gene-related peptide (CGRP) facilitates synaptic transmission between primary afferent neurons and spinal neurons by multiple mechanisms. CGRP receptors (CGRP-R) on terminals of primary afferent neurons increase the release of glutamate and other neuropeptides. CGRP-R on spinal neurons activate intracellular signaling pathways that increase the conductance of α-amino-3-hydroxy-5-methyl-4-isoxazolepropionate (AMPA) receptors activated by glutamate. CGRP in the synaptic space is degraded by an endopeptidase. Because CGRP is preferred over substance P (SP) as a substrate by this enzyme, the duration of SP and other tachykinins (e.g., neurokinin A, NKA) in the synapse is prolonged, increasing their activation of neurokinin 1 (NK1) receptors

mRNA for CGRP receptor proteins, a high degree of overlap exists in the distribution of CGRP and RCP immunoreactivity in dorsal root ganglion neurons and axons in the superficial regions of the dorsal horn. (Pokabla et al. 2002; Ma et al. 2003). This relationship suggests the occurrence of CGRP autoreceptors on dorsal root ganglion neurons (Fig. 1). In addition to autocrine regulation, the possibility of paracrine regulation of the adaptive cellular biological function of primary afferent neurons is supported by expression of CGRP receptor markers on non-CGRP-immunoreactive cell bodies of primary afferent neurons.

A change in the density of CGRP receptors in the dorsal horn of the spinal cord could have implications for the long-term contribution of CGRP to central sensitization following peripheral injury. Most receptors exhibit rapid downregulation following increased receptor activation, and this phenomenon is observed in NK1 receptors 24 h after treatment of spinal neurons with SP (Seybold and Abrahams 1995). However, in spite of the rapid and persistent release of CGRP in the spinal cord following induction of peripheral inflammation (see above), high-affinity CGRP binding is maintained in the dorsal spinal cord until 4 days later, and then decreases only transiently (Galeazza et al. 1992). The level of RCP immunoreactivity in the spinal cord increases within 2 h of induction of peripheral inflammation

(Ma et al. 2003), and the increase in expression of this protein may contribute to maintaining the pool of functional CGRP receptors. It remains to be determined whether an increase also occurs in RAMP1, which can increase the capacity of functional CGRP receptors (Zhang et al. 2007).

3.5 Contribution of CGRP Receptors to the Induction of Central Sensitization

The role of CGRP in spinal cord physiological function is beginning to be resolved with the aid of sophisticated genetic and electrophysiological tools. The role of CGRP in neurotransmission of nociception is indirect because CGRP causes no overt behavioral effect when injected by itself (Wiesenfeld-Hallin et al. 1984; Gamse and Saria 1986). Furthermore, nociception is not altered in α-CGRP (−/−) mice (Salmon et al. 1999; Zhang et al. 2001) or when expression of CGRP is downregulated in primary afferent neurons in adult mice by viral infection with antisense CGRP DNA (Tzabazis et al. 2007). However, behavioral and electrophysiological nociceptive responses are greater when they are evoked during high extracellular levels of CGRP in the spinal cord, such as those that occur following a pharmacological or pathophysiological manipulation. Intrathecal administration of CGRP causes acute hyperalgesia to mechanical stimuli (Oku et al. 1987; Sun et al. 2003). Likewise, a CGRP receptor antagonist blocks the increased synaptic current evoked in spinal dorsal horn neurons in vitro in a preparation obtained from rats with acutely inflamed joints (Bird et al. 2006). At the cellular level, these effects may be mediated by CGRP receptors at both pre- and postsynaptic sites as well as effects of CGRP in the extracellular space (Fig. 1). Early evidence suggested that CGRP receptors on the terminals of primary afferent neurons facilitate the release of excitatory amino acids and SP during neuronal firing (Oku et al. 1987; Ryu et al. 1988a; Kangrga and Randic 1990), which would have a feed-forward effect on nociceptor neurotransmission. Recent evidence, however, that treatment with CGRP does not increase the frequency of spontaneous postsynaptic currents in intracellular recordings of lamina II neurons (Bird et el. 2006) casts doubt on a presynaptic effect. Early data also indicated that CGRP has a postsynaptic effect in that it increases the excitability of spinal neurons (Ryu et al. 1988b; Murase et al. 1989). This mechanism is supported by findings that treatment with CGRP results in larger spontaneous postsynaptic currents in intracellular recordings from lamine II neurons (Bird et al. 2006). Colocalization of CGRP and α-amino-3-hydroxy-5-methyl-4-isoxazolepropionate (AMPA) receptor proteins on spinal dorsal horn neurons (Gu and Yu 2007) provides a morphological substrate for postsynaptic effects of CGRP, and evidence that phosphorylation of AMPA subunits by protein kinase A increases their insertion in the plasma membrane (Esteban et al. 2003) offers a cellular explanation for the increase in postsynaptic current. Finally, CGRP contributes to the development of central sensitization by competing with SP for catabolism by endopeptidases (Le Greves et al. 1985; Mao et al. 1992), resulting in prolonged extracellular concentrations of SP following release of the peptides from primary afferent neurons. This effect may contribute significantly to volume transmission of SP in that release of CGRP on one side of the spinal cord results in increased levels of SP on the contralateral side (Schaible et al. 1992). Therefore, pre- and postsynaptic effects as well as extracellular effects all support a role for CGRP in the development of central sensitization, which is clearly demonstrated by evidence that secondary hyperalgesia is blocked when peripheral inflammation is induced in α-CGRP (−/−) mice (Zhang et al. 2001).

3.6 *Contribution of CGRP Receptors to the Maintenance of Central Sensitization*

The CGRP receptor mediated phosphorylation events that facilitate induction of hyperalgesia continue to support central sensitization after hyperalgesia has developed. Intrathecal administration of a CGRP receptor antagonist blocks mechanically evoked nociceptive responses in animals after the development of hyperalgesia due to peripheral inflammation (Lofgren et al. 1997; Sun et al. 2003; Adwanikar et al. 2007). This implicates the continued activation of CGRP receptors in the maintenance of central sensitization by the continuous presence of extracellular CGRP. It is conceivable that increased expression of CGRP by primary afferent neurons (Donaldson et al. 1992; Galeazza et al. 1995) would maintain CGRP release in the face of increased nociceptor activity (Schaible et al. 1994). However, an equally profound contribution of CGRP to persistent central sensitization may be to increase the expression of genes for proteins that promote sensitization (Fig. 2). Increases in protein expression via gene transcription are controlled by transcription factors, and CGRP receptors couple to the phosphorylation of cAMP response element binding protein (CREB) to initiate cAMP response element (CRE)-dependent gene expression both in primary afferent neurons (Anderson and Seybold 2004) and in spinal neurons (Seybold et al. 2003b).

CRE-dependent gene expression is fundamental to long-term plasticity in the hippocampus and cerebellum, and most likely contributes to changes in proteins that maintain central sensitization. The occurrence of phosphorylated CREB (pCREB), the activated form of CREB, increases in the dorsal horn of the spinal cord in response to peripheral injection of chemicals that activate nociceptors (Ji and Rupp 1997; Messersmith et al. 1998; Anderson and Seybold 2000) and nerve injury (Ma and Quirion 2001; Miletic et al. 2002). A variety of protein kinases are able to phosphorylate CREB. The most documented is protein kinase A, which is activated by an increase in the level of cAMP following activation of adenylyl cyclase, but CREB can also be phosphorylated by Ca^{2+}/calmodulin-dependent protein kinase (CaMK) IV (Shaywitz and Greenberg 1999), which

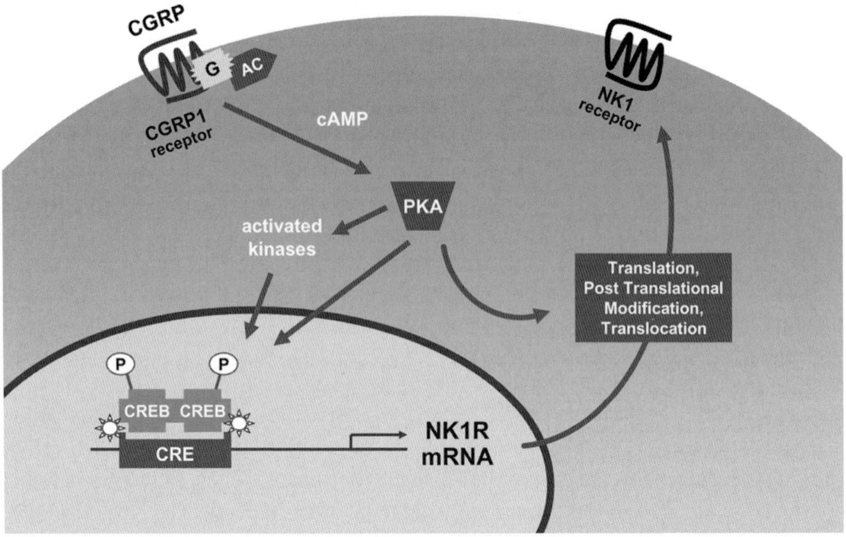

Fig. 2 CGRP increases gene expression by a cyclic AMP (cAMP)-dependent pathway. CGRP1 receptors are G protein coupled receptors that activate adenylyl cyclase, which generates cAMP. cAMP activates protein kinase A (PKA), which can activate other kinases as well. A significant downstream event following activation of PKA is the phosphorylation of the transcription factor cAMP response element binding protein (CREB). When phosphorylated, CREB binds to a cAMP response element site in the promoter region of genes in conjunction with accessory proteins, and gene transcription is initiated. This pathway occurs in dorsal root ganglion neurons as well as spinal neurons. One of the target genes whose expression is increased in spinal neurons is the NK1 receptor

is activated when the concentration of intracellular Ca^{2+} rises as a result of Ca^{2+} release from intracellular stores or influx of extracellular Ca^{2+} through voltage-gated Ca^{2+} channels (especially L-type channels; Mermelstein et al. 2000) or NMDA receptors. Thus, CGRP receptors may activate CREB through activating protein kinase A (Parsons and Seybold 1997), enhancing voltage-gated Ca^{2+} currents evoked by depolarization, or enhancing increases in intracellular Ca^{2+} evoked by other endogenous agonists. Other kinases have also been implicated, including phosphoinositol 3-kinase and Ras/extracellular-signal-regulated kinase (ERK; Lonze and Ginty 2002). ERK has been shown to be activated in the superficial region of the spinal cord in response to intense noxious stimuli (Ji et al. 1999). Not only is cross talk among these pathways implicated, but these pathways converge to activate CREB, indicating a high degree of signal integration.

Importantly, several genes for proteins that are known to promote hyperalgesia have binding sites for CREB within their promoter regions (Lonze and Ginty 2002), and these proteins increase in spinal neurons affected by peripheral inflammation: NK1 receptor (Abbadie et al. 1996; Honore et al. 1999), dynorphin (Iadarola et al. 1988; Ruda et al. 1988), cyclo-oxygenase (COX) 2 (Beiche et al. 1998; Samad et al. 2001; Seybold et al. 2003a) and neuronal nitric oxide synthase (NOS; Lam et al. 1996; Dolan et al. 2003). We have demonstrated regulation of the expression of NK1 receptors in spinal neurons by CGRP. We predicted that CGRP would increase the expression of NK1 receptor protein because the gene for the NK1 receptor has a CRE site within its promoter (Hershey et al. 1991) and CGRP receptors couple to production of cAMP in spinal neurons (Parsons and Seybold 1997), which may lead to phosphorylation of CREB. Furthermore, cAMP increases expression of NK1 receptors in primary cultures of rat spinal neurons (Abrahams et al. 1999). Direct evidence in support of this hypothesis is that CGRP increases the level of mRNA for the NK1 receptor as well as ^{125}I-SP binding in rat spinal neurons (Seybold et al. 2003b). CGRP regulation of NK1 receptor expression is likely mediated by CREB because CGRP increases pCREB immunoreactivity as well as CRE-dependent gene expression in rat spinal neurons. These data, generated in vitro, are compelling evidence for CGRP regulation of gene expression in spinal neurons, but it remains to be determined whether the same effects occur in vivo. Increased expression of NK1 receptors in spinal neurons may make significant contributions to the maintenance of central sensitization because lamina I neurons that express NK1 receptors are required for central sensitization (Khasabov et al. 2002) and hyperalgesia (Mantyh et al. 1997).

It is also important to consider that CGRP receptors on cell bodies of dorsal root and trigeminal ganglion neurons may contribute to changes in gene expression in nociceptors. CGRP is released from cell bodies of primary afferent neurons in vitro (Ulrich-Lai et al. 2001; Ouyang et al. 2005), and CGRP binding to dorsal root and trigeminal ganglion neurons (Edvinsson et al. 1997; Moreno et al. 1999; Segond von Banchet et al. 2002) is associated with functional CGRP receptors (Ryu et al. 1988a; Anderson and Seybold 2004). Because satellite cells surrounding cell bodies of neurons create a barrier to diffusion within dorsal root and trigeminal ganglia, CGRP regulation of gene transcription may occur predominately through autoreceptors. However, paracrine regulation may also be possible because the satellite cell barrier is not continuous (Allen and Kiernan 1994; Shinder and Devor 1994; Amir and Devor 1996), and the barrier may also be overcome by release of CGRP from "baskets" formed by primary afferent axons around individual cell bodies within ganglia (Garry et al. 1989; Quartu et al. 1990). Although CRE-dependent gene expression in dorsal root ganglion neurons has been linked to Ca^{2+} influx through voltage-dependent Ca^{2+} channels (Brosenitsch et al. 1998; Fields et al. 1997), the effect of CGRP on CRE-dependent gene expression is mediated solely by a protein kinase A dependent pathway (Anderson and Seybold 2004). Inhibition of ERK also blocks CGRP-dependent gene transcription, suggesting that activation of this enzyme is an intermediate step in the pathway (Anderson and Seybold 2004). Pronociceptive genes that contain CRE sites in their promoter regions and are increased in dorsal root ganglion neurons in response to peripheral inflammation include CGRP (Donaldson et al. 1992; Watson and Latchman 1995), SP (Donaldson et al. 1992; Morrison et al. 1994), and brain-derived neurotrophic factor (Shieh et al. 1998; Tao et al. 1998).

4 Neurokinin Receptors

4.1 Endogenous Ligands

Neurokinin receptors are activated by members of a family of peptides called tachykinins. Three tachykinins occur in the mammalian spinal cord: SP, neurokinin A (NKA) and neurokinin B (NKB). SP and NKA are encoded in the same precursor protein, preprotachykinin A (PPT-A), in an equal molar ratio. Approximately 30% of SP-immunoreactive varicosities in the superficial region of the dorsal horn remain following dorsal rhizotomy (Tuchscherer and Seybold 1989), indicating that although primary afferent neurons are the major source of SP input, a significant amount of SP release in this region also arises from descending and intrinsic sources (Hunt et al. 1981; Johansson et al. 1981). NKB is encoded in a different precursor protein, preprotachykinin B (Warden and Young 1988; Marksteiner et al. 1992), and is expressed by neurons intrinsic to the spinal cord (Ogawa et al. 1985). Projections from the hypothalamus to the spinal cord may also contribute to NKB released in the dorsal horn (Zhuo and Helke 1993).

4.2 Neurokinin Receptor Subtypes

On the basis of molecular, biochemical, and morphological evidence, NK1 and neurokinin 3 (NK3) receptors are the predominant neurokinin receptors in the spinal cord (McCarson and Krause 1994). SP has the highest affinity for the NK1 receptor expressed in spinal cords of naïve adult rats ($K_d = 400$ pM; Aanonsen et al. 1992). NKA is 250 times less potent than SP in competing for SP binding at the NK1 receptor, and NKB is 2,000 times less potent. Conversely, NKB has the highest affinity for the NK3 receptor (approximately 10 nM), whereas NKA has tenfold lower affinity and SP almost 100-fold lower affinity (Linden et al. 2000a). Both SP and NKA released from primary afferent neurons contribute to the activation of NK1 receptors following noxious stimulation of nociceptors (Trafton et al. 2001) and most likely activate NK3 receptors as well, given that their calculated effective concentrations for activating 50% of the NK3 receptors are 200 and 50 nM, respectively (Linden et al. 2000a). NKA has the highest affinity for neurokinin 2 (NK2) receptors. Although selective NK2 agonists and antagonists have effects on nociceptive processing at the level of the spinal cord (see later), limited biochemical evidence supports the occurrence of NK2 receptor protein in rat or mouse spinal cord. It is noteworthy that NKA released in the spinal cord has a long half-life (Duggan et al. 1990), which will contribute to accumulation of peptide for activation of multiple receptor subtypes and to its volume of distribution. Accumulation of released peptide in the extracellular space and activity of tachykinins at multiple neurokinin receptors must be taken into consideration in

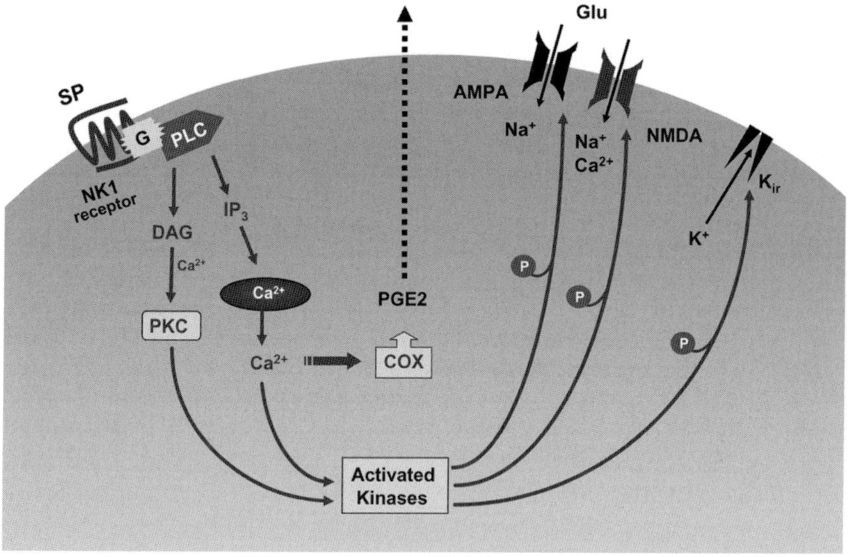

Fig. 3 NK1 receptors increase excitability of spinal neurons by multiple mechanisms. NK1 receptors are G protein coupled receptors that activate phospholipase C (PLC) in spinal neurons. PLC generates two second messengers that mediate the activation of multiple kinases. Protein kinase C (PKC) phosphorylates an inward rectifying K^+ channel, generating a slow excitatory postsynaptic potential. PKC also phosphorylates the NMDA receptor, decreasing the binding of the Mg^{2+} that blocks the channel at resting membrane potential and increasing its conductance. An increase in intracellular Ca^{2+} mediates activation of Ca^{2+}/calmodulin-dependent protein kinase II, which can phosphorylate the AMPA receptor, increasing its conductance. The increase in intracellular Ca^{2+} also activates cyclo-oxygenase (COX), generating prostaglandins (e.g., prostaglandin E_2, PGE2) which can diffuse across the plasma membrane and facilitate transmitter release from presynaptic terminals

understanding the pharmacological effects of endogenous tachykinins in central sensitization.

4.3 Signal Transduction of Neurokinin Receptors

All three neurokinin receptors (NK1, NK2, and NK3) are G protein coupled receptors (Fig. 3). When neurokinin receptors are stably expressed in cell lines, they couple to both phospholipase C and adenylyl cyclase (Nakajima et al. 1992; Takeda et al. 1992; Krause et al. 1997). Phospholipase C synthesizes diacylglycerol and inositol trisphosphate; adenylyl cyclase is responsible for the formation of cAMP. The ability of the NK1 receptor to generate inositol phosphates in neurons was confirmed in primary cultures of neonatal rat spinal cord (Parsons et al. 1995) which express NK1 receptors with biochemical properties comparable to those of adult spinal cord neurons (Stucky et al. 1993; Seybold and Abrahams 1995). However, tachykinins do not generate cAMP in this model (Parsons et al. 1995). Whether this is a developmental limitation of cultured neonatal rat spinal neurons or a true reflection of NK1 receptor coupling in neurons is not known.

Importantly, inositol trisphosphate mediates release of Ca^{2+} from intracellular stores in response to neurokinin receptor activation (Womack et al. 1988; Linden et al. 2000a; Trafton et al. 2001), and an increase in intracellular Ca^{2+} is required for the activation of several enzymes that contribute to central sensitization: CaMK, COX (the rate-limiting enzyme in the formation of prostanoids), and NOS (the rate-limiting enzyme in the formation of nitric oxide).

4.4 Regulation of Neurokinin Receptors

The regulation of neurokinin receptors has implications for the role of SP in the maintenance of central sensitization. Desensitization to the behavioral effects of SP occurs acutely in vivo following repeated intrathecal injection of the peptide (Moochhala and Sawynok 1984; Larson 1988). The desensitization can be attributed in part to internalization of NK1 receptors following activation by the ligand (Bowden et al. 1994). The time course of NK1 receptor internalization and recycling to the plasma membrane in neurons is 30–60 min (Southwell et al. 1996). After recycling, neuronal NK1 receptors retain their ability to bind peptide and undergo another round of endocytosis following a second exposure to SP (Southwell et al. 1998). Even though there is no change in receptor number after the receptor has had time to recycle to the cell surface, recycled receptor has a 50% lower affinity for SP. The lower affinity of the receptor results in a 50% decrease in binding of a low concentration of SP (Seybold and Abrahams 1995). This change persists for 24 h after a 1-h exposure to SP. Interestingly, cellular adaptation continues over the next 24 h, such that 48 h after a 1-h treatment with SP, SP binding is increased by 50% compared with the control. The increase in binding at 48 h is due to an increase in binding capacity (i.e., receptor number). Thus, exposure to SP contributes to time-dependent changes in NK1 receptor affinity and capacity. Whereas receptor internalization and decreases in affinity may be attributed to phosphorylation of the receptor following activation of protein kinase C downstream from phospholipase C, the sequence of biochemical events that contributes to the SP-mediated increase in receptor number has not been resolved.

Increased expression of NK1 receptor protein (Abbadie et al. 1996; Honore et al. 1999) and ligand binding (Stucky et al. 1993) occurs in the superficial region of the dorsal horn of the spinal cord in conjunction with peripheral inflammation. These changes are preceded by increases in NK1 receptor mRNA (McCarson and Krause

1994), but the stimuli that drive the change in mRNA are only partly resolved. The rat and human genes for the NK1 receptor exhibit a high degree of sequence homology (Gerard et al. 1991; Hershey et al. 1991), and a CRE occurs in the promoter regions. Following transfection of nonneuronal cell lines with the gene, NK1 mRNA increases as a consequence of pathways activated by cyclic AMP, phorbol esters (which activate protein kinase C), and Ca^{2+} (Krause et al. 1993). Because CGRP is released from primary afferent neurons during the development of peripheral inflammation (Galeazza et al. 1995), and CGRP receptors on spinal neurons couple to the generation of cAMP (see earlier), we tested the hypothesis that CGRP contributes to the expression of NK1 receptors in spinal neurons using the in vitro model of primary cultures of neonatal rat spinal cord. Indeed, treatment of spinal neurons in culture with CGRP results in a time dependent increase in SP binding that is preceded by an increase in NK1 receptor mRNA (Seybold et al. 2003b). The increase in NK1 receptor mRNA in neurons is most likely mediated by a protein kinase A dependent pathway that results in phosphorylation of CREB because activation of CGRP receptors increases CRE-dependent gene activity in spinal neurons and the change is blocked by inhibitors of protein kinase A. In vivo, pCREB immunoreactivity is increased in NK1 receptor immunoreactive neurons following peripheral injection of a noxious chemical (Anderson and Seybold 2000). Immunocytochemical studies confirmed that treatment with CGRP increases the occurrence of pCREB in neurons in spinal cord cultures, and biochemical analyses confirmed that CGRP does not activate CRE-dependent gene expression in non-neuronal cells isolated from neonatal spinal cord. In addition to CGRP, levels of prostaglandin (PG)-E2 increase in the spinal cord in response to noxious peripheral stimuli (Malmberg and Yaksh 1995; Sorkin and Moore 1996). Although PGE2 activates receptors, that like CGRP receptors couple to the generation of cAMP, treatment with PGE2 does not increase SP binding in spinal neurons (Seybold et al. 2003b). These data suggest that there is cellular or biochemical specificity in the neurochemical regulation of NK1 receptor expression.

Changes in NK3 receptor binding and gene expression also occur during the hyperalgesia that accompanies peripheral inflammation. Two days after peripheral injection of complete Freund's adjuvant (the earliest time point assayed), NK3 receptor binding is reduced by 50% in regions of the dorsal horn that receive projections from the primary afferent neurons that innervate the affected area (Linden et al. 2000b). NK3 receptor mRNA is increased in the dorsal horn as early as 12 h and persists through 4 days after injection of complete Freund's adjuvant (the latest time point assayed; McCarson and Krause 1994; Linden et al. 2000b), suggesting that the downregulation at 2 days occurs within the context of increased synthesis of the receptor. Whereas it is likely that the downregulation of NK3 receptor binding is a consequence of receptor activation, which endogenous tachykinins activate the NK3 receptor in this model has not been resolved. The decrease in NK3 receptor binding was associated with a 50% decrease in SP content in the same regions of the dorsal horn, but no change occurred in the amount of NKB peptide 2 (Linden et al. 2000b), another peptide synthesized from preprotachykinin B and therefore a marker for the expression of NKB (Marksteiner et al.

1992). The NKB peptide 2 data are difficult to interpret without additional biochemical context, but other studies have resolved that the decrease in SP content is associated with increased synthesis and release of the peptide (see earlier). Given that the relative potencies of SP and NKA (coreleased with SP) at NK3 receptors are in the nanomolar range (Linden et al. 2000a), these peptides must also be considered as candidates for activation of NK3 receptors during persistent inflammatory states.

4.5 Localization of Neurokinin Receptors in the Spinal Cord

4.5.1 NK1 Receptor

Data from radiohistochemical, immunohistochemical, and molecular approaches have established the occurrence of NK1 receptors in the spinal cord. Initial observations using radiohistochemistry demonstrated high levels of high-affinity SP binding sites in laminae I, II, and V (Charlton and Helke 1985; Mantyh et al. 1989), regions that overlap the distribution of SP-immunoreactive terminals (Hökfelt et al. 1977; Seybold and Elde 1980), terminals of nociceptors (Light and Perl 1979; Sugiura et al. 1986), and somatodendritic regions of spinothalamic tract neurons.

Whereas immunohistochemical studies at the levels of the light and electron microscopes offer greater resolution of the cellular localization of the receptor, importantly the data are consistent with reports from radiohistochemical studies. NK1 receptor immunoreactive dendrites and cells bodies occur in the highest density in lamina I of the rat spinal cord (Brown et al. 1995). Lamina II is largely devoid of NK1 receptor immunoreactivity, such that the next-highest density of immunoreactive cell bodies occurs in laminae III–V. The NK1 receptor immunoreactive neurons in the deeper laminae have superficially directed dendrites. A striking observation is the nearly continuous distribution of NK1 receptor immunoreactivity along the somatodendritic plasma membrane when only 15% of the area of the NK1 receptor immunoreactive plasma membrane is apposed by SP-immunoreactive terminals (Liu et al. 1994). Consequently, the extensive internalization of NK1 receptor immunoreactivity into endosomes in response to the application of noxious peripheral stimuli (Abbadie et al. 1997; Allen et al. 1997) provides morphological evidence in support of volume transmission for peptidergic transmitters in the dorsal horn of the spinal cord.

There is a noteworthy absence of NK1 receptor immunoreactive axon *terminals* in the spinal cord (Brown et al. 1995), suggesting that the receptor does not occur on the central processes of nociceptors. These data contrast with reports of NK1 receptor immunoreactivity on unmyelinated axons in glabrous skin of rat (Carlton et al. 1996) and localization of NK1 receptor mRNA to small dorsal root ganglion neurons using in situ hybridization (Li and Zhao 1998). We (unpublished observation) and others (McCarson 1999) have not detected NK1 receptor mRNA in dorsal root ganglia of naïve rats or those with peripheral inflammation using quantitative reverse transcription PCR or solution hybridization-nuclease protection assays, respectively, even though these same approaches detect levels of message in spinal neurons (McCarson and Krause 1994; Seybold et al. 2003b). Whether the negative data are due to low levels of sensitivity of the assays or the positive data reflect cross-reactivity of markers with other proteins remains to be resolved. Evidence that release of SP from peripheral terminals of primary afferent neurons is increased in NK1 (–/–) mice has been attributed to autoreceptors (Lever et al. 2003), but these data need to be interpreted with caution. The apparent decrease in inhibitory feedback in SP release in NK1 (–/–) mice could result from diminished NK1 receptor mediated release of secondary factors from nonneural cells in skin (Burbach et al. 2001; Liu et al. 2006).

Double-labeling studies provide significant insights into the projections of the lamina I neurons that express NK1 receptors. A very high proportion (80%) of lamina I projection neurons are immunoreactive for NK1 receptor protein (Todd et al. 2002), and these neurons terminate in the caudal level of the ventrolateral medulla (Spike et al. 2003), a region involved in descending modulation of nociception. It is noteworthy that the lamina I projection neurons that express NK1 receptors are critical to the development of hyperalgesia (Mantyh et al. 1997) and central sensitization (Khasabov et al. 2002) following persistent activation of nociceptors.

4.5.2 NK2 Receptor

Limited biochemical data support the pharmacological evidence for involvement of NK2 receptors in central processing of nociceptive information. Images generated in radiohistochemical studies show high-affinity NK2 receptor binding sites in superficial regions of the dorsal horn (Yashpal et al. 1990), and an increase in the density of binding sites following dorsal rhizotomy suggests a portion of the receptors are located postsynaptically (Yashpal et al. 1991). However, two laboratories failed to detect NK2 receptor mRNA in rat spinal cord (Tsuchida et al. 1990; Takeda and Krause 1991). These discrepancies may be attributed to induction of NK2 receptor expression in spinal cord cells (neurons, glial) in response to neuronal degeneration, splice variants of the NK2 receptor (Watling et al. 1993), or occurrence of NK2 receptors on central terminals of primary afferent neurons. However, NK2 receptor mRNA in dorsal root ganglion neurons has not been reported.

4.5.3 NK3 Receptor

With use of the same radiohistochemical, immunohistochemical, and molecular approaches, NK3 receptors have been localized to spinal neurons in the dorsal horn. In contrast to neurons that express the NK1 receptor, NK3 receptor immunoreactive neurons occur most densely within lamina II and fewer labeled neurons are distributed in lamina I (Seybold et al. 1997). This pattern is consistent with the distribution of high-affinity NK3 agonist binding (Mantyh et al. 1989; Linden et al. 2000b) such that NK3 receptors occur in a higher density than NK1 receptors within lamina II (substantia gelatinosa; Mantyh et al. 1989). At the cellular level, receptor immunoreactivity is localized to somatodendritic regions within individual neurons; no immunoreactivity is associated with dorsal root ganglia or axonal profiles. The occurrence of NK3 receptors on spinal neurons is supported by evidence of NK3 receptor mRNA detected by in situ hybridization (Ding et al. 1996) and solution hybridization-nuclease protection assays (McCarson and Krause 1994). Double-labeling studies demonstrate extensive codistribution of NK3 receptor immunoreactivity with NOS (more than 85%; Seybold et al. 1997). Electrophysiological and behavioral data support a functional relationship between NK3 receptors and nitric oxide at the level of the spinal cord (see later).

4.6 Contribution of Neurokinin Receptors to Development of Central Sensitization

Although intrathecal injection of SP in naïve rats evokes biting and scratching behaviors (Seybold et al. 1982), perception of a brief noxious stimulus does not require SP neurotransmission in the spinal cord. There is no change in nociceptive thresholds in mice when endogenous SP is eliminated by deleting the PPT-A gene responsible for synthesizing its precursor protein (Cao et al. 1998). Similarly, there are no changes in behavioral responses to brief noxious stimuli in NK1 receptor (−/−) mice (De Felipe et al. 1998), in rats in the presence of NK1 and NK3 receptor antagonists (Coderre and Melzack 1991; Malmberg and Yaksh 1992a; Picard et al. 1993; Linden and Seybold 1999), or when neurokinin receptors in rats are desensitized by repeated injection of SP intrathecally (Moochhala and Sawynok 1984; Sweeney and Sawynok 1986). There are conflicting data concerning effects of NK2 receptor antagonists (Fleetwood-Walker et al. 1990; Picard et al. 1993; Neugebauer et al. 1996). However, it must be noted that these results are based on measures of the *threshold* for perception of a stimulus as noxious. Data from preprotachykinin knockout mice (deletion of SP and NKA) support a role for SP and/or NKA in the perception of *graded* noxious stimuli in the range of moderate to intense (Cao et al. 1998). Evidence that more NK1 receptor internalization occurs with increasingly persistent and intense noxious stimuli (Allen et al. 1997) is consistent with the differential release of endogenous tachykinins with stimulus strength. Therefore, when data from studies with neurokinin receptor antagonists are interpreted, it is important to consider whether the stimuli would evoke release of endogenous tachykinins.

Relevant to central sensitization, there are many examples of hyperalgesia that persists after the biting and scratching behaviors evoked by spinal delivery of SP have subsided. The earliest include a decrease in the tail flick latency in response to noxious heat (Moochhala and Sawynok 1984) and lower threshold for withdrawal in response to a pressure stimulus (Sweeney and Sawynok 1986). Data from a variety of experimental models support a role for neurokinin receptors (especially NK1) in spinal mechanisms that contribute to the development of hyperalgesia in response to stimuli that would evoke robust responses from nociceptors (Cridland and Henry 1988; Yamamoto and Yaksh 1991; Yashpal et al. 1993; Ren et al. 1996; Sluka et al. 1997). These data are complemented by effects of NK1, NK2, and NK3 receptor agonists on excitability of spinal neurons. The contribution of each receptor will be described separately.

4.6.1 NK1 Receptor

Considerable evidence indicates that SP evokes central sensitization directly by increasing the excitability of spinal neurons (Henry 1976; Randic and Miletic 1977; Parsons et al. 1996; Liu and Sandkuhler 1997), and indirectly by facilitating the activation of NMDA receptors on these neurons (Randic et al. 1990; Dougherty and Willis 1991; Urban et al. 1994; Guo et al. 2002). Spinal neurons that are excited by noxious thermal (Henry 1976), mechanical (Randic and Miletic 1977), or chemical (Wright and Roberts 1980) stimuli are excited by SP. Specifically, SP causes a slow excitatory postsynaptic potential that facilitates activation of spinal nociceptive neurons by noxious peripheral stimuli (Henry 1976; Randic and Miletic 1977; Randić and Urbán 1987). At the cellular level, these effects are mediated by release of SP from presynapic terminals. SP-immunoreactive terminals occur on cell bodies of neurons in laminae I and V of the spinal cord, regions where nociceptors are known to terminate (Light and Perl 1979; Sugiura et al. 1986). Furthermore, SP-containing terminals occur more frequently presynaptic to neurons that are activated by noxious stimuli compared with those activated solely by innocuous stimuli (De Koninck et al. 1992).

SP has the highest affinity for NK1 receptors, and pharmacological as well as morphological evidence supports the conclusion that NK1 receptors mediate effects of endogenous SP. NK1 receptor immunoreactivity occurs on dendrites and cell bodies of neurons in the dorsal horn of the spinal cord, and these receptors undergo internalization in response to application of persistent noxious stimuli that release endogenous SP (Allen et al. 1997). Moreover, persistent activation of C-fibers by electrical current or chemical stimuli is sufficient to cause sensitization of dorsal horn neurons in vivo, and electrophysiological recordings demonstrate that spinal delivery of NK1 receptor antagonists decreases the facilitated responses of dorsal horn neurons to innocuous stimuli following induction of central sensitization (Laird et al. 1993; Dougherty et al. 1994). Importantly, NK1 receptors may also contribute to the *maintenance* of enhanced spinal cord activity. Two days after hyperalgesia develops in response to peripheral injection of complete Freund's adjuvant, spinal administration of an NK1 receptor antagonist is sufficient to reverse the increased activity in the electrically evoked nociceptive flexor reflex

(Parsons et al. 1996). An important component of these data is that the long latency activity of the reflex (1–2 min) is decreased by the NK1 receptor antagonist but not the short latency activity (0–5 s), which is consistent with the functional role of NK1 receptors in modulating synaptic transmission. However, these data are contrary to evidence that inflammation still induces persistent hyperalgesia when there is a functional deletion of either the precursor for SP [PPT-A (−/−) mice; Cao et al. 1998] or the NK1 receptor [NK1 (−/−) mice; De Felipe et al. 1998]. One reason for the discrepancy in the data among these models may be that data on the nociceptive flexor reflex are generated in a spinalized preparation which eliminates input from descending systems. Alternatively, developmental adaptation may contribute to a lack of effect of gene deletions on the occurrence of hyperalgesia by increasing the role of NKB in PPT-A (−/−) mice or other neurokinin receptors in NK1 (−/−) mice in central sensitization (see below).

NK1 receptors on spinal neurons couple to the activation of phospholipase C, which generates two intracellular messengers, diacylglycerol and inositol trisphosphate (Fig. 3). These messengers evoke downstream effects of activation of protein kinase C and release of Ca^{2+} from intracellular stores. Both signaling pathways may contribute to central sensitization. A protein kinase C dependent pathway is likely responsible for decreasing currents through K^{+} channels (Takano et al. 1996; Rojas et al. 2008), thereby generating the slow excitatory postsynaptic potential evoked by SP activation of NK1 receptors. The depolarization of the plasma membrane by NK1 receptor agonists may contribute to enhancement of NMDA receptor activity (Dougherty and Willis 1991; Rusin et al. 1992, 1993) by releasing the Mg^{2+} blockade of the ligand-gated cation channel (Mayer et al. 1984). In addition, the NMDA receptor has a consensus sequence for phosphorylation by protein kinase C (Moriyoshi et al. 1991). Phorbol esters, which directly activate protein kinase C, increase current through NMDA receptors (Chen and Huang 1992) and increase responses of dorsal horn neurons to NMDA (Gerber et al. 1989). However, evidence that spinally administered NMDA and NK1 receptor antagonists additively attenuate hyperalgesia associated with acute inflammation (Ren et al. 1996) supports a role for NK1 receptor mediated mechanisms that are independent of NMDA receptors. In addition to depolarization of the membrane, the release of Ca^{2+} from intracellular stores following activation of NK1 receptors may result in the activation of CaMK II via phosphorylation. Increased phosphorylation of CaMK II occurs in the dorsal horn of the spinal cord in a model of acute central sensitization (Fang et al. 2002), and spinal treatment with a CaMK II inhibitor prevents the increase in excitability of dorsal horn neurons in acute central sensitization. Furthermore, CaMK II dependent phosphorylation of the GluR1 subunit of the AMPA receptor at an amino acid known to increase conductance of the receptor channel occurs in conjunction with central sensitization. Thus, activation of NK1 receptors can contribute to central sensitization through multiple intracellular pathways.

One intracellular signaling pathway on which NK1 receptors and NMDA receptors converge is the generation of prostaglandins by COX. Two lines of evidence support the involvement of spinally generated prostaglandins in hyperalgesia.

Injection of PGE2 into the intrathecal space causes thermal and mechanical hyperalgesia in rodents (Taiwo and Levine 1986; Uda et al. 1990; Minami et al. 1994b). Conversely, spinal administration of nonsteroidal anti-inflammatory drugs (NSAIDs) attenuates thermal and mechanical hyperalgesia (Malmberg and Yaksh 1992a; Seibert et al. 1994) as well as behavioral responses to peripheral injection of formalin (Malmberg and Yaksh 1992b, 1995). The decrease in hyperalgesia following spinal delivery of NSAIDs is paralleled by a decrease in evoked firing of dorsal horn neurons (Chapman and Dickenson 1992; Jurna et al. 1992). Products of COX also have a role in maintaining central sensitization. Spinal delivery of an NSAID reduces the duration of the electrically evoked nociceptive flexor reflex 2 days after peripheral inflammation is induced by complete Freund's adjuvant (Seybold et al. 2003a).

In addition to peptides, PGE2 is released in the spinal cord in response to noxious thermal and chemical stimuli (Malmberg and Yaksh 1995), as well as in response to electrical stimulation of C-fibers (Sorkin and Moore 1996). Evidence that inhibitors of COX attenuate firing of spinal neurons in response to persistent noxious mechanical stimuli in naïve animals (Pitcher and Henry 1999; 2001) indicates that prostaglandins also have a role in encoding the intensity of a stimulus at the level of the spinal cord. Moreover, the release of PGE2 in the spinal cord is facilitated during peripheral inflammation (Sorkin and Moore 1996). Involvement of SP in the generation of prostaglandins at the level of the spinal cord is supported by evidence that intrathecal injection of SP evokes the release of PGE2 in the spinal cord (Hua et al. 1999). Furthermore, spinal administration of a COX2 inhibitor blocks the thermal hyperalgesia evoked by intrathecal administration of SP (Yaksh et al. 2001). However, it is difficult to conclude whether these effects of SP are independent of its facilitation of NMDA receptor activity because NMDA receptor agonists give the same results in comparable experimental paradigms (Yamamoto and Sakashita 1998; Svensson et al. 2003).

It is important to consider that SP-evoked release of prostaglandins in the spinal cord could account for effects on central terminals of primary afferent neurons attributed to SP in vivo (Fig. 4). The highest density of NK1 receptors in the dorsal horn occurs in superficial laminae (Stucky et al. 1993), and this distribution overlaps with the distribution of binding sites for PGE2 (Matsumura et al. 1992) and prostaglandin I_2 (Matsumura et al. 1995). A presynaptic site for prostaglandin receptors is supported by evidence that PGE2 and prostaglandin I_2 facilitate release of peptides from primary afferent neurons (Andreeva and Rang 1993; Vasko et al. 1994), as well as evidence that binding sites for the prostaglandins in superficial laminae of the dorsal horn decrease with degeneration of central terminals of primary afferent neurons following the lesion of dorsal roots (Matsumura et al. 1995). Thus, prostaglandins likely serve as retrograde signaling molecules at nociceptive synapses in the spinal cord, resulting in a feed-forward pathway for release of transmitters from primary afferent neurons. This possibility is supported by evidence that spinal administration of an NMDA receptor antagonist attenuates the hyperalgesia evoked by PGE2 administered by the same route (Minami et al. 1994a; Park et al. 2000).

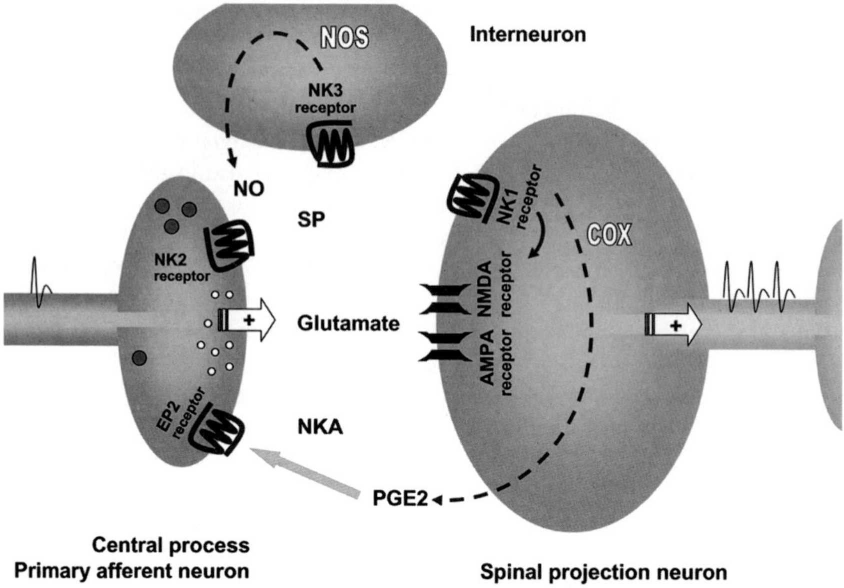

Fig. 4 Tachykinins released from primary afferent neurons contribute to central sensitization by activating different neurokinin receptors on different populations of neurons in the superficial regions of the dorsal horn of the spinal cord. Activation of NK1 receptors on spinal projection neurons results in a larger conductance of ions through AMPA and NMDA receptors activated by glutamate. In addition, NK1 receptors contribute to an increase in the synthesis of prostaglandins (e.g., PGE2) by COX. PGE2 can diffuse across the plasma membrane and activate prostaglandin receptors (e.g., EP2) on central terminals of nociceptors to increase transmitter release in response to action potentials. Activation of presynaptic neurokinin 2 receptors may have a similar effect. Activation of neurokinin 3 receptors on interneurons initiates an intracellular process that results in the activation of nitric oxide synthase and the generation of nitric oxide, which can also diffuse across the plasma membrane. Nitric oxide promotes hyperalgesia, but the mechanism is not known. It is likely that SP and NKA released from primary afferent neurons in response to persistent, intense noxious stimuli activate all three subtypes of neurokinin receptors expressed among these neurons

4.6.2 NK2 Receptor

Spinal injection of an NK2 receptor antagonist delays the development of secondary thermal hyperalgesia following induction of inflammation in the knee joint (Sluka et al. 1997). Moreover, spinal administration of NK2 receptor antagonists may reverse hyperalgesia *after* it has developed. NK2 receptor antagonists attenuate the activity of dorsal horn neurons when delivered within minutes following induction of central sensitization by the peripheral injection of a noxious chemical (Munro et al. 1993). Even more significantly, spinal administration of an NK2 receptor antagonist reduces the increased excitability of dorsal horn neurons several hours after development of inflammation in the knee (Neugebauer et al. 1996), and an NK2 receptor antagonist is still efficacious in decreasing excitability of spinal neurons 2 days after induction of inflammation in the paw (Jia and Seybold 1997).

The later time point is of particular significance because it exceeds the period during which phosphorylation of membrane proteins alone can account for changes in cellular activity.

The cellular site of action of NK2 agonists has not been resolved, and this review will defend the hypothesis that presynaptic NK2 receptors contribute to the effects of this class of neurokinin receptor agonists (Fig. 4). Data from a variety of experimental approaches suggest that tachykinins have effects on primary afferent neurons. In electrophysiological recordings of cutaneous nociceptors from adult rats in vitro, a supramaximal concentration of SP (10 μM) increases the response of C-fibers to chemical stimuli (Kessler et al. 1992). Whereas recent evidence implicates NK1 receptors on keratinocytes in modulating transduction of somatic stimuli (Burbach et al. 2001; Liu et al. 2006), the possibility of a direct action of tachykinins on primary afferent neurons is supported by evidence that superfusion with SP (0.1–1 μM) opens a nonselective cation channel (Inoue et al. 1995) and increases the concentration of free intracellular Ca^{2+} in neurons cultured from neonatal dorsal root ganglia (Bowie et al. 1994). It must be noted, though, that these responses require concentrations of SP that exceed saturation of NK1 receptors, making it unlikely that NK1 receptors mediate the effects.

Unlike the doubtful occurrence of NK1 or NK3 receptors on primary afferent neurons, the possibility of NK2 receptors, or some other tachykinin receptor, cannot be excluded. Pharmacological data support the hypothesis that the functional effects of tachykinins on primary afferent neurons are mediated by NK2 receptors because NKA is generally more potent than SP in evoking responses in primary afferent neurons (Kangrga and Randic 1990, Inoue et al. 1995), which is consistent with the order of potency of these peptides at NK2 receptors. Morphological evidence for NK2 receptors on primary afferent neurons is indirect, in that the distribution of NK2 binding sites in the superficial laminae of the dorsal horn of the spinal cord overlaps the pattern of termination of small-diameter primary afferent fibers (Yashpal et al. 1990). The most compelling evidence is from electrophysiological studies of isolated dorsal root ganglion neurons: a selective NK2 receptor agonist but not NK1 or NK3 agonists mimics the increased excitability evoked in dorsal root ganglion neurons by SP and NKA (Sculptoreanu and de Groat 2007). Therefore, physiological effects of endogenous SP and NKA on primary afferent neurons may be mediated by NK2 receptors. A presynaptic site of action of NK2 receptors would complement the contributions of NK1 and NK3 receptors on spinal neurons to central sensitization.

4.6.3 NK3 Receptor

NK3 receptor agonists facilitate a spinally mediated nociceptive reflex in the rat independent of other spinal neurokinin receptors (Linden et al. 1999; Linden and Seybold 1999). Indeed, in contrast to NK1 receptor agonists, there is no direct effect of an NK3 receptor agonist on membrane potential in electrophysiological recordings from adult rat spinal cord in vivo (Cumberbatch et al. 1995). Because NK3 receptor immunoreactivity is colocalized with NOS in neurons within substantia gelatinosa of the dorsal horn, and nitric oxide at the level of the spinal cord promotes hyperalgesia (Kitto et al. 1992; Malmberg and Yaksh 1993), we hypothesized that augmentation of a nociceptive reflex in the presence of an NK3 receptor agonist is mediated by nitric oxide (Fig. 4). Pretreatment with a competitive substrate of NOS, L-NAME (N^{G}-nitro-L-arginine methyl ester), attenuates the effect of an NK3 agonist, providing evidence in support of this hypothesis (Linden et al. 1999).

At the cellular level, NK3 receptor agonists couple to the activation of NOS through the release of Ca^{2+} from intracellular stores (Linden et al. 2000a). Although SP and NKA have lower potency than NKB in generating this response at NK3 receptors, their effective concentrations are still within the nanomolar range, suggesting that they may contribute to the generation of nitric oxide in vivo. Thus, in addition to NMDA receptors, which were first implicated in the generation of nitric oxide at the level of the spinal cord (Kitto et al. 1992; Malmberg and Yaksh 1993), activation of NK3 receptors must also be considered.

NK3 receptors in the spinal cord may preferentially promote thermal hyperalgesia. Spinal administration of an NK3 receptor agonist decreases the latency of withdrawal to a noxious thermal stimulus, but has no effect on responses to a noxious mechanical stimulus in unrestrained rats (Linden and Seybold 1999). Conversely, systemic administration of an NK3 receptor agonist blocks the development of thermal hyperalgesia in response to peripheral injection of complete Freund's adjuvant (Zaratin et al. 2000). Although we cannot exclude that one reason for the stimulus-dependent effects is that responses to a thermal stimulus were measured at the threshold for a response and responses to the mechanical stimulus were measured with a suprathreshold stimulus (50% response in control condition), intrathecal administration of a comparable dose of SP increased the response to the mechanical stimulus (Linden and Seybold 1999). Thus, the lack of effect of the NK3 receptor agonist on mechanical nociception was not because we were beyond the linear range of the assay. Furthermore, other investigations support a functional relationship between nitric oxide and thermal hyperalgesia (Meller and Gebhart 1994; Inoue et al. 1997).

4.7 Neurokinin Receptors and Gene Expression

There is evidence that a variety of transcription factors are activated in spinal neurons in conjunction with hyperalgesia (e.g., CREB, see earlier; fos, Hunt et al. 1987; jun, Messersmith et al. 1998; nuclear factor κB, Chan et al. 2000), but little is known about the intercellular messengers that initiate the process of activation. We are interested in the possibility that the transcription factor nuclear factor of activated T cells (NFAT) has a role in increasing the expression of pronociceptive genes in the spinal cord. NFAT is hypothesized to play a role in long-term changes in synaptic activity during development as well as in learning and memory

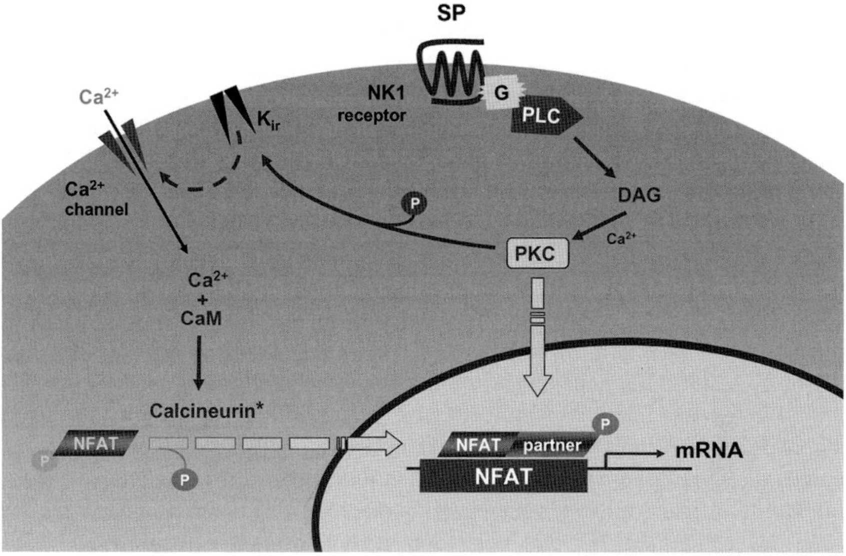

Fig. 5 NK1 receptors on spinal neurons activate gene transcription by a nuclear factor of activated T cells (NFAT)-dependent mechanism. Activation of the NFAT promoter requires the coincident binding of two proteins: the transcription factor NFAT and a nuclear partner (e.g., AP1). Phosphorylated NFAT is restricted to the cytoplasm, so the protein must be dephosphorylated in order for it to enter the nucleus, where it can bind to the NFAT promoter. The nuclear partner must be phosphorylated in order for it to bind to the NFAT promoter. Activation of NK1 receptors on spinal neurons initiates this process by activating PKC. PKC phosphorylates the nuclear partner and also phosphorylates an inward rectifying K^+ channel. Phosphorylation of the K^+ channel decreases its conductance, resulting in depolarization of the plasma membrane. The depolarization of the membrane opens L-type voltage-dependent Ca^{2+} channels, causing an influx of extracellular Ca^{2+}. The higher Ca^{2+} concentration in the cytoplasm promotes the activation of calcineurin, which *de*phosphorylates NFAT in the cytoplasm, thereby allowing it to move into the nucleus to initiate gene transcription

in the mature nervous system (Graef et al. 1999). Under basal conditions, NFAT resides in the cytoplasm. A sustained increase in intracellular Ca^{2+} activates calcineurin, which dephosphorylates NFAT, unmasking a sequence that promotes translocation of NFAT to the nucleus, where it binds DNA with a nuclear partner (e.g., AP-1) to initiate gene transcription (Fig. 5; reviewed by Graef et al. 2001). Termination of transcriptional activity occurs when NFAT is rephosphorylated, resulting in its return to the cytoplasm. In hippocampal neurons, NFAT-dependent gene transcription is activated by influx of Ca^{2+} through voltage-gated Ca^{2+} channels (Graef et al. 1999) as well as release of Ca^{2+} from intracellular stores following activation of TrkB receptors (Groth and Mermelstein 2003). Effects of TrkB receptor activation are mediated by phospholipase C. Given that neurokinin receptors couple to phospholipase C (Parsons et al. 1995, Linden et al. 2000a), and that the distribution of calcineurin-immunoreactive neurons

(Strack et al. 1996) overlaps that of NK1 and NK3 receptors in the superficial laminae of the dorsal horn (Abbadie et al. 1996, Seybold et al. 1997), we predicted that neurokinin receptors also couple to NFAT-dependent gene transcription in spinal neurons.

NFAT exists in multiple isoforms (Rao et al. 1997). NFATc-4 mRNA is distributed among dorsal root ganglion neurons and throughout the spinal cord (Groth et al. 2007), and immunocytochemical studies confirmed that NFATc-4 occurs in spinal neurons that are immunoreactive for NK1 receptor (Seybold et al. 2006). Although NFATc-4 was the focus of our studies, the possibility of the occurrence of other isoforms in these regions cannot be excluded. Treatment of primary cultures of neonatal rat neurons with SP increases NFAT-dependent gene expression with a potency of approximately 1 nM, which is consistent with the potency of SP in activating phospholipase C in this same model (Parsons et al. 1995). Selective NK1 receptor antagonists block the effect of SP, and NKA is tenfold less potent than SP in generating NFAT-dependent gene expression, which is consistent with their order of potency in activating NK1 receptors. When the activity of either protein kinase C or calcineurin is blocked with a selective enzyme inhibitor, the effect of SP on gene expression is reduced. These data are consistent with the requirement for two coincident events for the activation of NFAT-dependent gene transcription. Although NK1 receptors couple to the release of Ca^{2+} from intracellular stores in spinal neurons (Womack et al. 1988), the influx of extracellular Ca^{2+} is required for NK1 receptor mediated activation of NFAT. The slow depolarization evoked by activation of NK1 receptors is most likely responsible for the influx of Ca^{2+} through L-type Ca^{2+} channels that is required for the activation of calcineurin in spinal neurons.

5 Summary

Increased efficacy of synaptic signaling between nociceptors and spinal neurons contributes to central sensitization that underlies hyperalgesia. Peptidergic neurotransmission is an important component of this adaptive process, and SP and CGRP released from terminals of primary afferent neurons contribute to the development and maintenance through complementary cellular mechanisms. CGRP receptors on primary afferent and spinal neurons couple to the generation of the intracellular messenger cAMP. Activation of presynaptic CGRP receptors facilitates transmitter release and activation of postsynaptic receptors increases glutamate activation of AMPA receptors, culminating in increased firing of spinal neurons which is reflected as central sensitization. Neurokinin receptors on spinal neurons couple to phospholipase C and the generation of two intracellular messengers whose downstream effects include depolarizing the membrane by closing potassium channels and increasing the conductance of NMDA receptors. These modifications of channel function are sufficient to increase the firing of neurons in response to a synaptic event, yet activation of neurokinin receptors enhances the process of synaptic transmission further by generating retrograde synaptic messengers (prostaglandins and nitric oxide) that increase transmitter release from central terminals of primary afferent neurons. Therefore, the *development* of central sensitization is mediated by sequences of events that feed forward to strengthen synaptic transmission by multiple mechanisms. Although NK1, NK2, and NK3 receptors are associated with different aspects of these events and may be differentially localized among populations of neurons that participate in transmission of nociceptive information through the spinal cord, the possibility that all endogenous tachykinins may activate each neurokinin receptor following intense or persistent firing of nociceptors suggests all three receptors participate in the induction of central sensitization. The *maintenance* of central sensitization is accomplished by the increased production of enzymes, receptors, and ion channels that underlie processes to increase synaptic strength. Receptors for CGRP and SP contribute to these changes in gene expression through different intracellular pathways that culminate in the activation of different transcription factors.

The consequences of activation of receptors for CGRP and SP delineated in this review illustrate cellular mechanisms underlying central sensitization. These effects have particular significance for the induction of central sensitization following peripheral injury and the maintenance of central sensitization in inflammatory pain when the synthesis and release of CGRP and SP by primary afferent neurons is increased. The activation of additional peptide receptors at the level of the spinal cord adds redundancy and another level of complexity to therapeutic strategies to manage neuropathic pain, but the roles of CGRP and SP in central sensitization have been clearly established. CGRP and SP continue to serve as prototypical examples of the roles of peptides in central sensitization.

References

Aanonsen LM, Kajander KC, Bennett GJ, Seybold VS (1992) Autoradiographic analysis of ^{125}I-substance P binding in rat spinal cord following chronic constriction injury of the sciatic nerve. Brain Res 596:259–268

Abbadie C, Brown JL, Mantyh PW, Basbaum AI (1996) Spinal cord substance P receptor immunoreactivity increases in both inflammatory and nerve injury models of persistent pain. Neuroscience 70:201–209

Abbadie C, Trafton J, Liu H, Mantyh PW, Basbaum AI (1997) Inflammation increases the distribution of dorsal horn neurons that internalize the neurokinin-1 receptor in response to noxious and non-noxious stimulation. J Neurosci 17:8049–8060

Abrahams LG, Reutter MA, McCarson KE, Seybold VS (1999) Cyclic AMP regulates the expression of neurokinin1 receptors by neonatal rat spinal neurons in culture. J Neurochem 73:50–58

Adwanikar H, Ji G, Li W, Doods H, Willis WD, Neugebauer V (2007) Spinal CGRP1 receptors contribute to supraspinally organized pain behavior and pain-related sensitization of amygdala neurons. Pain 132:53–66

Agnati LF, Leo G, Zanardi A, Genedani S, Rivera A, Fuxe K, Guidolin D (2006) Volume transmission and wiring transmission from cellular to molecular networks: history and perspectives. Acta Physiol 187:329–344

Allen DT, Kiernan JA (1994) Permeation of proteins from the blood into peripheral nerves and ganglia. Neuroscience 59:755–764

Allen BJ, Rogers SD, Ghilardi JR, Menning PM, Kuskowski MA, Basbaum AI, Simone DA, Mantyh PW (1997) Noxious cutaneous thermal stimuli induce a graded release of endogenous substance P in the spinal cord: imaging peptide action in vivo. J Neurosci 17:5921–5927

Amara SG, Jonas V, Rosenfeld MG, Ong ES, Evans RM (1982) Alternative RNA processing in calcitonin gene expression generates mRNAs encoding different polypeptide products. Nature 298:240–244

Amara SG, Arriza JL, Leff SE, Swanson LW, Evans RM, Rosenfeld MG (1985) Expression in brain of a messenger RNA encoding a novel neuropeptide homologous to calcitonin gene-related peptide. Science 229:1094–1097

Amir R, Devor M (1996) Chemically mediated cross-excitation in rat dorsal root ganglia. J Neurosci 16:4733–4741

Anderson LE, Seybold VS (2000) Phosphorylated cAMP response element binding protein increases in neurokinin-1 receptor-immunoreactive neurons in rat spinal cord in response to formalin-induced nociception. Neurosci Lett 283:29–32

Anderson LE, Seybold VS (2004) Calcitonin gene-related peptide regulates gene transcription in primary afferent neurons. J Neurochem 91:1417–1429

Andreeva L, Rang HP (1993) Effect of bradykinin and prostaglandins on the release of calcitonin gene-related peptide-like immunoreactivity from the rat spinal cord in vitro. Br J Pharmacol 108:185–190

Beiche F, Brune K, Geisslinger G, Goppelt-Struebe M (1998) Expression of cyclooxygenase isoforms in the rat spinal cord and their regulation during adjuvant-induced arthritis. Inflamm Res 47:482–487

Bird GC, Han JS, Fu Y, Adwanikar H, Willis WD, Neugebauer V (2006) Pain-related synaptic plasticity in spinal dorsal horn neurons: role of CGRP. Mol Pain 2:31

Bowden JJ, Garland AM, Baluk P, Lefevre P, Grady EF, Vigna SR, Bunnett NW, McDonald DM (1994) Direct observation of substance P-induced internalization of neurokinin 1 (NK1) receptors at sites of inflammation. Proc Natl Acad Sci USA 91:8964–8968

Bowie D, Feltz P, Schlichter R (1994) Subpopulations of neonatal rat sensory neurons express functional neurotransmitter receptors which elevate intracellular calcium. Neuroscience 58:141–149

Brosenitsch TA, Salgado-Commissariat D, Kunze DL, Katz DM (1998) A role for L-type calcium channels in developmental regulation of transmitter phenotype in primary sensory neurons. J Neurosci 18:1047–1055

Brown JL, Liu H, Maggio JE, Vigna SR, Mantyh PW, Basbaum AI (1995) Morphological characterization of substance P receptor-immunoreactive neurons in the rat spinal cord and trigeminal nucleus caudalis. J Comp Neurol 356:327–344

Burbach GJ, Kim KH, Zivony AS, Kim A, Aranda J, Wright S, Naik SM, Caughman SW, Ansel JC, Armstrong CA (2001) The neurosensory tachykinins substance P and neurokinin A directly induce keratinocyte nerve growth factor. J Invest Dermatol 117:1075–1082

Cao YQ, Mantyh PW, Carlson EJ, Gillespie AM, Epstein CJ, Basbaum AI (1998) Primary afferent tachykinins are required to experience moderate to intense pain. Nature 392:390–394

Carlton SM, Zhou S, Coggeshall RE (1996) Localization and activation of substance P receptors in unmyelinated axons of rat glabrous skin. Brain Res 734:103–108

Chan CF, Sun WZ, Lin JK, Lin-Shiau SY (2000) Activation of transcription factors of nuclear factor kappa B, activator protein-1 and octamer factors in hyperalgesia. Eur J Pharmacol 402:61–68

Chapman V, Dickenson AH (1992) The spinal and peripheral roles of bradykinin and prostaglandins in nociceptive processing in the rat. Eur J Pharmacol 219:427–433

Charlton CG, Helke CJ (1985) Characterization and segmental distribution of ^{125}I-Bolton-Hunter-labeled substance P binding sites in rat spinal cord. J Neurosci 5:1293–1299

Chen L, Huang LY (1992) Protein kinase C reduces Mg^{2+} block of NMDA-receptor channels as a mechanism of modulation. Nature 356:521–523

Coderre TJ, Melzack R (1991) Central neural mediators of secondary hyperalgesia following heat injury in rats: neuropeptides and excitatory amino acids. Neurosci Lett 131:71–74
Cook AJ, Woolf CJ, Wall PD, McMahon SB (1987) Dynamic receptive field plasticity in rat spinal cord dorsal horn following C-primary afferent input. Nature 325:151–153
Cridland RA, Henry JL (1988) Facilitation of the tail-flick reflex by noxious cutaneous stimulation in the rat: antagonism by a substance P analogue. Brain Res 462:15–21
Cumberbatch MJ, Chizh BA, Headley PM (1995) Modulation of excitatory amino acid responses by tachykinins and selective tachykinin receptor agonists in the rat spinal cord. Br J Pharmacol 115:1005–1012
De Felipe C, Herrero JF, O'Brien JA, Palmer JA, Doyle CA, Smith AJ, Laird JM, Belmonte C, Cervero F, Hunt SP (1998) Altered nociception, analgesia and aggression in mice lacking the receptor for substance P. Nature 392:394–397
De Koninck Y, Ribeiro-da-Silva A, Henry JL, Cuello AC (1992) Spinal neurons exhibiting a specific nociceptive response receive abundant substance P-containing synaptic contacts. Proc Natl Acad Sci USA 89: 5073–5077
Ding YQ, Shigemoto R, Takada M, Ohishi H, Nakanishi S, Mizuno N (1996) Localization of the neuromedin K receptor (NK3) in the central nervous system of the rat. J Comp Neurol 364:290–310
Dolan S, Kelly JG, Huan M, Nolan AM (2003) Transient up-regulation of spinal cyclooxygenase-2 and neuronal nitric oxide synthase following surgical inflammation. Anesthesiology 98:170–180
Donaldson LF, Harmar AJ, McQueen DS, Seckl JR (1992) Increased expression of preprotachykinin, calcitonin gene-related peptide, but not vasoactive intestinal peptide messenger RNA in dorsal root ganglia during the development of adjuvant monoarthritis in the rat. Molec Brain Res 16:143–149
Dougherty PM, Willis WD (1991) Enhancement of spinothalamic neuron responses to chemical and mechanical stimuli following combined micro-iontophoretic application of *N*-methyl-D-aspartic acid and substance P. Pain 47:85–93
Dougherty PM, Palecek J, Palecková V, Willis WD (1994) Neurokinin 1 and 2 antagonists attenuate the responses and NK1 antagonists prevent the sensitization of primate spinothalamic tract neurons after intradermal capsaicin. J Neurophysiol 72:1464–1475
Duggan AW, Hendry IA, Morton CR, Hutchison WD, Zhao ZQ (1988) Cutaneous stimuli releasing immunoreactive substance P in the dorsal horn of the cat. Brain Res 451:261–273
Duggan AW, Hope PJ, Jarrott B, Schaible HG, Fleetwood-Walker SM (1990) Release, spread and persistence of immunoreactive neurokinin A in the dorsal horn of the cat following noxious cutaneous stimulation. Studies with antibody microprobes. Neuroscience 35:195–202
Duggan AW, Riley RC, Mark MA, MacMillan SJ, Schaible HG (1995) Afferent volley patterns and the spinal release of immunoreactive substance P in the dorsal horn of the anaesthetized spinal cat. Neuroscience 65:849–858
Durham PL (2004) CGRP receptor antagonists: a new choice for acute treatment of migraine? Curr Opin Investig Drugs 5:731–735
Edvinsson L (2005) Clinical data on the CGRP antagonist BIBN4096BS for treatment of migraine attacks. CNS Drug Rev 11:69–76
Edvinsson L, Cantera L, Jansen-Olesen I, Uddman R (1997) Expression of calcitonin gene-related peptide1 receptor mRNA in human trigeminal ganglia and cerebral arteries. Neurosci Lett 229:209–211
Esteban JA, Shi SH, Wilson C, Nuriya M, Huganir RL, Malinow R (2003) PKA phosphorylation of AMPA receptor subunits controls synaptic trafficking underlying plasticity. Nat Neurosci 6:136–143
Evans BN, Rosenblatt MI, Mnayer LO, Oliver KR, Dickerson IM (2000) CGRP-RCP, a novel protein required for signal transduction at calcitonin gene-related peptide and adrenomedullin receptors. J Biol Chem 275:31438–31443
Fang L, Wu J, Lin Q, Willis WD (2002) Calcium-calmodulin-dependent protein kinase II contributes to spinal cord central sensitization. J Neurosci 22:4196–204

Fields RD, Eshete F, Stevens B, Itoh K (1997) Action potential-dependent regulation of gene expression: temporal specificity in Ca^{2+}, cAMP-responsive element binding proteins, and mitogen-activated protein kinase signaling. J Neurosci 17:7252–7266

Fleetwood-Walker SM, Mitchell R, Hope PJ, El-Yassir N, Molony V, Bladon CM (1990) The involvement of neurokinin receptor subtypes in somatosensory processing in the superficial dorsal horn of the cat. Brain Res 519:169–182. Erratum in: Brain Res (1992) 579:357

Galeazza MT, O'Brien TD, Johnson KH, Seybold VS (1991) Islet amyloid polypeptide (IAPP) competes for two binding sites of CGRP. Peptides 12:585–491

Galeazza MT, Stucky CL, Seybold VS (1992) Changes in [^{125}I]hCGRP binding in rat spinal cord in an experimental model of acute, peripheral inflammation. Brain Res 591:198–208

Galeazza MT, Garry MG, Yost HJ, Strait KA, Hargreaves KM, Seybold VS (1995) Plasticity in the synthesis and storage of substance P and calcitonin gene-related peptide in primary afferent neurons during peripheral inflammation. Neuroscience 66:443–458

Gamse R, Saria A (1986) Nociceptive behavior after intrathecal injections of substance P, neurokinin A and calcitonin gene-related peptide in mice. Neurosci Lett 70:143–147

Garry MG, Hargreaves KM (1992) Enhanced release of immunoreactive CGRP and substance P from spinal dorsal horn slices occurs during carrageenan inflammation. Brain Res 582:139–142

Garry MG, Miller KE, Seybold VS (1989) Lumbar dorsal root ganglia of the cat: a quantitative study of peptide immunoreactivity and cell size. J Comp Neurol 284:36–47

Gerard NP, Garraway LA, Eddy RL Jr, Shows TB, Iijima H, Paquet JL, Gerard C (1991) Human substance P receptor (NK-1): organization of the gene, chromosome localization, and functional expression of cDNA clones. Biochemistry 30:10640–10646

Gerber G, Kangrga I, Ryu PD, Larew JS, Randic M (1989) Multiple effects of phorbol esters in the rat spinal dorsal horn. J Neurosci 9:3606–3617

Graef IA, Mermelstein PG, Stankunas K, Neilson JR, Deisseroth K, Tsien RW, Crabtree GR (1999) L-type calcium channels and GSK-3 regulate the activity of NF-ATc4 in hippocampal neurons. Nature 401:703–708

Graef IA, Chen F, Crabtree GR (2001) NFAT signaling in vertebrate development. Curr Opin Genet Dev 11:505–512

Groth RD, Mermelstein PG (2003) Brain-derived neurotrophic factor activation of NFAT (nuclear factor of activated T cells)-dependent transcription: a role for the transcription factor NFATc4 in neurotrophin-mediated gene expression. J Neurosci 23:8125–8134

Groth RD, Coicou LG, Mermelstein PG, Seybold VS (2007) Neurotrophin activation of NFAT-dependent transcription contributes to the regulation of pro-nociceptive genes. J Neurochem 102:1162–1174

Gu XL, Yu LC (2007) The colocalization of CGRP receptor and AMPA receptor in the spinal dorsal horn neuron of rat: a morphological and electrophysiological study. Neurosci Lett 414:237–241

Guo W, Zou S, Guan Y, Ikeda T, Tal M, Dubner R, Ren K (2002) Tyrosine phosphorylation of the NR2B subunit of the NMDA receptor in the spinal cord during the development and maintenance of inflammatory hyperalgesia. J Neurosci 22:6208–6217

Henry JL (1976) Effects of substance P on functionally identified units in cat spinal cord. Brain Res 114:439–451

Hershey AD, Dykema PE, Krause JE (1991) Organization, structure and expression of the gene encoding the rat substance P receptor. J Biol Chem 266:4366–4374

Hill R (2000) NK1 (substance P) receptor antagonists – why are they not analgesic in humans? Trends Pharmacol Sci 21:244–246

Hökfelt T, Ljungdahl A, Terenius L, Elde R, Nilsson G (1977) Immunohistochemical analysis of peptide pathways possibly related to pain and analgesia: enkephalin and substance P. Proc Natl Acad Sci USA 74:3081–3085

Honore P, Menning PM, Rogers SD, Nichols ML, Basbaum AI, Besson JM, Mantyh PW (1999) Spinal substance P receptor expression and internalization in acute, short-term, and long-term inflammatory pain states. J Neurosci 19:7670–7678

Hua XY, Chen P, Marsala M, Yaksh TL (1999) Intrathecal substance P-induced thermal hyperalgesia and spinal release of prostaglandin E2 and amino acids. Neuroscience 89:525–534

Hunt SP, Kelly JS, Emson PC, Kimmel JR, Miller RJ, Wu JY (1981) An immunohistochemical study of neuronal populations containing neuropeptides or gamma-aminobutyrate within the superficial layers of the rat dorsal horn. Neuroscience 6:1883–1898

Hunt SP, Pini A, Evan G (1987) Induction of c-fos-like protein in spinal cord neurons following sensory stimulation. Nature 328:632–634

Hylden JL, Nahin RL, Traub RJ, Dubner R (1989) Expansion of receptive fields of spinal lamina I projection neurons in rats with unilateral adjuvant-induced inflammation: the contribution of dorsal horn mechanisms. Pain 37:229–243

Iadarola MJ, Brady LS, Draisci G, Dubner R (1988) Enhancement of dynorphin gene expression in spinal cord following experimental inflammation: stimulus specificity, behavioral parameters and opioid receptor binding. Pain 35:313–326

Inagaki S, Kito S, Kubota Y, Girgis S, Hillyard CJ, MacIntyre I (1986) Autoradiographic localization of calcitonin gene-related peptide binding sites in human and rat brains. Brain Res 374:287–298

Inoue K, Nakazawa K, Inoue K, Fujimori K (1995) Nonselective cation channels coupled with tachykinin receptors in rat sensory neurons. J Neurophysiol 73:736–742

Inoue T, Mashimo T, Shibuta S, Yoshiya I (1997) Intrathecal administration of a new nitric oxide donor, NOC-18, produces acute thermal hyperalgesia in the rat. J Neurol Sci 153:1–7

Ji RR, Rupp F (1997) Phosphorylation of transcription factor CREB in rat spinal cord after formalin-induced hyperalgesia: relationship to c-fos induction. J Neurosci 17:1776–1785

Ji RR, Baba H, Brenner GJ, Woolf CJ (1999) Nociceptive-specific activation of ERK in spinal neurons contributes to pain hypersensitivity. Nat Neurosci 2:1114–1119

Ji RR, Kohno T, Moore KA, Woolf CJ (2003) Central sensitization and LTP: do pain and memory share similar mechanisms? Trends Neuro Sci 26:696–705

Jia YP, Seybold VS (1997) Spinal NK2 receptors contribute to the increased excitability of the nociceptive flexor reflex during persistent peripheral inflammation. Brain Res 751:169–174

Johansson O, Hökfelt T, Pernow B, Jeffcoate SL, White N, Steinbusch HW, Verhofstad AA, Emson PC, Spindel E (1981) Immunohistochemical support for three putative transmitters in one neuron: coexistence of 5-hydroxytryptamine, substance P- and thyrotropin releasing hormone-like immunoreactivity in medullary neurons projecting to the spinal cord. Neuroscience 6:1857–1881

Juaneda C, Dumont Y, Quirion R (2000) The molecular pharmacology of CGRP and related peptide receptor subtypes. Trends Pharmacol Sci 21:432–438

Jurna I, Spohrer B, Bock R (1992) Intrathecal injection of acetylsalicylic acid, salicylic acid and indomethacin depresses C fibre-evoked activity in the rat thalamus and spinal cord. Pain 49:249–256

Kangrga I, Randic M (1990) Tachykinins and calcitonin gene-related peptide enhance release of endogenous glutamate and aspartate from the rat spinal dorsal horn slice. J Neurosci 10:2026–2038

Kessler W, Kirchhoff C, Reeh PW, Handwerker HO (1992) Excitation of cutaneous afferent nerve endings in vitro by a combination of inflammatory mediators and conditioning effect of substance P. Exp Brain Res 91:467–476

Khasabov SG, Rogers SD, Ghilardi JR, Peters CM, Mantyh PW, Simone DA (2002) Spinal neurons that possess the substance P receptor are required for the development of central sensitization. J Neurosci 22:9086–9098

Kitto KF, Haley JE, Wilcox GL (1992) Involvement of nitric oxide in spinally mediated hyperalgesia in the mouse. Neurosci Lett 148:1–5

Krause JE, Bu JY, Takeda Y, Blount P, Raddatz R, Sachais BS, Chou KB, Takeda J, McCarson K, DiMaggio D (1993) Structure, expression and second messenger-mediated regulation of the human and rat substance P receptors and their genes. Regul Pept 46:59–66

Krause JE, Staveteig PT, Mentzer JN, Schmidt SK, Tucker JB, Brodbeck RM, Bu JY, Karpitskiy VV (1997) Functional expression of a novel human neurokinin-3 receptor homolog that binds [^{3}H]senktide and [^{125}I-MePhe7]neurokinin B, and is responsive to tachykinin peptide agonists. Proc Natl Acad Sci USA 94:310–315

Kruger L, Mantyh PW, Sternini C, Brecha NC, Mantyh CR (1988) Calcitonin gene-related peptide (CGRP) in the rat central nervous system: patterns of immunoreactivity and receptor binding sites. Brain Res 463:223–244

Laird J (2001) Gut feelings about tachykinins NK1 receptor antagonists. Trends Pharmacol Sci 22:169

Laird JM, Hargreaves RJ, Hill RG (1993) Effect of RP 67580, a non-peptide neurokinin1 receptor antagonist, on facilitation of a nociceptive spinal flexion reflex in the rat. Br J Pharmacol 109:713–718

Lam HH, Hanley DF, Trapp BD, Saito S, Raja S, Dawson TM, Yamaguchi H (1996) Induction of spinal cord neuronal nitric oxide synthase (NOS) after formalin injection in the rat hind paw. Neurosci Lett 210:201–204

Larson AA (1988) Desensitization to intrathecal substance P in mice: possible involvement of opioids. Pain 32:367–374

Lazar P, Reddington M, Streit W, Raivich G, Kreutzberg GW (1991) The action of calcitonin gene-related peptide on astrocyte morphology and cyclic AMP accumulation in astrocyte cultures from neonatal rat brain. Neurosci Lett 130:99–102

Le Greves P, Nyberg F, Terenius L, Hökfelt T (1985) Calcitonin gene-related peptide is a potent inhibitor of substance P degradation. Eur J Pharmacol 115:309–311

Lee SE, Kim JH (2007) Involvement of substance P and calcitonin gene-related peptide in development and maintenance of neuropathic pain from spinal nerve injury model of rat. Neurosci Res 58:245–249

Lever IJ, Grant AD, Pezet S, Gerard NP, Brain SD, Malcangio M (2003) Basal and activity-induced release of substance P from primary afferent fibres in NK1 receptor knockout mice: evidence for negative feedback. Neuropharmacology 45:1101–1110

Li HS, Zhao ZQ (1998) Small sensory neurons in the rat dorsal root ganglia express functional NK-1 tachykinin receptor. Eur J Neurosci 10:1292–1299

Light AR, Perl ER (1979) Spinal termination of functionally identified primary afferent neurons with slowly conducting myelinated fibers. J Comp Neurol 186:133–150

Linden DR, Seybold VS (1999) Spinal neurokinin3 receptors mediate thermal but not mechanical hyperalgesia via nitric oxide. Pain 80:309–317

Linden DR, Jia YP, Seybold VS (1999) Spinal neurokin3 receptors facilitate the nociceptive flexor reflex via a pathway involving nitric oxide. Pain 80:301–308

Linden DR, Chell MJ, El-Fakahany EE, Seybold VS (2000a) Neurokinin(3) receptors couple to the activation of neuronal nitric-oxide synthase in stably transfected Chinese hamster ovary cells. J Pharmacol Exp Ther 293:559–568

Linden DR, Reutter MA, McCarson KE, Seybold VS (2000b) Time-dependent changes in neurokinin(3) receptors and tachykinins during adjuvant-induced peripheral inflammation in the rat. Neuroscience 98:801–811

Liu X, Sandkuhler J (1997) Characterization of long-term potentiation of C-fiber-evoked potentials in spinal dorsal horn of adult rat: essential role of NK1 and NK2 receptors. J Neurophysiol 78:1973–1982

Liu H, Brown JL, Jasmin L, Maggio JE, Vigna SR, Mantyh PW, Basbaum AI (1994) Synaptic relationship between substance P and the substance P receptor: light and electron microscopic characterization of the mismatch between neuropeptides and their receptors. Proc Natl Acad Sci USA 91:1009–1013

Liu JY, Hu JH, Zhu QG, Li FQ, Sun HJ (2006) Substance P receptor expression in human skin keratinocytes and fibroblasts. Br J Dermatol 155:657–662

Lofgren O, Yu LC, Theodorsson E, Hansson P, Lundeberg T (1997) Intrathecal CGRP(8–37) results in a bilateral increase in hindpaw withdrawal latency in rats with a unilateral thermal injury. Neuropeptides 31:601–607

Lonze BE, Ginty DD (2002) Function and regulation of CREB family transcription factors in the nervous system. Neuron 35:605–623

Lundberg JM, Rudehill A, Sollevi A, Fried G, Wallin G (1989) Co-release of neuropeptide Y and noradrenaline from pig spleen in vivo: importance of subcellular storage, nerve impulse frequency and pattern, feedback regulation and resupply by axonal transport. Neuroscience. 28:475–486

Ma W, Chabot JG, Powell KJ, Jhamandas K, Dickerson IM, Quirion R (2003) Localization and modulation of calcitonin gene-related peptide-receptor component protein-immunoreactive cells in the rat central and peripheral nervous systems. Neuroscience 120:677–694

Ma W, Quirion R (2001) Increased phosphorylation of cyclic AMP response element-binding protein (CREB) in the superficial dorsal horn neurons following partial sciatic nerve ligation. Pain 93:295–301

Malmberg AB, Yaksh TL (1992a) Hyperalgesia mediated by spinal glutamate or substance P receptor blocked by spinal cyclooxygenase inhibition. Science 257:1276–1279

Malmberg AB, Yaksh TL (1992b) Antinociceptive actions of spinal nonsteroidal anti-inflammatory agents on the formalin test in the rat. J Pharmacol Exp Ther 263:136–146

Malmberg AB, Yaksh TL (1993) Spinal nitric oxide synthesis inhibition blocks NMDA-induced thermal hyperalgesia and produces antinociception in the formalin test in rats. Pain 54:291–300

Malmberg AB, Yaksh TL (1995) Cyclooxygenase inhibition and the spinal release of prostaglandin E2 and amino acids evoked by paw formalin injection: a microdialysis study in unanesthetized rats. J Neurosci 15:2768–2776

Mantyh PW, Gates T, Mantyh CR, Maggio JE (1989) Autoradiographic localization and characterization of tachykinin receptor binding sites in the rat brain and peripheral tissues. J Neurosci 9:258–279

Mantyh PW, Rogers SD, Honore P, Allen BJ, Ghilardi JR, Li J, Daughters RS, Lappi DA, Wiley RG, Simone DA (1997) Inhibition of hyperalgesia by ablation of lamina I spinal neurons expressing the substance P receptor. Science 278:275–279

Mao J, Coghill RC, Kellstein DE, Frenk H, Mayer DJ (1992) Calcitonin gene-related peptide enhances substance P-induced behaviors via metabolic inhibition: in vivo evidence for a new mechanism of neuromodulation. Brain Res 574:157–163

Marksteiner J, Sperk G, Krause JE (1992) Distribution of neurons expressing neurokinin B in the rat brain: immunohistochemistry and in situ hybridization. J Comp Neurol 317:341–356

Matsumura K, Watanabe Y, Imai-Matsumura K, Connolly M, Koyama Y, Onoe H, Watanabe Y (1992) Mapping of prostaglandin E2 binding sites in rat brain using quantitative autoradiography. Brain Res 581:292–298

Matsumura K, Watanabe Y, Onoe H, Watanabe Y (1995) Prostacyclin receptor in the brain and central terminals of the primary sensory neurons: an autoradiographic study using a stable prostacyclin analogue [^{3}H]iloprost. Neuroscience 65:493–503

Mayer ML, Westbrook GL, Guthrie PB (1984) Voltage-dependent block by Mg^{2+} of NMDA responses in spinal cord neurones. Nature 309:261–263

McCarson KE (1999) Central and peripheral expression of neurokinin-1 and neurokinin-3 receptor and substance P-encoding messenger RNAs: peripheral regulation during formalin-induced inflammation and lack of neurokinin receptor expression in primary afferent sensory neurons. Neuroscience 93:361–370

McCarson KE, Krause JE (1994) NK-1 and NK-3 type tachykinin receptor mRNA expression in the rat spinal cord dorsal horn is increased during adjuvant or formalin-induced nociception. J Neurosci 1994 14:712–720

McCarthy PW, Lawson SN (1989) Cell type and conduction velocity of rat primary sensory neurons with substance P-like immunoreactivity. Neuroscience 28:745–753

McCarthy PW, Lawson SN (1990) Cell type and conduction velocity of rat primary sensory neurons with calcitonin gene-related peptide-like immunoreactivity. Neuroscience 34:623–632

McLatchie LM, Fraser NJ, Main MJ, Wise A, Brown J, Thompson N, Solari R, Lee MG, Foord SM (1998) RAMPs regulate the transport and ligand specificity of the calcitonin-receptor-like receptor. Nature 393:333–339

Meller ST, Gebhart GF (1994) Spinal mediators of hyperalgesia. Drugs 47:10–20

Mermelstein PG, Bito H, Deisseroth K, Tsien RW (2000) Critical dependence of cAMP response element-binding protein phosphorylation on L-type calcium channels supports a selective response to EPSPs in preference to action potentials. J Neurosci 20:266–273

Messersmith DJ, Kim DJ, Iadarola MJ (1998) Transcription factor regulation of prodynorphin gene expression following rat hindpaw inflammation. Mol Brain Res 53:260–269

Miletic G, Pankratz MT, Miletic V (2002) Increases in the phosphorylation of cyclic AMP response element binding protein (CREB) and decreases in the content of calcineurin accompany thermal hyperalgesia following chronic constriction injury in rats. Pain 99:493–500

Minami T, Nishihara I, Uda R, Ito S, Hyodo M, Hayaishi O (1994a) Involvement of glutamate receptors in allodynia induced by prostaglandins E2 and F2 alpha injected into conscious mice. Pain 57:225–231

Minami T, Uda R, Horiguchi S, Ito S, Hyodo M, Hayaishi O (1994b) Allodynia evoked by intrathecal administration of prostaglandin E2 to conscious mice. Pain 57:217–223

Moochhala SM, Sawynok J (1984) Hyperalgesia produced by intrathecal substance P and related peptides: desensitization and cross desensitization. Br J Pharmacol 82:381–388

Moreno MJ, Cohen Z, Stanimirovic DB, Hamel E (1999) Functional calcitonin gene-related peptide type 1 and adrenomedullin receptors in human trigeminal ganglia, brain vessels, and cerebromicrovascular or astroglial cells in culture. J Cereb Blood Flow Metab 19:1270–1278

Moreno MJ, Terrón JA, Stanimirovic DB, Doods H, Hamel E (2002) Characterization of calcitonin gene-related peptide (CGRP) receptors and their receptor-activity-modifying proteins (RAMPs) in human brain microvascular and astroglial cells in culture. Neuropharmacology 42:270–280

Moriyoshi K, Masu M, Ishii T, Shigemoto R, Mizuno N, Nakanishi S (1991) Molecular cloning and characterization of the rat NMDA receptor. Nature 354:31–37

Morrison CF, McAllister J, Dobson SP, Mulderry PK, Quinn JP (1994) An activator element within the preprotachykinin-A promoter. Mol Cell Neurosci 5:165–175

Morton CR, Hutchison WD (1989) Release of sensory neuropeptides in the spinal cord: studies with calcitonin gene-related peptide and galanin. Neuroscience 31:807–815

Mulderry PK Ghatei MA, Spokes RA, Jones PM, Pierson AM, Hamid QA, Kanse S, Amara SG, Burrin JM, Legon S et al (1988) Differential expression of alpha-CGRP and beta-CGRP by primary sensory neurons and enteric autonomic neurons of the rat. Neuroscience 25:195–205

Munro FE, Fleetwood-Walker SM, Parker RM, Mitchell R (1993) The effects of neurokinin receptor antagonists on mustard oil-evoked activation of rat dorsal horn neurons. Neuropeptides 25:299–305

Murase K, Ryu PD, Randic M (1989) Excitatory and inhibitory amino acids and peptide-induced responses in acutely isolated rat spinal dorsal horn neurons. Neurosci Lett 103:56–63

Nakajima Y, Tsuchida K, Negishi M, Ito S, Nakanishi S (1992) Direct linkage of three tachykinin receptors to stimulation of both phosphatidylinositol hydrolysis and cyclic AMP cascades in transfected Chinese hamster ovary cells. J Biol Chem. 267:2437–2442

Neugebauer V, Schaible HG (1990) Evidence for a central component in the sensitization of spinal neurons with joint input during development of acute arthritis in cat's knee. J Neurophysiol 64:299–311

Neugebauer V, Rumenapp P, Schaible HG (1996) The role of spinal neurokinin-2 receptors in the processing of nociceptive information from the joint and in the generation and maintenance of inflammation-evoked hyperexcitability of dorsal horn neurons in the rat. Eur J Neurosci 8:249–260

Noguchi K, Senba E, Morita Y, Sato M, Tohyama M (1990) Co-expression of alpha-CGRP and beta-CGRP mRNAs in the rat dorsal root ganglion cells. Neurosci Lett 108:1–5

O'Brien C, Woolf CJ, Fitzgerald M, Lindsay RM, Molander C (1989) Differences in the chemical expression of rat primary afferent neurons which innervate skin, muscle or joint. Neuroscience 32:493–502

Ogawa T, Kanazawa I, Kimura S (1985) Regional distribution of substance P, neurokinin alpha and neurokinin beta in rat spinal cord, nerve roots and dorsal root ganglia, and the effects of dorsal root section or spinal transection. Brain Res 359:152–157

Oku R, Satoh M, Fujii N, Otaka A, Yajima H, Takagi H (1987) Calcitonin gene-related peptide promotes mechanical nociception by potentiating release of substance P from the spinal dorsal horn in rats. Brain Res 403:350–354

Oliver KR, Kane SA, Salvatore CA, Mallee JJ, Kinsey AM, Koblan KS, Keyvan-Fouladi N, Heavens RP, Wainwright A, Jacobson M, Dickerson IM, Hill RG (2001) Cloning, characterization and central nervous system distribution of receptor activity modifying proteins in the rat. Eur J Neurosci 14:618–628

Ouyang K, Zheng H, Qin X, Zhang C, Yang D, Wang X, Wu C, Zhou Z, Cheng H (2005) Ca^{2+} sparks and secretion in dorsal root ganglion neurons. Proc Natl Acad Sci USA 102:12259–12264

Park YH, Shin CY, Lee TS, Huh IH, Sohn UD (2000) The role of nitric oxide and prostaglandin E2 on the hyperalgesia induced by excitatory amino acids in rats. J Pharm Pharmacol 52:431–436

Parsons AM, Seybold VS (1997) Calcitonin gene-related peptide induces the formation of second messengers in primary cultures of neonatal rat spinal cord. Synapse 26:235–242

Parsons AM, el-Fakahany EE, Seybold VS (1995) Tachykinins alter inositol phosphate formation, but not cyclic AMP levels, in primary cultures of neonatal rat spinal neurons through activation of neurokinin receptors. Neuroscience 68:855–865

Parsons AM, Honda CN, Jia YP, Budai D, Xu XJ, Wiesenfeld-Hallin Z, Seybold VS (1996) Spinal NK1 receptors contribute to the increased excitability of the nociceptive flexor reflex during persistent peripheral inflammation. Brain Res 739:263–275

Perry MJ, Lawson SN (1998) Differences in expression of oligosaccharides, neuropeptides, carbonic anhydrase and neurofilament in rat primary afferent neurons retrogradely labelled via skin, muscle or visceral nerves. Neuroscience 85:293–310

Picard P, Boucher S, Regoli D, Gitter BD, Howbert JJ, Couture R (1993) Use of non-peptide tachykinin receptor antagonists to substantiate the involvement of NK1 and NK2 receptors in a spinal nociceptive reflex in the rat. Eur J Pharmacol 232:255–261

Pitcher GM, Henry JL (1999) Mediation and modulation by eicosanoids of responses of spinal dorsal horn neurons to glutamate and substance P receptor agonists: results with indomethacin in the rat in vivo. Neuroscience 93:1109–1121

Pitcher GM, Henry JL (2001) Meloxicam selectively depresses the afterdischarge of rat spinal dorsal horn neurones in response to noxious stimulation. Neurosci Lett 305:45–48

Pokabla MJ, Dickerson IM, Papka RE (2002) Calcitonin gene-related peptide-receptor component protein expression in the uterine cervix, lumbosacral spinal cord, and dorsal root ganglia. Peptides 23:507–514

Poyner D (1995) Pharmacology of receptors for calcitonin gene-related peptide and amylin. Trends Pharmacol Sci 16:424–428

Quartu M, Floris A, Del Fiacco M (1990) Substance P- and calcitonin gene-related peptide-like immunoreactive pericellular baskets in human trigeminal ganglion. Basic Appl Histochem 34:177–181

Randic M, Miletic V (1977) Effects of substance P in cat dorsal horn neurons activated by noxious stimuli. Brain Res 128:164–169

Randić M, Urbán L (1987) Slow excitatory transmission in rat spinal dorsal horn and the effects of capsaicin. Acta Physiol Hung 69:375–392
Randic M, Hecimovic H, Ryu PD (1990) Substance P modulates glutamate-induced currents in acutely isolated rat spinal dorsal horn neurones. Neurosci Lett 117:74–80
Rao A, Luo C, Hogan PG (1997) Transcription factors of the NFAT family: regulation and function. Annu Rev Immunol 15:707–747
Ren K, Iadarola MJ, Dubner R (1996) An isobolographic analysis of the effects of *N*-methyl-D-aspartate and NK1 tachykinin receptor antagonists on inflammatory hyperalgesia in the rat. Br J Pharmacol 117:196–202
Rojas A, Su J, Yang L, Lee M, Cui N, Zhang X, Fountain D, Jiang C (2008) Modulation of the heteromeric Kir4.1–Kir5.1 channel by multiple neurotransmitters via Galphaq-coupled receptors. J Cell Physiol 214:84–95
Rosenfeld MG, Mermod JJ, Amara SG, Swanson LW, Sawchenko PE, Rivier J, Vale WW, Evans RM (1983) Production of a novel neuropeptide encoded by the calcitonin gene via tissue-specific RNA processing. Nature 304:129–135
Ruda MA, Iadarola MJ, Cohen LV, Young WS 3rd (1988) In situ hybridization histochemistry and immunohistochemistry reveal an increase in spinal dynorphin biosynthesis in rat model of peripheral inflammation and hyperalgesia. Proc Natl Acad Sci USA 85:622–626
Rusin KI, Ryu PD, Randic M (1992) Modulation of excitatory amino acid responses in rat dorsal horn neurons by tachykinins. J Neurophysiol 68:265–286
Rusin KI, Bleakman D, Chard PS, Randic M, Miller RJ (1993) Tachykinins potentiate *N*-methyl-D-aspartate responses in acutely isolated neurons from the dorsal horn. J Neurochem 60: 952–960
Ryu PD, Gerber G, Murase K, Randic M (1988a) Calcitonin gene-related peptide enhances calcium current of rat dorsal root ganglion neurons and spinal excitatory synaptic transmission. Neurosci Lett 89:305–312
Ryu PD, Gerber G, Murase K, Randic M (1988b) Actions of calcitonin gene-related peptide on rat spinal dorsal horn neurons. Brain Res 441:357–361
Salmon AM, Damaj I, Sekine S, Picciotto MR, Marubio L, Changeux JP (1999) Modulation of morphine analgesia in alphaCGRP mutant mice. Neuroreport 10:849–854
Samad TA, Moore KA, Sapirstein A, Billet S, Allchorne A, Poole S, Bonventre JV, Woolf CJ (2001) Interleukin-1 beta-mediated induction of Cox-2 in the CNS contributes to inflammatory pain hypersensitivity. Nature 410:471–475
Schaible HG, Jarrott B, Hope PJ, Duggan AW (1990) Release of immunoreactive substance P in the spinal cord during development of acute arthritis in the knee joint of the cat: a study with antibody microprobes. Brain Res 529:214–223
Schaible HG, Hope PJ, Lang CW, Duggan AW (1992) Calcitonin gene-related peptide causes intraspinal spreading of substance P released by peripheral stimulation. Eur J Neurosci 4:750–757
Schaible HG, Freudenberger U, Neugebauer V, Stiller RU (1994) Intraspinal release of immunoreactive calcitonin gene-related peptide during development of inflammation in the joint in vivo – a study with antibody microprobes in cat and rat. Neuroscience 62:1293–1305
Sculptoreanu A, de Groat WC (2007) Neurokinins enhance excitability in capsaicin-responsive DRG neurons. Exp Neurol 205:92–100
Segond von Banchet G, Pastor A, Biskup C, Schlegel C, Benndorf K, Schaible HG (2002) Localization of functional calcitonin gene-related peptide binding sites in a subpopulation of cultured dorsal root ganglion neurons. Neuroscience 110:131–145
Seibert K, Zhang Y, Leahy K, Hauser S, Masferrer J, Perkins W, Lee L, Isakson P (1994) Pharmacological and biochemical demonstration of the role of cyclooxygenase 2 in inflammation and pain. Proc Natl Acad Sci USA 91:12013–12017
Seybold VS, Abrahams LG (1995) Characterization and regulation of neurokinin1 receptors in primary cultures of rat neonatal spinal neurons. Neuroscience 69:1263–1273

Seybold V, Elde R (1980) Immunohistochemical studies of peptidergic neurons in the dorsal horn of the spinal cord. J Histochem Cytochem 28:367–370

Seybold VS, Hylden JLK, Wilcox GL (1982) Intrathecal substance P and somatostatin in rats: Behaviors indicative of sensation. Peptides 3:49–54

Seybold VS, Grkovic I, Portbury AL, Ding YQ, Shigemoto R, Mizuno N, Furness JB, Southwell BR (1997) Relationship of NK3 receptor-immunoreactivity to subpopulations of neurons in rat spinal cord. J Comp Neurol 381:439–448

Seybold VS, Jia YP, Abrahams LG (2003a) Cyclo-oxygenase-2 contributes to central sensitization in rats with peripheral inflammation. Pain 105:47–55

Seybold VS, McCarson KE, Mermelstein PG, Groth RD, Abrahams LG (2003b) Calcitonin gene-related peptide regulates expression of neurokinin1 receptors by rat spinal neurons. J Neurosci 23:1816–1824

Seybold VS, Coicou LG, Groth RD, Mermelstein PG (2006) Substance P initiates NFAT-dependent gene expression in spinal neurons. J Neurochem 97:397–407

Shaywitz AJ, Greenberg ME (1999) CREB: a stimulus-induced transcription factor activated by a diverse array of extracellular signals. Annu Rev Biochem 68:821–861

Shieh PB, Hu SC, Bobb K, Timmusk T, Ghosh A (1998) Identification of a signaling pathway involved in calcium regulation of BDNF expression. Neuron 20:727–740

Shinder V, Devor M (1994) Structural basis of neuron-to-neuron cross-excitation in dorsal root ganglia. J Neurocytol 23:515–531

Sluka KA, Milton MA, Willis WD, Westlund KN (1997) Differential roles of neurokinin 1 and neurokinin 2 receptors in the development and maintenance of heat hyperalgesia induced by acute inflammation. Br J Pharmacol 120:1263–1273

Sorkin LS, Moore JH (1996) Evoked release of amino acids and prostanoids in spinal cords of anesthetized rats: changes during peripheral inflammation and hyperalgesia. Am J Ther 3:268–275

Southwell BR, Woodman HL, Murphy R, Royal SJ, Furness JB (1996) Characterisation of substance P-induced endocytosis of NK1 receptors on enteric neurons. Histochem Cell Biol 106:563–571

Southwell BR, Seybold VS, Woodman HL, Jenkinson KM, Furness JB (1998) Quantitation of neurokinin 1 receptor internalization and recycling in guinea-pig myenteric neurons. Neuroscience 87:925–931

Spike RC, Puskár Z, Andrew D, Todd AJ (2003) A quantitative and morphological study of projection neurons in lamina I of the rat lumbar spinal cord. Eur J Neurosci 18:2433–2448

Strack S, Wadzinski BE, Ebner FF (1996) Localization of the calcium/calmodulin-dependent protein phosphatase, calcineurin, in the hindbrain and spinal cord of the rat. J Comp Neurol 375:66–76

Stucky CL, Galeazza MT, Seybold VS (1993) Time-dependent changes in Bolton-Hunter-labeled ^{125}I-substance P binding in rat spinal cord following unilateral adjuvant-induced peripheral inflammation. Neuroscience 57:397–409

Sugiura Y, Lee CL, Perl ER (1986) Central projections of identified, unmyelinated (C) afferent fibers innervating mammalian skin. Science 234:358–361

Sun RQ, Lawand NB, Willis WD (2003) The role of calcitonin gene-related peptide (CGRP) in the generation and maintenance of mechanical allodynia and hyperalgesia in rats after intradermal injection of capsaicin. Pain 104:201–208

Sun RQ, Tu YJ, Lawand NB, Yan JY, Lin Q, Willis WD (2004) Calcitonin gene-related peptide receptor activation produces PKA- and PKC-dependent mechanical hyperalgesia and central sensitization. J Neurophysiol 92:2859–2866

Svensson CI, Hua XY, Protter AA, Powell HC, Yaksh TL (2003) Spinal p38 MAP kinase is necessary for NMDA-induced spinal PGE(2) release and thermal hyperalgesia. Neuroreport 14:1153–1157

Sweeney MI, Sawynok J (1986) Evidence that substance P may be a modulator rather than a transmitter of noxious mechanical stimulation. Can J Physiol Pharmacol 64:1324–1327

Taiwo YO, Levine JD (1986) Indomethacin blocks central nociceptive effects of PGF2 alpha. Brain Res 373:81–84

Takano K, Yasufuku-Takano J, Kozasa T, Singer WD, Nakajima S, Nakajima Y (1996) Gq/11 and PLC-beta 1 mediate the substance P-induced inhibition of an inward rectifier K^+ channel in brain neurons. J Neurophysiol 76:2131–2136

Takeda Y, Krause JE (1991) Pharmacological and molecular biological studies on the diversity of rat tachykinin NK-2 receptor subtypes in rat CNS, duodenum, vas deferens, and urinary bladder. Ann N Y Acad Sci 632:479–482

Takeda Y, Blount P, Sachais BS, Hershey AD, Raddatz R, Krause JE (1992) Ligand binding kinetics of substance P and neurokinin A receptors stably expressed in Chinese hamster ovary cells and evidence for differential stimulation of inositol 1,4,5-trisphosphate and cyclic AMP second messenger responses. J Neurochem 59:740–745

Tao X, Finkbeiner S, Arnold DB, Shaywitz AJ, Greenberg ME (1998) Ca^{2+} influx regulates BDNF transcription by a CREB family transcription factor-dependent mechanism. Neuron 20:709–726

Todd AJ, Puskar Z, Spike RC, Hughes C, Watt C, Forrest L (2002) Projection neurons in lamina I of rat spinal cord with the neurokinin 1 receptor are selectively innervated by substance p-containing afferents and respond to noxious stimulation. J Neurosci 22:4103–4113

Trafton JA, Abbadie C, Basbaum AI (2001) Differential contribution of substance P and neurokinin A to spinal cord neurokinin-1 receptor signaling in the rat. J Neurosci 21:3656–3664

Tschopp FA, Tobler PH, Fischer JA (1985) Calcitonin gene-related peptide and its binding sites in the human central nervous system and pituitary. Proc Natl Acad Sci USA 82:248–252

Tsuchida K, Shigemoto R, Yokota Y, Nakanishi S (1990) Tissue distribution and quantitation of the mRNAs for three rat tachykinin receptors. Eur J Biochem 193:751–757

Tuchscherer MM, Seybold VS (1989) A quantitative study of the coexistence of peptides in varicosities within the superficial laminae of the dorsal horn of the rat spinal cord. J Neurosci 9:195–205

Tzabazis AZ, Pirc G, Votta-Velis E, Wilson SP, Laurito CE, Yeomans DC (2007) Antihyperalgesic effect of a recombinant herpes virus encoding antisense for calcitonin gene-related peptide. Anesthesiology 106:1079–1080

Uda R, Horiguchi S, Ito S, Hyodo M, Hayaishi O (1990) Nociceptive effects induced by intrathecal administration of prostaglandin D_2, E_2, or $F_{2\alpha}$ to conscious mice. Brain Res 510:26–32

Ulrich-Lai YM, Flores CM, Harding-Rose CA, Goodis HE, Hargreaves KM (2001) Capsaicin-evoked release of immunoreactive calcitonin gene-related peptide from rat trigeminal ganglion: evidence for intraganglionic neurotransmission. Pain 91:219–226

Urban AL and Fox AJ (2000) NK_1 receptor antagonists – are they really without effect in the pain clinic? Trends Pharmacol Sci 12:462–464

Urban L, Thompson SWN, Dray A (1994) Modulation of spinal excitability: co-operation between neurokinin and excitatory amino acid neurotransmitters. Trends Neurosci 17:432–438

Vasko MR, Campbell WB, Waite KJ (1994) Prostaglandin E2 enhances bradykinin-stimulated release of neuropeptides from rat sensory neurons in culture. J Neurosci 14:4987–4997

Verhage M, McMahon HT, Ghijsen WE, Boomsma F, Scholten G, Wiegant VM, Nicholls DG (1991) Differential release of amino acids, neuropeptides, and catecholamines from isolated nerve terminals. Neuron 6:517–524

Villar MJ, Cortés R, Theodorsson E, Wiesenfeld-Hallin Z, Schalling M, Fahrenkrug J, Emson PC, Hökfelt T (1989) Neuropeptide expression in rat dorsal root ganglion cells and spinal cord after peripheral nerve injury with special reference to galanin. Neuroscience 33:587–604

Wall PD, Woolf CJ (1984) Muscle but not cutaneous C-afferent input produces prolonged increases in the excitability of the flexion reflex in the rat. J Physiol 356:443–458

Warden MK, Young WS 3rd (1988) Distribution of cells containing mRNAs encoding substance P and neurokinin B in the rat central nervous system. J Comp Neurol 272:90–113

Watling KJ, Guard S, Krause JE, Takeda Y, Quirion R, Zarnegar R, Pain D, Franks R (1993) On the presence of NK2 receptor subtypes in peripheral and central tissues. Regul Pept 46:311–313

Watson A, Latchman D (1995) The cyclic AMP response element in the calcitonin/calcitonin gene-related peptide gene promoter is necessary but not sufficient for its activation by nerve growth factor. J Biol Chem 270:9655–9660

Wiesenfeld-Hallin Z, Hokflet T, Lundberg JM, Forssmann WG, Reinecke M, Tschopp FA, Fischer JA (1984) Immunoreactive calcitonin gene-related peptide and substance P coexist in sensory neurons to the spinal cord and interact in spinal behavioral responses of the rat. Neurosci Lett 52:199–204

Womack MD, MacDermott AB, Jessell TM (1988) Sensory transmitters regulate intracellular calcium in dorsal horn neurons. Nature 334:351–353. Erratum in: Nature (1988) 335:744

Woolf CJ, King AE (1990) Dynamic alterations in the cutaneous mechanoreceptive fields of dorsal horn neurons in the rat spinal cord. J Neurosci 10:2717–2726

Wright DM, Roberts MH (1980) Responses of spinal neurones to a substance P analogue, noxious pinch and bradykinin. Eur J Pharmacol 64:165–167

Yaksh TL, Jessell TM, Gamse R, Mudge AW, Leeman SE (1980) Intrathecal morphine inhibits substance P release from mammalian spinal cord in vivo. Nature 286:155–157

Yaksh TL, Dirig DM, Conway CM, Svensson C, Luo ZD, Isakson PC (2001) The acute anti-hyperalgesic action of nonsteroidal, anti-inflammatory drugs and release of spinal prostaglandin E2 is mediated by the inhibition of constitutive spinal cyclooxygenase-2 (COX-2) but not COX-1. J Neurosci 21:5847–5853

Yamamoto T, Sakashita Y (1998) COX-2 inhibitor prevents the development of hyperalgesia induced by intrathecal NMDA or AMPA. Neuroreport 9:3869–3873

Yamamoto T, Yaksh TL (1991) Stereospecific effects of a nonpeptidic NK1 selective antagonist, CP-96,345: antinociception in the absence of motor dysfunction. Life Sci 49:1955–1963

Yashpal K, Dam TV, Quirion R (1990) Quantitative autoradiographic distribution of multiple neurokinin binding sites in rat spinal cord. Brain Res 506:259–266

Yashpal K, Dam TV, Quirion R (1991) Effects of dorsal rhizotomy on neurokinin receptor subtypes in the rat spinal cord: a quantitative autoradiographic study. Brain Res 552:240–247

Yashpal K, Radhakrishnan V, Coderre TJ, Henry JL (1993) CP-96,345, but not its stereoisomer, CP-96,344, blocks the nociceptive responses to intrathecally administered substance P and to noxious thermal and chemical stimuli in the rat. Neuroscience 52:1039–1047

Zaratin P, Angelici O, Clarke GD, Schmid G, Raiteri M, Carità F, Bonanno G (2000) NK3 receptor blockade prevents hyperalgesia and the associated spinal cord substance P release in monoarthritic rats. Neuropharmacology 39:141–149

Zhang X, Ji RR, Arvidsson J, Lundberg JM, Bartfai T, Bedecs K, Hökfelt T (1996) Expression of peptides, nitric oxide synthase and NPY receptor in trigeminal and nodose ganglia after nerve lesions. Exp Brain Res 111:393–404

Zhang L, Hoff AO, Wimalawansa SJ, Cote GJ, Gagel RF, Westlund KN (2001) Arthritic calcitonin/alpha calcitonin gene-related peptide knockout mice have reduced nociceptive hypersensitivity. Pain 89:265–273

Zhang Z, Winborn CS, Marquez de Prado B, Russo AF (2007) Sensitization of calcitonin gene-related peptide receptors by receptor activity-modifying protein-1 in the trigeminal ganglion. J Neurosci 27:2693–2703

Zhuo H, Helke CJ (1993) Neurokinin B peptide-2 neurons project from the hypothalamus to the thoracolumbar spinal cord of the rat. Neuroscience 52:1019–1028

Part III
Current and Future Treatment Strategies Targeting Sensory Nerves

Opioids and Sensory Nerves

Christoph Stein and Christian Zöllner

Contents

Abstract This chapter reviews the expression and regulation of opioid receptors in sensory neurons and the interactions of these receptors with endogenous and exogenous opioid ligands. Inflammation of peripheral tissues leads to increased synthesis and axonal transport of opioid receptors in dorsal root ganglion neurons. This results in opioid receptor upregulation and enhanced G protein coupling at peripheral sensory nerve terminals. These events are dependent on neuronal electrical activity, and on production of proinflammatory cytokines and nerve growth factor within the inflamed tissue. Together with the disruption of the perineurial barrier, these factors lead to an

C. Stein (✉)
Klinik für Anaesthesiologie und operative Intensivmedizin, Freie Universität Berlin, Charité – Campus Benjamin Franklin, 12200 Berlin, Germany
christoph.stein@charite.de

B.J. Canning and D. Spina (eds.), *Sensory Nerves*,
Handbook of Experimental Pharmacology 194, DOI: 10.1007/978-3-540-79090-7_14,

enhanced analgesic efficacy of peripherally active opioids. The major local source of endogenous opioid ligands (e.g. β-endorphin) is leukocytes. These cells contain and upregulate signal-sequence-encoding messenger RNA of the β-endorphin precursor proopiomelanocortin and the entire enzymatic machinery necessary for its processing into the functionally active peptide. Opioid-containing immune cells extravasate using adhesion molecules and chemokines to accumulate in inflamed tissues. Upon stressful stimuli or in response to releasing agents such as corticotropin-releasing factor, cytokines, chemokines, and catecholamines, leukocytes secrete opioids. Depending on the cell type, this release is contingent on extracellular Ca^{2+} or on inositol triphosphate receptor triggered release of Ca^{2+} from endoplasmic reticulum. Once secreted, opioid peptides activate peripheral opioid receptors and produce analgesia by inhibiting the excitability of sensory nerves and/or the release of proinflammatory neuropeptides. These effects occur without central untoward side effects such as depression of breathing, clouding of consciousness, or addiction. Future aims include the development of peripherally restricted opioid agonists, selective targeting of opioid-containing leukocytes to sites of painful injury, and the augmentation of peripheral opioid peptide and receptor synthesis.

Keywords opioid peptides, peripheral, opioid receptors, immune cells, peripheral analgesia, immune cells, inflammation, pain, cytokines, chemokines, secretory pathways, G-protein coupled receptor signaling, receptor recycling, opioid tolerance, endorphin, enkephalin, dynorphin, endomorphin, arthritis

1 Introduction

Peripheral sensory neurons express opioid receptors and opioid peptides, and the function of these neurons can be modulated by endogenous opioids derived from immune cells or by opioid drugs. This scenario has evolved from studies on mechanisms of inflammatory pain and its inhibition. Opioids are the most powerful drugs for severe pain but their use is hampered by side effects such as depression of breathing, nausea, clouding of consciousness, constipation, addiction, and tolerance (Zöllner and Stein 2007). Thus, the development of opioid drugs lacking such effects has always been a major goal in pain research. The discovery of opioid receptors on sensory nerves has now put this goal within reach. Moreover, in the course of these investigations modulatory opioid effects on inflammation and wound healing were detected (Tegeder and Geisslinger 2004). These latter effects have sparked intense interest in light of the pressing need for novel anti-inflammatory therapies (Ledford 2007). Following studies on the local application of conventional opioids in peripheral damaged tissue, a new generation of opioid drugs unable to pass the blood-brain-barrier is now emerging, thus avoiding centrally mediated unwanted effects (Brower 2000; Stein et al. 2003). Endogenous opioid peptides binding to peripheral opioid receptors have been identified within skin and subcutaneous tissue, particularly in inflammatory cells. This has led to new directions of research, for example, the selective targeting of opioid peptide containing cells to sites of painful injury, the augmentation of opioid synthesis by gene transfer, and the inhibition of inflammation by peripherally acting opioids (Stein et al. 2003; Machelska 2007; Rittner et al. 2008).

Tissue destruction, abnormal immune reactivity, and/or nerve injury are frequently associated with an inflammatory response. Within peripheral damaged tissue (such as skin, muscles, joints, and viscera), primary sensory neurons transduce noxious mechanical, chemical, or heat stimuli into action potentials. The cell bodies of these neurons are located in the trigeminal and dorsal root ganglia (DRG) and give rise to myelinated (Aδ) and small-diameter unmyelinated axons (C-fibers, "nociceptors"). The latter are particularly sensitive to capsaicin, a ligand at the transient receptor potential vanilloid-1 (TRPV1) channel, and are considered the dominant fibers in clinical pain. After synaptic transmission and modulation within the sensory neuron and spinal cord, nociceptive signals reach the brain, where they are finally perceived as "pain," within the context of cognitive and environmental factors (Woolf and Salter 2000).

For many years attention was focused on the characterization of proinflammatory and proalgesic effects elicited by the myriad of mediators occurring in injured tissue (see Part II of this volume). Concurrently, however, endogenous mechanisms counteracting pain and inflammation are in the ascendancy. In the periphery, such effects are produced by interactions between leukocyte-derived opioid peptides and opioid receptors on peripheral nociceptor endings, by anti-inflammatory cytokines, and by cannabinoids (Stein et al. 2003; Rittner et al. 2005, 2008). This chapter will focus on the localization, trafficking, and function of peripheral opioid receptors, on the production and release of opioid peptides from inflammatory cells, and on analgesia, tolerance, anti-inflammatory, and wound-healing effects brought about by peripherally acting opioids.

2 Opioid Receptors

2.1 Opioid Receptor Types

Early binding studies and bioassays defined three main types of opioid receptors in the central nervous system, the μ-, δ-, and κ-receptors. Additional receptor types were proposed (e.g., σ, ε, orphanin) but are currently not considered "classical" opioid receptors (Kieffer and Gaveriaux-Ruff 2002). The identification of complementary DNA confirmed only three genes and allowed for the study of individual opioid receptor types with regard to pharmacological profile, intracellular effector coupling, anatomical distribution, and regulation of expression. Opioid receptors belong to the family of seven transmembrane G protein coupled receptors (GPCR) and show 50–70% homology between their genes (Evans et al. 1992; Kieffer et al. 1992; Meng et al. 1993; Wang et al. 1993). Additional pharmacological subtypes may result from alternative splicing, posttranslational modifications, or receptor oligomerization. Opioid receptors are expressed by central and peripheral neurons, by neuroendocrine (pituitary, adrenals), immune, and ectodermal cells (Zöllner and Stein 2007).

2.2 Signal Transduction and Recycling

The signaling pathways of opioid receptors are well characterized. After the ligand binds at the receptor, conformational changes allow intracellular coupling of mainly $G_{i/o}$ proteins to the C-terminus of opioid receptors. At the $G\alpha$ subunit, GDP is replaced by GTP and dissociation of the trimeric G protein complex into $G\alpha$ and $G\beta\gamma$ subunits ensues. Subsequently these subunits can inhibit adenylyl cyclase and thereby cyclic adenosine monophosphate (cAMP) production, and/or directly interact with K^+, Ca^{2+}, and other ion channels in the membrane (Fig. 1). Ion

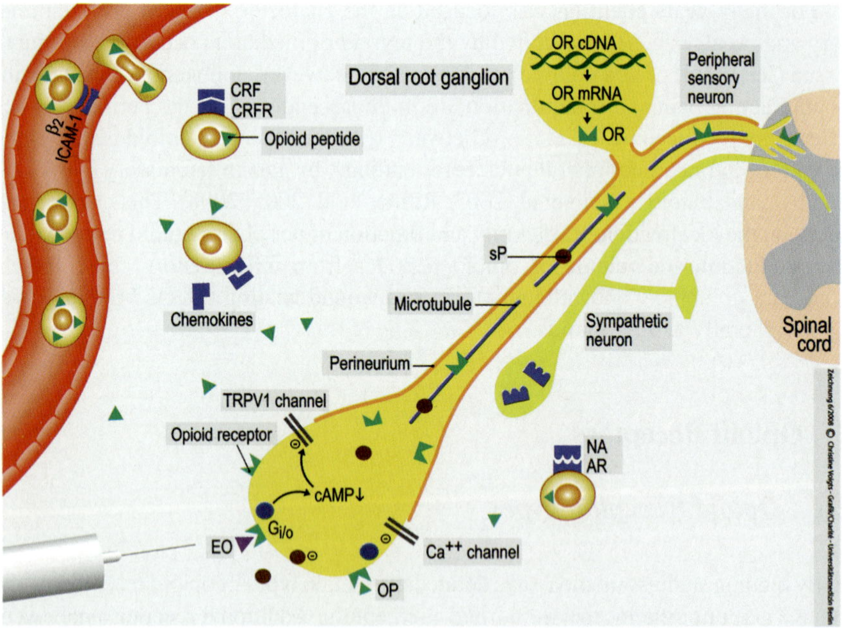

Fig. 1 Opioid peptide containing circulating leukocytes extravasate upon activation of adhesion molecules (e.g., intercellular adhesion molecule-1, integrin β_2) and chemotaxis by chemokines. Subsequently, these leukocytes are stimulated by stress or releasing agents to secrete opioid peptides. For example, corticotropin-releasing factor (CRF), chemokines and noradrenaline (released from sympathetic neurons) can elicit opioid release by activating their respective receptors (CRF receptors; adrenergic receptors) on leukocytes. Exogenous opioids (symbolized by a *syringe*) or endogenous opioid peptides (*green triangles*) bind to opioid receptors that are synthesized in dorsal root ganglia and transported along intraaxonal microtubules to peripheral (and central) terminals of sensory neurons. The subsequent inhibition of ion channels (e.g., transient receptor potential vanilloid-1, Ca^{2+}) and of substance P release results in antinociceptive effects

channels are mainly regulated via Gβγ subunits (Herlitze et al. 1996). All three opioid receptors modulate various N-, T- and P/Q-type Ca^{2+}channels, and suppress Ca^{2+} influx and the excitation and/or neurotransmitter release in many neuronal systems. A prominent example is the inhibition of substance P (a pronociceptive and proinflammatory neuropeptide) release from central and peripheral terminals of sensory neurons (Yaksh 1988; Kondo et al. 2005). At the postsynaptic membrane, opioid receptors mediate hyperpolarization by opening K^+ channels, thereby preventing excitation and/or propagation of action potentials (Zöllner and Stein 2007). Various enzymes such as phosphokinase C and GPCR kinases can phosphorylate opioid receptors, leading to increased affinity for intracellular arrestin molecules. Arrestin-receptor complexes lead to opioid receptor desensitization by preventing G protein coupling and promote internalization via clathrin-dependent pathways (Law et al. 2000). Recycling of opioid receptors to the plasma membrane promotes rapid resensitization of signal transduction, whereas targeting to lysosomes leads to proteolytic downregulation. It was suggested that GPCR-associated sorting proteins modulate lysosomal sorting and functional downregulation (Whistler et al. 2002). Additional opioid-modulated pathways involve *N*-methyl-D-aspartate receptors, mitogen-activated protein kinase, and phospholipase C (Zöllner and Stein 2007).

2.3 *Opioid Receptors on Peripheral Sensory Neurons*

In the late 1980s evidence began to accumulate that antinociceptive effects can be mediated by opioid receptors located on peripheral sensory neurons (Bartho et al. 1990; Stein et al. 1990b; Stein 1993, 1995). Opioid receptors are expressed in small-, medium-, and large-diameter DRG neurons (Mansour et al. 1994; Buzas and Cox 1997; Chen et al. 1997; Coggeshall et al. 1997; Zhang et al. 1998a, c; Wang and Wessendorf 2001; Silbert et al. 2003; Rau et al. 2005; Gendron et al. 2006), they are coexpressed with prototypical sensory neuropeptides such as substance P and calcitonin-gene-related peptide (CGRP) (Minami et al. 1995; Li et al. 1998; Zhang et al. 1998b, c; Ständer et al. 2002; Mousa et al. 2007a, b), they are transported to the peripheral nerve terminals (Hassan et al. 1993; Li et al. 1996; Mousa et al. 2001), and they are coupled to $G_{i/o}$ proteins that inhibit adenylyl cyclase and modulate ion channels (Zöllner et al. 2003, 2008). The decrease of Ca^{2+} currents, but not the modulation of K^+ channels, appears to be a major mechanism for the inhibition of sensory neuron functions (Akins and McCleskey 1993). Recently, G protein coupled inwardly rectifying K^+ channels and μ-opioid receptors were colocalized on sensory nerve endings in the epidermis (Khodorova et al. 2003), but no direct evidence of functional coupling or modulation of K^+ channels in DRG neurons has been provided so far. However, opioid receptors on DRG neurons suppress tetrodotoxin-resistant Na^+ and nonselective cation currents (Ingram and Williams 1994; Gold and Levine 1996), as well as TRPV1 currents via $G_{i/o}$ and the cAMP pathway (Endres-Becker et al. 2007). As a result, opioid agonists can attenuate the excitability of nociceptors, the propagation of action potentials, and the release of proinflammatory neuropeptides (substance P, CGRP) from central and peripheral nociceptor terminals. Particularly within injured tissue, these events lead to antinociceptive and anti-inflammatory effects (see later).

2.4 *Plasticity of Peripheral Opioid Receptors*

2.4.1 Ontogeny

The ontogeny of opioid receptors has been examined in the central and peripheral nervous system during pre- and postnatal development. With use of radioligand binding and in situ hybridization techniques, μ-, δ-, and κ-receptor expression was found to be distinct at all ages. Prenatally, the expression of δ-receptor lags behind that of μ- and κ-receptors in the brain (Zhu et al. 1998). However, in mouse DRG neurons the first opioid receptor expressed is the δ-receptor at embryonic day 12.5, followed by the μ-receptor (embryonic day 13.5) and the κ-receptor (embryonic day 17.5) (Zhu et al. 1998). A greater proportion of rat DRG neurons immunoreactive for μ- and δ-receptors was found before postnatal day 7 than at postnatal day 21 (κ-receptor was not examined) (Beland and Fitzgerald 2001). Moreover, during the first postnatal week both opioid receptors were detected in cells of all sizes but by postnatal day 21 expression was restricted to small- and medium-diameter cells, suggesting a selective downregulation in nonnociceptive neurons (Beland and Fitzgerald 2001). The transcription factor Runx1 was suggested to suppress postnatal μ-receptor expression in a subset of nociceptive mouse DRG neurons (Chen et al. 2006).

2.4.2 Influence of Inflammation

Painful inflammation of peripheral tissue (of varying duration) has been most extensively studied as a regulatory stimulus of opioid receptor plasticity in adult sensory neurons. Both the systemic and the local application of μ-, δ-, and κ-receptor agonists elicits significantly more pronounced analgesic effects in injured than in noninjured tissue of animals and humans (Stein 1993, 1995; Stein et al. 2003). This intriguing finding has stimulated extensive research into the underlying mechanisms.

Peripheral inflammation can induce differential upregulation of opioid receptor messenger RNA (mRNA) and protein in DRG neurons. In complete Freund's adjuvant induced paw inflammation, μ-receptor mRNA displays a biphasic upregulation (at 2 and 96 h), whereas mRNA for δ-receptors remains unchanged, and κ-receptor mRNA shows a peak at 12 h (Pühler et al. 2004, 2006). In parallel, μ- and κ-receptor binding is upregulated. The upregulation is related to neuronal electrical activity (Pühler et al. 2004), to cytokine production in the inflamed tissue

(Pühler et al. 2006), and may be mediated by cytokine-induced binding of transcription factors to opioid receptor gene promoters (Kraus et al. 2001). Not surprisingly, a short-lasting (30-min) inflammatory stimulus (intraperitoneal acetic acid) does not change opioid receptor expression on sensory nerve terminals (Labuz et al. 2007). Thus, the expression of opioid receptors changes depending on the receptor type and the duration of inflammation. μ-Receptors were most extensively studied and were consistently shown to be upregulated (Ji et al. 1995; Zhang et al. 1998a; Mousa et al. 2002; Ballet et al. 2003; Zöllner et al. 2003; Pühler et al. 2004; Shaqura et al. 2004). It was shown that the upregulation of μ-opioid binding sites in DRG is due to an increase in both the number of neurons expressing μ-receptors and the number of μ-receptors per neuron, while the affinity of opioid agonists to μ-receptors remained unchanged (Zöllner et al. 2003). In addition, G protein coupling of opioid receptors in DRG neurons is augmented by subcutaneous inflammation (Zöllner et al. 2003; Shaqura et al. 2004).

Bradykinin, a typical inflammatory mediator, was found to stimulate the trafficking of intracellular δ-receptors to the plasma membrane of cultured DRG neurons (Patwardhan et al. 2005). Furthermore, bradykinin pretreatment of these neurons led to more potent inhibition of CGRP release and of cAMP accumulation by μ- and δ-agonists (Patwardhan et al. 2005; Berg et al. 2007b). The μ-agonist effect was dependent on integrins colocalized with μ-opioid receptors in the DRG membrane (Berg et al. 2007a). Similarly, painful paw inflammation and activation of sensory neurons by capsaicin were shown to enhance membrane recruitment as well as ligand-induced internalization of δ-receptors in DRG neurons (Gendron et al. 2006; Zhang et al. 2006).

Subsequent to the opioid receptor upregulation in DRG, the peripherally directed axonal transport of opioid receptors is augmented (Hassan et al. 1993; Ji et al. 1995; Mousa et al. 2001; Pühler et al. 2004). The axonal transport is stimulated by cytokines and nerve growth factor produced within the peripheral inflamed tissue (Jeanjean et al. 1995; Mousa et al. 2007b) and results in increased density of opioid receptors at peripheral nerve terminals (Stein et al. 1990b). Inflammation is also accompanied by a sprouting of opioid-receptor-bearing peripheral sensory nerve terminals (Mousa et al. 2001) and by a disrupted perineural barrier facilitating the access of opioid agonists to their receptors (Antonijevic et al. 1995). In addition, low pH can increase opioid agonist efficacy, presumably by altering the interaction of opioid receptors with G proteins (Rasenick and Childers 1989; Selley et al. 1993; Vetter et al. 2006). All of these mechanisms likely contribute to the increased antinociceptive efficacy of opioids in inflamed tissue. In line with these findings, clinical studies have shown that the proximal perineural application of opioids along intact (noninjured) nerves (e.g., axillary plexus) does not reliably produce analgesic effects (Picard et al. 1997).

2.4.3 Influence of Nerve Damage

Mechanical nerve injury resulting in neuropathic pain is another condition influencing opioid receptors in sensory neurons. Different animal models (e.g., partial nerve ligation, axotomy) have been examined with variable results. For example, at 2 and 14 days after chronic constriction injury of the sciatic nerve (a partial ligation with preferential ischemic degeneration of large myelinated fibers but relative preservation of unmyelinated fibers) μ-receptor protein was upregulated in DRG and accumulated proximal and distal to the lesion, indicating anterograde and retrograde axonal transport. At 14 days μ-receptors were also increased in distal small surviving axons and in small sprouting axons at and distal to this lesion (Truong et al. 2003). Similarly, on day 14 following partial sciatic nerve ligation an upregulation of δ-receptors was shown in DRG and in sciatic nerve (Kabli and Cahill 2007) and 14 days after partial saphenous nerve ligation an upregulation of μ-receptors was found in DRG and in paw skin (Walczak et al. 2005). A few studies found downregulation of DRG μ-receptors at 7 days (Rashid et al. 2004) or 16 days after partial sciatic nerve ligation (Pol et al. 2006), as well as after peripheral axotomy (Zhang et al. 1998c).

2.4.4 Sympathetic Neurons

Opioid receptor expression in sympathetic postganglionic neurons has also been suggested. However, neither opioid receptor mRNA nor protein has been detected in such neurons (Coggeshall et al. 1997; Wenk and Honda 1999; Ständer et al. 2002; Mousa et al. 2007a). Moreover, chemical sympathectomy with 6-hydroxydopamine did not change the expression of opioid receptors in the DRG or the peripheral analgesic effects of μ-, δ-, and κ-receptor agonists in a model of inflammatory pain (Zhang et al. 1998a; Zhou 1998).

3 Opioid Peptides

The endogenous ligands of opioid receptors are derived from the three precursor proteins proopiomelanocortin (POMC), proenkephalin (PENK), and prodynorphin. Appropriate processing yields the major representative opioid peptides β-endorphin, Met-enkephalin and dynorphin A, respectively. These peptides and their derivatives exhibit different affinities and selectivities for the μ-receptors (β-endorphin, Met-enkephalin), δ-receptors (enkephalins, β-endorphin), and κ-receptors (dynorphin). Two additional endogenous opioid peptides have been isolated from bovine brain: endomorphin-1 and endomorphin-2. Both peptides are considered highly selective μ-receptor ligands but their precursors are not known yet (Fichna et al. 2007).

3.1 Opioid Peptides in Sensory Neurons

Evidence for the presence of opioid peptides in sensory neurons began to accumulate in the 1980s. Several reports demonstrated immunoreactive dynorphins (Przewlocki et al. 1983; Weihe et al. 1985; Sweetnam et al. 1986; Gibbins et al. 1987) and enkephalins (Przewlocki et al. 1983; Quartu and Del Fiacco 1994; Bergström et al. 2006) in DRG and in peripheral sensory neurons. These peptides were shown to be transported towards central and peripheral nerve terminals and were demonstrated in cutaneous nerves (Gibbins et al. 1987; Crowe et al. 1994; Carlton and Coggeshall 1997). With regard to mRNA, only one study detected PENK mRNA in intermediate-sized DRG neurons (Pohl et al. 1994), but neither PENK nor prodynorphin mRNA was found in DRG of normal or polyarthritic rats by others (Calza et al. 1998). Endomorphins were also described in sensory nerves (Martin-Schild et al. 1998; Pierce et al. 1998; Mousa et al. 2002). It was suggested that these opioid peptides can exert (auto-) modulation of sensory nerve function, but direct evidence has not been provided so far.

3.2 Opioid Peptides in Immune Cells

The discovery that opioid receptors on sensory nerves are upregulated during subcutaneous inflammation prompted the search for endogenous ligands within inflamed tissue. POMC-related opioid peptides have been found in leukocytes of many vertebrates and invertebrates (Smith 2003). Earlier studies described several truncated POMC mRNAs, but more recently a full-length transcript encoding all three POMC exons was shown in rat mononuclear leukocytes (Lyons and Blalock 1997; Sitte et al. 2007). POMC transcripts containing the signal sequence necessary for correct routing into the regulated secretory pathway are upregulated in lymphocytes from rats with painful paw inflammation (Sitte et al. 2007) and the enzymes (prohormone convertases, carboxypeptidase) required for proteolytic processing of POMC are expressed in leukocytes (Mousa et al. 2004). PENK mRNA, Met-enkephalin, and the appropriate enzymes for posttranslational processing of PENK have also been detected in human and rodent leukocytes (Vindrola et al. 1994; LaMendola et al. 1997). Deletion of the gene coding for PENK resulted in the complete absence of Met-enkephalin both in the brain and in T cells, strongly indicating that this peptide derives from the same precursor in the nervous and immune systems (Hook et al. 1999). Finally, dynorphin and endomorphins have been demonstrated in immune cells (Mousa et al. 2002; Chadzinska et al. 2005). Opioid peptide containing cells include granulocytes, monocytes/macrophages, and lymphocytes (Przewlocki et al. 1992; Cabot et al. 1997; Mousa et al. 2001; Rittner et al. 2001, 2007b; Labuz et al. 2006; Zöllner et al. 2008). Recently, T lymphocytes were postulated to mediate analgesia via β-endorphin expression in the visceral system (Verma-Gandhu et al. 2006) and keratinocyte-derived β-endorphin was proposed to mediate peripheral antinociception in noninflamed skin (Khodorova et al. 2003; Ibrahim et al. 2005).

3.3 Migration of Opioid-Containing Cells to Inflamed Tissue

The recruitment of leukocytes from the circulation into inflammatory sites involves a well-orchestrated set of events. This begins with rolling along the endothelial cell wall mediated predominantly by selectins. Then leukocytes are activated by chemokines that are released from endothelial and inflammatory cells and are presented on the endothelium. This leads to the upregulation and increased avidity of integrins which mediate the firm adhesion of leukocytes to endothelial cells via, e.g., intercellular adhesion molecule-1 (ICAM-1). Finally, leukocytes transmigrate through the endothelium mediated by, e.g., platelet-endothelial cell adhesion molecule-1 (von Andrian and Mackay 2000).

In inflamed rat paws L-selectin, integrin β_2, and the CXC chemokine receptor 2 (CXCR2) are coexpressed by opioid-containing leukocytes (Mousa et al. 2000; Brack et al. 2004b; Machelska et al. 2004). Pretreatment with a selectin blocker, antibodies against ICAM-1, against integrins α_4 and β_2, or against the chemokines CXCL1 and CXCL2/3 substantially decreases the number of opioid-containing immune cells accumulating in the inflamed tissue (Machelska et al. 1998, 2002, 2004; Brack et al. 2004b). In addition, this cell recruitment is dependent on neurokinin-1 receptors (Rittner et al. 2007a) and might be regulated by adhesion to neurons (Hua et al. 2006). Finally, the migration of opioid-containing leukocytes into injured tissue appears to be modulated by central mechanisms. For example, intrathecally administered morphine, in a dose producing analgesia, decreases the number of β-endorphin containing leukocytes in inflamed rat paws (Schmitt et al. 2003). This was confirmed in a clinical study using epidural analgesia in patients undergoing surgery (Heurich et al. 2007). Thus, an effective central inhibition of pain apparently signals a reduced need for recruitment of opioid-containing cells to injured tissues.

3.4 Release of Opioid Peptides from Immune Cells

As in the pituitary, corticotropin-releasing factor (CRF) and interleukin (IL)-1β can stimulate secretion of opioid peptides from leukocytes in a receptor-specific and calcium-dependent manner (Schäfer et al. 1994; Cabot et al. 1997, 2001). Several other mediators have been recognized as potent releasing agents of opioid peptides from immune cells. For example, activation of CXCR2 on granulocytes leads to release of β-endorphin and Met-enkephalin, which is dependent on inositol triphosphate receptor triggered release of Ca^{2+} from endoplasmic reticulum, (partially) on phosphoinositol 3-kinase and on p38 mitogen-activated protein kinase (Rittner et al. 2006b, 2007b). Furthermore, noradrenaline stimulates release of β-endorphin from leukocytes in an adrenergic receptor-specific manner (Kavelaars et al. 1990; Binder et al. 2004). The endogenous source of noradrenaline is sympathetic nerve fibers located in proximity to these cells (Binder et al. 2004). Opioid peptide containing immune cells coexpress adrenergic receptors, chemokine receptors, as well as CRF receptors and IL-1β receptors (Mousa et al. 1996, 2003; Binder et al. 2004). Moreover, these cells package opioids into vesicular structures that are translocated to the membrane upon stimulation (Mousa et al. 2004; Rittner et al. 2007b; Zöllner et al. 2008). In granulocytes these structures have been identified as primary (azurophil) granules (Rittner et al. 2007b). Thus, opioid release from immune cells is consistent with the regulated secretory pathway, similar to neuroendocrine cells.

4 Modulation of Pain and Inflammation

4.1 Exogenous Opioid Agonists

Earlier attempts to demonstrate peripheral opioid analgesia in noninjured tissue produced controversial results, but subsequent studies in models of pathological pain were more successful (Stein 1993; Stein et al. 2003). In models of peripheral inflammation, the local injection of low, systemically inactive doses of μ-, δ-, and κ-agonists produced analgesia that was dose-dependent, stereospecific, and reversible by selective opioid antagonists (Stein et al. 1989; Stein 1993). Potent antinociception was also shown in models of nerve damage and of visceral, thermal, bone, and cancer pain (Stein et al. 2003; Baamonde et al. 2005; Obara et al. 2007; Zöllner and Stein 2007). In addition, anti-inflammatory effects were demonstrated in different models of somatic and visceral inflammation. Possible underlying mechanisms include a reduced release of proinflammatory neuropeptides or cytokines, and a diminished expression of adhesion molecules (Stein et al. 2001; Philippe et al. 2003; Tegeder and Geisslinger 2004; Chakass et al. 2007; Straub et al. 2008). These findings stimulated the development of novel opioid ligands acting exclusively in the periphery without central side effects (DeHaven-Hudkins and Dolle 2004; Riviere 2004; Fürst et al. 2005; Bileviciute-Ljungar et al. 2006). A common approach is the use of hydrophilic compounds with minimal capability to cross the blood–brain-barrier. Among the first compounds were the μ-agonist loperamide (originally known as an antidiarrheal drug) and the κ-agonist asimadoline (Machelska et al. 1999). Peripheral restriction was also achieved with newly developed arylacetamide and peptidic κ-agonists (Stein et al. 2003; Riviere 2004). Several studies indicate that a large proportion (about 50–80%) of the analgesic effects produced by systemically administered opioids can be mediated by peripheral opioid receptors (Craft et al. 1995; Reichert et al. 2001; Shannon and

Lutz 2002; Fürst et al. 2005; Labuz et al. 2007). In addition, human studies have shown that opioid agonists that do not readily cross the blood–brain barrier (e.g., morphine 6-glucuronide) can have the same analgesic efficacy as conventional opioids (Tegeder et al. 2003; Hanna et al. 2005; Dahan et al. 2008).

4.2 Exogenous Stimulation of Opioid Release from Inflammatory Cells

When injected into inflamed subcutaneous tissue, all the releasing agents mentioned in Sect. 3.4 can produce analgesic effects. Depending on the stage and type of inflammation, these effects are mediated by different opioid peptides (Schäfer et al. 1994; Machelska et al. 2003; Mousa et al. 2003; Binder et al. 2004; Brack et al. 2004b; Labuz et al. 2006). Immunosuppression with cyclosporine A, depletion of granulocytes, blockade of chemokines (CXCL1, CXCL2/3), or anti-selectin and anti-ICAM-1 treatments significantly reduce opioid-containing cells and antinociception (Schäfer et al. 1994; Machelska et al. 1998, 2002; Brack et al. 2004b; Rittner 2006, CXCR2). Conversely, the impaired antinociception following immunosuppression can be restored by transfer of allogenic lymphocytes (Hermanussen et al. 2004) or granulocytes (Rittner et al. 2006b). In line with these findings, the isolated recruitment of granulocytes does not induce pain in noninflamed tissue (Rittner et al. 2006a), and CRF (Hargreaves et al. 1989), IL-6, and tumor necrosis factor α (Czlonkowski et al. 1993) administered into inflamed tissue produce opioid-mediated analgesia.

In this context it is important to note that in noninflamed tissue, cytokines such as IL-1α, IL-1β, IL-6, and tumor necrosis factor α were found to induce hyperalgesia (Cunha and Ferreira 2003). Also, several chemokines were described as inducing pain or decreasing the analgesic effects of other compounds (Oh et al. 2001; Szabo et al. 2002). Noradrenaline had no effect or increased pain behavior (Binder et al. 2004). The most obvious explanation for these findings is that noninflamed tissue does not contain opioid-producing immune cells. Hence, short of immune cells bearing their receptors, these agents now act on different targets, e.g., neurons or blood vessels. It is therefore not surprising that a given agent can produce different effects depending on the presence or absence of inflammation. Another recent finding in noninflamed tissue is that activation of keratinocytes by endothelin agonists and cannabinoid agonists can lead to release of β-endorphin, which then acts on opioid receptors on primary afferent neurons to inhibit nociception (Khodorova et al. 2003; Ibrahim et al. 2005).

4.3 Endogenous Stimulation of Opioid Release from Inflammatory Cells

Stress is a natural stimulus triggering inhibition of pain (Willer et al. 1981; Terman et al. 1984). In rats with unilateral hindpaw inflammation stress induced by cold water, swimming elicits potent antinociception in inflamed but not in the contralateral noninflamed paws (Stein et al. 1990a; Machelska et al. 2003). Whereas at early stages of the inflammatory response (several hours) both peripheral and central opioid receptors contribute, at later stages (several days) endogenous analgesia is mediated exclusively by peripheral opioid receptors (Stein et al. 1990a, b; Machelska et al. 2003). Thus, peripheral opioid mechanisms of pain control become more prevalent with the duration and severity of inflammation. The most prominent opioid peptide involved is β-endorphin but Met-enkephalin, dynorphin, and endomorphins also contribute (Stein et al. 1990a; Machelska et al. 2003; Labuz et al. 2006). Endogenous triggers of swim-stress-induced analgesia are locally produced CRF and sympathetic nerve-derived catecholamines (Schäfer et al. 1996; Machelska et al. 2003; Binder et al. 2004).

Stress-induced analgesia can be abolished by cyclosporine A, whole body irradiation, or depletion of monocytes/macrophages (Stein et al. 1990b; Przewlocki et al. 1992; Brack et al. 2004c). Since L-selectin, integrin β_2, and CXCR2 are expressed by opioid-containing leukocytes (Mousa et al. 2000; Brack et al. 2004b; Machelska et al. 2004), pretreatment with selectin blockers, antibodies against ICAM-1, integrins, or the chemokines CXCL1 and CXCL2/3 substantially decreases the number of opioid cells and abolishes endogenous peripheral opioid analgesia (Machelska et al. 1998, 2002, 2004; Brack et al. 2004b). Stress-induced analgesia is also decreased by blockade of neural cell adhesion molecule, presumably by preventing the adhesion of opioid-containing cells to peripheral nerves in inflamed tissue (Hua et al. 2006). Thus, adhesion molecules apparently modulate pain via extravasation of opioid-containing immune cells and/or their adhesion to sensory neurons. In addition, the migration of opioid cells and endogenous analgesia within peripheral injured tissue appear to be influenced by central mechanisms (see earlier) (Schmitt et al. 2003; Heurich et al. 2007).

Importantly, in models of inflammation (Sitte et al. 2007) and bone cancer (Baamonde et al. 2006), as well as in humans undergoing knee surgery (Stein et al. 1993), the local injection of opioid receptor antagonists into injured tissue was shown to exacerbate pain. This strongly indicates that opioid peptides are continuously released and counteract hyperalgesia elicited by the many known proinflammatory agents present in inflammation (Rittner et al. 2005, 2008). Thus, even though hyperalgesia typically prevails in inflamed tissue, this hyperalgesia would be much more severe if opioid peptides were not present and tonically released at the same time.

A future challenge is to identify factors that increase homing of opioid-containing cells to injured tissue. For example, we showed that hematopoietic growth factors mobilized granulocytes in the blood but produced only a minor increase in the number of opioid-containing leukocytes in inflamed paws, and no change of CRF- or stress-induced antinociception (Brack et al. 2004a). Increasing the recruitment of opioid-containing cells with local injections of CXCL2/3 did not result in stronger antinociception either. Most probably this was a result of the relatively low number of neuronal opioid receptors at the respective (early) stage of tissue injury (Brack et al. 2004a). Indeed, our previous studies had shown that intrinsic analgesia increases with the duration of inflammation, in parallel with the number of opioid-containing leukocytes, with the number of peripheral opioid receptors, and with the efficacy of opioid receptor-G protein coupling in sensory neurons (Mousa et al. 2001; Rittner et al. 2001; Zöllner et al. 2003).

4.4 Opioid Tolerance

Long-term opioid treatment can result in the eventual loss of opioid receptor activated function (i.e., desensitization). Three mechanisms are associated with desensitization of GPCRs: (1) receptor phosphorylation, (2) receptor internalization and/or sequestration, and (3) receptor downregulation (i.e., a reduced total number of receptors). Opioid receptors are substrates for second messenger kinases (e.g., protein kinase C) and for GPCR kinases. Opioid receptor phosphorylation by these kinases increases the affinity for arrestin molecules. Arrestin–receptor complexes sterically prevent coupling between receptor and G proteins and promote internalization via clathrin-dependent pathways (Law et al. 2000). Agonist-induced internalization of the receptor via the endocytic pathway has been thought to contribute directly to tolerance by decreasing the number of opioid receptors on the cell surface. However, more recent studies have shown that morphine fails to promote endocytosis of opioid receptors in cultured cells (Eisinger et al. 2002) and native neurons (Sternini et al. 1996), although it is highly efficient in inducing tolerance in vivo (Hanninen et al. 1996). Moreover, increased endocytosis and recycling of opioid receptors was shown to dramatically decrease opioid tolerance (Koch et al. 2005). These findings led to the current concept that desensitization and receptor internalization prevent the development of tolerance.

Experimental studies on tolerance are often performed in the absence of painful tissue injury, which precludes extrapolation to the clinical situation. Recently we showed that rats undergoing prolonged treatment with morphine do not develop signs of tolerance at peripheral μ-opioid receptors in the presence of painful paw inflammation. In DRG neurons of these animals, internalization of μ-receptors was significantly increased, and G protein coupling of μ-receptors as well as inhibition of cAMP accumulation were preserved. However, opioid receptor internalization and signaling were reduced and tolerance was restored when endogenous opioid peptides in inflamed tissue were removed by antibodies or by depleting opioid-producing granulocytes, monocytes, and lymphocytes with cyclophosphamide (Zöllner et al. 2008). These data indicate that the continuous availability of endogenous opioids in inflamed tissue increases recycling and preserves signaling of μ-receptors in sensory neurons, and thereby counteracts the development of peripheral opioid tolerance. These findings infer that the use of peripherally acting opioid agonists for the prolonged treatment of inflammatory pain is not necessarily accompanied by opioid tolerance.

5 Clinical Implications and Perspectives

Peripheral mechanisms of opioid analgesia have gained recognition in the clinical setting. Opioid receptors have been demonstrated on peripheral terminals of sensory nerves in human synovia (Stein et al. 1996; Mousa et al. 2007a), dermal and epidermal nerve fibers (Ständer et al. 2002), and dental pulp (Jaber et al. 2003). That such receptors mediate analgesia has been amply demonstrated in patients with various types of pain (e.g., in chronic rheumatoid arthritis and osteoarthritis, oral mucositis, bone pain, after dental, laparoscopic, urinary bladder, and knee surgery) (Sawynok 2003; Stein et al. 2003; Kopf et al. 2006). One of the most extensively studied and most successful applications is the intraarticular injection of morphine into inflamed knee joints (Stein et al. 1991, 1999; Likar et al. 1997; Kalso et al. 2002; American Society of Anesthesiologists Task Force on Acute Pain Management 2004; http://www.guideline.gov). Novel peripherally restricted κ-agonists have been investigated in humans with chronic painful pancreatitis (Eisenach et al. 2003). Opioid peptides were found in human subcutaneous and synovial cells, mast cells, granulocytes, lymphocytes, and macrophages. The prevailing peptides are β-endorphin and Met-enkephalin, but dynorphin and endomorphins were also detected (Stein et al. 1993, 1996; Likar et al. 2004, 2007; Heurich et al. 2007; Mousa et al. 2007a; Rittner et al. 2007b; Straub et al. 2008). Furthermore, in patients undergoing knee surgery, blocking intraarticular opioid receptors by the local administration of naloxone resulted in significantly increased postoperative pain (Stein et al. 1993). These findings suggest that in a stressful (e.g., postoperative) situation, opioids are tonically released in inflamed tissue and activate peripheral opioid receptors to attenuate clinical pain. In addition, CRF receptors are coexpressed with β-endorphin in synovial inflammatory cells and the intraarticular application of CRF can transiently reduce postoperative pain (Likar et al. 2007). Apparently, endogenous immune-cell-derived opioids do not interfere with exogenous agonists since intraarticular morphine is an equally potent analgesic in patients with and without opioid-producing inflammatory synovial cells (Stein et al. 1996; Likar et al. 2004). Similar to the findings of our animal studies (Zöllner et al. 2008), this suggests that immune-cell-derived opioids do not produce cross-tolerance to morphine, but rather prevent the development of tolerance at peripheral opioid receptors.

These findings provide new insights into intrinsic mechanisms of pain control and open up novel strategies to develop drugs and alternative approaches to treatment of pain and inflammation. Immunocompromised patients (e.g., in AIDS, cancer, diabetes) frequently suffer from painful neuropathies. These can be associated with intra-

and perineural inflammation, with reduced intraepidermal nerve fiber density, and with low $CD4^+$ lymphocyte counts (Polydefkis et al. 2003). Thus, it may be interesting to investigate the opioid production/release and the migration of opioid-containing leukocytes in these patients. The important role of adhesion molecules and chemokines in the trafficking of opioid-containing cells indicates that antiadhesion or anti-chemokine strategies for the treatment of inflammatory diseases may, in fact, carry a significant risk to exacerbate pain. It would be highly desirable to identify stimulating factors and strategies that selectively attract opioid-producing cells, augment opioid peptide production, and/or increase peripheral opioid receptor numbers in damaged tissue. Studies using various gene therapeutic approaches are under way (Mata et al. 2002; Pohl et al. 2003; Beutler et al. 2005; Kyrkanides et al. 2007). A further interesting question is whether immune-derived opioid peptides and exogenous opioids interact in a synergistic fashion. Undoubtedly, peripherally acting opioid agonists would be most attractive because of their lack of central side effects (respiratory depression, nausea, dysphoria, addiction, tolerance) and of typical adverse effects of nonsteroidal anti-inflammatory drugs (gastric erosions, ulcers, bleeding, diarrhea, renal toxicity, thromboembolic complications).

Acknowledgements This work was supported by grants from the Deutsche Forschungsgemeinschaft (KFO 100) and the International Anesthesia Research Society.

References

Akins PT, McCleskey EW (1993) Characterization of potassium currents in adult rat sensory neurons and modulation by opioids and cyclic AMP. Neuroscience 56:759–769

American Society of Anesthesiologists Task Force on Acute Pain Management (2004) Practice guidelines for acute pain management in the perioperative setting: an updated report by the American Society of Anesthesiologists Task Force on Acute Pain Management. Anesthesiology 100:1573–1581

Antonijevic I, Mousa SA, Schäfer M, Stein C (1995) Perineurial defect and peripheral opioid analgesia in inflammation. J Neurosci 15:165–172

Baamonde A, Lastra A, Juarez L, Garcia V, Hidalgo A, Menendez L (2005) Effects of the local administration of selective mu-, delta- and kappa-opioid receptor agonists on osteosarcoma-induced hyperalgesia. Naunyn Schmiedebergs Arch Pharmacol 372:213–219

Baamonde A, Lastra A, Juarez L, Garcia-Suarez O, Meana A, Hidalgo A, Menendez L (2006) Endogenous beta-endorphin induces thermal analgesia at the initial stages of a murine osteosarcoma. Peptides 27:2778–2785

Ballet S, Conrath M, Fischer J, Kaneko T, Hamon M, Cesselin F (2003) Expression and G-protein coupling of mu-opioid receptors in the spinal cord and dorsal root ganglia of polyarthritic rats. Neuropeptides 37:211–219

Bartho L, Stein C, Herz A (1990) Involvement of capsaicin-sensitive neurones in hyperalgesia and enhanced opioid antinociception in inflammation. Naunyn Schmiedebergs Arch Pharmacol 342:666–670

Beland B, Fitzgerald M (2001) Mu- and delta-opioid receptors are downregulated in the largest diameter primary sensory neurons during postnatal development in rats. Pain 90: 143–150

Berg KA, Zardeneta G, Hargreaves KM, Clarke WP, Milam SB (2007a) Integrins regulate opioid receptor signaling in trigeminal ganglion neurons. Neuroscience 144:889–897

Berg KA, Patwardhan AM, Sanchez TA, Silva YM, Hargreaves KM, Clarke WP (2007b) Rapid modulation of mu-opioid receptor signaling in primary sensory neurons. J Pharmacol Exp Ther 321:839–847

Bergström J, Ahmed M, Li J, Ahmad T, Kreicbergs A, Spetea M (2006) Opioid peptides and receptors in joint tissues: study in the rat. J Orthop Res 24:1193–1199

Beutler AS, Banck MS, Walsh CE, Milligan ED (2005) Intrathecal gene transfer by adeno-associated virus for pain. Curr Opin Mol Ther 7:431–439

Bileviciute-Ljungar I, Spetea M, Guo Y, Schutz J, Windisch P, Schmidhammer H (2006) Peripherally mediated antinociception of the mu-opioid receptor agonist 2-[(4,5α-epoxy-3-hydroxy-14β-methoxy-17-methylmorphinan-6β-yl)amino]acetic acid (HS-731) after subcutaneous and oral administration in rats with carrageenan-induced hindpaw inflammation. J Pharmacol Exp Ther 317:220–227

Binder W, Mousa SA, Sitte N, Kaiser M, Stein C, Schäfer M (2004) Sympathetic activation triggers endogenous opioid release and analgesia within peripheral inflamed tissue. Eur J Neurosci 20:92–100

Brack A, Rittner HL, Machelska H, Beschmann K, Sitte N, Schäfer M, Stein C (2004a) Mobilization of opioid-containing polymorphonuclear cells by hematopoietic growth factors and influence on inflammatory pain. Anesthesiology 100:149–157

Brack A, Rittner HL, Machelska H, Leder K, Mousa SA, Schafer M, Stein C (2004b) Control of inflammatory pain by chemokine-mediated recruitment of opioid-containing polymorphonuclear cells. Pain 112:229–238

Brack A, Labuz D, Schiltz A, Rittner HL, Machelska H, Schafer M, Reszka R, Stein C (2004c) Tissue monocytes/macrophages in inflammation: hyperalgesia versus opioid-mediated peripheral antinociception. Anesthesiology 101:204–211

Brower V (2000) New paths to pain relief. Nat Biotechnol 18:387–391

Buzas B, Cox BM (1997) Quantitative analysis of mu- and delta-opioid receptor gene expression in rat brain and peripheral ganglia using competitive polymerase chain reaction. Neuroscience 76:479–489

Cabot PJ, Carter L, Gaiddon C, Zhang Q, Schäfer M, Loeffler JP, Stein C (1997) Immune cell-derived β-endorphin: production, release and control of inflammatory pain in rats. J Clin Invest 100:142–148

Cabot PJ, Carter L, Schäfer M, Stein C (2001) Methionine-enkephalin- and dynorphin A-release from immune cells and control of inflammatory pain. Pain 93:207–212

Calza L, Pozza M, Zanni M, Manzini CU, Manzini E, Hokfelt T (1998) Peptide plasticity in primary sensory neurons and spinal cord during adjuvant-induced arthritis in the rat: an immunocytochemical and in situ hybridization study. Neuroscience 82:575–589

Carlton SM, Coggeshall RE (1997) Immunohistochemical localization of enkephalin in peripheral sensory axons in the rat. Neurosci Lett 221:121–124

Chadzinska M, Starowicz K, Scislowska-Czarnecka A, Bilecki W, Pierzchala-Koziec K, Przewlocki R, Przewlocka B, Plytycz B (2005) Morphine-induced changes in the activity of proopiomelanocortin and prodynorphin systems in zymosan-induced peritonitis in mice. Immunol Lett 101:185–192

Chakass D, Philippe D, Erdual E, Dharancy S, Malapel M, Dubuquoy C, Thuru X, Gay J, Gaveriaux-Ruff C, Dubus P, Mathurin P, Kieffer BL, Desreumaux P, Chamaillard M (2007) Mu-opioid receptor activation prevents acute hepatic inflammation and cell death. Gut 56:974–981

Chen JJ, Dymshitz J, Vasko MR (1997) Regulation of opioid receptors in rat sensory neurons in culture. Mol Pharmacol 51:666–673

Chen CL, Broom DC, Liu Y, de Nooij JC, Li Z, Cen C, Samad OA, Jessell TM, Woolf CJ, Ma Q (2006) Runx1 determines nociceptive sensory neuron phenotype and is required for thermal and neuropathic pain. Neuron 49:365–377

Coggeshall RE, Zhou S, Carlton SM (1997) Opiate receptors on peripheral sensory axons. Brain Res 764:126–132

Craft RM, Henley SR, Haaseth RC, Hruby VJ, Porreca F (1995) Opioid antinociception in a rat model of visceral pain: systemic versus local drug administration. J Pharmacol Exp Ther 275:1535–1542

Crowe R, Parkhouse N, McGrouther D, Burnstock G (1994) Neuropeptide-containing nerves in painful hypertrophic human scar tissue. Br J Dermatol 130:444–452

Cunha FQ, Ferreira SH (2003) Peripheral hyperalgesic cytokines. Adv Exp Med Biol 521:22–39

Czlonkowski A, Stein C, Herz A (1993) Peripheral mechanisms of opioid antinociception in inflammation: involvement of cytokines. Eur J Pharmacol 242:229–235

Dahan A, van Dorp E, Smith T, Yassen A (2008) Morphine-6-glucuronide (M6G) for postoperative pain relief. Eur J Pain 12:403–411

DeHaven-Hudkins DL, Dolle RE (2004) Peripherally restricted opioid agonists as novel analgesic agents. Curr Pharm Des 10:743–757

Eisenach JC, Carpenter R, Curry R (2003) Analgesia from a peripherally active κ-opioid receptor agonist in patients with chronic pancreatitis. Pain 101:89–95

Eisinger DA, Ammer H, Schulz R (2002) Chronic morphine treatment inhibits opioid receptor desensitization and internalization. J Neurosci 22:10192–10200

Endres-Becker J, Heppenstall PA, Mousa SA, Labuz D, Oksche A, Schäfer M, Stein C, Zöllner C (2007) Mu-opioid receptor activation modulates transient receptor potential vanilloid 1 (TRPV1) currents in sensory neurons in a model of inflammatory pain. Mol Pharmacol 71:12–18

Evans CJ, Keith DE Jr, Morrison H, Magendzo K, Edwards RH (1992) Cloning of a delta-opioid receptor by functional expression. Science 258:1952–1955

Fichna J, Janecka A, Costentin J, Do Rego JC (2007) The endomorphin system and its evolving neurophysiological role. Pharmacol Rev 59:88–123

Fürst S, Riba P, Friedmann T, Timar J, Al-Khrasani M, Obara I, Makuch W, Spetea M, Schutz J, Przewlocki R, Przewlocka B, Schmidhammer H (2005) Peripheral versus central antinociceptive actions of 6-amino acid-substituted derivatives of 14-*O*-methyloxymorphone in acute and inflammatory pain in the rat. J Pharmacol Exp Ther 312:609–618

Gendron L, Lucido AL, Mennicken F, O'Donnell D, Vincent JP, Stroh T, Beaudet A (2006) Morphine and pain-related stimuli enhance cell surface availability of somatic delta-opioid receptors in rat dorsal root ganglia. J Neurosci 26:953–962

Gibbins IL, Furness JB, Costa M (1987) Pathway-specific patterns of the co-existence of substance P, calcitonin gene-related peptide, cholecystokinin and dynorphin in neurons of the dorsal root ganglia of the guinea pig. Cell Tissue Res 248:417–437

Gold MS, Levine JD (1996) DAMGO inhibits prostaglandin E_2-induced potentiation of a TTX-resistant Na^+ current in rat sensory neurons in vitro. Neurosci Lett 212:83–86

Hanna MH, Elliott KM, Fung M (2005) Randomized, double-blind study of the analgesic efficacy of morphine-6-glucuronide versus morphine sulfate for postoperative pain in major surgery. Anesthesiology 102:815–821

Hanninen A, Salmi M, Simell O, Andrew D, Jalkanen S (1996) Recirculation and homing of lymphocyte subsets: dual homing specificity of beta 7-integrin(high)-lymphocytes in nonobese diabetic mice. Blood 88:934–944

Hargreaves KM, Dubner R, Costello AH (1989) Corticotropin releasing factor (CRF) has a peripheral site of action for antinociception. Eur J Pharmacol 170:275–279

Hassan AHS, Ableitner A, Stein C, Herz A (1993) Inflammation of the rat paw enhances axonal transport of opioid receptors in the sciatic nerve and increases their density in the inflamed tissue. Neuroscience 55:185–195

Herlitze S, Garcia DE, Mackie K, Hille B, Scheuer T, Catterall WA (1996) Modulation of Ca^{2+} channels by G-protein beta gamma subunits. Nature 380:258–262

Hermanussen S, Do M, Cabot PJ (2004) Reduction of beta-endorphin-containing immune cells in inflamed paw tissue corresponds with a reduction in immune-derived antinociception: reversible by donor activated lymphocytes. Anesth Analg 98:723–729

Heurich M, Mousa SA, Lenzner M, Morciniec P, Kopf A, Welte M, Stein C (2007) Influence of pain treatment by epidural fentanyl and bupivacaine on homing of opioid-containing leukocytes to surgical wounds. Brain Behav Immun 21:544–552

Hook S, Camberis M, Prout M, Konig M, Zimmer A, Van Heeke G, Le Gros G (1999) Preproenkephalin is a Th2 cytokine but is not required for Th2 differentiation in vitro. Immunol Cell Biol 77:385–390

Hua S, Hermanussen S, Tang L, Monteith GR, Cabot PJ (2006) The neural cell adhesion molecule antibody blocks cold water swim stress-induced analgesia and cell adhesion between lymphocytes and cultured dorsal root ganglion neurons. Anesth Analg 103:1558–1564

Ibrahim MM, Porreca F, Lai J, Albrecht PJ, Rice FL, Khodorova A, Davar G, Makriyannis A, Vanderah TW, Mata HP, Malan TP Jr (2005) CB2 cannabinoid receptor activation produces antinociception by stimulating peripheral release of endogenous opioids. Proc Natl Acad Sci USA 102:3093–3098

Ingram SL, Williams JT (1994) Opioid inhibition of Ih via adenylyl cyclase. Neuron 13:179–186

Jaber L, Swaim WD, Dionne RA (2003) Immunohistochemical localization of mu-opioid receptors in human dental pulp. J Endod 29:108–110

Jeanjean AP, Moussaoui SM, Maloteaux J-M, Laduron PM (1995) Interleukin-1β induces long-term increase of axonally transported opiate receptors and substance P. Neuroscience 68:151–157

Ji R-R, Zhang Q, Law P-Y, Low HH, Elde R, Hökfelt T (1995) Expression of μ-, δ-, and κ-opioid receptor-like immunoreactivities in rat dorsal root ganglia after carrageenan-induced inflammation. J Neurosci 15:8156–8166

Kabli N, Cahill CM (2007) Anti-allodynic effects of peripheral delta-opioid receptors in neuropathic pain. Pain 127:84–93

Kalso E, Smith L, McQuay HJ, Moore RA (2002) No pain, no gain: clinical excellence and scientific rigour – lessons learned from IA morphine. Pain 98:269–275

Kavelaars A, Ballieux RE, Heijnen CJ (1990) In vitro beta-adrenergic stimulation of lymphocytes induces the release of immunoreactive beta-endorphin. Endocrinology 126:3028–3032

Khodorova A, Navarro B, Jouaville LS, Murphy JE, Rice FL, Mazurkiewicz JE, Long-Woodward D, Stoffel M, Strichartz GR, Yukhananov R, Davar G (2003) Endothelin-B receptor activation triggers an endogenous analgesic cascade at sites of peripheral injury. Nat Med 9:1055–1061

Kieffer BL, Gaveriaux-Ruff C (2002) Exploring the opioid system by gene knockout. Prog Neurobiol 66:285–306

Kieffer BL, Befort K, Gaveriaux-Ruff C, Hirth CG (1992) The delta-opioid receptor: isolation of a cDNA by expression cloning and pharmacological characterization. Proc Natl Acad Sci USA 89:12048–12052

Koch T, Widera A, Bartzsch K, Schulz S, Brandenburg LO, Wundrack N, Beyer A, Grecksch G, Hollt V (2005) Receptor endocytosis counteracts the development of opioid tolerance. Mol Pharmacol 67:280–287

Kondo I, Marvizon JC, Song B, Salgado F, Codeluppi S, Hua XY, Yaksh TL (2005) Inhibition by spinal mu- and delta-opioid agonists of afferent-evoked substance P release. J Neurosci 25:3651–3660

Kopf A, Schmidt S, Stein C (2006) Topical administration of analgesics. In: Bruera E, Higginson IJ, Ripamonti C, von Gunten CF (eds) Textbook of palliative medicine. Hodder Arnold, London, pp 450–457

Kraus J, Borner C, Giannini E, Hickfang K, Braun H, Mayer P, Hoehe MR, Ambrosch A, Konig W, Höllt V (2001) Regulation of mu-opioid receptor gene transcription by interleukin-4 and influence of an allelic variation within a STAT6 transcription factor binding site. J Biol Chem 276:43901–43908

Kyrkanides S, Fiorentino PM, Miller JN, Gan Y, Lai YC, Shaftel SS, Puzas JE, Piancino MG, O'Banion MK, Tallents RH (2007) Amelioration of pain and histopathologic joint abnormalities in the Col1-IL-1beta(XAT) mouse model of arthritis by intraarticular induction of mu-opioid receptor into the temporomandibular joint. Arthritis Rheum 56:2038–2048

Labuz D, Berger S, Mousa SA, Zöllner C, Rittner HL, Shaqura MA, Segovia-Silvestre T, Przewlocka B, Stein C, Machelska H (2006) Peripheral antinociceptive effects of exogenous and immune cell-derived endomorphins in prolonged inflammatory pain. J Neurosci 26:4350–4358

Labuz D, Mousa SA, Schafer M, Stein C, Machelska H (2007) Relative contribution of peripheral versus central opioid receptors to antinociception. Brain Res 1160:30–38

LaMendola J, Martin SK, Steiner DF (1997) Expression of PC3, carboxypeptidase E and enkephalin in human monocyte-derived macrophages as a tool for genetic studies. FEBS Lett 404:19–22

Law PY, Wong YH, Loh HH (2000) Molecular mechanisms and regulation of opioid receptor signaling. Annu Rev Pharmacol Toxicol 40:389–430

Ledford H (2007) Fever pitch. Nature 450:600–601

Li JL, Kaneko T, Mizuno N (1996) Effects of peripheral nerve ligation on expression of mu-opioid receptor in sensory ganglion neurons: an immunohistochemical study in dorsal root and nodose ganglion neurons of the rat. Neurosci Lett 214:91–94

Li JL, Ding YQ, Li YQ, Li JS, Nomura S, Kaneko T, Mizuno N (1998) Immunocytochemical localization of mu-opioid receptor in primary afferent neurons containing substance P or calcitonin gene-related peptide. A light and electron microscope study in the rat. Brain Res 794:347–352

Likar R, Schäfer M, Paulak F, Sittl R, Pipam W, Schalk H, Geissler D, Bernatzky G (1997) Intraarticular morphine analgesia in chronic pain patients with osteoarthritis. Anesth Analg 84:1313–1317

Likar R, Mousa SA, Philippitsch G, Steinkellner H, Koppert W, Stein C, Schäfer M (2004) Increased numbers of opioid expressing inflammatory cells do not affect intra-articular morphine analgesia. Br J Anaesth 93:375–380

Likar R, Mousa SA, Steinkellner H, Koppert W, Philippitsch G, Stein C, Schafer M (2007) Involvement of intra-articular corticotropin-releasing hormone in postoperative pain modulation. Clin J Pain 23:136–142

Lyons PD, Blalock JE (1997) Pro-opiomelanocortin gene expression and protein processing in rat mononuclear leukocytes. J Neuroimmunol 78:47–56

Machelska H (2007) Targeting of opioid-producing leukocytes for pain control. Neuropeptides 41:355–363

Machelska H, Cabot PJ, Mousa SA, Zhang Q, Stein C (1998) Pain control in inflammation governed by selectins. Nat Med 4:1425–1428

Machelska H, Pflüger M, Weber W, Piranvisseh-Volk M, Daubert JD, Dehaven R, Stein C (1999) Peripheral effects of the kappa-opioid agonist EMD 61753 on pain and inflammation in rats and humans. J Pharmacol Exp Ther 290:354–361

Machelska H, Mousa SA, Brack A, Schopohl JK, Rittner HL, Schäfer M, Stein C (2002) Opioid control of inflammatory pain regulated by intercellular adhesion molecule-1. J Neurosci 22:5588–5596

Machelska H, Schopohl JK, Mousa SA, Labuz D, Schafer M, Stein C (2003) Different mechanisms of intrinsic pain inhibition in early and late inflammation. J Neuroimmunol 141:30–39

Machelska H, Brack A, Mousa SA, Schopohl JK, Rittner HL, Schafer M, Stein C (2004) Selectins and integrins but not platelet-endothelial cell adhesion molecule-1 regulate opioid inhibition of inflammatory pain. Br J Pharmacol 142:772–780

Mansour A, Fox CA, Burke S, Meng F, Thompson RC, Akil H, Watson SJ (1994) Mu, delta, and kappa-opioid receptor mRNA expression in the rat CNS: an in situ hybridization study. J Comp Neurol 350:412–438

Martin-Schild S, Gerall AA, Kastin AJ, Zadina JE (1998) Endomorphin-2 is an endogenous opioid in primary sensory afferent fibers. Peptides 19:1783–1789

Mata M, Glorioso JC, Fink DJ (2002) Targeted gene delivery to the nervous system using herpes simplex virus vectors. Physiol Behav 77:483–488

Meng F, Xie GX, Thompson RC, Mansour A, Goldstein A, Watson SJ, Akil H (1993) Cloning and pharmacological characterization of a rat kappa-opioid receptor. Proc Natl Acad Sci USA 90:9954–9958

Minami M, Maekawa K, Yabuuchi K, Satoh M (1995) Double in situ hybridization study on coexistence of mu-, delta- and kappa-opioid receptor mRNAs with preprotachykinin A mRNA in the rat dorsal root ganglia. Brain Res Mol Brain Res 30:203–210

Mousa SA, Schäfer M, Mitchell WM, Hassan AHS, Stein C (1996) Local upregulation of corticotropin- releasing hormone and interleukin-1 receptors in rats with painful hindlimb inflammation. Eur J Pharmacol 311:221–231

Mousa SA, Machelska H, Schäfer M, Stein C (2000) Co-expression of beta-endorphin with adhesion molecules in a model of inflammatory pain. J Neuroimmunol 108:160–170

Mousa SA, Zhang Q, Sitte N, Ji R, Stein C (2001) beta-Endorphin-containing memory-cells and mu-opioid receptors undergo transport to peripheral inflamed tissue. J Neuroimmunol 115:71–78

Mousa SA, Machelska H, Schäfer M, Stein C (2002) Immunohistochemical localization of endomorphin-1 and endomorphin-2 in immune cells and spinal cord in a model of inflammatory pain. J Neuroimmunol 126:5–15

Mousa SA, Bopaiah CP, Stein C, Schafer M (2003) Involvement of corticotropin-releasing hormone receptor subtypes 1 and 2 in peripheral opioid-mediated inhibition of inflammatory pain. Pain 106:297–307

Mousa SA, Shakibaei M, Sitte N, Schäfer M, Stein C (2004) Subcellular pathways of beta-endorphin synthesis, processing, and release from immunocytes in inflammatory pain. Endocrinology 145:1331–1341

Mousa SA, Straub RH, Schafer M, Stein C (2007a) Beta-endorphin, Met-enkephalin and corresponding opioid receptors within synovium of patients with joint trauma, osteoarthritis and rheumatoid arthritis. Ann Rheum Dis 66:871–879

Mousa SA, Cheppudira BP, Shaqura M, Fischer O, Hofmann J, Hellweg R, Schafer M (2007b) Nerve growth factor governs the enhanced ability of opioids to suppress inflammatory pain. Brain 130:502–513

Obara I, Makuch W, Spetea M, Schutz J, Schmidhammer H, Przewlocki R, Przewlocka B (2007) Local peripheral antinociceptive effects of 14-*O*-methyloxymorphone derivatives in inflammatory and neuropathic pain in the rat. Eur J Pharmacol 558:60–67

Oh SB, Tran PB, Gillard SE, Hurley RW, Hammond DL, Miller RJ (2001) Chemokines and glycoprotein120 produce pain hypersensitivity by directly exciting primary nociceptive neurons. J Neurosci 21:5027–5035

Patwardhan AM, Berg KA, Akopain AN, Jeske NA, Gamper N, Clarke WP, Hargreaves KM (2005) Bradykinin-induced functional competence and trafficking of the delta-opioid receptor in trigeminal nociceptors. J Neurosci 25:8825–8832

Philippe D, Dubuquoy L, Groux H, Brun V, Chuoi-Mariot MT, Gaveriaux-Ruff C, Colombel JF, Kieffer BL, Desreumaux P (2003) Anti-inflammatory properties of the mu-opioid receptor support its use in the treatment of colon inflammation. J Clin Invest 111:1329–1338

Picard PR, Tramer MR, McQuay HJ, Moore RA (1997) Analgesic efficacy of peripheral opioids (all except intra-articular): a qualitative systematic review of randomised controlled trials. Pain 72:309–318

Pierce TL, Grahek MD, Wessendorf MW (1998) Immunoreactivity for endomorphin-2 occurs in primary afferents in rats and monkey. Neuroreport 9:385–389

Pohl M, Collin E, Bourgoin S, Conrath M, Benoliel JJ, Nevo I, Hamon M, Giraud P, Cesselin F (1994) Expression of preproenkephalin A gene and presence of Met-enkephalin in dorsal root ganglia of the adult rat. J Neurochem 63:1226–1234

Pohl M, Meunier A, Hamon M, Braz J (2003) Gene therapy of chronic pain. Curr Gene Ther 3:223–238

Pol O, Murtra P, Caracuel L, Valverde O, Puig MM, Maldonado R (2006) Expression of opioid receptors and c-fos in CB1 knockout mice exposed to neuropathic pain. Neuropharmacology 50:123–132

Polydefkis M, Griffin JW, McArthur J (2003) New insights into diabetic polyneuropathy. JAMA 290:1371–1376

Przewlocki R, Gramsch C, Pasi A, Herz A (1983) Characterization and localization of immunoreactive dynorphin, alpha-neoendorphin, met-enkephalin and substance P in human spinal cord. Brain Res 280:95–103

Przewlocki R, Hassan AHS, Lason W, Epplen C, Herz A, Stein C (1992) Gene expression and localization of opioid peptides in immune cells of inflamed tissue. Functional role in antinociception. Neuroscience 48:491–500
Pühler W, Zollner C, Brack A, Shaqura MA, Krause H, Schafer M, Stein C (2004) Rapid upregulation of mu-opioid receptor mRNA in dorsal root ganglia in response to peripheral inflammation depends on neuronal conduction. Neuroscience 129:473–479
Pühler W, Rittner HL, Mousa SA, Brack A, Krause H, Stein C, Schafer M (2006) Interleukin-1 beta contributes to the upregulation of kappa-opioid receptor mRNA in dorsal root ganglia in response to peripheral inflammation. Neuroscience 141:989–998
Quartu M, Del Fiacco M (1994) Enkephalins occur and colocalize with substance P in human trigeminal ganglion neurones. Neuroreport 5:465–468
Rasenick MM, Childers SR (1989) Modification of G_s-stimulated adenylate cyclase in brain membranes by low *p*H pretreatment: correlation with altered guanine nucleotide exchange. J Neurochem 53:219–225
Rashid MH, Inoue M, Toda K, Ueda H (2004) Loss of peripheral morphine analgesia contributes to the reduced effectiveness of systemic morphine in neuropathic pain. J Pharmacol Exp Ther 309:380–387
Rau KK, Caudle RM, Cooper BY, Johnson RD (2005) Diverse immunocytochemical expression of opioid receptors in electrophysiologically defined cells of rat dorsal root ganglia. J Chem Neuroanat 29:255–264
Reichert JA, Daughters RS, Rivard R, Simone DA (2001) Peripheral and preemptive opioid antinociception in a mouse visceral pain model. Pain 89:221–227
Rittner HL, Brack A, Machelska H, Mousa SA, Bauer M, Schäfer M, Stein C (2001) Opioid peptide-expressing leukocytes: identification, recruitment, and simultaneously increasing inhibition of inflammatory pain. Anesthesiology 95:500–508
Rittner HL, Machelska H, Stein C (2005) Leukocytes in the regulation of pain and analgesia. J Leukoc Biol 78:1215–1222
Rittner HL, Mousa SA, Labuz D, Beschmann K, Schafer M, Stein C, Brack A (2006a) Selective local PMN recruitment by CXCL1 or CXCL2/3 injection does not cause inflammatory pain. J Leukoc Biol 79:1022–1032
Rittner HL, Labuz D, Schaefer M, Mousa SA, Schulz S, Schafer M, Stein C, Brack A (2006b) Pain control by CXCR2 ligands through Ca^{2+}-regulated release of opioid peptides from polymorphonuclear cells. FASEB J 20:2627–2629
Rittner HL, Lux C, Labuz D, Mousa SA, Schafer M, Stein C, Brack A (2007a) Neurokinin-1 receptor antagonists inhibit the recruitment of opioid-containing leukocytes and impair peripheral antinociception. Anesthesiology 107:1009–1017
Rittner HL, Labuz D, Richter JF, Brack A, Schafer M, Stein C, Mousa SA (2007b) CXCR1/2 ligands induce p38 MAPK-dependent translocation and release of opioid peptides from primary granules in vitro and in vivo. Brain Behav Immun 21:1021–1032
Rittner HL, Brack A, Stein C (2008) The other side of the medal: How chemokines promote analgesia. Neurosci Lett 437:203–208
Riviere PJ (2004) Peripheral kappa-opioid agonists for visceral pain. Br J Pharmacol 141:1331–1334
Sawynok J (2003) Topical and peripherally acting analgesics. Pharmacol Rev 55:1–20
Schäfer M, Carter L, Stein C (1994) Interleukin-1β and corticotropin-releasing-factor inhibit pain by releasing opioids from immune cells in inflamed tissue. Proc Natl Acad Sci USA 91:4219–4223
Schäfer M, Mousa SA, Zhang Q, Carter L, Stein C (1996) Expression of corticotropin-releasing factor in inflamed tissue is required for intrinsic peripheral opioid analgesia. Proc Natl Acad Sci USA 93:6096–6100
Schmitt TK, Mousa SA, Brack A, Schmidt DK, Rittner HL, Welte M, Schäfer M, Stein C (2003) Modulation of peripheral endogenous opioid analgesia by central afferent blockade. Anesthesiology 98:195–202

Selley DE, Breivogel CS, Childers SR (1993) Modification of G protein-coupled functions by low *p*H pretreatment of membranes from NG108-15 cells: increase in opioid agonist efficacy by decreased inactivation of G proteins. Mol Pharmacol 44:731–741

Shannon HE, Lutz EA (2002) Comparison of the peripheral and central effects of the opioid agonists loperamide and morphine in the formalin test in rats. Neuropharmacology 42:253–261

Shaqura MA, Zöllner C, Mousa SA, Stein C, Schäfer M (2004) Characterization of mu-opioid receptor binding and G protein coupling in rat hypothalamus, spinal cord, and primary afferent neurons during inflammatory pain. J Pharmacol Exp Ther 308:712–718

Silbert SC, Beacham DW, McCleskey EW (2003) Quantitative single-cell differences in mu-opioid receptor mRNA distinguish myelinated and unmyelinated nociceptors. J Neurosci 23:34–42

Sitte N, Busch M, Mousa SA, Labuz D, Rittner H, Gore C, Krause H, Stein C, Schafer M (2007) Lymphocytes upregulate signal sequence-encoding proopiomelanocortin mRNA and beta-endorphin during painful inflammation in vivo. J Neuroimmunol 183:133–145

Smith EM (2003) Opioid peptides in immune cells. Adv Exp Med Biol 521:51–68

Ständer S, Gunzer M, Metze D, Luger T, Steinhoff M (2002) Localization of mu-opioid receptor 1A on sensory nerve fibers in human skin. Regul Pept 110:75–83

Stein C (1993) Peripheral mechanisms of opioid analgesia. Anesth Analg 76:182–191

Stein C (1995) The control of pain in peripheral tissue by opioids. N Engl J Med 332:1685–1690

Stein C, Millan MJ, Shippenberg TS, Peter K, Herz A (1989) Peripheral opioid receptors mediating antinociception in inflammation. Evidence for involvement of mu, delta and kappa receptors. J Pharmacol Exp Ther 248:1269–1275

Stein C, Gramsch C, Herz A (1990a) Intrinsic mechanisms of antinociception in inflammation. Local opioid receptors and β-endorphin. J Neurosci 10:1292–1298

Stein C, Hassan AH, Przewlocki R, Gramsch C, Peter K, Herz A (1990b) Opioids from immunocytes interact with receptors on sensory nerves to inhibit nociception in inflammation. Proc Natl Acad Sci USA 87:5935–5939

Stein C, Comisel K, Haimerl E, Yassouridis A, Lehrberger K, Herz A, Peter K (1991) Analgesic effect of intraarticular morphine after arthroscopic knee surgery. N Engl J Med 325:1123–1126

Stein C, Hassan AHS, Lehrberger K, Giefing J, Yassouridis A (1993) Local analgesic effect of endogenous opioid peptides. Lancet 342:321–324

Stein C, Pflüger M, Yassouridis A, Hoelzl J, Lehrberger K, Welte C, Hassan AHS (1996) No tolerance to peripheral morphine analgesia in presence of opioid expression in inflamed synovia. J Clin Invest 98:793–799

Stein A, Yassouridis A, Szopko C, Helmke K, Stein C (1999) Intraarticular morphine versus dexamethasone in chronic arthritis. Pain 83:525–532

Stein C, Machelska H, Schäfer M (2001) Peripheral analgesic and anti-inflammatory effects of opioids. Z Rheumatol 60:416–424

Stein C, Schäfer M, Machelska H (2003) Attacking pain at its source: new perspectives on opioids. Nat Med 9:1003–1008

Sternini C, Spann M, Anton B, Keith DE Jr, Bunnett NW, von Zastrow M, Evans C, Brecha NC (1996) Agonist-selective endocytosis of mu-opioid receptor by neurons in vivo. Proc Natl Acad Sci USA 93:9241–9246

Straub RH, Wolff C, Fassold A, Hofbauer R, Chover-Gonzalez A, Richards LJ, Jessop DS (2008) Anti-inflammatory role of endomorphins in osteoarthritis, rheumatoid arthritis, and adjuvant-induced polyarthritis. Arthritis Rheum 58:456–466

Sweetnam PM, Wrathall JR, Neale JH (1986) Localization of dynorphin gene product-immunoreactivity in neurons from spinal cord and dorsal root ganglia. Neuroscience 18:947–955

Szabo I, Chen XH, Xin L, Adler MW, Howard OM, Oppenheim JJ, Rogers TJ (2002) Heterologous desensitization of opioid receptors by chemokines inhibits chemotaxis and enhances the perception of pain. Proc Natl Acad Sci USA 99:10276–10281

Tegeder I, Geisslinger G (2004) Opioids as modulators of cell death and survival–unraveling mechanisms and revealing new indications. Pharmacol Rev 56:351–369

Tegeder I, Meier S, Burian M, Schmidt H, Geisslinger G, Lotsch J (2003) Peripheral opioid analgesia in experimental human pain models. Brain 126:1092–1102
Terman GW, Shavit Y, Lewis JW, Cannon JT, Liebeskind JC (1984) Intrinsic mechanisms of pain inhibition: activation by stress. Science 226:1270–1277
Truong W, Cheng C, Xu QG, Li XQ, Zochodne DW (2003) Mu-opioid receptors and analgesia at the site of a peripheral nerve injury. Ann Neurol 53:366–375
Verma-Gandhu M, Bercik P, Motomura Y, Verdu EF, Khan WI, Blennerhassett PA, Wang L, El-Sharkawy RT, Collins SM (2006) $CD4^+$ T-cell modulation of visceral nociception in mice. Gastroenterology 130:1721–1728
Vetter I, Kapitzke D, Hermanussen S, Monteith GR, Cabot PJ (2006) The effects of *p*H on beta-endorphin and morphine inhibition of calcium transients in dorsal root ganglion neurons. J Pain 7:488–499
Vindrola O, Mayer AMS, Citera G, Spitzer JA, Espinoza LR (1994) Prohormone convertases PC2 and PC3 in rat neutrophils and macrophages. Neuropeptides 27:235–244
von Andrian UH, Mackay CR (2000) T-cell function and migration. Two sides of the same coin. N Engl J Med 343:1020–1034
Walczak JS, Pichette V, Leblond F, Desbiens K, Beaulieu P (2005) Behavioral, pharmacological and molecular characterization of the saphenous nerve partial ligation: a new model of neuropathic pain. Neuroscience 132:1093–1102
Wang H, Wessendorf MW (2001) Equal proportions of small and large DRG neurons express opioid receptor mRNAs. J Comp Neurol 429:590–600
Wang JB, Imai Y, Eppler CM, Gregor P, Spivak CE, Uhl GR (1993) Mu-opiate receptor: cDNA cloning and expression. Proc Natl Acad Sci USA 90:10230–10234
Weihe E, Hartschuh W, Weber E (1985) Prodynorphin opioid peptides in small somatosensory primary afferents of guinea pig. Neurosci Lett 58:347–352
Wenk HN, Honda CN (1999) Immunohistochemical localization of delta-opioid receptors in peripheral tissues. J Comp Neurol 408:567–579
Whistler JL, Enquist J, Marley A, Fong J, Gladher F, Tsuruda P, Murray SR, Von Zastrow M (2002) Modulation of postendocytic sorting of G protein-coupled receptors. Science 297:615–620
Willer JC, Dehen H, Cambier J (1981) Stress-induced analgesia in humans: endogenous opioids and naloxone-reversible depression of pain reflexes. Science 212:689–691
Woolf CJ, Salter MW (2000) Neuronal plasticity: increasing the gain in pain. Science 288: 1765–1769
Yaksh TL (1988) Substance P release from knee joint afferent terminals: modulation by opioids. Brain Res 458:319–324
Zhang Q, Schäfer M, Elde R, Stein C (1998a) Effects of neurotoxins and hindpaw inflammation on opioid receptor immunoreactivities in dorsal root ganglia. Neuroscience 85:281–291
Zhang X, Bao L, Arvidsson U, Elde R, Hökfelt T (1998b) Localization and regulation of the delta-opioid receptor in dorsal root ganglia and spinal cord of the rat and monkey: evidence for association with the membrane of large dense-core vesicles. Neuroscience 82:1225–1242
Zhang X, Bao L, Shi TJ, Ju G, Elde R, Hökfelt T (1998c) Down-regulation of mu-opioid receptors in rat and monkey dorsal root ganglion neurons and spinal cord after peripheral axotomy. Neuroscience 82:223–240
Zhang X, Bao L, Guan JS (2006) Role of delivery and trafficking of delta-opioid peptide receptors in opioid analgesia and tolerance. Trends Pharmacol Sci 27:324–329
Zhou L, Zhang Q, Stein C, Schäfer M (1998) Contribution of opioid receptors on primary afferent versus sympathetic neurons to peripheral opioid analgesia. J Pharmacol Exp Ther 286 (2):1000–1006
Zhu Y, Hsu MS, Pintar JE (1998) Developmental expression of the mu-, kappa-, and delta-opioid receptor mRNAs in mouse. J Neurosci 18:2538–2549
Zöllner C, Stein C (2007) Opioids. Handb Exp Pharmacol 177:31–63

The Pharmacology of Voltage-Gated Sodium Channels in Sensory Neurones

Reginald J. Docherty and Clare E. Farmer

Contents

Abstract Voltage-gated sodium channels (VGSCs) are vital for the normal functioning of most excitable cells. At least nine distinct functional subtypes of VGSCs are recognized, corresponding to nine genes for their pore-forming α-subunits. These have different developmental expression patterns, different tissue distributions in the adult and are differentially regulated at the cellular level by

R.J. Docherty (✉)
Neurorestoration Group, Wolfson CARD, King's College London, London SE1 9RT, UK
reginald.docherty@kcl.ac.uk

B.J. Canning and D. Spina (eds.), *Sensory Nerves*,
Handbook of Experimental Pharmacology 194, DOI: 10.1007/978-3-540-79090-7_15,

receptor-coupled cell signalling systems. Unsurprisingly, VGSC blockers are found to be useful as drugs in diverse clinical applications where excessive excitability of tissue leads to pathological dysfunction, e.g. epilepsy or cardiac tachyarrhythmias. The effects of most clinically useful VGSC blockers are use-dependent, i.e. their efficacy depends on channel activity. In addition, many natural toxins have been discovered that interact with VGSCs in complex ways and they have been used as experimental probes to study the structure and function of the channels and to better understand how drugs interact with the channels. Here we have attempted to summarize the properties of VGSCs in sensory neurones, discuss how they are regulated by cell signalling systems and we have considered briefly current concepts of their physiological function. We discuss in detail how drugs and toxins interact with archetypal VGSCs and where possible consider how they act on VGSCs in peripheral sensory neurones. Increasingly, drugs that block VGSCs are being used as systemic analgesic agents in chronic pain syndromes, but the full potential for VGSC blockers in this indication is yet to be realized and other applications in sensory dysfunction are also possible. Drugs targeting VGSC subtypes in sensory neurones are likely to provide novel systemic analgesics that are tissue-specific and perhaps even disease-specific, providing much-needed novel therapeutic approaches for the relief of chronic pain.

Keywords Voltage-gated sodium channel, Local anaesthetic, Anticonvulsant, Antiarrhythmic, Tetrodotoxin, Pain, Hyperalgesia, Analgesic

Abbreviations

BTX	Batrachotoxin
DRG	Dorsal root ganglion
IFM	Isoleucine, phenylalanine and methionine
MAPK	Mitogen-activated protein kinase
PKA	Protein kinase A
PKC	Protein kinase C
STX	Saxitoxin
TTX	Tetrodotoxin
TTXR	Tetrodotoxin resistant
TTXS	Tetrodotoxin sensitive
VGSC	Voltage-gated sodium channel

1 Introduction

Voltage-gated sodium channels (VGSCs) are expressed throughout the animal kingdom and are vital for the normal function of most excitable cells. Several excellent broad-ranging reviews concerning their structure and function are available (Catterall 2000; Yu and Catterall 2003; Catterall et al. 2005). Some blockers of

VGSCs have been licensed for use as medicines for several decades, while others, as components of natural products, have been in use for centuries. Drugs that target VGSCs and the assay technology used to discover them or to study their effects have been reviewed recently from a medicinal chemistry perspective (Anger et al. 2001; Kyle and Ilyin 2006). The three mainstream categories of clinically useful drugs are antiarrhythmics for the treatment of cardiac dysfunction, anticonvulsants for epilepsy, and local anaesthetics for regional anaesthesia (Catterall 1987; Ragsdale et al. 1996). The boundaries between these categories are vague at best and most clinically used drugs appear in more than one category. As a rule, the classification of a given VGSC blocker reflects its longest-standing or most common use. The usefulness of VGSC blockers as systemic analgesics, especially to treat chronic pain, is now widely recognized (Lai et al. 2004; Wood et al. 2004; Amir et al. 2006; Cummins et al. 2007) and other indications are emerging, such as multiple sclerosis (Waxman 2006; Smith 2007), asthma (Hunt et al. 2004) and even the metastasis of tumour cells (Fraser et al. 2003).

Tissue selectivity of VGSC blockers is a highly desirable therapeutic goal to improve the side-effect profile and clinical efficacy of existing drugs and to target new applications. For example, selective blockers of sensory neurone VGSCs would be expected to provide novel, safe and much needed analgesics for a wide variety of sensory dysfunctions including chronic pain. In this review we describe some current ideas concerning how drugs interact with VGSCs in general and consider how the drugs act on peripheral sensory neurones in particular.

1.1 VGSC Structure

The mammalian neuronal sodium channel consists of a primary α-subunit of approximately 260 kDa associated with one or more β-subunits of 33–36 kDa (Hartshorne and Catterall 1981, 1984; Hartshorne et al. 1984; Messner and Catterall 1985; Morgan et al. 2000; Yu et al. 2003). The α-subunit is composed of four homologous domains (D1-D4) each containing six α-helical transmembrane segments (S1–S6) connected by alternating intracellular and extracellular loops with large intracellular N and C termini (Fig. 1). There are large extracellular loops between S5 and S6 in each domain which dip back into the membrane to form a pore loop (P loop). The short lipophilic stretches that partly penetrate the membrane to form the P loops are termed the "SS1 and SS2 regions". The four domains are connected by three large intracellular loops and are positioned in the membrane with the P loops facing each other forming the extracellular mouth of the ion-conducting pore. The S6 segments from each domain line the intracellular mouth of the pore and form its inner vestibule (Guy and Seetharamulu 1986).

Expression of the α-subunit alone in cells is enough to produce a functional channel (Goldin et al. 1986); however, expression of one or more auxiliary β-subunits appears to be required for appropriate channel expression and normal current gating kinetics. Four β-subunits (β1–β4) have been identified and α-subunits will associate with one of β1 or β3 plus one of β2 or β4 in vivo through

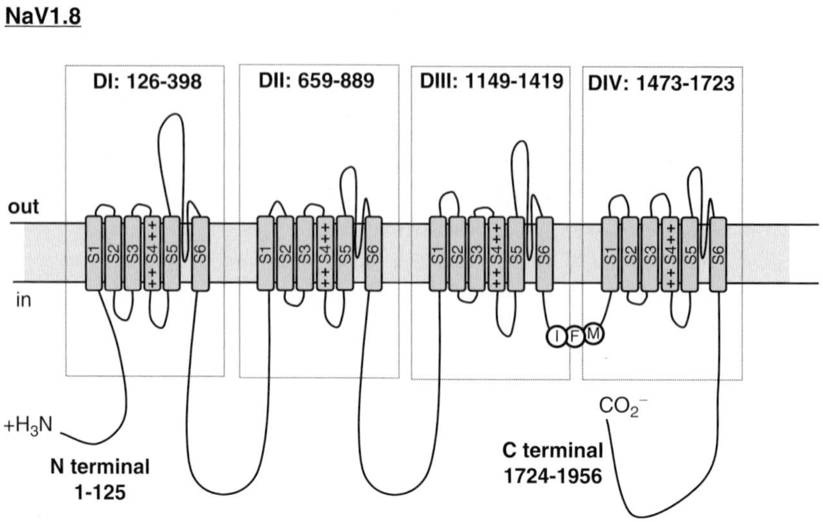

Fig. 1 The α-subunit of a voltage-gated sodium channel (VGSC). The diagram shows the proposed secondary structure of the α-subunit based on the original diagram designed by Noda (1993) for $Na_V1.2$. Each of four domains (designated D1–D4) contains six membrane-spanning α-helical regions (S1–S6) of 19–27 amino acids in length joined by short (four to 19 amino acids) connecting loops. The loop between S5 and S6 in each domain (54–100 amino acids) dips back into the membrane to form the outer pore and selectivity filter. The lipophilic sections of the S5–S6 loop that form the "sides" of the loop, partly traversing the membrane, are referred to as the SS1 and SS2 regions. Positive charges in the S4 regions are highlighted to indicate the proposed voltage-sensing regions and the isoleucine, phenylalanine and methionine motif in the D3–D4 linker, of importance for channel inactivation, is also highlighted. A more complete diagram indicating conserved motifs in the channels can be found in Ekberg and Adams (2006). The amino acid ranges that contribute to the different regions of the protein given here are for $Na_V1.8$

covalent (β2 and β4) or non-covalent (β1 and β3) bonding (Isom et al. 1992, 1995; Morgan et al. 2000; Yu et al. 2003). Cloning of β-subunits revealed a single transmembrane segment with small intracellular and large glycosylated extracellular domains which are thought to act like cell adhesion molecules by binding to extracellular matrix proteins and probably play a role in cell-cell interactions, or in the localization and clustering of the sodium channel protein in the membrane (Yu et al. 2003; Isom et al. 1992, 1995; Srinivasan et al. 1998; Morgan et al. 2000; Ratcliffe et al. 2001; Lai and Jan 2006). All four β-subunits are expressed to varying degrees in sensory neurones (Oh et al. 1995; Yu et al. 2003), with β3 being the dominant subunit expressed in small-diameter neurones (Shah et al. 2000). Limited published information is available concerning the pharmacology of the β-subunits and most known drugs that interact with VGSCs do so by binding to the α-subunit, so it is here that we have focused our attention.

1.2 VGSC Function

The characteristic features underlying VGSC function have been described as selective ion conductance, voltage-dependent activation and subsequent rapid inactivation (Hille 2001). Within the cell membrane, VGSCs typically cycle through three main functional states moving from resting to open to inactivated and then back to a resting state.

Ion selectivity of the VGSC is conferred by the presence of two specific amino acid residues in each domain located in the P loops that form the extracellular mouth of the pore. These residues form negatively charged inner and outer rings that act as an ion-selectivity filter, allowing the positively charged sodium ions to enter the mouth of the pore. Voltage-dependent activation of the VGSC is achieved by voltage sensors located in the highly conserved S4 transmembrane segments. Positively charged amino acid residues located at every third position in these segments are normally stabilized in the membrane by interacting with nearby negatively charged residues. Depolarization produces changes in the transmembrane electric field which release these charges, causing the S4 segments to spiral outwards, generating a conformational change which opens the pore. This process was termed the "sliding helix model" (Catterall 1986) or the "helical screw model" (Guy and Seetharamulu 1986) when first proposed.

Inactivation of VGSCs occurs following activation and opening of the channels and prevents further ion movement through the pore. This allows full repolarization of the action potential to occur during subsequent openings of voltage-gated potassium channels. Inactivation of VGSCs allows the cells to support repetitive action potential firing, with the time course of inactivation contributing to the frequency at which thc neurones can fire. Fast inactivation occurs over milliseconds via a "hinged lid mechanism" where an intracellular portion of the channel protein occludes the pore by binding to a docking region. A critical sequence of three hydrophobic amino acids – isoleucine, phenylalanine and methionine (IFM) – which forms the docking particle has been located on the loop between D3 and D4 (West et al. 1992).

2 Classification, Distribution and Proposed Function of VGSC α-Subunits in Peripheral Sensory Neurones

At present, nine functional VGSC α-subunit isoforms have been described, giving rise to nine sodium channel subtypes termed "$Na_V1.1$–$Na_V1.9$". These channels have specific tissue distributions. All VGSCs except $Na_V1.4$ are found in adult sensory neurones, but most attention in this tissue has focused on $Na_V1.1$, $Na_V1.3$, $Na_V1.6$, $Na_V1.7$, $Na_V1.8$ and $Na_V1.9$. A useful pharmacological distinction between two classes of sodium channel is made using the specific VGSC neurotoxin tetrodotoxin (TTX). The majority of VGSC isoforms are blocked by nanomolar concentrations of TTX and are termed "TTX-sensitive (TTXS) channels". These channels give rise to rapidly activating and inactivating sodium currents (Ikeda et al. 1986; Roy and Narahashi 1992). However, $Na_V1.5$, $Na_V1.8$ and $Na_V1.9$ are relatively resistant to the toxin and produce TTX-resistant (TTXR) currents, of which $Na_V1.8$ typically activates and inactivates slowly (Roy and Narahashi 1992), whereas $Na_V1.9$ appears to produce a persistent TTXR current (Dib-Hajj et al. 2002). The interaction of TTX with the sodium channel will be examined in detail herein.

Several excellent reviews have appeared recently that summarize current knowledge of localization and function of sodium channel subtypes in dorsal root ganglia (DRG) and of plasticity of expression and function, especially in pain states (see, e.g., Lai et al. 2004; Wood et al. 2004; Amir et al. 2006; Cummins et al. 2007). The following is a brief account.

2.1 *Na_V1.1*

Expression of Na_V1.1 messenger RNA has been shown in cells of all sizes in the DRG, with the highest expression in large-diameter cells and a lower expression in small nociceptive somata (Black et al. 1996). The function of the TTXS current that this channel could produce in sensory neurones has not yet been elucidated; however, it is probable that Na_V1.1 will contribute to the production of TTXS action potentials in large-diameter DRG cells.

2.2 *Na_V1.2*

A common sodium channel in rat brain, Na_V1.2 is also expressed in DRG neurones (Felts et al. 1997), but details of its contribution to sensory function are lacking.

2.3 *Na_V1.3*

Na_V1.3 is expressed in fetal neural tissue and at birth its expression is down-regulated (Felts et al. 1997). In the adult brain and in sensory neurones the channel is re-expressed when tissue is injured (Waxman et al. 1994). It is thought to underlie a rapidly repriming (recovers from inactivation quickly) TTXS current and could be an important motor for spontaneous firing of action potentials in damaged neurones and neuromae (Cummins and Waxman 1997). It is therefore an important drug target for neuropathic pain.

2.4 *Na_V1.4*

Skeletal muscle cells express Na_V1.4, but of all of the VGSC channel subtypes this is the least likely to be important for sensory neurone mechanisms.

2.5 *Na_V1.5*

The cardiac VGSC Na_V1.5 is expressed in sensory neurones. Its role in sensation is not defined, but it has been argued that it is expressed in rat DRG neurones and contributes to TTXR current (Renganathan et al. 2002). In the mouse a splice variant, $Na_V1.5a$, may be the dominant form (Kerr et al. 2007).

2.6 $Na_V1.6$

$Na_V1.6$ is the predominant TTXS VGSC subtype found at the nodes of Ranvier of large myelinated sensory fibres where it underlies the upstroke of the action potentials that propagate along the axon by saltatory conduction (Caldwell et al. 2000). It is also found in most large and medium cell bodies in the DRG, with a lower expression in small-diameter cell bodies (Black et al. 1996). Black et al. (2002) have shown expression of $Na_V1.6$ along unmyelinated fibres and have suggested that it contributes to action potential generation in these fibres. $Na_V1.6$ may be a substrate for a persistent TTXS current that can be recorded from DRG neurones (Baker 2000; Rush et al. 2005).

2.7 $Na_V1.7$

Expression of $Na_V1.7$ is widespread in peripheral sensory neurones. It has been shown in all classes of neurone in the DRG but appears more common in the somata of small-diameter nociceptive neurones, where it may be responsible for the majority of TTXS current recorded in these cells (Black et al. 1996; Cummins et al. 2007). One of the biophysical features of $Na_V1.7$ is its ability to produce a slowly inactivating inward current in response to small depolarizations around the membrane potential. As a result of this, $Na_V1.7$ is likely to contribute towards setting the threshold for cell firing. Aside from the cell body, expression is also high in the neurites of nociceptive neurones (Toledo-Aral et al. 1997), located at the peripheral end of the neurone where painful stimuli are detected and, therefore, $Na_V1.7$ is likely to play a major role in the initial transmission of pain signals to the nervous system. Recognition of the role of gain-of-function mutations in $Na_V1.7$ in the aetiology of congenital pain syndromes (Dib-Hajj et al. 2005) and loss-of-function mutations in congenital insensitivity to pain (Cox et al. 2006; Goldberg et al. 2007) has focused special attention on this subtype.

2.8 $Na_V1.8$ and $Na_V1.9$

The TTXR channels $Na_V1.8$ and $Na_V1.9$ are restricted primarily to the cell bodies and terminals of small-diameter nociceptive neurones in the DRG and trigeminal ganglion and consequently are considered to play an important role in nociceptive processing (Padilla et al. 2007; Cummins et al. 2007). Upregulation of expression of both channel types contributes to hyperalgesia in inflammation, but the role of the channels in neuropathic pain states is more controversial. Studies in $Na_V1.8$ knockout mice have suggested that the channel is responsible for the majority of sodium current underlying the initial rapid depolarization of the action potential in these nociceptive cell bodies (Renganathan et al. 2001). The persistent current carried by $Na_V1.9$ is activated close to the resting membrane potential and is likely to be involved in setting the membrane potential and boosting the response to subthreshold inputs in the DRG (Dib-Hajj et al. 2002). Expression of $Na_V1.8$ and $Na_V1.9$ is also seen along the axon in unmyelinated fibres, but their contribution towards action potential generation in these fibres is unclear since TTX normally blocks axonal conduction even in C fibres (Farrag et al. 2002). $Na_V1.8$ is attributed to a role in spike-frequency adaptation whereby the contribution of $Na_V1.8$ to repeated action potentials is diminished by accumulation of slow time-dependent inactivation leading to a progressive reduction in excitability (Blair and Bean 2003) and a similar process may be involved in frequency-dependent regulation of conduction velocity in C fibre terminal axons (De Col et al. 2008). The inactivation properties of $Na_V1.8$ are relatively resistant to change when the neurones are cooled compared with TTXS channel subtypes, which has led to the interesting suggestion that $Na_V1.8$ may help to maintain the excitability of nociceptor terminals at low temperatures, allowing the continuance of the perception of pain sensation in such conditions (Zimmermann et al. 2007).

3 Modulation of VGSCs in Sensory Neurones by Receptor Signalling Systems

VGSCs are subject to modulation by receptors coupled to intracellular signalling systems which primarily act to phosphorylate specific residues on the α-subunit through the action of cytoplasmic protein kinases. The functional effects of phosphorylation appear to depend on both the subtype of channel that is phosphorylated and the cell type containing the channel. The two major protein kinases that have been shown to target the VGSC are protein kinase A (PKA) and protein kinase C (PKC), both of which are activated by G protein mediated second messenger systems. The second messenger pathways involved are common to many G protein coupled receptors, implying that a wide range of compounds, endogenous or otherwise, have the potential to cause phosphorylation of VGSCs via cell signalling systems. The specific amino acid residues that are phosphorylated by PKA and PKC are located primarily on the linker between domains 1 and 2. In rat brain VGSCs, PKA phosphorylates four serine residues at positions 573, 610, 623 and 687 (rat brain nomenclature), whereas PKC phosphorylates serines at positions 554, 573 and 576 as well as serine 1506 in the linker between D3 and D4 which forms the inactivation gate (Murphy et al. 1993; Cantrell et al. 2002).

Agents that activate PKA or PKC in sensory neurones have been shown to cause a general enhancement of sodium channel activity. In acute cultures of DRG neurones, application of hyperalgesic agents such as prostaglandin E_2 (see Fig. 2a), adenosine, and 5-hydroxytryptamine have been shown to increase TTXR current amplitude in a cyclic AMP (cAMP) and PKA dependent manner (England et al. 1996; Gold et al. 1996; Cardenas et al. 2001). Activation of PKA accelerates fast inactivation of TTXR but delays entry into slow inactivated states (Docherty and Farrag 2006). The effect of these hyperalgesic agents on the TTXR current is likely to play an important role in sensitizing nociceptive neurones during inflammatory pain states. In these experiments the likely target for phosphorylation is $Na_V1.8$, which will most likely be responsible for carrying most of the TTXR current recorded. Indeed specific cAMP-mediated phosphorylation of the $Na_V1.8$ channel at amino acid residues on the D1–D2 linker has been shown to produce a similar increase in $Na_V1.8$-mediated current amplitude (Fitzgerald et al. 1999). As well as acute effects, channel expression is also upregulated by inflammatory mediators (Gould et al. 1998). Interestingly, the NSAID ibuprofen has been shown to inhibit this, implicating cyclo-oxygenase products in long-term as well as acute regulation of channel activity (Gould et al. 2004).

As with PKA, activation of PKC in isolated DRG neurones leads to an increase in TTXR sodium current amplitude (Gold et al. 1998). In particular, PKC has been shown to cause an increase in activity of the $Na_V1.9$ VGSC subtype which produces

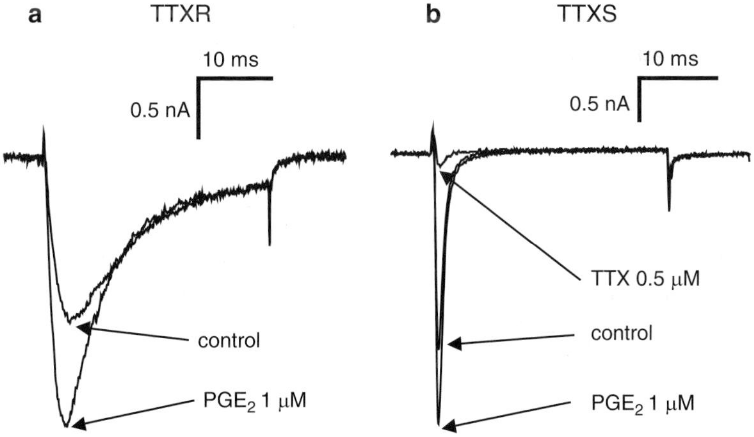

Fig. 2 The effect of prostaglandin E_2 (PGE_2) on VGSC current in voltage-clamped rat dorsal root ganglion neurones. Currents are evoked during 30-ms voltage steps to −10 mV from a holding potential of −90 mV. The recording method is as described in Docherty and Farrag (2006). The increase in current amplitude that occurs about 6 min after application of 1 μM PGE_2 is shown in (**a**) and that which occurs about 3 min after application of 1 μM PGE_2 is shown in **b**. In **a** the currents were recorded in the presence of 0.5 μM tetrodotoxin (TTX) throughout so this is a TTX-resistant current. In (**b**) the currents were identified as TTX-sensitive by their characteristic rapid kinetics and this was confirmed by applying 0.5 μM TTX to the current after it had been enhanced by application of PGE_2

a persistent TTXR current (Baker 2005) that is G protein regulated (Ostman et al. 2008). The actions of these two protein kinases on sensory neuronal VGSCs appear to be somewhat cooperative as an inhibition of PKC activity has been shown to significantly reduce the enhancing effect of PKA on TTXR current in the DRG (Gold et al. 1998). Similarly, in nodose neurones, potentiation of $Na_V1.8$ currents by PKC activation is inhibited by PKA inhibitors and 8-bromo-cAMP appears to act through both PKA and PKC (Matsumoto et al. 2007).

In CNS neurones, phosphorylation by either PKC or PKA inhibits VGSCs (Chahine et al. 2005) perhaps by modulating slow inactivated states (Chen et al. 2006b). These studies imply that the peripheral TTXR and CNS TTXS subtypes are modulated in opposing ways by channel phosphorylation. One might expect that TTXS currents in peripheral sensory neurones would be inhibited by phosphorylation also. Interestingly, 5-hydroxytryptamine , which is an inflammatory mediator, enhances TTXS currents as well as TTXR currents in sensory neurones (Cardenas et al. 2001) and the same is true for prostaglandin E_2 (Fig. 2b). Not only TTXR current (see above) but also TTXS current in DRG neurones is increased by PKA activation and the overall rate of development of slow inactivation is slowed (Docherty and Farrag 2006). Vijayaragavan et al. (2004) have shown that $Na_V1.7$, which is probably the predominant TTXS subtype in small DRG neurones, is inhibited by phosphorylation when heterologously expressed in *Xenopus* oocytes, but $Na_V1.8$ is enhanced in the same expression system, which suggests that modulation is subtype-specific. Conceivably the PKA-mediated enhancement of TTXS currents in DRG is due to a different VGSC subtype. $Na_V1.1$ and $Na_V1.2$ are inhibited by PKA (Li et al. 1992; Smith and Goldin 1996, 1998) and $Na_V1.4$ is not expressed in DRG, so if the PKA effect is subtype-specific presumably $Na_V1.3$ and $Na_V1.6$ are the most likely candidates. On the other hand, Smith and Goldin (2000) have shown that although PKA can inhibit VGSCs by phosphorylating consensus sites in the D1–D2 linker, additional PKA activity (when these sites are already phosphorylated) causes enhancement of activity which has been attributed to an indirect mechanism, i.e. due to phosphorylation of another protein, a mechanism that also occurs in cardiac $Na_V1.5$ channels (Frohnwieser et al. 1995). It is possible that the enhancing effects of phosphorylation on DRG VGSCs are indirect via a similar unidentified protein in DRG (e.g. cytoskeletal proteins or another kinase, see below) that is itself activated by PKA phosphorylation. Several potential protein interactions with $Na_V1.8$ have been identified and discussed (Wood et al. 2004).

Although most research to date has focused on sodium channel phosphorylation by PKA and PKC, other signalling pathways may also be able to acutely modulate sodium channel function. Recent attention has focused on the p38 mitogen activated protein kinase (MAPK) signalling pathway and its acute modulation of sodium channel activity. Activation of p38 MAPK has been shown to phosphorylate the TTXS $Na_V1.6$ channel at a site in the domain 1–2 linker, and this produces a reduction in sodium current density with no effect on the voltage-dependence of activation or inactivation (Wittmack et al. 2005). The p38 MAPK pathway is a common intracellular pathway for many inflammatory cytokines and interestingly application of tumour necrosis factor α onto DRG neurones produced an increase in TTXR sodium currents by a p38 MAPK-dependent mechanism (Jin and Gereau 2006). This sodium channel modulation by tumour necrosis factor-α appears to contribute to hyperexcitability of primary sensory neurones and production of hyperalgesia. Signalling via p38 has been identified as a downstream path for PKC and PKA signalling mechanisms in adipose fibroblasts (Chen et al. 2007), so it may be a good candidate for an indirect mediator of increases of VGSC activity produced by PKA activation in DRG neurones, although this hypothesis is as yet untested.

4 Drugs and Toxins Acting at VGSCs in Sensory Neurones

4.1 Local Anaesthetics

Local anaesthetics, at sufficiently high concentration, block completely the generation and conduction of action potentials in all nerve cells and their axons. When injected close to a nerve of interest they eliminate sensation arising from the territory that the sensory fibres innervate. They do so by binding to and blocking VGSCs in the nerve axons and terminals. To achieve this kind of nerve block, or to anaesthetize an area of skin by infiltration of local anaesthetic into the area, high concentrations are injected locally – about 10–100 mM for lidocaine, which is one of the most widely used drugs. At lower systemic concentrations, about 1–100 μM, lidocaine produces much more subtle effects on excitability and conduction of action potentials. This is especially important in the heart, where local anaesthetics are administered systemically and used clinically to control (but not block) action potential generation and conduction in cardiac tissues to regularize heart rate and rhythm in pathological cardiac arrhythmias. By analogy, relatively low doses of local anaesthetics (or antiarrhythmics, see later) administered systemically have the potential to be used to reduce excitability of peripheral nociceptive sensory neurones, without completely blocking them. Clinical studies have shown that local anaesthetics can be used in this way as an effective treatment for intractable neuropathic pain and although this therapeutic application has considerable merit (McLeane 2007), it is controversial (Carroll 2007). Strangely, although lidocaine has a fairly short plasma half-life, the analgesic effect produced by an intravenous infusion of lidocaine can last for several weeks (McLeane 2007).

Lidocaine is used as a local anaesthetic and antiarrhythmic and can also be used as an anticonvulsant (Sugai 2007), although its use in this application is uncommon. Indeed, it has proconvulsant effects at high systemic concentrations (DeToledo 2000). It has been used widely to study the mechanism of block of VGSCs by local anaesthetics in a variety of tissues. The mechanism has been studied in considerable detail and is complex. It is difficult to analyse the dose-dependence of the effects of lidocaine by conventional pharmacological analyses because of the phenomenon of "use-dependence" (Courtney 1975) whereby the effectiveness of a given concentration of local anaesthetic increases the more the tissue is stimulated (i.e. "used"). This means that lidocaine yields a range of EC_{50} values for block of sodium currents from about 10 μM to 1 mM depending on whether the system is highly active or relatively inactive, respectively. To explain the phenomenon of "use-dependence", Hille (1977) took the concept of "state-dependent" binding that had been developed for potassium channel blockers by Armstrong (1971) and applied it to VGSCs to create an ingenious model that has been widely accepted called the "modulated receptor hypothesis". This model has been tested and reviewed extensively and a good discussion of the details can be found in Hille (2001), and in the recent review by Nau and Wang (2004). Essentially, the model suggests that VGSCs exhibit a specific binding site for local anaesthetics that has an affinity that depends on the state of the channel. As VGSCs cycle through their resting, open and inactivated states during the upstroke of an action potential, the affinity of the local anaesthetic binding site changes such that lidocaine binds more avidly to open and inactivated states. If this cycle is repeated frequently relative to the rate at which lidocaine dissociates from its binding site, there will be an accumulation of blocked channels that manifests itself as a use-dependent blocking action. The binding site for local anaesthetics has been located to the inner mouth of the channel pore (Ragsdale et al. 1994). Here, two key amino acids have been identified, a phenylalanine and a tyrosine, in a highly conserved region of the D4S6 region of the VGSC (F1711 and Y1718 in rat $Na_V1.8$), that are critical for local anaesthetic binding. These are present in equivalent positions in all of the mammalian VGSCs, so the site of local anaesthetic block is likely to be similar in all subtypes, although fine details of the mechanism of block may differ. Apart from these, several other residues have been identified that contribute to the local anaesthetic binding site (for a comprehensive discussion and references see Nau and Wang 2004).

Lidocaine is a weak base ($pK_a = 7.9$) and at physiological pH of 7.4 it exists as a mixture of a predominantly (about 70%) protonated form and a neutral form. It is thought that the neutral form of the local anaesthetics can access the binding site via a hydrophobic pathway, i.e. by passing through the lipid membrane from outside the cell, but the charged form must negotiate a hydrophilic pathway by entering the inner vestibule of the channel pore from the cytosol. Experiments using benzocaine – a hydrophobic analogue of lidocaine that is uncharged – suggest that the binding of the neutral form of lidocaine is of relatively low affinity and probably accounts for the "tonic" block of VGSCs in their resting state. Benzocaine does not show the use-dependent blocking action that is characteristic of lidocaine or similar local anaesthetics that are weak bases (Starmer et al. 1984). By contrast, experiments with QX314 and QX222, where the basic amine group has been quaternized to produce permanently charged analogues of lidocaine, have shown that these compounds must be applied to the cytosolic surface of most VGSCs to be effective and exert virtually no resting or tonic block but they are strongly use-dependent (Narahashi et al. 1972; Strichartz 1973; Hille 1991). Presumably, the intramolecular juxtaposition of the residues involved in binding changes when the channel opens and inactivates in such a way that high affinity binding of the charged form is favoured. QX314 requires channels to be opened and not inactivated to access the local anaesthetic binding site, so it seems that the binding site is also "guarded" by the channel gates, at least for charged local anaesthetics. A "guarded-receptor" hypothesis that complements the modulated-receptor hypothesis but favours the view that access to the receptor rather than an affinity change is the major determinant of state-dependent binding was developed by Starmer et al. (1984). To further complicate matters, if the channel gates close after the drug has bound, the bound drug molecule can become trapped inside the channel (Strichartz 1973). With respect to access to the local anaesthetic binding, site $Na_V1.5$ is an exception to this pattern since QX314 can block this channel – the cardiac subtype – from either side of the membrane (Alpert et al. 1989). Interestingly, a critical residue in the outer mouth of the channel that protects $Na_V1.5$ from block by TTX (C374 in rat $Na_V1.5$, see below) is required to enable the extracellular block of $Na_V1.5$ by QX314 (Sunami et al. 2000), but the equivalent residue in $Na_V1.8$ (S356 in rat) that confers TTX resistance in this channel isoform (see below) does not render the channel sensitive to extracellular QX314 (Leffler et al. 2005; Binshtok et al. 2007). This is important because even though not all the VGSC isoforms have been tested systematically for sensitivity to extracellular QX314, the result implies that the cardiac channel alone exhibits this property.

Apart from the obvious complexity of the binding of local anaesthetics to VGSCs, it remains unclear how conductance block is actually achieved when the local anaesthetic is bound. The local anaesthetic molecule may occlude the channel pore physically or by electrostatic effects or it may stabilize the channel in a non-conducting (inactivated) state or both. Local anaesthetics can change profoundly the voltage-dependence of inactivation and slow the rate of recovery from inactivated states, so it seems certain that this mechanism at least contributes to the reduced conductance (Hille 1991; Nau and Wang 2004). Both fast inactivation (Hille 1991; Nau and Wang 2004) and slower closed-state inactivation (Balser et al. 1996) conformations have been implicated. There is evidence that local anaesthetic block is severely compromised in mutant channels that have been made inactivation-deficient by mutation of the IFM motif of the D3–D4 linker region of the molecule that is responsible for fast inactivation (Bennett et al. 1995). In these mutant channels the lack of fast inactivation has been used to reveal an open-channel blocking mechanism (Wang et al. 1987, 2004; Grant et al. 2000). This open-channel block may involve an electrostatic repulsion of Na^+ ions (Lipkind and Fozzard 2005; McNulty et al. 2007; Ahern et al. 2008). Recently, Armstrong (2007) proposed a model of VGSC function that suggests that closed-state inactivation requires that the S4 voltage sensor regions of D3 and D4 are in the "activated" position (with additional movement of D1S4 and D2S4 being required for opening), the conformations of which are stabilized by lidocaine (Sheets and Hanck 2007), thus linking conformational changes associated with activation to closed-state inactivation and lidocaine binding. The rates of association and dissociation of individual compounds to the local anaesthetic binding site relative to the kinetics of state transitions in the channel may have an impact on the details of the blocking mechanism for a given compound (Grant et al. 2000), e.g. whether stabilization of fast or slow inactivated states or open- or closed-channel block dominates. Thus, despite the emergence of a common molecular model it may not be possible to generalize across all local anaesthetic compounds and channel isoforms with respect to the fine details of channel block.

There is some evidence that selectivity of action of drugs acting at the local anaesthetic binding site is possible between sodium channel isoforms in sensory neurones. A range of EC_{50} values for lidocaine from about 100 to 1,300 μM has been reported for TTXR (potentially comprising $Na_V1.8$ and $Na_V1.9$) currents (Roy and Narahashi 1992; Brau and Elliott 1998; Brau et al. 2001; Scholz et al. 1998; Gold and Thut 2001; Weiser 2006; Docherty and Farrag 2006). An even wider range of EC_{50} values from about 10 to 1,000 μM are reported for the sensitivity of TTXS currents (potentially comprising $Na_V1.1$, $Na_V1.2$, $Na_V1.3$, $Na_V1.6$ and $Na_V1.7$) to lidocaine (Brau et al. 2001; Roy and Narahashi 1992; Brau and Elliott 1998; Scholz et al. 1998; Gold and Thut 2001; Weiser 2006; Docherty and Farrag 2006). There is also evidence for a persistent current in large sensory neurones that is relatively sensitive to lidocaine (Baker 2000). Since both TTXS and TTXR VGSCs show plasticity of expression in sensory neurones (Lai et al. 2004; Rush et al. 2007) it could be that cell preparation and culture conditions in different laboratories, which necessarily involve damage to the tissue, have resulted in different "mixes" of channel isoforms in their preparations and this underlies the differences in sensitivity of currents to lidocaine (and presumably to other local anaesthetics). Despite the reported differences in lidocaine sensitivity of some isoforms (Chevrier et al. 2004), this is probably an optimistic view. It is more likely that the differences are due to differences in experimental recording conditions. For example, lidocaine sensitivity is proportional to extracellular Na^+ concentration, which is often reduced in voltage-clamp experiments to a variable extent (see the discussion by Weiser 2006) and, although bound lidocaine cannot be protonated from the cytoplasm (Hille 2001), the intracellular pH will nevertheless affect the relative proportion of neutral to protonated lidocaine in the cytoplasm, and this too varies. Even quite small changes in holding potential may change the level of resting closed state inactivation, which will have a profound effect on lidocaine sensitivity – especially for TTXS currents, which have a more negative voltage-dependence for closed-state inactivation (Docherty and Farrag 2006). PKA-induced phosphorylation causes a modest increase in lidocaine sensitivity of TTXR in situ (Docherty et al. 2006), which may also introduce a variable. Leffler et al. (2007) have shown that differences in the sensitivity to lidocaine between TTXS currents and the $Na_V1.8$ TTXR isoform are largely due to differences in state-dependent binding rather than due to differences in the local anaesthetic binding site per se. Interestingly, Sheets and Hanck (2007) have shown that mutations of human $Na_V1.7$ associated with erythromelalgia leads to a reduced sensitivity to lidocaine when the mutation occurs within the local anaesthetic binding region, but not otherwise, predicting genotype-specific lidocaine resistance.

At first sight, QX314 and other charged analogues of lidocaine cannot be used to target sensory neurones since they cannot access the local anaesthetic binding site from the extracellular space (except in the heart, see earlier). This view has been overturned recently. Lim et al. (2007) demonstrated very convincingly that QX314 provoked a long-lasting local anaesthetic effect in vivo using a range of animal models of pain. Binshtok et al. (2007) also demonstrated analgesic effects of QX314 but they took a different approach by using capsaicin to provide a nociceptor-specific portal for entry of QX314 into the cytosol of sensory neurones. TRPV1, the capsaicin-activated non-specific cation channel has a pore that can accommodate a molecule as large as QX314 and allow it to enter cells. Binshtok et al. (2007) showed that a combination of capsaicin with QX314 provokes a nociceptor-specific block of VGSCs that results in analgesia. Since TRPV1 activity is implicated in the cause of some chronic inflammatory and neuropathic pain syndromes (Szallasi et al. 2006), it may even be possible to use QX314 or similar analogues to treat such conditions, as Lim et al. (2007) have done, without the need for concomitant application of a TRPV1 agonist since TRPV1 channels would presumably be spontaneously active. This opens a whole new approach to the use of local anaesthetics to treat chronic pain. Weak bases such as lidocaine are predominantly charged at low pH and they are thought to be ineffective in inflammatory conditions where extracellular pH is low because the charged protonated species cannot enter the cell and reach the high-affinity binding site via the cytosol (see above). Where TRPV1 is active, as is the case in some forms of chronic pain, this restriction may no longer apply and this could explain why low systemic concentrations of lidocaine are effective in some forms of chronic pain. If charged lidocaine (or QX314) becomes trapped in the cells, it may also explain why the effect of lidocaine in these cases outlasts its availability in the plasma (McLeane 2007).

4.2 *Antiarrhythmic Drugs*

Antiarrhythmic drugs are used clinically for the treatment of cardiac arrhythmias which are caused by abnormal electrical activity in the heart. Class I antiarrhythmics target the TTXR cardiac VGSC ($Na_V1.5$), where they produce inhibition of the channel. This typically acts to slow the rate of depolarization during the initial upstroke of the action potential in the cardiac muscle cell, which has the effect of reducing excitability in the heart. The drugs found in this class of antiarrhythmics all display state-dependent binding, a phenomenon described earlier for the actions of local anaesthetics, where drugs bind preferentially to a particular functional state of the sodium channel, usually the open or inactivated state. As a result of this, class I antiarrhythmics display use-dependent inhibition of VGSCs whereby drug binding accumulates during high-frequency activity such as that which occurs during tachyarrhythmias, but normal heart activity is relatively unaffected. Paradoxically, because class I drugs affect conduction pathways in the heart, they and other VGSC blockers all have the potential to provoke arrhythmias in normal cardiac tissue, which is a significant problem for drug development in other applications such as anticonvulsant therapy or analgesia. Class I antiarrhythmics are further classified into three subclasses – Ia, Ib and Ic – depending on the speed of their binding kinetics. The rate of binding to the sodium channel, and subsequently dissociating from it, is fast for class Ib drugs, slow for class Ic drugs and intermediate for class Ia drugs.

4.2.1 Class Ia

Quinidine, procainamide and disopyramide are examples of class Ia antiarrhythmics. These drugs all inhibit sodium channels through an open-channel block whereby they bind to the channel pore whilst it is in the open, activated state and prevent the passage of sodium ions through the channel.

4.2.2 Class Ib

The prototypical class Ib antiarrhythmic is lidocaine, but other common drugs in this class include mexiletine and tocainide, which have longer-lasting effects and are orally available. The molecular mechanism is essentially the same as for lidocaine discussed earlier.

4.2.3 Class Ic

The most common class Ic antiarrhythmic is flecainide, but this group also includes propafenone. These drugs act in a manner similar to the class Ia drugs, inhibiting the sodium channel through an open-channel block. Class Ic drugs have a particular propensity to provoke proarrhythmic effects, which restricts their usefulness (Pratt and Moye 1990).

For all subclasses of class I antiarrhythmics the binding site on the sodium channel is located on the intracellular side of the pore, and, similarly to local anaesthetics, the drugs must access it through either a hydrophilic pathway, e.g. the channel pore, or a hydrophobic membrane-delimited pathway (see earlier). Although the class Ib drugs bind to the local anaesthetic receptor described previously, it is likely that the binding site for the class Ia and Ic drugs overlaps with this (Ragsdale et al. 1996). Indeed the two amino acid residues that are critical for lidocaine binding (see earlier) have been shown to be important for block by several class I antiarrhythmic agents of different subclasses. Additionally, residues in the sodium channel selectivity filter located on the extracellular side of the pore are thought to be important in controlling access of antiarrhythmic drugs to the intracellular binding site of $Na_V1.5$ (Sasaki et al. 2004).

Owing to their known blockade of cardiac sodium channels, and the high level of homology between sodium channel α-subunits, it is not surprising that class I antiarrhythmics also target VGSCs in sensory neurones. Consequently, some of the class I agents apart from lidocaine may be useful as treatments for peripheral neuropathic pain syndromes (Chabal et al. 1989; Challapalli et al. 2005). The use-dependence of the drugs is likely to be especially important when treating neuropathic pain, as it should allow them to potently inhibit the hyperexcitability of sensory neurones that underlies the pain while sparing normal sensation. Mexiletine and flecainide are probably the best-studied examples in this context and are discussed in the following sections. In addition, a recent study by Tzeng et al. (2007) has shown a local-anaesthetic-type action of quinidine, mexiletine and flecainide following localized injections.

4.2.4 Mexiletine

In small DRG neurones, application of the VGSC opener veratridine causes depolarization and subsequent release of substance P. Mexiletine has been shown to prevent this release of substance P, suggesting it will block sodium channels in the DRG (Akada et al. 2006). More specifically, mexiletine has been shown to block TTXR sodium currents recorded in small rat DRG neurones in a tonic and use-dependent manner (Brau et al. 2001; Weiser 2006), and will also block TTXR current passing through human $Na_V1.8$ channels expressed in a neuroblastoma cell line (Dekker et al. 2005). However, it should be noted that blockade is not restricted to TTXR channels, as blockade of TTXS channels has also been shown (Weiser 2006; Ragsdale et al. 1996).

The efficacy of mexiletine has been tested in several animal models of neuropathic pain where it can reduce behavioural hyperalgesia and allodynia. Following a chronic constriction injury in the rat, systemic mexiletine has been shown to suppress spontaneous firing and burst firing in peripheral sensory nerve without affecting normal conduction (Nakamura and Atsuta 2005). Mexiletine can also inhibit sensory neuronal-mediated reflex responses to noxious bladder distension in the rat (Su et al. 2007). In humans, mexiletine has been useful clinically as a treatment for painful diabetic neuropathy, usually when standard treatments such as tricyclic antidepressants have proved ineffective or to be poorly tolerated (Jarvis and Coukell 1998). Painful diabetic neuropathy is a complication of diabetes where peripheral nerves can become damaged, leading to symptoms of sensory dysfunction including neuropathic pain. The sodium channel blocking ability of mexiletine can provide relief by suppressing pathological spontaneous firing and elevated neuronal excitability in peripheral sensory neurones. However, mexiletine is a CNS penetrant drug and it is probable that effects on sodium channels in both the CNS and the peripheral nervous system contribute to its analgesic effect.

4.2.5 Flecainide

The class Ic agent flecainide has also been shown to block sensory neuronal sodium channels. Recent clinical trials support its use as an analgesic (Von Gunten et al. 2007). When applied to small DRG neurones, flecainide produced a tonic and use-dependent inhibition of TTXR sodium currents (Osawa et al. 2004). Work in our laboratory has also shown that flecainide will produce a tonic and use-dependent block of peripheral sensory nerve compound action potentials in both large myelinated mechanosensory A fibres and small unmyelinated nociceptive C fibres (Fig. 3). The sodium channels underlying the A fibre action potentials will be of the TTXS subtype and so it is clear that flecainide can inhibit both TTXR and TTXS sodium channel subtypes in sensory neurones. Animal and human clinical studies have also suggested a potential analgesic effect of flecainide in neuropathic pain syndromes (Dunlop et al. 1988; Ichimata et al. 2001a, b). For example, intravenous administration of flecainide to rats following a chronic constriction injury of the sciatic nerve suppressed ectopic firing in peripheral neurones and also reduced behavioural signs of neuropathic pain (Ichimata et al. 2001a). However, the use of class Ic antiarrhythmics in humans carries additional clinical issues as a consequence of results obtained from the cardiac arrhythmia suppression trial. This

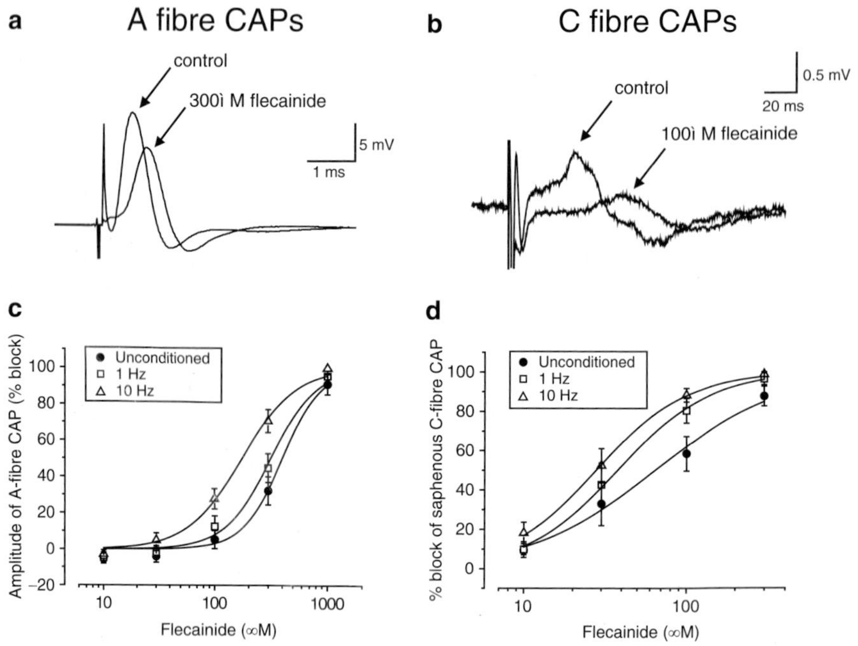

Fig. 3 The effect of flecainide on sensory nerve compound action potential conduction in the rat. The effect of extracellular application of flecainide on the conduction of saphenous nerve compound action potentials in the rat was measured using an in vitro grease-gap recording method (Docherty et al. 2005). Flecainide produced a tonic block of both (**a**) the A fibre and (**b**) the C fibre compound action potentials. The graphs show dose-response curves for the inhibitory effect of flecainide in (**c**) A fibres and (**d**) C fibres with the unconditioned data set representing tonic inhibition. After trains of impulses had been applied to the nerve at 1 and 10 Hz, the potency of flecainide inhibition was increased, as shown by the leftward shift in the dose response curves in **c** and **d**. The data clearly highlight the use-dependent action of the open-channel blocker flecainide

clinical trial revealed a fatally proarrhythmic effect of encainide and flecainide in humans compared with a placebo (Pratt and Moye 1990).

4.3 Anticonvulsants

Blockade of VGSCs is an effective method of suppressing the abnormal neuronal activity underlying epileptic seizures, making sodium channel blockers a useful therapeutic tool in many forms of epilepsy. Commonly used anticonvulsants include phenytoin, carbamazepine, lamotrigine and valproate, and these drugs typically display potent voltage- and use-dependent activities at the VGSC which allow them to target the high frequency activity or long depolarizations that are associated with seizures, without affecting normal brain function. However, these drugs have increasingly been used in the treatment of other pathological conditions where suppression of neuronal excitability is beneficial, most notably in neuropathic pain which arises from injury to sensory nerves (Rogawski and Löscher 2004). Indeed carbamazepine, one of the most commonly used anticonvulsants, was originally developed to treat the neuropathic pain condition trigeminal neuralgia, and still remains the first line treatment for the condition (Spina and Perugi 2004).

The target for several of these anticonvulsant drugs was shown to be the VGSC by the use of batrachotoxin (BTX)-displacement assays (Willow and Catterall 1982; Willow et al. 1985; Cheung et al. 1992). The effective displacement of BTX suggested that the anticonvulsant binding site was likely to be at, or very close to, the "site 2" toxin binding site (see later). It is now known that anticonvulsant drugs target a common receptor site on the VGSC (Kuo 1998) and they bind to the channel in a manner similar to local anaesthetics, which themselves bind with some overlap to the "site 2" receptor (Nau and Wang 2004). Anticonvulsants show state-dependent binding whereby they preferentially bind to the inactivated state of the sodium channel and this feature contributes towards their voltage- and use-dependent activities. Amino acid residues in the S6 segments of domains 3 and 4 that have been proven to be important for local anaesthetic binding are also required for anticonvulsant binding (Ragsdale et al. 1996; Yarov-Yarovoy et al. 2001), and Liu et al. (2003) further identified residues in D4S6 which seem to be required for the binding of lamotrigine.

Binding of anticonvulsant drugs stabilizes the VGSC in the inactivated state and subsequently reduces the number of channels that are available for activation. Electrophysiologically, VGSCs blocked by anticonvulsants show reduced current sizes, a hyperpolarizing shift in the voltage-dependence of inactivation and a slowed recovery from inactivation (Lang et al. 1993; Kuo and Lu 1997; Ragsdale et al. 1991; Matsuki et al. 1984). However, compared with local anaesthetics, anticonvulsants tend to show slower onset rates of binding and this is particularly true for phenytoin (Kuo and Bean 1994). A slow binding rate means that long depolarizations (that can be observed during seizure activity) will be selectively targeted by anticonvulsants, as depolarizations associated with normal brain function are likely to be too brief to allow significant drug binding. The slow rate of antiepileptic unbinding relative to the recovery of the VGSC from inactivation underlies their use-dependent activity.

4.3.1 Anticonvulsants and Neuropathic Pain

It may be unsurprising that anticonvulsant drugs are also effective in the treatment of neuropathic pain as characteristic features of neuropathic pain are hyperexcitable neurones and the production of spontaneous ectopic firing –electrical events not dissimilar to those occurring in the brain in epilepsy. In addition, sufferers of neuropathic pain frequently respond poorly to conventional opioid or NSAID treatments, making the use of anticonvulsants particularly valuable. As mentioned previously, one of the primary uses of anticonvulsants is in the treatment of trigeminal neuralgia, where carbamazepine has been used since the 1960s, although other anticonvulsants also show some efficacy in this condition (Rogawski and Löscher 2004). A comprehensive review of the effects of anticonvulsants in the treatment of neuropathic pain has recently been provided by Eisenberg et al. (2007); however, the clinical usefulness of lamotrigine in neuropathic pain conditions has also recently been challenged (Wiffen and Rees 2007). It is worth considering that, although suppression of ectopic firing is a valuable mechanism for the treatment of both epilepsy and neuropathic pain, an important downstream effect of the sodium channel blockade caused by anticonvulsants may be suppression of excitatory neurotransmitter release, which would help to further dampen transmission of electrical impulses.

It is likely that the analgesic properties of anticonvulsants arise from actions at both central and peripheral sites. Given their efficacy in epilepsy, the drugs are obviously CNS-penetrant and can act on the TTXS VGSC subtypes found centrally. Indeed lamotrigine has been shown to act at the level of the dorsal horn to suppress nociceptive signalling (Blackburn-Munro and Fleetwood-Walker 1997). However, anticonvulsants can also act directly on the cell bodies and axons of primary sensory neurones. Phenytoin and carbamazepine will block both TTXS and TTXR currents in DRG neurones (Song et al. 1996; Rush and Elliott 1997; Cardenas et al. 2006), although it has been suggested that TTXR blockade by carbamazepine only occurs at concentrations that are higher than those clinically effective (Brau et al. 2001). A new analogue of phenytoin – α-hydroxyphenylamide – has been shown to block TTXS and TTXR sodium currents in small DRG neurones from the rat with a higher potency than phenytoin itself. This compound also produced an antihyperalgesic action following a chronic constriction injury to the sciatic nerve in the rat with a marked reduction in side effects when compared with phenytoin (Ko et al. 2006). Action potentials recorded in peripheral sensory neurones can also be inhibited by anticonvulsants – both electrically stimulated impulses and ectopic firing as a result of nerve injury (Schwarz and Grigat 1989; Guven et al. 2006; Ritter et al. 2007). Ectopic firing is commonly observed in neuropathic pain syndromes and significantly contributes to the production of pain (Devor 2006) and consequently it is an important pharmacological target. Anticonvulsants can also act as local analgesic agents at the peripheral terminals of nociceptive neurones. Direct injection of phenytoin or carbamazepine into the paw of a rat has been shown to increase the length of time a noxious thermal insult can be applied to the paw, interestingly at doses that are several orders of magnitude lower than that of the local anaesthetic agent lidocaine (Todorovic et al. 2003).

4.3.2 Anticonvulsants and Persistent Sodium Current

In addition to effects on transient sodium currents, anticonvulsants have also been shown to block persistent sodium currents in CNS neurones at therapeutic concentrations, and may selectively target the persistent current fraction (Segal and Douglas 1997; Gebhardt et al. 2001; Taverna et al. 1998; Sun et al. 2007). Although this is thought to provide benefit in epilepsy by suppressing repetitive firing, it could potentially be a beneficial property in the treatment of neuropathic pain. The sodium channel subtype $Na_V1.9$ is localized to nociceptive neurones and produces a non-inactivating TTXR sodium current (Dib-Hajj et al. 2002) which could be a target for antiepileptic drugs. In addition, carbamazepine and topiramate have been shown to inhibit the persistent sodium current observed following expression of $Na_V1.3$ sodium channels in human embryonic kidney cells (Sun et al. 2007). The $Na_V1.3$ subtype is particularly of interest as it is upregulated in peripheral sensory neurones in several different animal models of nerve injury that produce neuropathic pain (Black et al. 1999; Kim et al. 2001; Lindia et al. 2005). At present an increased persistent current in peripheral sensory neurones attributable to $Na_V1.3$ has not been reported in these models but, interestingly, following spinal cord injury a non-inactivating current is observed in second-order nociceptive neurones in the dorsal horn that is postulated to be due to increased $Na_V1.3$ expression (Lampert et al. 2006).

4.4 Toxins and Related Drugs

Catterall has produced a classification of six toxin binding sites on VGSCs that has provided an invaluable framework for studying the pharmacological properties of the channels in relation to their structure and function (Cestele and Catterall 2000). The TTX binding site "site 1" and the BTX binding site "site 2" are the most extensively studied. Other major classes of toxins that have been shown to associate with distinct binding sites on VGSCs are the α-toxins of scorpion venom, some sea anemone toxins and spider toxins (peptides acting at "site 3"), the β-scorpion toxins (peptides acting at "site 4"), brevetoxins and ciguatoxins ("site 5") and δ-conotoxins ("site 6"). An extended classification has been suggested (Zlotkin 1999; Anger et al. 2001) to include the natural pyrethroid insecticides and DDT analogues ("site 7"), *Conus striatus* toxin and *Goniopora* coral toxin (peptides acting at "site 8") and the local anaesthetic binding site ("site 9"). Many other natural toxins and synthetic compounds are known to affect VGSC activity, but their binding sites in relation to this scheme have not yet been established definitively.

4.4.1 "Site 1" Toxins: TTX and Saxitoxin

The neurotoxins that bind to "site 1" are the structurally related compounds TTX and saxitoxin (STX), as well as the peptide μ-conotoxins. These toxins produce a highly specific block of VGSCs.

TTX has been used widely as an experimental tool for the classification of VGSCs, particularly those found in sensory neurones (see earlier). TTX is produced by bacteria that are symbiotic partners to a wide variety of organisms but is found most famously in fish of the *Tetraodon* family (puffer fish), where it is concentrated in the liver, ovaries, intestines and skin. STX is produced by certain marine dinoflagellates (algae) but is often found concentrated in shellfish which feed on the algae and, as a consequence, it is the primary toxin responsible for paralytic shellfish poisoning. TTX and STX are structurally distinct molecules (Anger et al. 2001) but produce a remarkably similar inhibition of sodium channels as they share some common features known to be important for binding to the VGSC. Specifically, they both contain at least one guanidinium group (three nitrogens surrounding a central carbon), which is positively charged at physiological pH and they both also contain several hydroxyl (–OH) groups.

The neurotoxin binding "site 1" is located within the extracellular pore of the VGSC and is composed of two rings of predominantly negatively charged amino acids. The positively charged guanidinium ions of the toxins are attracted to these negative residues and form an electrostatic interaction with them which has the effect of "plugging" the channel. The toxin can be stabilized by formation of hydrogen bonds between its hydroxyl groups and oxygens found in the pore of the channel (Hille 1975; Lipkind and Fozzard 1994; Choudhary et al. 2003; Scheib et al. 2006). In contrast to the local anaesthetics, antiarrhythmics and anticonvulsants described earlier, TTX or STX can access its binding site on the VGSC directly from the extracellular side and binding is less dependent on channel gating, thus it can block resting, open and inactivated sodium channels. However, in a manner similar to state-dependent drugs, a use-dependent mechanism of action of TTX and STX has been demonstrated (Lönnendonker 1994). Two separate theories exist as to the mechanism underlying this feature of the neurotoxins. Firstly, the presence of a low-affinity and a high-affinity TTX binding site has been postulated, with the increased affinity arising through a conformational change associated with channel activation (Patton and Goldin 1991). The second theory, which can reportedly also account for all the biophysical properties of the first theory, is the trapped ion mechanism (Salgado et al. 1986; Conti et al. 1996). Under this scheme, cations present in the extracellular solution can enter the pore of the resting channel and become trapped, which has the effect of inhibiting toxin binding through electrostatic repulsion. The opening of channels allows the cations to escape into the intracellular space, and therefore permits stronger toxin binding, which can then accumulate over successive channel openings. Thus, in this model the affinity of the binding site is not altered with channel gating.

The specific residues that form the two rings of the binding site were identified by mutagenesis studies (Terlau et al. 1991) and shown to reside in the SS2 regions of the four sodium channel domains. Within each SS2 linker there were two critical residues, located at the same position in each domain and mainly negatively charged, which were proposed to form an inner and an outer ring in the channel pore. For the rat brain sodium channel ($Na_V1.2$) the inner ring comprises residues D384 in domain 1, E942 in domain 2, K1422 in domain 3 and A1714 in domain 4 (DEKA motif). The respective residues making up the outer ring are E387, E945, D1426 and D1717. Interestingly, reducing the negative charge of these rings not only affected toxin binding but also produced a reduction in single-channel conductance, thus suggesting that cation selectivity of the channel was also affected (Terlau et al. 1991). Indeed it is now well established that these two rings of amino acids comprise the ion selectivity filter of the VGSC, and TTX has been a vital tool in probing this region of the channel.

Although TTX and STX are highly specific sodium channel blockers, the concentration required for block differs across the various VGSC subtypes. As described, the nine VGSC subtypes can be classified into two groups by their sensitivity to TTX, with blocking concentrations being in the nanomolar range for the TTXS channels ($Na_V1.1$, $Na_V1.2$, $Na_V1.3$, $Na_V1.4$, $Na_V1.6$ and $Na_V1.7$) and in the micromolar range for the TTXR channels ($Na_V1.5$, $Na_V1.8$ and $Na_V1.9$). The structural determinant of TTX resistance has been located as a single amino acid residue found directly adjacent to the inner-ring residue in domain I. In TTXS channels this residue is a tyrosine or phenylalanine, but in TTXR channels it is a cysteine or serine (Sivilotti et al. 1997; Heinemann et al. 1992; Satin et al. 1992). However, it is unclear at present how this residue interacts with TTX to determine its blocking ability. One distinguishing structural feature between the two classes is that tyrosine and phenylalanine residues contain aromatic ring structures in their side chains which are not present in serine or cysteine residues. Various interactions between TTX and these residues have been proposed which include the formation of hydrogen bonds between the guanidinium group and tyrosine in $Na_V1.4$ (Satin et al. 1992), hydrophobic interactions between tyrosine or phenylalanine and a non-polar region of the TTX molecule (Lipkind and Fozzard 1994; Sivilotti et al. 1997) or, more recently, steric interactions between the TTX guanidinium group, the critical residue of domain 1 and a second residue in domain 2 (Scheib et al. 2006).

These toxins are particularly useful for studying peripheral sensory neurones which contain both TTXS and TTXR subtypes in specific distributions. The neuronal TTXR subtypes ($Na_V1.8$ and $Na_V1.9$) are localized largely to nociceptive C fibres and their associated small-diameter cell bodies in the DRG, trigeminal and nodose ganglia and consequently they play an important role in the transmission of nociceptive signals (Cummins et al. 2007). The activity of these channels can be studied in isolation from the TTXS subtypes that are coexpressed in nociceptive neurones by application of concentrations of TTX which block TTXS channels but not TTXR channels. Axonal conduction in the purely TTXS-containing Aβ fibres, which transmit mechanosensory information, can be inhibited at low concentrations of TTX, whereas conduction in C fibres is more resistant (Farrag et al. 2002). Owing to their role in pain processing, the TTXR channels are an attractive target for novel analgesic therapies, and much effort is being employed to try and discover clinically effective TTXR-specific pharmacological agents (see later).

4.4.2 "Site 1" Toxins: μ-Conotoxins

μ-Conotoxins are short peptides, around 22 amino acids in length, which have been isolated from the venom of various types of cone snail (Ekberg et al. 2008). They contain several residues that are positively charged at physiological pH and which are important for the attraction of the peptide to the negatively charged residues of the selectivity filter. In particular, they have a conserved arginine at position 13 or 14 which provides a guanidinium group, and it is this residue which appears to be most critical for channel block (Sato et al. 1991; Becker et al. 1992; Shon et al. 1998; Hui et al. 2002; Keizer et al. 2003). Blockade of sodium current through the channel is thought to be achieved by a combination of physical occlusion of the pore with electrostatic repulsion of the cation by the positive charges of the toxin molecule (Hui et al. 2002). These toxins are much larger than TTX and STX and while they interact at binding site 1, they are also likely to interact at other positions in the sodium channel. Residues that are important for TTX resistance in the VGSC appear not to be involved in the action of the μ-conotoxins, suggesting their site of action overlaps with that of TTX, rather than matching it exactly (Stephan et al. 1994).

At least 12 different μ-conotoxins have been described to date, but as cone snail venoms contain hundreds of different peptides it is likely that more will be identified. They appear to show some subtype selectivity towards VGSCs that does not follow that seen with TTX and STX. For example, one group of μ-conotoxins, which includes GIIIA, GIIIB and GIIIC, are highly effective blockers of the skeletal muscle sodium channel $Na_V1.4$ (Ekberg et al. 2008). However, and of particular interest to this review, several of the μ-conotoxins, including SmIIIA, SIIIA and KIIIA, are selective inhibitors of TTXR VGSCs. To date, most of these studies on isoform-specificity of μ-conotoxins have been performed in amphibious preparations (mainly frog tissue); however, Wang et al. (2006) have shown that the μ-conotoxin SIIIA is able to block TTXR sodium currents in rat DRG neurones with little effect on TTXS currents. The actions of KIIIA were examined in a mammalian system by Zhang et al. (2007), who found that, contrary to the results observed in the frog, KIIIA inhibited TTXS VGSCs to a greater extent than TTXR VGSCs in mouse DRG neurones. Administration of KIIIA also provided analgesic properties in the formalin model of inflammatory pain, presumably as a result of its VGSC inhibition (Zhang et al. 2007). At the amino acid level, the basis of the isoform-specificity of μ-conotoxins is thought to be related to specific residues in the S5–S6 linker in D2 of the VGSC as well as differences in toxin structure and composition (Li et al. 2003). The actions of μ-conotoxins on mammalian sodium channels are of current interest and could become clinically useful, particularly if non-toxic subtype-specific blockers of TTXR sodium channels could be identified.

4.4.3 "Site 2" Toxins

The "site 2" toxins are characterized by a common binding locus on VGSCs (Cestele and Catterall 2000). They are a chemically diverse group of compounds that include BTX from the poison dart frog and grayanotoxin, veratridine and aconitine, which are derived from various plants. All of the compounds are reputed to increase activity of VGSCs and they are often described as sodium channel "agonists". Estimates of potency vary widely according to the species, preparation and assay, but in general BTX is by far the most potent, having an EC_{50} or K_d in the submicromolar range, with grayanotoxin, veratridine and aconitine having EC_{50} or K_d usually in the 10–100-μM range (Ulbricht 1998). Concoctions that contain type II toxins have been used as poisons for millennia but they may also have medicinal uses. Extracts of *Liliaceae* (false hellebore) and aconite (wolfsbane, monkshood) containing, respectively, veratridine and aconitine are described in nineteenth century materia medica texts as anodynes for use in neuralgia – aconitine in particular is credited with powerful analgesic properties (Craig 1887). Topically applied BTX provokes numbness that has been attributed to a depolarizing block of action potential conduction in peripheral sensory neurones (Bosmans et al. 2004) and veratridine has been shown to cause a use-dependent block of action potential conduction that is moderately selective for C fibres (Schneider et al. 1991). Whatever the mechanism, the therapeutic use of the compounds has fallen into decline, presumably because they have many dangerous side effects, including cardiotoxicity. In recent, more enlightened, times the "site 2" toxins have been exploited as molecular probes for studying VGSCs (Ulbricht 1998; Cestele and Catterall 2000; Wang and Wang 2003). As for the local anaesthetics described above, most of the detailed information concerning the molecular biology of the binding determinants for the type II toxins and the biophysics of their functional interaction with the receptor comes from studies on VGSCs in excitable cells other than sensory neurones (Hille 2001; Wang and Wang 2003). The "site 2" toxins share a binding locus in the inner vestibule of VGSCs that overlaps partly with the local anaesthetic binding site (Wang and Wang 2003; Wang et al. 2007) and might also overlap with the receptor for the IFM motif of the inactivation particle of the D3–D4 linker (Narahashi 1986; Ghatpande et al. 1997). The site of this inactivation docking receptor probably incorporates residues at the intracellular extremes of D1S6, D2S6 and D4S6 (Yarov-Yarovoy et al. 2002). Since the compounds are lipophilic, they would be expected to approach their binding locus via the lipid phase (Hille 1991), but there is evidence that they approach the channel via a cytosolic pathway analogous to the "hydrophilic" local anaesthetic route (Li et al. 2002). Nevertheless, where there are residues in common with binding sites for other chemicals, e.g. local anaesthetics, the toxins may interact with a different aspect of the residues (Wang and Wang 2003), so it remains unclear whether local anaesthetics compete directly with "site 2" toxins for binding or whether their interaction is allosteric. Similarly to local anaesthetics, binding of the "site 2" toxins is state-dependent, such that the channel must be in the open conformation and not inactivated for binding (Hille 2001). The mechanisms for BTX and veratridine are probably very similar. When bound, the toxin changes the voltage-dependence of opening to more negative potentials so that the channels do not deactivate (return to the closed state) except at very negative potentials and nor do they inactivate – presumably because the toxin prevents the docking of the D3–D4 linker inactivation particle. The channels therefore remain open and conducting until the drug dissociates and allows the channel to inactivate and deactivate or both. A compelling picture of BTX binding and its consequential effects on gating is provided in Wang and Wang (2003). The drug-bound open channels also lose their selectivity for Na^+ ions and behave like non-selective cation channels and, importantly, channel conductance is reduced. The degree to which net sodium conductance is reduced differs between the toxins, with BTX having least conductance block, veratridine having more and aconitine having the most.

Differences between the effects of "site 2" toxins on sodium channel subtypes in sensory neurones have not been explored systematically, but given the chemical diversity of the compounds such differences would not be surprising and subtype-selective differences have been noted elsewhere, at least for aconitine (Wright 2002). BTX has qualitatively similar effects on the sensory neurone $Na_V1.8$ VGSC (Bosmans et al. 2004) as it does in other tissues. In sensory neurones the TTXS currents respond to veratridine in a way that looks very similar to that previously reported for skeletal muscle or brain channels, but the extent of the negative shift of the activation of the VGSCs may be somewhat less in sensory neurones (Farrag et al. 2008). The effect of veratridine on TTXR VGSCs in sensory neurones is qualitatively similar but much less impressive than the effect on TTXS (Campos et al. 2004), the difference having been attributed to a more rapid drug dissociation of veratridine from the TTXR channels that allows slow inactivation of channels to accumulate during prolonged depolarization (Farrag et al. 2008). This explains why veratridine does not provoke a TTX-resistant response in sensory neurones or other cells that are not voltage-clamped despite the presence of TTXR VGSCs (Vickery et al. 2004; Benjamin et al. 2006; Liu et al. 2006). BTX may prove to be a better chemical probe for the "site 2" binding locus of TTXR channels in mammalian sensory neurones (Bosmans et al. 2004) that could be used in non-electrophysiological cell-based assays. In frog DRG neurones, grayanotoxin has been shown to be selective for TTXR channels (Yakehiro et al. 2000) but it is not known whether the compound can discriminate equally well between TTXR and TTXS channels in mammalian neurones. There is little published information available on the effects of aconitine on sodium channels in sensory neurones, but data from our laboratory suggest aconitine acts more like a simple blocker of VGSCs in DRG, at least for TTXR. The effect of aconitine is quite distinct from that of veratridine. We have found in rat DRG that at 100 μM the dominant effect of

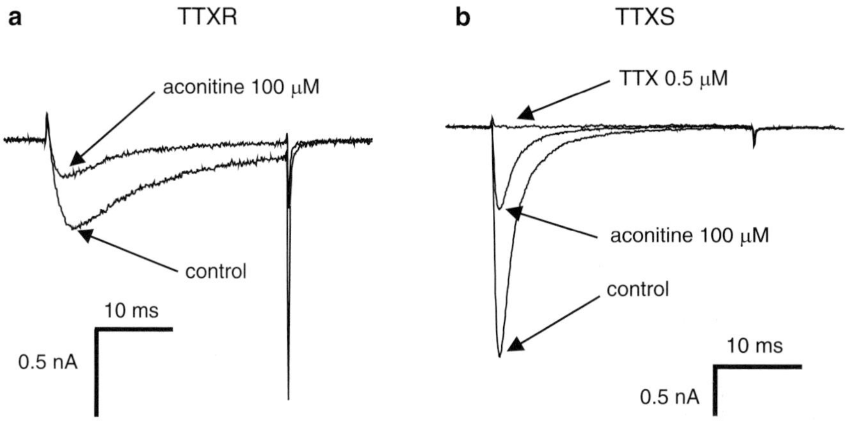

Fig. 4 The effect of aconitine on VGSC current in voltage-clamped rat dorsal root ganglion neurones. Currents are evoked during 30-ms voltage steps to -10 mV from a holding potential of -90 mV. The recording methods are as described in Farrag et al. (2005). The decrease in current amplitude that occurs following rapid application of 100 μM aconitine is shown. In (**a**) the currents were recorded in the presence of 0.5 μM TTX throughout, so this is a TTX-resistant current. In (**b**) the currents were identified as TTX-sensitive by their characteristic rapid kinetics and this was confirmed by applying 0.5 μM TTX to the residual current after it had been depressed by application of aconitine

aconitine is inhibitory in both TTXR and TTXS currents (Fig. 4). There is a very small negative shift in the threshold for activation of TTXS currents but no significant difference in the voltage-dependence of TTXR and no effect on inactivation rates or persistence of current for either TTXS or TTXR (K.J. Farrag and R.J. Docherty, unpublished observations).

Ralfinamide (NW-1029), a compound identified from a BTX binding displacement assay, binds presumably to "site 2" and has promising analgesic properties (Veneroni et al. 2003). It has been shown to be a blocker of both TTXS and TTXR VGSCs in DRG neurones (Stummann et al. 2005) but has a preferential effect on excitability of nociceptive (capsaicin-sensitive) sensory neurones (Yamane et al. 2007).

4.4.4 "Sites 3–9" Toxins and Drugs

Experiments with toxins acting at "site 3" have been important for establishing a link between the conformational changes that occur in VGSCs during activation and inactivation. The extracellular loop linking D4S3 and D4S4 is a critical component of "site 3" binding (Cestele and Catterall 2000). The actions of scorpion toxins, including the α-toxins that act at "site 3", have been reviewed recently (Bosmans and Tytgat 2007). In general, toxins acting at "site 3" enhance VGSC activity by slowing or reducing inactivation. Chen et al. (2002) showed that the scorpion α-toxin Lqh-3 was 100-fold more potent as an enhancer of $Na_V1.7$ over

$Na_V1.2$, whereas Lqh-2, another peptide from the same venom, had a 20-fold preference the other way round. $Na_V1.8$ is resistant to Lqh toxin, which is attributed to a four amino acid extension in the D4S3–D4S4 linker region of $Na_V1.8$ (Saab et al. 2002). Maertens et al. (2006) showed that another scorpion toxin, OD1, is 250-fold more potent as an enhancer of $Na_V1.7$ over $Na_V1.3$ and is relatively inactive against $Na_V1.8$. They also showed that a classic α-toxin (AahII) and an α-like toxin (BmK M1 or BmK I) have a similar, albeit less dramatic, preference for $Na_V1.7$ over other sensory neurone TTXS channels and are inactive against $Na_V1.8$. Chen et al. (2005) have also demonstrated selective effects of BmK I on TTXS and TTXR VGSCs in rat DRG neurones. Given the recent evidence that $Na_V1.7$ is a major mediator of pain signalling (see earlier), these results point to the α-toxin component of scorpion, sea anemone (Ständker et al. 2006) and spider venoms (Xiao et al. 2005) as having a major contribution to the production of pain associated with stings or bites.

Another component of scorpion venom, the β-toxins, are distinguished from α-toxins by binding to a different site, "site 4", located in the D2S4 region (Cestele and Catterall 2000; Campos et al. 2007). The scorpion β-toxins shift sodium channel activation to more negative values but reduce overall conductance (Cestele and Catterall 2000). It is difficult to predict what would be the net effect of β-toxins on excitability in neurones and little information is available concerning their effects on sensory neurones or the sodium channel subtypes that are expressed in sensory neurones. A β-like toxin from the Asian scorpion *Buthus martensi* Karsch (Goudet et al. 2002), BmK abT, has been shown to prolong action potential duration and increase VGSC currents in rat DRG neurones, but details of the mechanism are not known (Ye et al. 2000). Recently a scorpion β-toxin from *Tityus zulianus* was shown to select for $Na_V1.4$ (skeletal muscle) over $Na_V1.5$ (cardiac) and was inactive against $Na_V1.7$ (Leipold et al. 2006). The extent to which β-toxins contribute to pain and other sensory symptoms of scorpion toxins is therefore unclear. Another toxin from *Buthus* – BmK AS-1 – has been shown to be an analgesic and an inhibitor of sensory neurone VGSCs (Tan et al. 2001). Though not structurally related to either the α-toxin or the β-toxin group, BmK AS-1 has β-toxin-like effects on DRG VGSCs, but the emphasis of the effect is on inhibition (Chen et al. 2006a, b). Two toxins from tarantula venom – ProTxI and ProTxII – that are non-selective inhibitors of VGSCs (Middleton et al. 2002) have been suggested to act at "site 4" (but see Smith et al. 2007). In contrast to most other peptide toxins from a variety of sources, ProTxI and ProTxII are distinguished by their ability to block TTXR isoforms, including sensory neurone $Na_V1.8$ (Priest et al. 2007).

The "site 5" toxins, ciguatoxin in particular, provoke a range of effects in humans, including pain and paresthesia (Cameron et al. 1991), that are consistent with enhancement or activation of VGSCs in sensory nerves (Pearn 2001). Brevetoxin has been shown to have effects on TTXS VGSCs in sensory neurones from nodose ganglion (Jeglitsch et al. 1998) that are quite similar to those of the "type 2" toxins, including a shift in activation to more negative potentials and inhibition of inactivation. But the binding site, which is probably the same as that for ciguatoxin (Lombet et al. 1987), is at an intramembrane site involving residues on the extracellular ends of D1S6 and D4S5 (Trainer et al. 1994; Cestele and Catterall 2000). In DRG, ciguatoxin has distinct effects on TTXS and TTXR currents. TTXS currents are affected as expected and adopt a continuously conducting state at near resting membrane potentials, but the voltage-dependence of TTXR is unaffected. The main effect on TTXR is an acceleration of repriming from an inactivated state (Strachan et al. 1999).

Apart from the μ-conotoxins that act at "site 1" discussed already, *Conus* species produce many other classes of toxins, including the δ-conus toxin, which slows inactivation of $Na_V1.4$ by binding to "site 6", which is in the D4S4 region, probably partly overlapping "site 3" (Leipold et al. 2005; Ekberg et al. 2008), but these have not been tested on mammalian sensory neurones so far as we are aware. Other *Conus* toxins may bind to "site 8", which is relatively poorly defined at present.

The natural pyrethroid insecticides and synthetic analogues such as DDT are said to bind to "site 7" (Zlotkin 1999). Pyrethroids differentially modulate TTXS and TTXR sodium currents in sensory neurones, having a preferential action on TTXR. Their effects are quite similar to those of BTX and veratridine in that they slow inactivation and shift activation to more hyperpolarized potentials (Tatebayashi and Narahashi 1994; Tabarean and Narahashi 2001). They do so by binding to a distinct site incorporating residues in D2S5, D3S6 and the D2S4–D2S5 linker regions (O'Reilly et al. 2006). Structure-activity studies suggest subtle differences occur in the ways in which a range of commercial pyrethroids interact with $Na_V1.8$ channels (Choi and Soderlund 2006). It has been suggested that enhancement of activity of $Na_V1.8$ by pyrethroids may underlie the paresthesia that can occur when skin is exposed to commercial compounds (Choi and Soderlund 2006).

4.5 Other Drugs

Many new or known drugs of other classes have been found to block VGSCs and have been attributed with analgesic properties. For example, the NK1 receptor antagonist (+/−) CP96345 was shown to provoke a use-dependent block of VGSCs in rat brain that was not associated with any change in voltage-dependence of activation or inactivation and was attributed to an open channel blocking mechanism (Caeser et al. 1993). Other drugs include crobenetine (BIII 890 CL), a use-dependent VGSC blocker developed for the treatment of stroke (Dekker et al. 2005); vinpocetine, a nootropic derivative of a *Vinca* alkaloid (Zhou et al. 2003); fluphenazine, a neuroleptic (Zhou et al. 2006; Dong et al. 2008); ifenprodil, an NMDA antagonist (Tanahashi et al. 2007); ambroxol, a mucolytic agent and expectorant (Weiser 2006); and several antidepressant agents (Dick et al. 2007). Several other analgesic compounds have appeared from drug discovery programmes that have VGSC blocking activity as their primary screen. Ralfinamide (NW-1029) was mentioned earlier as a possible "site 2" binding agent that has marked frequency-dependent blocking properties (Stummann et al. 2005; Yamane et al. 2007) but whether this compound binds at "site 2" or influences BTX binding by an allosteric effect is not known. Several other drugs with an action qualitatively similar to that of ralfinamide have appeared recently. PPPA, is an analogue of the anticonvulsant V102862 (Ilyin et al. 2006) and is relatively potent but not very selective. A series of cyclopentane dicarboxamides (Shao et al. 2005), including CDA54 (Brochu et al. 2006), have been discovered using a high-throughput fluorescence resonant energy transfer assay. They are VGSC blockers and are selective for neuropathic pain and discriminate to a small extent between VGSC subtypes in DRG. Butyl 2-(4-[1.1′-biphenyl]-4-yl-1*H*-imidazol-2-yl)ethylcarbamate, a structurally distinct compound identified from BTX binding displacement assays and veratridine-induced cytotoxicity screening is, like CDA54, an antihyperalgesic rather than an analgesic, but electrophysiological analysis and information on channel selectivity is not yet available (Liberatore et al. 2007). M58373 was identified in a veratridine-induced substance P release assay and has been shown to possess analgesic properties attributed to block of VGSCs, but further development was abandoned owing to unwanted cardiac side effects (Akada et al. 2006). These discoveries reflect the emergence of new classes of VGSC blockers that are targeted at pathological pain states.

A series of benzazepinone compounds, also discovered using a fluorescence resonant energy transfer based assay system, have been described as frequency-dependent blockers of $Na_V1.7$ and have oral analgesic activity in neuropathic pain models. It is claimed that compounds with some selectivity for $Na_V1.7$ have been discovered within this series and there exists the potential for achieving further subtype selectivity using compounds of the same class (Williams et al. 2007).

Finally, A-803567 is an especially interesting compound since this shows a strong preference for blocking TTXR $Na_V1.8$, including the human isoforms, over a range of other subtypes, including $Na_V1.2$, $Na_V1.3$, $Na_V1.5$ and $Na_V1.7$. This compound is the most convincing candidate produced so far of a small-molecule inhibitor that is selective for TTXR channels. It causes a negative shift in the inactivation voltage dependence of channels without affecting their voltage-dependence of activation but, interestingly, the compound has no apparent use-dependence when tested in excitability studies. This compound is a potent analgesic in animal models and a promising candidate for clinical development as an analgesic for chronic pain syndromes.

5 Conclusion

Clearly, there are a great many potential binding sites for drugs on VGSCs that may be discrete, overlap or interact by allosteric mechanisms. Drugs and toxins that interact with VGSCs are legion and are structurally diverse (Anger et al. 2001; Kyle and Ilyin 2006). Amongst this diversity, the prospects are good for the eventual development of blockers that can select for sensory neurone VGSCs by activity-dependent mechanisms or by subtype selectivity or both; both would probably be best. Potentially, VGSC blockers could be used to treat any peripherally generated paresthesias, but chronic pain syndromes represent the greatest unmet medical need in sensory dysfunction and are probably the most attractive target from a clinical or a commercial point of view. Recent discoveries include novel compounds with selectivity for sensory neurone sodium channels and for either $Na_V1.7$, the principal component of TTXS currents in nociceptive neurones, or for $Na_V1.8$, the principal component of TTXR currents. Other targets such as $Na_V1.3$ and $Na_V1.9$ are inviting prospects. At the very least the development of these novel compounds will provide much needed tools to better define the roles of VGSC in sensation and they would furnish clinicians with much needed, improved, better-targeted and safer pharmaceuticals to alleviate pain.

References

Ahern CA, Eastwood AL, Dougherty DA, Horn RA (2008) Electrostatic contributions of aromatic residues in the local anesthetic receptor of voltage-gated sodium channels. Circ Res 102:86–94

Akada Y, Ogawa S, Amano K, Fukudome Y, Yamasaki F, Itoh M, Yamamoto I (2006) Potent analgesic effects of a putative sodium channel blocker M58373 on formalin-induced and neuropathic pain in rats. Eur J Pharmacol 536:248–255

Alpert LA, Fozzard HA, Hanck DA, Makielski JC (1989) Is there a second external lidocaine binding site on mammalian cardiac cells? Am J Physiol 257:H79–H84

Amir R, Argoff CE, Bennett GJ, Cummins TR, Durieux ME, Gerner P, Gold MS, Porreca F, Strichartz GR (2006) The role of sodium channels in chronic inflammatory and neuropathic pain. J Pain 7(Suppl 3):S1–S29

Anger T, Madge DJ, Mulla M, Riddall D (2001) Medicinal chemistry of neuronal voltage-gated sodium channel blockers. J Med Chem 44:115–137

Armstrong CM (1971) Interaction of tetraethyammonium ion derivatives with the potassium channels of giant axons. J Gen Physiol 58:413–437

Armstrong CM (2007) Na channel inactivation from open and closed states. Proc Natl Acad Sci USA 103:17991–17996

Baker MD (2000) Selective block of late Na^+ current by local anaesthetics in rat large sensory neurones. Br J Pharmacol 129:1617–1626

Baker MD (2005) Protein kinase C mediates up-regulation of tetrodotoxin-resistant, persistent Na^+ current in rat and mouse sensory neurones. J Physiol 567:851–867

Balser JR, Nuss HB, Romashko DN, Marban E, Tomaselli GF (1996) Functional consequences of lidocaine binding to slow-inactivated sodium channels. J Gen Physiol 107:643–658

Becker S, Prusak-Sochaczewski E, Zamponi G, Beck-Sickinger AG, Gordon RD, French RJ (1992) Action of derivatives of mu-conotoxin GIIIA on sodium channels. Single amino acid substitutions in the toxin separately affect association and dissociation rates. Biochemistry 31:8229–8238

Benjamin ER, Pruthi F, Olanrewaju S, Ilyin VI, Crumley G, Kutlina E, Valenzano KJ, Woodward RM (2006) State-dependent compound inhibition of $Na_V1.2$ sodium channels using the FLIPR Vm dye: on-target effects of diverse pharmacological agents. J Biomol Screen 11:29–39

Bennett PB, Valenzuela C, Chen LQ, Kallen RG (1995) On the molecular nature of the lidocaine receptor of cardiac Na^+ channels. Modification of block by alterations in the alpha-subunit III–IV interdomain. Circ Res 77:584–592

Binshtok AM, Bean BP, Wolff CJ (2007) Inhibition of nociceptors by entry of impermeant sodium channel blockers. Nature 449:607–610

Black JA, Dib-Hajj S, McNabola K, Jeste S, Rizzo MA, Kocsis JD, Waxman SG (1996) Spinal sensory neurons express multiple sodium channel alpha-subunit mRNAs. Brain Res Mol Brain Res 43:117–131

Black JA, Cummins TR, Plumpton C, Chen YH, Hormuzdiar W, Clare JJ, Waxman SG (1999) Upregulation of a silent sodium channel after peripheral, but not central, nerve injury in DRG neurons. J Neurophysiol 82:2776–2785

Black JA, Renganathan M, Waxman SG (2002) Sodium channel $Na_V1.6$ is expressed along nonmyelinated axons and it contributes to conduction. Brain Res Mol Brain Res 105:19–28

Blackburn-Munro G, Fleetwood-Walker SM (1997) The effects of Na^+ channel blockers on somatosensory processing by rat dorsal horn neurones. Neuroreport 8:1549–1554

Blair NT, Bean BP (2003) Role of tetrodotoxin-resistant Na^+ current slow inactivation in adaptation of action potential firing in small-diameter dorsal root ganglion neurons. J Neurosci 23:10338–10350

Bosmans F, Tytgat J (2007) Voltage-gated sodium channel modulation by scorpion alpha-toxins. Toxicon 49:142–158

Bosmans F, Maertens C, Verdonck F, Tytgat J (2004) The poison dart frog's batrachotoxin modulates $Na_V1.8$. FEBS Lett 577:245–248

Brau ME, Elliott JR (1998) Local anaesthetic effects on tetrodotoxin-resistant Na^+ currents in rat dorsal root ganglion neurons. Eur J Anaesthesiol 15:80–88

Brau ME, Dreimann M, Oischewski A, Vogel W, Hempelmann G (2001) Effect of drugs used for neuropathic pain management on tetrodotoxin-resistant Na^+ currents in rat sensory neurons. Anesthesiology 94:137–144

Brochu RM, Dick IE, Tarpley JW, McGowan E, Gunner D, Herrington J, Shao PP, Ok D, Li C, Parsons WH, Stump GL, Regan CP, Lynch JJ Jr, Lyons KA, McManus OB, Clark S, Ali Z, Kaczorowski GJ, Martin WJ, Priest BT (2006) Block of peripheral nerve sodium channels selectively inhibits features of neuropathic pain in rats. Mol Pharmacol 69:823–832

Caeser M, Seabrook GR, Kemp JA (1993) Block of voltage-dependent sodium currents by the substance P receptor antagonist (+/−)-CP-96,345 in neurones cultured from rat cortex. Br J Pharmacol 109:918–924

Caldwell JH, Schaller KL, Lasher RS, Peles E, Levinson SR (2000) Sodium channel $Na_V1.6$ is localized at nodes of Ranvier, dendrites, and synapses. Proc Natl Acad Sci USA 97:5616–5620

Cameron J, Flowers AE, Capra MF (1991) Electrophysiological studies on ciguatera poisoning in man (part II). J Neurol Sci 101:93–97

Campos FV, Moreira TH, Beirão PSL, Cruz JS (2004) Veratridine modifies the TTX-resistant Na^+ channels in rat vagal afferent neurons. Toxicon 43:401–406

Campos FV, Chanda B, Beirão PS, Bezanilla F (2007) beta-Scorpion toxin modifies gating transitions in all four voltage sensors of the sodium channel. J Gen Physiol 130:257–268

Cantrell AR, Tibbs VC, Yu FH, Murphy BJ, Sharp EM, Qu Y, Catterall WA, Scheuer T (2002) Molecular mechanism of convergent regulation of brain Na^+ channels by protein kinase C and protein kinase A anchored to AKAP-15. Mol Cell Neurosci 21:63–80

Cardenas LM, Cardenas CG, Scroggs RS (2001) 5HT increases excitability of nociceptor-like rat dorsal root ganglion neurons via cAMP-coupled TTX-resistant Na^+ channels. J Neurophysiol 86:241–248

Cardenas CA, Cardenas CG, de Armandi AJ, Scroggs RS (2006) Carbamazepine interacts with a slow inactivation state of $Na_V1.8$-like sodium channels. Neurosci Lett 408:129–134

Carroll I (2007) Intravenous lidocaine for neuropathic pain: diagnostic utility and therapeutic efficacy. Curr Pain Headache Rep 11:20–24

Catterall WA (1987) Common modes of drug action on Na^+ channels: local anesthetics, antiarrhymics and anticonvulsants. Trends Pharmacol Sci 8:57–65

Catterall WA (1986) Voltage-dependent gating of sodium channels: correlating structure and function. Trends Neurosci 9:7–10

Catterall WA (2000) From ionic currents to molecular mechanisms: the structure and function of voltage-gated sodium channels. Neuron 26:13–25
Catterall WA, Goldin AL, Waxman SG (2005) International Union of Pharmacology. XLVII. Nomenclature and structure-function relationships of voltage-gated sodium channels. Pharmacol Rev 57:397–409
Cestele S, Catterall WA (2000) Molecular mechanisms of neurotoxin action on voltage-gated sodium channels. Biochimie 82:883–892
Chabal C, Russell LC, Burchiel KJ (1989) The effect of intravenous lidocaine, tocainide, and mexiletine on spontaneously active fibers originating in rat sciatic neuromas. Pain 38:333–338
Chahine M, Ziane R, Vijayaragavan K, Okamura Y (2005) Regulation of Na v channels in sensory neurons. Trends Pharmacol Sci 26:496–502
Challapalli V, Tremont-Lukats IW, McNicol ED, Lau J, Carr DB (2005) Systemic administration of local anesthetic agents to relieve neuropathic pain. Cochrane Database Syst Rev 4:CD003345
Chen H, Lu SQ, Leipold E, Gordon D, Hansel A, Heinemann SH (2002) Differential sensitivity of sodium channels from the central and peripheral nervous system to the scorpion toxins Lqh-2 and Lqh-3. Eur J Neurosci 16:767–770
Chen J, Tan ZY, Zhao R, Feng XH, Shi J, Ji YH (2005) The modulation effects of BmK I, an alpha-like scorpion neurotoxin on voltage-gated Na^+ currents in rat dorsal root ganglion neurons. Neurosci Lett 390:66–71
Chen J, Feng XH, Shi J, Tan ZY, Bai ZT, Liu T, Ji YH (2006a) The anti-nociceptive effect of BmK AS, a scorpion active polypeptide, and the possible mechanism on specifically modulating voltage-gated Na^+ currents in primary afferent neurons. Peptides 27:2182–2192
Chen Y, Yu FH, Surmeier DJ, Scheuer T, Catterall WA (2006b) Neuromodulation of Na^+ channel slow inactivation via cAMP-dependent protein kinase and protein kinase C. Neuron 49:409–420
Chen D, Reierstad S, Lin Z, Lu M, Brooks C, Li N, Innes J, Bulun SE (2007) Prostaglandin E_2 induces breast cancer related aromatase promoters via activation of p38 and c-Jun NH_2-terminal kinase in adipose fibroblasts. Cancer Res 67:8914–8922
Cheung H, Kamp D, Harris E (1992) An in vitro investigation of the action of lamotrigine on neuronal voltage-activated sodium channels. Epilepsy Res 13(2):107–12
Chevrier P, Vijayaragavan K, Chahine M (2004) Differential modulation of $Na_V1.7$ and $Na_V1.8$ peripheral nerve sodium channels by the local anaesthetic lidocaine. Br J Pharmacol 142:576–584
Choi JS, Soderlund DM (2006) Structure-activity relationships for the action of 11 pyrethroid insecticides on rat Na_v 1.8 sodium channels expressed in *Xenopus* oocytes. Toxicol Appl Pharmacol 211:233–244
Choudhary G, Yotsu-Yamashita M, Shang L, Yasumoto T, Dudley SC Jr (2003) Interactions of the C-11 hydroxyl of tetrodotoxin with the sodium channel outer vestibule. Biophys J 84:287–294
Conti F, Gheri A, Pusch M, Moran O (1996) Use dependence of tetrodotoxin block of sodium channels: a revival of the trapped-ion mechanism. Biophys J 71:1295–1312
Courtney KR (1975) Mechanism of frequency-dependent inhibition of sodium currents in from myelinated nerve by the lidocaine derivative GEA 968. J Pharm Exp Ther 195:225–236
Cox JJ, Reimann F, Nicholas AK, Thornton G, Roberts E, Springell K, Karbani G, Jafri H, Mannan J, Raashid Y, Al-Gazali L, Hamamy H, Valente EM, Gorman S, Williams R, McHale DP, Wood JN, Gribble FM, Woods CG (2006) An SCN9A channelopathy causes congenital inability to experience pain. Nature 444:894–898
Craig W (1887) Manual of materia medica and therapeutics, 5th edn. Livingstone, Edinburgh
Cummins TR, Waxman SG (1997) Downregulation of tetrodotoxin-resistant sodium currents and upregulation of a rapidly repriming tetrodotoxin-sensitive sodium current in small spinal sensory neurons after nerve injury. J Neurosci 17:3503–3514
Cummins TR, Sheets PL, Waxman SG (2007) The roles of sodium channels in nociception: Implications for mechanisms of pain. Pain 131:243–257

De Col R, Messlinger K, Carr RW (2008) Conduction velocity is regulated by sodium channel inactivation in unmyelinated axons innervating the rat cranial meninges. J Physiol 586:1089–1103

Dekker LV, Daniels Z, Hick C, Elsegood K, Bowden S, Szestak T, Burley JR, Southan A, Cronk D, James IF (2005) Analysis of human $Na_V1.8$ expressed in SH-SY5Y neuroblastoma cells. Eur J Pharmacol 528:52–58

DeToledo JC (2000) Lidocaine and seizures. Ther Drug Monit 22:320–322

Devor M (2006) Sodium channels and mechanisms of neuropathic pain. J Pain 7(Suppl 1):S3–S12

Dib-Hajj S, Black JA, Cummins TR, Waxman SG (2002) NaN/$Na_V1.9$: a sodium channel with unique properties. Trends Neurosci 25:253–259

Dib-Hajj SD, Rush AM, Cummins TR, Hisama FM, Novella S, Tyrrell L, Marshall L, Waxman SG (2005) Gain-of-function mutation in $Na_V1.7$ in familial erythromelalgia induces bursting of sensory neurons. Brain 128:1847–1854

Dick IE, Brochu RM, Purohit Y, Kaczorowski GJ, Martin WJ, Priest BT (2007) Sodium channel blockade may contribute to the analgesic efficacy of antidepressants. J Pain 8:315–324

Docherty RJ, Farrag KJ (2006) The effect of dibutyryl cAMP on tetrodotoxin-sensitive and -resistant voltage-gated sodium currents in rat dorsal root ganglion neurons and the consequences for their sensitivity to lidocaine. Neuropharmacology 51:1047–1057

Docherty RJ, Charlesworth G, Farrag K, Bhattacharjee A, Costa S (2005) The use of the rat isolated vagus nerve for functional measurements of the effect of drugs in vitro. J Pharm Tox Methods 51:235–242

Dong XW, Jia Y, Lu SX, Zhou X, Cohen-Williams M, Hodgson R, Li H, Priestley T (2008) The antipsychotic drug, fluphenazine, effectively reverses mechanical allodynia in rat models of neuropathic pain. Psychopharmacology 195:559–568

Dunlop R, Davies RJ, Hockley J, Turner P (1988) Analgesic effects of oral flecainide. Lancet 331:420–421

Eisenberg E, River Y, Shifrin A, Krivoy N (2007) Antiepileptic drugs in the treatment of neuropathic pain. Drugs 67:1265–1289

Ekberg J, Adams DJ (2006) Neuronal voltage-gated sodium channel subtypes: key roles in inflammatory and neuropathic pain. Int J Biochem Cell Biol. 38:2005–2010

Ekberg J, Craik DJ, Adams DJ (2008) Conotoxin modulation of voltage-gated sodium channels. Int J Biochem Cell Biol 40(11):2363–2368. doi:10.1016/j.biocel.2007.08.017

England S, Bevan S, Docherty RJ (1996) PGE2 modulates the tetrodotoxin-resistant sodium current in neonatal rat dorsal root ganglion neurones via the cyclic AMP-protein kinase A cascade. J Physiol 495:429–440

Farrag KJ, Costa SK, Docherty RJ (2002) Differential sensitivity to tetrodotoxin and lack of effect of prostaglandin E2 on the pharmacology and physiology of propagated action potentials. Br J Pharmacol 135:1449–1456

Farrag KJ, Bhattacharjee A, Docherty RJ (2008) A comparison of the effects of veratridine on tetrodotoxin-sensitive and tetrodotoxin-resistant sodium channels in isolated rat dorsal root ganglion neurons. Pflugers Arch 455:929–938

Felts PA, Yokoyama S, Dib-Hajj S, Black JA, Waxman SG (1997) Sodium channel alpha-subunit mRNAs I, II, III, NaG, Na6 and hNE (PN1): different expression patterns in developing rat nervous system. Brain Res Mol Brain Res 45:71–82

Fitzgerald EM, Okuse K, Wood JN, Dolphin AC, Moss SJ (1999) cAMP-dependent phosphorylation of the tetrodotoxin-resistant voltage-dependent sodium channel SNS. J Physiol 516:433–446

Fraser SP, Salvador V, Manning EA, Mizal J, Altun S, Raza M, Berridge RJ, Djamgoz MB (2003) Contribution of functional voltage-gated Na^+ channel expression to cell behaviors involved in the metastatic cascade in rat prostate cancer: I. Lateral motility. J Cell Physiol 195:479–487

Frohnwieser B, Weigl L, Schreibmayer W (1995) Modulation of cardiac sodium channel isoform by cyclic AMP dependent protein kinase does not depend on phosphorylation of serine 1504 in the cytosolic loop interconnecting transmembrane domains III and IV. Pflugers Arch 430:751–753

Gebhardt C, Breustedt JM, Nöldner M, Chatterjee SS, Heinemann U (2001) The antiepileptic drug losigamone decreases the persistent Na^+ current in rat hippocampal neurons. Brain Res 920:27–31

Ghatapande AS, Sikdar SK (1997) Competition for binding between veratridine and KIFMK: an open channel blocking peptide of the RIIA sodium channel. J Membr Biol 160:177–182

Gold MS, Thut PD (2001) Lithium increases potency of lidocaine-induced block of voltage-gated Na^+ currents in rat sensory neurons in vitro. J Pharmacol Exp Ther 299:705–711

Gold MS, Reichling DB, Shuster MJ, Levine JD (1996) Hyperalgesic agents increase a tetrodotoxin-resistant Na^+ current in nociceptors. Proc Natl Acad Sci USA 93:1108–1112

Gold MS, Levine JD, Correa AM (1998) Modulation of TTX-R INa by PKC and PKA and their role in PGE2-induced sensitization of rat sensory neurons in vitro. J Neurosci 18:10345–10355

Goldberg YP, MacFarlane J, MacDonald ML, Thompson J, Dube MP, Mattice M, Fraser R, Young C, Hossain S, Pape T, Payne B, Radomski C, Donaldson G, Ives E, Cox J, Younghusband HB, Green R, Duff A, Boltshauser E, Grinspan GA, Dimon JH, Sibley BG, Andria G, Toscano E, Kerdraon J, Bowsher D, Pimstone SN, Samuels ME, Sherrington R, Hayden MR (2007) Loss-of-function mutations in the $Na_V1.7$ gene underlie congenital indifference to pain in multiple human populations. Clin Genet 71:311–319

Goldin AL, Snutch T, Lubbert H, Dowsett A, Marshall J, Auld V, Downey W, Fritz LC, Lester HA, Dunn R (1986) Messenger RNA coding for only the alpha subunit of the rat brain Na channel is sufficient for expression of functional channels in *Xenopus* oocytes. Proc Natl Acad Sci USA 83:7503–7507

Goudet C, Chi C-W, Tytgat J (2002) An overview of toxins and genes from the venom of the Asian scorpion *Buthus martensi Karsch*. Toxicon 40:1239–1258

Gould HJ 3rd, England JD, Liu ZP, Levinson SR (1998) Rapid sodium channel augmentation in response to inflammation induced by complete Freund's adjuvant. Brain Res 802:69–74

Gould HJ 3rd, England JD, Soignier RD, Nolan P, Minor LD, Liu ZP, Levinson SR, Paul D (2004) Ibuprofen blocks changes in Na_v 1.7 and Na_V 1.8 sodium channels associated with complete Freund's adjuvant-induced inflammation in rat. J Pain 5:270–280

Grant AO, Chandra R, Keller C, Carboni M, Starmer CF (2000) Block of wild-type and inactivation deficient sodium channels IFM/QQQ stably expressed in mammalian cells. Biophysical J 79:3019–3035

Guven M, Bozdemir H, Gunay I, Sarica Y, Kahraman I, Koc F (2006) The actions of lamotrigine and levetiracetam on the conduction properties of isolated rat sciatic nerve. Eur J Pharmacol 553:129–134

Guy HR, Seetharamulu P (1986) Molecular model of the action potential sodium channel. Proc Natl Acad Sci USA 83:508–512

Hartshorne RP, Catterall WA (1981) Purification of the saxitoxin receptor of the sodium channel from rat brain. Proc Natl Acad Sci USA 78:4620–4624

Hartshorne RP, Catterall WA (1984) The sodium channel from rat brain. Purification and subunit composition. J Biol Chem 259:1667–1675

Hartshorne RP, Messner DJ, Coppersmith JC, Catterall WA (1984) The saxitoxin receptor of the sodium channel from rat brain. Evidence for two nonidentical beta subunits. J Biol Chem 257:13888–13891

Heinemann SH, Terlau H, Imoto K (1992) Molecular basis for pharmacological differences between brain and cardiac sodium channels. Pflugers Arch 422:90–92

Hille B (1975) The receptor for tetrodotoxin and saxitoxin. A structural hypothesis. Biophys J 15:615–619

Hille B (1977) Local anesthetics: hydrophilic and hydrophobic pathways for the drug receptor reaction. J Gen Physiol 69:497–515

Hille B (2001) Ion channels of excitable membranes, 3rd edn. Sinauer, Sunderland

Hui K, Lipkind G, Fozzard HA, French RJ (2002) Electrostatic and steric contributions to block of the skeletal muscle sodium channel by mu-conotoxin. J Gen Physiol 119:45–54

Hunt LW, Frigas E, Butterfield JH, Kita H, Blomgren J, Dunnette SL, Offord KP, Gleich GJ (2004) Treatment of asthma with nebulized lidocaine: a randomized, placebo-controlled study. J Allergy Clin Immunol 113:853–859

Ichimata M, Ikebe H, Yoshitake S, Hattori S, Iwasaka H, Noguchi T (2001a) Analgesic effects of flecainide on postherpetic neuralgia. Int J Clin Pharmacol Res 21:15–19

Ichimata M, Kitano T, Ikebe H, Iwasaka H, Noguchi T (2001b) Flecainide reverses neuropathic pain and suppresses ectopic nerve discharge in rats. Neuroreport 12:1869–1873

Ikeda SR, Scholfield GG, Weight FF (1986) Na^+ and Ca^{2+} currents of acutely isolated adult rat nodose ganglion cells. J Neurophysiol 55:527–539

Ilyin VI, Pomonis JD, Whiteside GT, Harrison JE, Pearson MS, Mark L, Turchin PI, Gottshall S, Carter RB, Nguyen P, Hogenkamp DJ, Olanrewaju S, Benjamin E, Woodward RM (2006) Pharmacology of 2-[4-(4-chloro-2-fluorophenoxy)phenyl]-pyrimidine-4-carboxamide: a potent, broad-spectrum state-dependent sodium channel blocker for treating pain states. J Pharmacol Exp Ther 318:1083–1093

Isom LL, De Jongh KS, Patton DE, Reber BF, Offord J, Charbonneau H, Walsh K, Goldin AL, Catterall WA (1992) Primary structure and functional expression of the beta 1 subunit of the rat brain sodium channel. Science 256:839–842

Isom LL, Ragsdale DS, De Jongh KS, Westenbroek RE, Reber BF, Scheuer T, Catterall WA (1995) Structure and function of the beta 2 subunit of brain sodium channels, a transmembrane glycoprotein with a CAM motif. Cell 83:433–442

Jarvis B, Coukell AJ (1998) Mexiletine. A review of its therapeutic use in painful diabetic neuropathy. Drugs 56:691–707

Jeglitsch G, Rein K, Baden DG, Adams DJ (1998) Brevetoxin-3 (PbTx-3) and its derivatives modulate single tetrodotoxin-sensitive sodium currents in rat sensory neurons. J Pharmacol Exp Ther 284:516–525

Jin X, Gereau RW 4th (2006) Acute p38-mediated modulation of tetrodotoxin-resistant sodium channels in mouse sensory neurons by tumor necrosis factor-alpha. J Neurosci 26:246–255

Keizer DW, West PJ, Lee EF, Yoshikami D, Olivera BM, Bulaj G, Norton RS (2003) Structural basis for tetrodotoxin-resistant sodium channel binding by mu-conotoxin SmIIIA. J Biol Chem 278:46805–46813

Kerr NC, Gao Z, Holmes FE, Hobson SA, Hancox JC, Wynick D, James AF (2007) The sodium channel $Na_V1.5a$ is the predominant isoform expressed in adult mouse dorsal root ganglia and exhibits distinct inactivation properties from the full-length $Na_V1.5$ channel. Mol Cell Neurosci 35:283–291

Kim CH, Oh Y, Chung JM, Chung K (2001) The changes in expression of three subtypes of TTX sensitive sodium channels in sensory neurons after spinal nerve ligation. Brain Res Mol Brain Res 95, 153–161

Ko SH, Jochnowitz N, Lenkowski PW, Batts TW, Davis GC, Martin WJ, Brown ML, Patel MK (2006) Reversal of neuropathic pain by alpha-hydroxyphenylamide: a novel sodium channel antagonist. Neuropharmacology 50:865–873

Kuo CC (1998) A common anticonvulsant binding site for phenytoin, carbamazepine, and lamotrigine in neuronal Na^+ channels. Mol Pharmacol 54:712–721

Kuo CC, Bean BP (1994) Slow binding of phenytoin to inactivated sodium channels in rat hippocampal neurons. Mol Pharmacol 46:716–725

Kuo CC, Lu L (1997) Characterization of lamotrigine inhibition of Na^+ channels in rat hippocampal neurones. Br J Pharmacol 121:1231–1238

Kyle DJ, Ilyin VI (2006) Sodium channel blockers. J Med Chem 50:2583–2588

Lai HC, Jan LY (2006) The distribution and targeting of neuronal voltage-gated ion channels. Nat Rev Neurosci 7:548–562

Lai J, Porreca F, Hunter JC, Gold MS (2004) Voltage-gated sodium channels and hyperalgesia. Ann Rev Pharmacol Toxicol 44:371–397

Lampert A, Hains BC, Waxman SG (2006) Upregulation of persistent and ramp sodium current in dorsal horn neurons after spinal cord injury. Exp Brain Res 174:660–666

Lang DG, Wang CM, Cooper BR (1993) Lamotrigine, phenytoin and carbamazepine interactions on the sodium current present in N4TG1 mouse neuroblastoma cells. J Pharmacol Exp Ther 266(2):829–835

Leffler A, Herzog RI, Dib-Hajj SD, Waxman SG, Cummins TR (2005) Pharmacological properties of neuronal TTX-resistant sodium channels and the role of a critical serine pore residue. Pflugers Arch 451:454–463

Leffler A, Reiprich A, Mohapatra DP, Nau C (2007) Use-dependent block by lidocaine but not by amitriptyline is more pronounced in tetrodotoxin (TTX)-resistant than in TTX-sensitive Na^+ channels. J Pharm Exp Ther 320:354–364

Leipold E, Hansel A, Olivera BM, Terlau H, Heinemann SH (2005) Molecular interaction of delta-conotoxins with voltage-gated sodium channels. FEBS Lett 579:3881–3884

Leipold E, Hansel A, Borges A, Heinemann SH (2006) Subtype specificity of scorpion beta-toxin Tz1 interaction with voltage-gated sodium channels is determined by the pore loop of domain 3. Mol Pharmacol 70:340–347

Li M, West JW, Lai Y, Scheuer T, Catterall WA (1992) Functional modulation of brain sodium channels by cAMP-dependent phosphorylation. Neuron 8:1151–1159

Li HL, Hadid D, Ragsdale DS (2002) The batrachotoxin receptor on the voltage-gated sodium channel is guarded by the channel activation gate. Mol Pharmacol 61:905–912

Li RA, Ennis IL, Xue T, Nguyen HM, Tomaselli GF, Goldin AL, Marbán E (2003) Molecular basis of isoform-specific micro-conotoxin block of cardiac, skeletal muscle, and brain Na^+ channels. J Biol Chem 278:8717–8724

Liberatore AM, Schulz J, Favre-Guilmard C, Pommier J, Lannoy J, Pawlowski E, Barthelemy MA, Huchet M, Auguet M, Chabrier PE, Bigg D (2007) Butyl 2-(4-[1.1′-biphenyl]-4-yl-1*H*-imidazol-2-yl)ethylcarbamate, a potent sodium channel blocker for the treatment of neuropathic pain. Bioorg Med Chem Lett 17:1746–1749

Lindia JA, Kohler MG, Martin WJ, Abbadie C (2005) Relationship between sodium channel $Na_V1.3$ expression and neuropathic pain behavior in rats. Pain 117:145–153

Lim TKY, MacLeod BA, Ries CR, Schwartz SKW (2007) The quaternary lidocaine derivative, QX-314, produces long-lasting local anesthesia in animal models in vivo. Anesthesiology 107:305–311

Lipkind GM, Fozzard HA (1994) A structural model of the tetrodotoxin and saxitoxin binding site of the Na^+ channel. Biophys J 66:1–13

Lipkind GM, Fozzard HA (2005) Molecular modeling of local anesthetic drug binding by voltage-gated sodium currents. Mol Pharmacol 68:1611–1622

Liu G, Yarov-Yarovoy V, Nobbs M, Clare JJ, Scheuer T, Catterall WA (2003) Differential interactions of lamotrigine and related drugs with transmembrane segment IVS6 of voltage-gated sodium channels. Neuropharmacology 44:413–422

Liu CJ, Priest BT, Bugianesi RM, Dulski PM, Felix JP, Dick IE, Brochu RM, Knaus H-G, Middleton RE, Kaczorowski GJ, Slaughter RS, Garcia ML, Kohler MG (2006) A high-capacity membrane potential FRET-based assay for $Na_V1.8$ channels. Assay Drug Dev Technol 4:37–48

Lombet A, Bidard JN, Lazdunski M (1987) Ciguatoxin and brevetoxins share a common receptor site on the neuronal voltage-dependent Na^+ channel. FEBS Lett 219:355–359

Lönnendonker U (1994) Use dependence of guanidinium toxins in frog myelinated nerve: evidence for features of native voltage-gated sodium channels. Prog Neurobiol 42:359–374

Maertens C, Cuypers E, Amininasab M, Jalali A, Vatanpour H, Tytgat J (2006) Potent modulation of the voltage-gated sodium channel $Na_V1.7$ by OD1, a toxin from the scorpion *Odonthobuthus doriae*. Mol Pharmacol 70:405–414

Matsuki N, Quandt FN, Ten Eick RE, Yeh JZ (1984) Characterization of the block of sodium channels by phenytoin in mouse neuroblastoma cells. J Pharmacol Exp Ther 228:523–530

Matsumoto S, Yoshida S, Ikeda M, Tanimoto T, Saiki C, Takeda M, Shima Y, Ohta H (2007) Effect of 8-bromo-cAMP on the tetrodotoxin-resistant sodium ($Na_V1.8$) current in small-diameter nodose ganglion neurones. Neuropharmacology 52:904–924

McLeane G (2007) Intravenous lidocaine: an outdated or underutilized treatment for pain. J Palliat Med 10:798–805

McNulty MM, Edgerton GB, Shah RD, Hanck DA, Fozzard HA, Lipkind GM (2007) Charge at the lidocaine binding site residue Phe-1759 affects permeation in human cardiac voltage-gated sodium channels. J Physiol 581:741–755

Messner DJ, Catterall WA (1985) The sodium channel from rat brain. Separation and characterization of subunits. J Biol Chem 260:10597–10604

Middleton RE, Warren VA, Kraus RL, Hwang JC, Liu CJ, Dai G, Brochu RM, Kohler MG, Gao YD, Garsky VM, Bogusky MJ, Mehl JT, Cohen CJ, Smith MM (2002) Two tarantula peptides inhibit activation of multiple sodium channels. Biochemistry 41:14734–14747

Morgan K, Stevens EB, Shah B, Cox PJ, Dixon AK, Lee K, Pinnock RD, Hughes J, Richardson PJ, Mizuguchi K, Jackson AP (2000) Beta 3: an additional auxiliary subunit of the voltage-sensitive sodium channel that modulates channel gating with distinct kinetics. Proc Natl Acad Sci USA 97:2308–2313

Murphy BJ, Rossie S, De Jongh KS, Catterall WA (1993) Identification of the sites of selective phosphorylation and dephosphorylation of the rat brain Na^+ channel alpha subunit by cAMP-dependent protein kinase and phosphoprotein phosphatases. J Biol Chem 268:27355–27362

Nakamura S, Atsuta Y (2005) Effect of sodium channel blocker (mexiletine) on pathological ectopic firing pattern in a rat chronic constriction nerve injury model. J Orthop Sci 10:315–320

Narahashi T (1986) Toxins that modulate the sodium channel gating mechanism. Ann N Y Acad Sci 479:133–151

Narahashi T, Frazier DT, Moore JW (1972) Comparison of tertiary and quaternary amine local anesthetics in their ability to depress membrane ionic conductances. J Neurobiol 3:267–276

Nau C, Wang GK (2004) Interactions of local anesthetics with voltage-gated Na^+ channels. J Membr Biol 201:1–8

Noda M (1993) Structure and function of sodium channels. Ann N Y Acad Sci 707:20–37

Oh Y, Sashihara S, Black JA, Waxman SG (1995) Na^+ channel beta 1 subunit mRNA: differential expression in rat spinal sensory neurons. Brain Res Mol Brain Res 30:357–61

O'Reilly AO, Khambay BP, Williamson MS, Field LM, Wallace BA, Davies TG (2006) Modelling insecticide-binding sites in the voltage-gated sodium channel. Biochem J 396:255–263

Osawa Y, Oda A, Iida H, Tanahashi S, Dohi S (2004) The effects of class Ic antiarrhythmics on tetrodotoxin-resistant Na^+ currents in rat sensory neurons. Anesth Analg 99:464–471

Ostman JAR, Nassar MA, Wood JN, Baker MD (2008) GTP up-regulated persistent Na^+ current and enhanced nociceptor excitability require $Na_V1.9$. J Physiol 586:1077–1087

Padilla F, Couble ML, Coste B, Maingret F, Clerc N, Crest M, Ritter AM, Magloire H, Delmas P (2007) Expression and localization of the $Na_V1.9$ sodium channel in enteric neurons and in trigeminal sensory endings: implication for intestinal reflex function and orofacial pain. Mol Cell Neurosci 35:138–152

Patton DE, Goldin AL (1991) A voltage-dependent gating transition induces use-dependent block by tetrodotoxin of rat IIA sodium channels expressed in *Xenopus* oocytes. Neuron 7:637–647

Pearn J (2001) Neurology of ciguatera. J Neurol Neurosurg Psychiatr 70:4–8

Pratt CM, Moye LA (1990) The cardiac arrhythmia suppression trial: background, interim results and implications. Am J Cardiol 65:20B–29B

Priest BT, Blumenthal KM, Smith JJ, Warren VA, Smith MM (2007) ProTx-I and ProTx-II: gating modifiers of voltage-gated sodium channels. Toxicon 49:194–201

Ragsdale DS, Scheuer T, Catterall WA (1991) Frequency and voltage-dependent inhibition of type IIA Na^+ channels, expressed in a mammalian cell line, by local anesthetic, antiarrhythmic, and anticonvulsant drugs. Mol Pharmacol 40:756–65

Ragsdale DS, McPhee JC, Scheuer T, Catterall WA (1994) Molecular determinants of state-dependent block of Na^+ channels by local anaesthetics. Science 265:1724–1728

Ragsdale DS, McPhee JC, Scheuer T, Catterall WA (1996) Common molecular determinants of local anesthetic, antiarrhythmic, and anticonvulsant block of voltage-gated Na^+ channels. Proc Natl Acad Sci USA 93:9270–9275

Ratcliffe CF, Westenbroek RE, Curtis R, Catterall WA (2001) Sodium channel beta1 and beta3 subunits associate with neurofascin through their extracellular immunoglobulin-like domain. J Cell Biol 154:427–434

Renganathan M, Cummins TR, Waxman SG (2001) Contribution of $Na_V1.8$ sodium channels to action potential electrogenesis in DRG neurons. J Neurophysiol 86:629–640

Renganathan M, Dib-Hajj S, Waxman SG (2002) $Na_V1.5$ underlies the 'third TTX-R sodium current' in rat small DRG neurons. Brain Res Mol Brain Res 106:70–82

Ritter AM, Ritchie C, Martin WJ (2007) Relationship between the firing frequency of injured peripheral neurons and inhibition of firing by sodium channel blockers. J Pain 8:287–295

Rogawski MA, Löscher W (2004) The neurobiology of antiepileptic drugs for the treatment of nonepileptic conditions. Nat Med 10:685–692

Roy ML, Narahashi T (1992) Differential properties of tetrodotoxin-sensitive and tetrodotoxin-resistant sodium channels in rat dorsal root ganglion neurons. J Neurosci 12:2104–2111

Rush AM, Elliott JR (1997) Phenytoin and carbamazepine: differential inhibition of sodium currents in small cells from adult rat dorsal root ganglia. Neurosci Lett 226:95–98

Rush AM, Dib-Hajj SD, Waxman SG (2005) Electrophysiological properties of two axonal sodium channels, $Na_V1.2$ and $Na_V1.6$, expressed in mouse spinal sensory neurones. J Physiol 564:803–815

Rush AM, Cummins TR, Waxman SG (2007) Multiple sodium channels and their roles in electrogenesis within dorsal root ganglion neurons. J Physiol 579:1–14

Saab CY, Cummins TR, Dib-Hajj SD, Waxman SG (2002) Molecular determinant of $Na_V1.8$ sodium channel resistance to the venom from the scorpion *Leiurus quinquestraitus hebraeus*. Neurosci Lett 331:79–82

Salgado VL, Yeh JZ, Narahashi T (1986) Use- and voltage-dependent block of the sodium channel by saxitoxin. Ann N Y Acad Sci 479:84–95

Sasaki K, Makita N, Sunami A, Sakurada H, Shirai N, Yokoi H, Kimura A, Tohse N, Hiraoka M, Kitabatake A (2004) Unexpected mexiletine responses of a mutant cardiac Na^+ channel implicate the selectivity filter as a structural determinant of antiarrhythmic drug access. Mol Pharmacol 66:330–336

Satin J, Kyle JW, Chen M, Bell P, Cribbs LL, Fozzard HA, Rogart RB (1992) A mutant of TTX-resistant cardiac sodium channels with TTX-sensitive properties. Science 256:1202–1205

Sato K, Ishida Y, Wakamatsu K, Kato R, Honda H, Ohizumi Y, Nakamura H, Ohya M, Lancelin JM, Kohda D, Inagaki F (1991) Active site of mu-conotoxin GIIIA, a peptide blocker of muscle sodium channels. J Biol Chem 266:16989–16991

Scheib H, McLay I, Guex N, Clare JJ, Blaney FE, Dale TJ, Tate SN, Robertson GM (2006) Modelling the pore structure of voltage-gated sodium channels in closed, open, and fast-inactivated conformation reveals details of site 1 toxin and local anesthetic binding. J Mol Model 12:813–822

Scholz A, Kuboyama N, Hempelmann G, Vogel W (1998) Complex blockade of TTX-resistant Na^+ currents by lidocaine and bupivacaine reduce firing frequency in DRG neurons. J Neurophysiol 79:1746–1754

Schwarz JR, Grigat G (1989) Phenytoin and carbamazepine: potential- and frequency-dependent block of Na currents in mammalian myelinated nerve fibers. Epilepsia 30:286–294

Schneider M, Datta S, Strichartz G (1991) A preferential inhibition of impulses in C-fibers of the rabbit vagus nerve by veratridine, an activator of sodium channels. Anaesthesiology 74:270–280

Segal MM, Douglas AF (1997) Late sodium channel openings underlying epileptiform activity are preferentially diminished by the anticonvulsant phenytoin. J Neurophysiol 77:3021–3034

Shah BS, Stevens EB, Gonzalez MI, Bramwell S, Pinnock RD, Lee K, Dixon AK (2000) Beta3, a novel auxiliary subunit for the voltage-gated sodium channel, is expressed preferentially in sensory neurons and is upregulated in the chronic constriction injury model of neuropathic pain. Eur J Neurosci 12:3985–3990

Shao PP, Ok D, Fisher MH, Garcia ML, Kaczorowski GJ, Li C, Lyons KA, Martin WJ, Meinke PT, Priest BT, Smith MM, Wyvratt MJ, Ye F, Parsons WH (2005) Novel cyclopentane dicarboxamide sodium channel blockers as a potential treatment for chronic pain. Bioorg Med Chem Lett 15:1901–1907

Sheets MF, Hanck DA (2007) Outward stabilization of the S4 segments in domains III and IV enhances lidocaine block of sodium channels. J Physiol 582:317–334

Shon KJ, Olivera BM, Watkins M, Jacobsen RB, Gray WR, Floresca CZ, Cruz LJ, Hillyard DR, Brink A, Terlau H, Yoshikami D (1998) mu-Conotoxin PIIIA, a new peptide for discriminating among tetrodotoxin-sensitive Na channel subtypes. J Neurosci 18:4473–4481

Sivilotti L, Okuse K, Akopian AN, Moss S, Wood JN (1997) A single serine residue confers tetrodotoxin insensitivity on the rat sensory-neuron-specific sodium channel SNS. FEBS Lett 409:49–52

Smith KJ (2007) Sodium channels and multiple sclerosis: roles in symptom production, damage and therapy. Brain Pathol 17:230–242

Smith RD, Goldin AL (1996) Phosphorylation of brain sodium channels in the I–II linker modulates channel function in *Xenopus* oocytes. J Neurosci 16:1965–1974

Smith RD, Goldin AL (1998) Functional analysis of the rat I sodium channel in *Xenopus* oocytes. J Neurosci 18:811–820

Smith RD, Goldin AL (2000) Potentiation of rat brain sodium channel currents by PKA in *Xenopus* oocytes involves the I–II linker. Am J Physiol Cell Physiol 278:C638–C645

Smith JJ, Cummins TR, Alphy S, Blumenthal KM (2007) Molecular interactions of the gating modifier toxin ProTx-II with $Na_V1.5$: implied existence of a novel toxin binding site coupled to activation. J Biol Chem 282:12687–12697

Song JH, Nagata K, Huang CS, Yeh JZ, Narahashi T (1996) Differential block of two types of sodium channels by anticonvulsants. Neuroreport 7:3031–3036

Spina E, Perugi G (2004) Antiepileptic drugs: indications other than epilepsy. Epileptic Disord 6:57–75

Srinivasan J, Schachner M, Catterall WA (1998) Interaction of voltage-gated sodium channels with the extracellular matrix molecules tenascin-C and tenascin-R. Proc Natl Acad Sci USA 95:15753–15757

Ständker L, Béress L, Garateix A, Christ T, Ravens U, Salceda E, Soto E, John H, Forssmann WG, Aneiros A (2006) A new toxin from the sea anemone *Condylactis gigantea* with effect on sodium channel inactivation. Toxicon 48:211–220

Starmer CF, Grant AO, Strauss HC (1984) Mechanisms of use-dependent block of sodium channels in excitable membranes by local anesthetics. Biophys J 46:15–27

Stephan MM, Potts JF, Agnew WS (1994) The microI skeletal muscle sodium channel: mutation E403Q eliminates sensitivity to tetrodotoxin but not to mu-conotoxins GIIIA and GIIIB. J Membr Biol 137:1–8

Strachan LC, Lewis RJ, Nicholson GM (1999) Differential actions of pacific ciguatoxin-1 on sodium channel subtypes in mammalian sensory neurons. J Pharmacol Exp Ther 288:379–388

Strichartz GR (1973) The inhibition of sodium currents in myelinated nerve by quaternary derivatives of lidocaine. J Gen Physiol 62:37–57

Stummann TC, Salvati P, Fariello RG, Faravelli L (2005) The anti-nociceptive agent ralfinamide inhibits tetrodotoxin-resistant and tetrodotoxin-sensitive Na^+ currents in dorsal root ganglion neurons. Eur J Pharmacol 510:197–208

Su X, Riedel ES, Leon LA, Laping NJ (2007) Pharmacologic evaluation of pressor and visceromotor reflex responses to bladder distension. Neurourol Urodyn 27:249–253

Sugai K (2007) Treatment of convulsive status epilepticus in infants and young children in Japan. Acta Neurol Scand Suppl 186:62–70

Sun GC, Werkman TR, Battefeld A, Clare JJ, Wadman WJ (2007) Carbamazepine and topiramate modulation of transient and persistent sodium currents studied in HEK293 cells expressing the $Na_V1.3$ alpha-subunit. Epilepsia 48:774–782

Sunami A, Glasser IW, Fozzard HA (2000) A critical residue for isoforms difference in tetrodotoxin affinity is a molecular determinant of the external path for local anesthetics in the cardiac sodium channel. Proc Nat Acad Sci USA 97:2326–2331

Szallasi A, Cruz F, Geppetti P (2006) TRPV1: a therapeutic target for novel analgesic drugs? Tr Mol Med 12:545–554

Tabarean IV, Narahashi T (2001) Kinetics of modulation of tetrodotoxin-sensitive and tetrodotoxin-resistant sodium channels by tetramethrin and deltamethrin. J Pharm Exp Ther 299:988–997

Tan ZY, Mao X, Xiao H, Zhao ZQ, Ji YH (2001) *Buthus martensi Karsch* agonist of skeletal muscle RyR-1, a scorpion active polypeptide: antinociceptive effect on rat peripheral nervous system and spinal cord, and inhibition of voltage-gated Na^+ currents in dorsal root ganglion neurons. Neurosci Lett 297:65–68

Tanahashi S, Iida H, Oda A, Osawa Y, Uchida M, Dohi S (2007) Effects of ifenprodil on voltage-gated tetrodotoxin-resistant Na^+ channels in rat sensory neurons. Eur J Anaesthesiol 24:782–788

Tatebayashi H, Narahashi T (1994) Differential mechanism of action of the pyrethroid tetramethrin on tetrodotoxin-sensitive and tetrodotoxin-resistant sodium channels. J Pharmacol Exp Ther 270:595–603

Taverna S, Mantegazza M, Franceschetti S, Avanzini G (1998) Valproate selectively reduces the persistent fraction of Na^+ current in neocortical neurons. Epilepsy Res 32:304–308

Terlau H, Heinemann SH, Stuhmer W, Pusch M, Conti F, Imoto K, Numa S (1991) Mapping the site of block by tetrodotoxin and saxitoxin of sodium channel II. FEBS Lett 293:93–96

Todorovic SM, Rastogi AJ, Jevtovic-Todorovic V (2003) Potent analgesic effects of anticonvulsants on peripheral thermal nociception in rats. Br J Pharmacol 140:255–260

Toledo-Aral JJ, Moss BL, He ZJ, Koszowski AG, Whisenand T, Levinson SR, Wolf JJ, Silos-Santiago I, Halegoua S, Mandel G (1997) Identification of PN1, a predominant voltage-dependent sodium channel expressed principally in peripheral neurons. Proc Natl Acad Sci USA 94:1527–1532

Trainer VL, Baden DG, Catterall WA (1994) Identification of peptide components of the brevetoxin receptor site of rat brain sodium channels. J Biol Chem 269:19904–19909

Tzeng JI, Cheng KI, Huang KL, Chen YW, Chu KS, Chu CC, Wang JJ (2007) The cutaneous analgesic effect of class I antiarrhythmic drugs. Anesth Analg 104:955–958

Ulbricht W (1998) Effects of veratridine on sodium currents and fluxes. Rev Physiol Biochem Pharmacol 133:1–54

Veneroni O, Maj R, Calabresi M, Faravelli L, Fariello RG, Salvati P (2003) Anti-allodynic effect of NW-1029, a novel Na^+ channel blocker, in experimental animal models of inflammatory and neuropathic pain. Pain 102:17–25

Vickery RG, Amagasu SM, Chang R, Mai N, Kauman E, Martin J, Hembrador J, O'Keefe MD, Gee C, Marquess D, Smith JA (2004) Comparison of the pharmacological properties of rat $Na_V1.8$ with Rat Na_V 1.2a and human $Na_V1.5$ voltage-gated sodium channel subtypes using a membrane potential sensitive dye and FLIPR. Receptors Channels 10:11–23

Vijayaragavan K, Boutjdir M, Chahine M (2004) Modulation of $Na_V1.7$ and $Na_V1.8$ peripheral nerve sodium channels by protein kinase A and protein kinase C. J Neurophysiol 91: 1556–1569

Von Gunten CF, Eappen S, Cleary JF, Taylor SG 4th, Moots P, Regevik N, Cleeland C, Cella D (2007) Flecainide for the treatment of chronic neuropathic pain: a Phase II trial. Palliat Med 21:667–672

Wang S-Y, Wang GK (2003) Voltage-gated sodium channels as primary targets of diverse lipid-soluble neurotoxins. Cell Signal 15:151–159

Wang GK, Brodwick MS, Eaton DC, Strichartz GR (1987) Inhibition of sodium currents by local anaesthetics in chloramine-T treated squid axons. The role of channel activation. J Gen Physiol 89:645–667

Wang S-Y, Mitchell J, Moczydlowski E, Wang GK (2004) Block of inactivation-deficient Na^+ channels by local anaesthetics in stably transfected mammalian cells: evidence for drug binding along the activation pathway. J Gen Physiol 124:691–701

Wang CZ, Zhang H, Jiang H, Lu W, Zhao ZQ, Chi CW (2006) A novel conotoxin from *Conus striatus*, mu-SIIIA, selectively blocking rat tetrodotoxin-resistant sodium channels. Toxicon 47:122–132

Wang S-Y, Tikhonov DB, Zhorov BS, Mitchell J, Wang GK (2007) Serine-401 as a batrachotoxin- and local anesthetic-sensing residue in the human cardiac Na^+ channel. Pflugers Arch 454: 277–287

Waxman SG (2006) Axonal conduction and injury in multiple sclerosis: the role of sodium channels. Nat Rev Neurosci 7:932–941

Waxman SG, Kocsis JD, Black JA (1994) Type III sodium channel mRNA is expressed in embryonic but not adult spinal sensory neurons, and is re-expressed following axotomy. J Neurophysiol 72:466–470

Weiser T (2006) Comparison of the effects of four Na^+ channel analgesics on TTX-resistant Na^+ currents in rat sensory neurons and recombinant $Na_V1.2$ channels. Neurosci Lett 395:179–184

West JW, Patton DE, Scheuer T, Wang Y, Goldin AL, Catterall WA (1992) A cluster of hydrophobic amino acid residues required for fast Na^+-channel inactivation. Proc Natl Acad Sci USA 89:10910–10914

Wiffen PJ, Rees J (2007) Lamotrigine for acute and chronic pain. Cochrane Database Syst Rev 2: CD006044

Williams BS, Felix JP, Priest BT, Brochu RM, Dai K, Hoyt SB, London C, Tang YS, Duffy JL, Parsons WH, Kaczorowski GJ, Garcia ML (2007) Characterization of a new class of potent inhibitors of the voltage-gated sodium channel $Na_V1.7$. Biochemistry 46:14693–14703

Willow M, Catterall WA (1982) Inhibition of binding of [^{3}H]batrachotoxinin A 20-alpha-benzoate to sodium channels by the anticonvulsant drugs diphenylhydantoin and carbamazepine. Mol Pharmacol 22:627–635

Willow M, Gonoi T, Catterall WA (1985) Voltage clamp analysis of the inhibitory actions of diphenylhydantoin and carbamazepine on voltage-sensitive sodium channels in neuroblastoma cells. Mol Pharmacol 27:549–558

Wittmack EK, Rush AM, Hudmon A, Waxman SG, Dib-Hajj SD (2005) Voltage-gated sodium channel $Na_V1.6$ is modulated by p38 mitogen-activated protein kinase. J Neurosci 25:6621–6630

Wood JN, Boorman JP, Okuse K, Baker MD (2004) Voltage-gated sodium channels and pain pathways. J Neurobiol 61:55–71

Wright SN (2002) Comparison of aconitine-modified human heart (hH1) and rat skeletal muscle (mu1) Na^+ channels: an important role for external Na^+ ions. J Physiol 538:759–771

Xiao Y, Tang J, Hu W, Xie J, Maertens C, Tytgat J, Liang S (2005) Jingzhaotoxin-I, a novel spider neurotoxin preferentially inhibiting cardiac sodium channel inactivation. J Biol Chem 280:12069–12076

Yakehiro M, Yuki T, Yamaoka K, Furue T, Mori Y, Imoto K, Seyama I (2000) An analysis of the variations in potency of gryanotoxin analogs in modifying frog sodium channels of different subtypes. Mol Pharmacol 58:692–700

Yamane H, de Groat WC, Sculptoreanu A (2007) Effects of ralfinamide, a Na^+ channel blocker, on firing properties of nociceptive dorsal root ganglion neurons of adult rats. Exp Neurol 208:63–72

Yarov-Yarovoy V, Brown J, Sharp EM, Clare JJ, Scheuer T, Catterall WA (2001) Molecular determinants of voltage-dependent gating and binding of pore-blocking drugs in transmembrane segment IIIS6 of the Na^+ channel alpha subunit. J Biol Chem 276:20–27

Yarov-Yarovoy V, McPhee JC, Idsvoog D, Pate C, Scheuer T, Catterall WA (2002) Role of amino acid residues in transmembrane segments IS6 and IIS6 of the Na^+ channel alpha subunit in voltage-dependent gating and drug block. J Med Chem 277:35393–35401

Ye JG, Wang CY, Li YJ, Tan ZY, Yan YP, Li C, Chen J, Ji YH (2000) Purification, cDNA cloning and function assessment of BmK abT, a unique component from the Old World scorpion species. FEBS Lett 479:136–140

Yu FH, Catterall WA (2003) Overview of the voltage-gated sodium channel family. Genome Biol 4:207

Yu FH, Westenbroek RE, Silos-Santiago I, McCormick KA, Lawson D, Ge P, Ferriera H, Lilly J, DiStefano PS, Catterall WA, Scheuer T, Curtis R (2003) Sodium channel beta4, a new disulfide-linked auxiliary subunit with similarity to beta2. J Neurosci 23:7577–7585

Zhang MM, Green BR, Catlin P, Fiedler B, Azam L, Chadwick A, Terlau H, McArthur JR, French RJ, Gulyas J, Rivier JE, Smith BJ, Norton RS, Olivera BM, Yoshikami D, Bulaj G (2007) Structure/function characterization of micro-conotoxin KIIIA, an analgesic, nearly irreversible blocker of mammalian neuronal sodium channels. J Biol Chem 282:30699–30706

Zhou X, Dong XW, Crona J, Maguire M, Priestley T (2003) Vinpocetine is a potent blocker of rat $Na_V1.8$ tetrodotoxin-resistant sodium channels. J Pharmacol Exp Ther 306:498–504

Zhou X, Dong XW, Priestley T (2006) The neuroleptic drug, fluphenazine, blocks neuronal voltage-gated sodium channels. Brain Res 1106:72–81

Zimmermann K, Leffler A, Babes A, Cendan CM, Carr RW, Kobayashi J, Nau C, Wood JN, Reeh PW (2007) Sensory neuron sodium channel $Na_V1.8$ is essential for pain at low temperatures. Nature 447:855–858

Zlotkin E (1999) The insect voltage-gated sodium channel as target of insecticides. Annu Rev Entemol 44:429–455

Role of Calcium in Regulating Primary Sensory Neuronal Excitability

T.D. Gover, T.H. Moreira, and D. Weinreich

Contents

Abstract The fundamental role of calcium ions (Ca^{2+}) in an excitable tissue, the frog heart, was first demonstrated in a series of classical reports by Sydney Ringer in the latter part of the nineteenth century (1882a, b; 1893a, b). Even so, nearly a

D. Weinreich (✉)
Department of Pharmacology and Experimental Therapeutics, University of Maryland School of Medicine, Room 4-002, Bressler Research Building, 655 West Baltimore Street, Baltimore, MD21201-1559, USA
dweinrei@umaryland.edu

B.J. Canning and D. Spina (eds.), *Sensory Nerves*,
Handbook of Experimental Pharmacology 194, DOI: 10.1007/978-3-540-79090-7_16,

century elapsed before it was proven that Ca^{2+} regulated the excitability of primary sensory neurons. In this chapter we review the sites and mechanisms whereby internal and external Ca^{2+} can directly or indirectly alter the excitability of primary sensory neurons: excitability changes being manifested typically by variations in shape of the action potential or the pattern of its discharge.

Keywords Voltage-dependent calcium channels, BK channels, IK channels, SK channels, Calcium-dependent currents, Extracellular calcium sensor, Intracellular calcium stores, Calcium ATPase, Sodium/calcium exchanger, Ryanodine receptor, Inositol triphosphate receptor, Spike frequency accommodation, Spike broadening

1 Introduction

The first direct demonstration that calcium ions (Ca^{2+}) can regulate excitability in mammalian primary sensory neurons was the observation of Ca^{2+}-dependent regenerative responses in rodent nodose ganglion neurons (NGNs) and dorsal root ganglion (DRG) neurons recorded in the absence of extracellular sodium (Na^{+}; Matsuda et al. 1976; Ransom and Holz 1977; Gallego and Eyzaguirre 1978). We now know that Ca^{2+} can influence the excitability of primary sensory neurons through a variety of distinct mechanisms. It can serve as a charge carrier through voltage-dependent Ca^{2+} channels (VDCC), leading to changes in membrane potential and alterations in the action potential waveform. Ca^{2+} influx via VDCC, or ligand-gated channels, or Ca^{2+} release from intracellular stores can activate cationic or anionic channels, leading to excitatory or inhibitory effects. Finally, Ca^{2+} can bind to Ca^{2+}-sensing proteins on the extracellular plasma membrane of primary sensory neurons to increase cationic currents (Conigrave et al. 2000; Undem et al. 2002).

Primary sensory neurons, like many other excitable cells, have evolved elaborate mechanisms to maintain intracellular Ca^{2+} concentration at nanomolar levels. These processes include Ca^{2+}-buffering proteins, Ca^{2+} exchangers and transport proteins in the endoplasmic reticulum (ER), mitochondria, and plasma membranes (Thayer et al. 2002). It has been demonstrated that interference with these systems can result in elevated cytoplasmic intracellular Ca^{2+} concentration, which in turn can lead to excitability changes via the Ca^{2+}-dependent mechanisms described above.

In this review, we examine the sites and mechanisms where internal and external Ca^{2+} alters the excitability of primary sensory neurons. Increases or decreases in excitability of primary sensory neurons can be brought about by direct and indirect actions of Ca^{2+}. Direct effects would include alterations in the resting membrane potential or resting membrane conductance. Ca^{2+} can indirectly affect excitability by modifying the conductance of K^{+} and Cl^{-} ions. Such effects often result in changes to the shape of the action potential and the pattern of firing, which in turn can alter the amount of neurotransmitter secreted from central and peripheral nerve terminals of the primary afferent neuron.

2 Morphology of Sensory Neurons

Primary sensory neurons are pseudo-unipolar cells consisting of a spheroidal cell body (somata), which produces a single axon (stem process) that extends from the cell body to a site of bifurcation (a distance ranging from a few microns to hundreds of microns), and peripherally and centrally projecting processes (Bird and Lieberman 1976). The somata of primary sensory neurons are housed in one of several ganglia present throughout the body: DRG and trigeminal ganglia (TG) in the case of somatosensory and some visceral sensory afferents and in vagal ganglia for primarily visceral sensory afferents. In this review, information about the role of Ca^{2+} and primary sensory neuron excitability will be drawn from literature studies on vagal primary afferents whose somata are located in the superior vagal ganglion or jugular ganglion and inferior vagal ganglion or nodose ganglion, and to a lesser degree from literature studies on DRG and TG neurons.

3 Biophysical and Pharmacological Properties of Voltage-Gated Calcium Channels

Most primary sensory neurons express at least three biophysical and pharmacologically distinct types of VDCC. VDCCs are transmembrane proteins that change their conformations in response to alterations in membrane voltage (Hille 2001). Upon membrane depolarization, VDCCs make a transition from a closed state to an open state that subsequently allows an influx of Ca^{2+}. In primary sensory neurons, and other neurons, VDCCs can be divided into two main groups on the basis of their voltage sensitivity: high voltage activated (HVA) and low voltage activated (LVA). As their names suggest, LVA VDCCs have gating thresholds in the range from -60 to -50 mV, while HVA VDCCs have thresholds in the range from -30 to -20 mV. LVA and HVA VDCCs can also be distinguished from one another by their sensitivity to drugs and toxins (Table 1).

VDCCs are formed by α_1 subunits that bestow all the channel's biophysical properties plus accessory subunits, α_2, β, δ, and γ, that serve to modulate the properties of the channel complex. Mimicking the nomenclature defining voltage-gated potassium channels, different VDCCs are classified by a letter-based nomenclature (Ertel et al. 2000). Ca_v represents the permeable ion with the subscript v denoting the principle physiological regulator, voltage. The numerical identifier denotes the Ca_v channel α_1 superfamily (1–3 at present) and the order of discovery of the α_1 subunit within the gene superfamily.

Table 1 Pharmacological and biophysical properties of voltage-dependent calcium channels in sensory neurons

Ca^{2+} current type	Ca^{2+} channel gene	Neuronal location	Antagonist	Biophysics properties	Sensory neuron type	Function
L-type	$Ca_V1.1$	Not present	Dihydropyridines; phenylalkylamines; benzothiazepines	g = 13–17 pS (Ba^{2+}) V_a = 8–14 mV τ_a = 50 ms at 10 mV V_h = −8 mV	Not present	
	$Ca_V1.2$	Cell bodies and proximal dendrites	Dihydropyridines; phenylalkylamines; benzothiazepines	g = 25 pS (Ba^{2+}) c = 9 pS (Ca^{2+}) V_a = −4 to−19 mV τ_a = 1 ms at 10 mV V_h = −50 to −60 mV (Ca^{2+})	Cochlea, organ of Corti	Regulating activity-dependent gene expression
	$Ca_V1.3$	Cell bodies and dendrites	Dihydropyridines; phenylalkylamines; benzothiazepines	g not established V_a = −15 to−20 mV τ_a < 1 ms at 10 mV V_h = −50 to −60 mV	Photoreceptor, auditory hair cells	Regulating activity-dependent gene expression
	$Ca_V1.4$	Retinal rod and bipolar cells	Dihydropyridines; phenylalkylamines; benzothiazepines	g not established V_a = −2.5 to −12 mV τ_a < 1 ms at V_{max} V_h = −9 to −27 mV (Ca^{2+})	Retinal photoreceptor, bipolar cell	Neurotransmitter release in retinal cell
P/Q-type	$Ca_V2.1$	Nerve terminal and dendrites	ω-Agatoxin IVA	g = 9 to 19 pS V_a = −5 mV for P V_a = −11 mV for Q τa = 2.2 ms at 10 mV V_h = −17.2 to −1.6 mV (Ba^{2+})	Large distribution	Neurotransmitter release

N-type	$Ca_V2.2$	Nerve terminal and dendrites	ω-Conotoxin-GVIA	$g = 20$ pS $V_a = -7.8$ mV $\tau_a = 3$ ms at 10 mV $V_h = -61$ mV	Large distribution	Sensation and transmission of pain, neurotransmitter release
R-type	$Ca_V2.3$	Cell bodies and dendrites	SNX-482	g not established $V_a = -29.1$ to 3 mV $\tau_a = 1.3$ ms at 0 mV $V_h = -71$ to -78.1 mV (Ba^{2+})	Large distribution	Neurotransmitter release, repetitive firing, posttetanic potentiation, long-term potentiation
T-type	$Ca_V3.1$	Cell bodies and dendrites	Mibefradil; kurtoxin	$g = 7.5$ pS $V_a = -46$ mV $\tau_a = 1$ at -10 mV $V_h = -73$ mV		Neuronal oscillation
	$Ca_V3.2$	Cell bodies and dendrites	Mibefradil; kurtoxin	$g = 9$ pS $V_a = -46$ mV $\tau_a = 2$ at -10 mV $V_h = -72$ mV	Olfactory bulb	Unknown
	$Ca_V3.3$	Cell bodies and dendrites	Mibefradil	$g = 11$ pS $V_a = -44$ mV $\tau_a = 7$ at -10 mV $V_h = -72$ mV	Olfactory bulb	Neuronal oscillation

Modified from Catterall et al. (2005)
g conductance, V_a activation, τ_a tall for activation, V_h inactivation

The different complement of VDCCs expressed by primary sensory neurons probably reflects the diverse sensory modalities transmitted by these cells (Scroggs and Fox 1992). For example, many primary afferent neurons with a nociceptive function have a hump on the falling phase of their action potential that is produced by a Ca^{2+} current (Fig. 1). The Ca^{2+} component of the action potential contributes to the primary sensory neuron excitability by prolonging the action potential duration and thus the time the neuron is depolarized. It also promotes more Ca^{2+} influx to trigger the activation of Ca^{2+}-dependent excitability changes (Scroggs and Fox 1992).

4 Calcium-Activated Currents

A rise in intracellular Ca^{2+} produced by an opening of VDCCs, release from intracellular Ca^{2+} stores, or Ca^{2+} influx through ligand-activated channels can activate K^+ or Cl^- currents on the plasma membrane. Ca^{2+}-activated K^+ currents ($I_{K(Ca)}$) can alter the excitability of primary sensory neurons by hyperpolarizing the membrane potential, altering the shape of the action potential, and by influencing the frequency and pattern of firing activity (Hille 2001). Ca^{2+}-activated Cl^- currents ($I_{Cl(Ca)}$) in primary sensory neurons can change neuronal excitability by depolarizing the membrane potential and by activating slow, depolarizing afterpotentials (Mayer 1985). In this section we describe how Ca^{2+}-activated currents affect the excitability of primary sensory neurons.

Three classes of Ca^{2+}-activated K^+ channels can be distinguished by their kinetics, single channel conductance, and pharmacological properties (for a review see, Sah and Faber 2002; Vogalis et al. 2003). These include large conductance Ca^{2+}-activated K^+ channels (BK, or maxi-K, channels, more than 200 pS), interme-

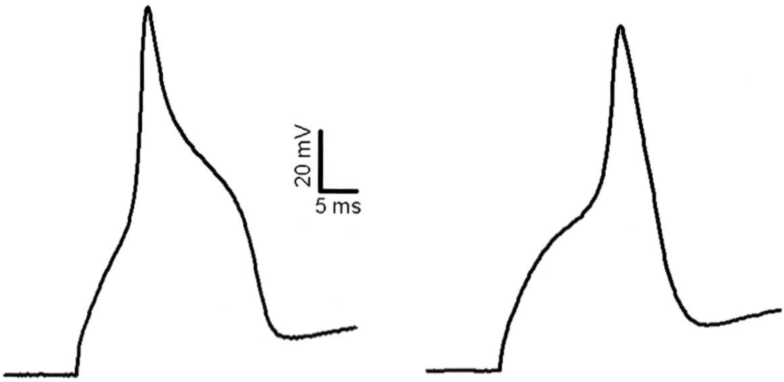

Fig. 1 Effect of Ca^{2+} on the duration of the action potential in a sensory neuron. The action potential on the *left* was recorded in normal physiological solution. The action potential on the *right* was recorded in a physiological solution containing nominally zero Ca^{2+}. Note the duration of the falling phase is substantially shortened in zero Ca^{2+}, indicating that the "hump" on the falling phase of the control action potential was due to a Ca^{2+} current

diate conductance Ca^{2+}-activated K^+ channels (IK channels, 10–60 pS), and small conductance Ca^{2+}-activated K^+ channels (SK channels, 2–20 pS). BK channels are voltage- and Ca^{2+}-sensitive, while IK and SK channels are only sensitive to increases in intracellular Ca^{2+}. Currents produced by BK, IK, and SK channels underlie various components of the action potential afterhyperpolarization (AHP; Figs. 2, 3). By controlling the magnitude and duration of the AHP, these channels play a fundamental role in controlling the pattern of action potential activity of primary sensory neurons (Fig. 3).

4.1 BK Channels

BK channels are activated by a synergistic rise in both cytoplasmic Ca^{2+} and membrane depolarization. BK, or $K_{Ca}1.1$, channels have been cloned (Adelman et al. 1992; Atkinson et al. 1992; see Salkoff et al. 2006 for a review). Interest in the role of BK channels in primary sensory neurons arises, in part, from the observations that BK channels have been shown to be located in small-diameter cells that are associated with nociceptive function (Li et al. 2007; Zhang et al. 2003). BK channels underlie a fast activating current that contributes to action potential repolarization and to a fast AHP in primary sensory neurons and many other types of neurons (Fowler et al. 1985; Christian et al. 1994; Zhang et al. 2003). Thus, by sculpting the action potential duration and the fast AHP duration and magnitude, BK channels can dramatically affect the excitability of sensory neurons. Blockade of BK channels by low-nanomolar concentrations of iberiotoxin or charybdotoxin, scorpion-derived neurotoxins, can increase action potential firing rates (Li et al. 2007), while opening of BK channels with NS1619 leads to reduced action potential firing (Zhang et al. 2003; Fox et al. 1997)

4.2 IK Channel

IK channels are present in both nociceptive and nonnociceptive primary sensory neurons (Hay and Kunze 1994; Mongan et al. 2005). IK channels are blocked by clotrimazole (10 μM), and are insensitive to apamin and low concentrations of tetraethylammonium chloride (5 mM). They display voltage-independence, exhibit single-channel conductance of 30–40 pS, and are 42–44% identical (amino acid substitutions) to channels of the SK family (Ishii et al. 1997; Vogalis et al. 2003). The *IK1/SK4/KCNN4* gene encodes IK channel K_{Ca} 3.1 (a.k.a IKCa1). Although these channels are present in primary sensory neurons, their role in controlling excitability remains to be determined. By contrast, there is evidence that IK channels can modulate excitability of intrinsic primary afferent enteric neurons (Neylon et al. 2004).

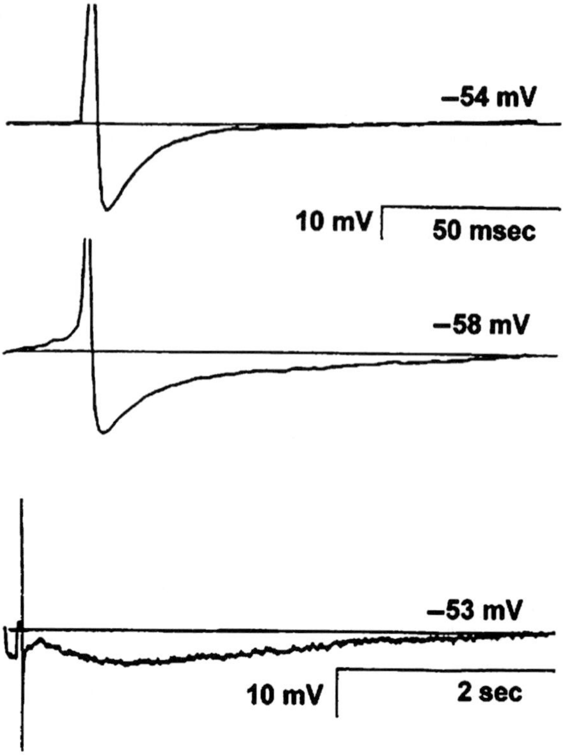

Fig. 2 Distinct types of action potential evoked after hyperpolarizations and their Ca^{2+} dependency recorded in primary sensory neurons. A single action potential can evoke three temporally distinct types of afterhyperpolarizations (AHP) in vagal sensory neurons of the rabbit. *Top trace*: A neuron with a single-component AHP lasting about 30 ms. This AHP is designated AHP_{fast}. All neurons have this short-duration AHP; it is usually Ca^{2+}-independent. *Middle trace*: Example of a neuron with a two-component AHP, an AHP_{fast} followed by a longer-lasting AHP (about 300 ms), the AHP_{medium}. In approximately half of the neurons, the AHP_{medium} is Ca^{2+}-dependent. *Bottom trace*: In a subset of C-fiber-type neurons, a slowly developing (hundreds of milliseconds) and long-lasting (2–15-s) AHP is observed. This slow AHP (AHP_{slow}) is always Ca^{2+}-dependent. The AHP_{slow} is preceded by an AHP_{fast} (downward deflection) and by an AHP_{medium}; it is noteworthy that the AHP_{slow} only begins many hundreds of milliseconds after the action potential (see Cordoba-Rodriquez et al. 1999 for details). Data were recorded at room temperature from adult neurons acutely isolated from rabbit vagal sensory ganglia. The *values depicted near the horizontal lines* are resting membrane potentials. The *calibration bar near thetop trace* also applies to the *middle trace*. Similar results have been recorded in guinea pig and ferret vagal ganglion neurons

4.3 SK Channels

Four SK channel family genes have been cloned, SK1, SK2, SK3, and SK4 (Bond et al. 2004). SK2 channels can mediate a medium-duration AHP (mAHP; decay time constant ranging between 100 and 200 ms) that controls the postspike

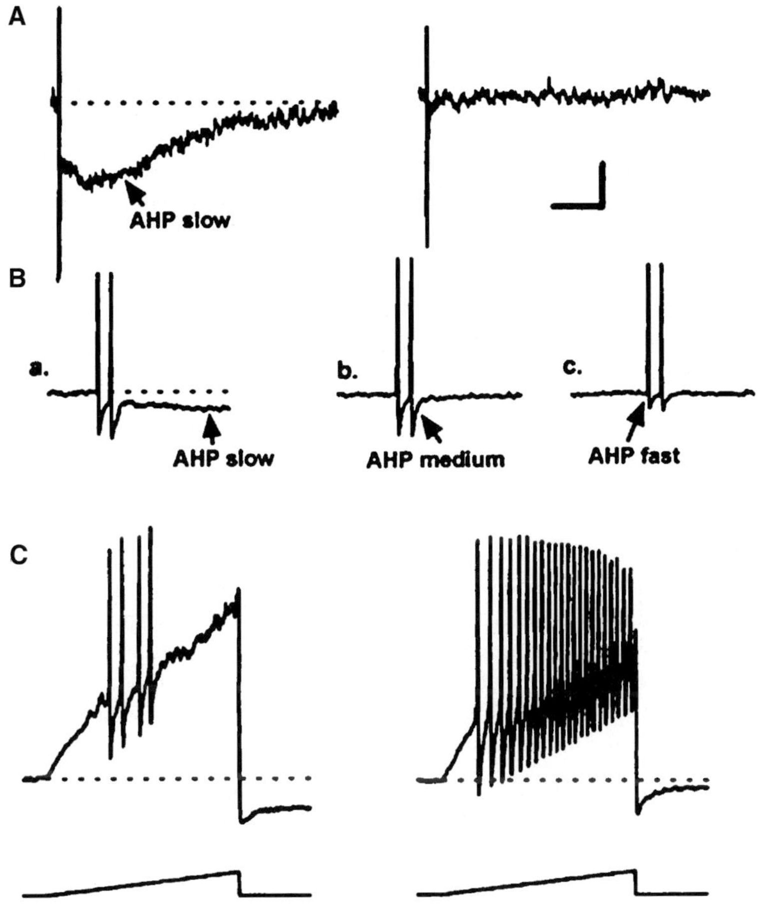

Fig. 3 The effects of blocking the AHP_{slow} on the excitability of a primary sensory neuron. Chelating intracellular Ca^{2+} with BAPTA abolishes the action potential evoked AHP_{slow} and increases the excitability of a primary vagal sensory neuron. (**A**) Bath-applied 1,2-bis(*O*-amino-phenoxy)ethane-*N,N,N′,N′*-tetraacetic acid (BAPTA)/acetomethylester (10 μM) blocks the AHP_{slow} within 5 min without changing the resting membrane potential or membrane input resistance. Action potentials were evoked by transmembrane depolarizing current pulses (4 nA, 1.5 ms, 10 Hz) and are truncated. (**B**) Responses recorded at a faster sweep speed to illustrate the kinetics of the AHP_{fast} and AHP_{medium}, which precede the AHP_{slow}. The AHP_{fast} is unaffected by 10 μM BAPTA (compare **a** with **b**). The Ca^{2+} dependence of the AHP_{medium} is illustrated in Bc, where the neuron is superfused with 100 μM $CdCl_2$ for 30 s, which blocks most of the AHP_{medium}. The residual component of the AHP recorded in $CdCl_2$, a nonspecific antagonist of voltage-dependent Ca^{2+} channels (VDCCs), is the AHP_{fast}, which is mediated by delayed rectifier K^+ channels. (**C**) Depression of the AHP_{slow} markedly increases neuronal excitability. The average action potential firing frequency induced by a current ramp protocol (1 nA, 2 s) increased from 1 to 5.5 Hz when the AHP_{slow} was blocked. Similar increase in excitability can be observed in the presence of bradykinin, prostaglandin D_2, histamine, or many other inflammatory autacoids. The *scale bar* represents 3 mV, 2 s in **A**, 15 mV, 0.25 s in **B**, and 15 mV, 0.5 s in **C**. The *dashed line* indicates the resting membrane potential (−60 mV). Resting membrane input resistance was 70 MΩ. All recordings were made in the same sensory neurons

refractory period and thus neuronal firing rate. In CNS neurons, the mAHP is blocked by subnanomolar concentrations of apamin (IC_{50} < 0.1 nM), a bee neurotoxin (Faber and Sah 2003). In vagal primary sensory neurons, the mAHP appears to be mediated by BK channels rather than SK channels because the mAHP is voltage-dependent, blocked by 5 mM tetraethylammonium, and it is unaffected by micromolar concentrations of apamin (Cordoba-Rodriquez et al. 1999).

SK channels were thought to underline a slow AHP (sAHP) that has a slow rise time (hundreds of milliseconds) and can persist for many seconds (Vogalis et al. 2003). Because the sAHP and the SK1 channels were apamin-insensitive, voltage-insensitive, and required Ca^{2+} influx via VDCCs, it was initially suggested that SK1 channels mediate the currents producing the sAHP (Marrion and Tavalin 1998). Subsequent observations revealed that SK1 channels are apamin-sensitive in mammalian cell lines and the sAHP is unaffected in mice lacking any of the SK channels (Shah and Haylett 2000; Bond et al. 2004).

In vagal primary sensory neurons, the sAHP rises to a peak over hundreds of milliseconds and can last up to 15 s following a single action potential (reviewed by Cordoba-Rodriguez et al. 1999). The slow kinetics of the sAHP is probably due to its dependence on Ca^{2+} release from ryanodine-sensitive ER Ca^{2+} pools (Cohen et al. 1997). When examined in different species of vagal afferents, the sAHP is distributed exclusively in C-type sensory neurons, including nociceptors (Undem et al. 1993; Cordoba-Rodriguez et al. 1999). The sAHP influences the excitability of primary afferents and controls action potential firing frequency over the physiological range 0.1–10 Hz (Fig. 3; Weinreich and Wonderlin 1987). The sAHP is also a major substrate for inflammatorymediator-mediated increases in afferent excitability. The excitatory affects of inflammatory mediators such as histamine (Jafri et al. 1997), serotonin (Christian et al. 1989), and prostaglandins (Undem et al. 1993; Gold et al. 1996) are mediated, in part, by inhibition of the sAHP.

4.4 Other Ca^{2+}-Activated Potassium Currents

A slow Ca^{2+}-dependent K^+ current that is distinct from the Ca^{2+}-activated K^+ currents associated with the sAHP has been characterized in primary vagal afferent neurons of the rabbit (Hoesch et al. 2004). This K^+ current is not activated by Ca^{2+} released from ryanodine-sensitive ER Ca^{2+} pools; rather, it is activated by Ca^{2+} released from inositol trisphosphate (IP_3)-sensitive ER Ca^{2+} pools. This current (I_{IP3}) is insensitive to apamin, iberiotoxin, and 8-bromoadenosine 3′,5′-cyclic monophosphate, common antagonists of known $I_{K(Ca)}$ responsible for the sAHP in primary sensory neurons. I_{IP3} is triggered by extracellular ATP through P2Y receptor activation (Hoesch et al. 2002). Because many other metabotropic receptors capable of triggering IP_3 formation are present in primary sensory neurons (Lee et al. 2004), it is likely that I_{IP3} may represent a pivotal Ca^{2+}-dependent mechanism for controlling membrane excitability in sensory neurons. However, a direct demonstration of the role of I_{IP3} in neuronal excitability has not yet been described.

4.5 Calcium-Dependent Chloride Currents

Many primary sensory neurons express Ca^{2+}-activated Cl^- currents ($I_{Cl(Ca)}$), including DRG neurons (Mayer 1985) and TG neurons (Bader et al. 1987; Schlichter et al. 1989) (reviewed by Scott et al. 1995; Frings et al. 2000; Hartzell et al. 2005). This current is responsible for a spike afterdepolarization (ADP). $I_{Cl(Ca)}$ is expressed in vagotomized NGNs (Lancaster et al. 2002) but its existence in normal NGNs has not been reported. In most adult primary sensory neurons, the Cl^- equilibrium potential is substantially more positive (about −30 mV) than the resting membrane potential (Deschenes et al. 1976; Gallagher et al. 1978; Sung et al. 2000). Consequently, when Cl^- channels open, Cl^- ions exit primary sensory neurons, producing an inward depolarizing current. Thus, activation of $I_{Cl(Ca)}$ in primary sensory neurons enhances neuronal excitability.

$I_{Cl(Ca)}$ is activated by a rise in intracellular Ca^{2+} in the range 0.2–5 μM. The rise in intracellular Ca^{2+} and subsequent activation of $I_{Cl(Ca)}$ can be evoked by Ca^{2+} influx via VDCCs (Scott et al. 1988), release of Ca^{2+} from intracellular stores (Currie and Scott 1992), and after activation of ionotrophic and metabotrophic receptors (Sung et al. 2000; Oh and Weinreich 2004). A physiological consequences of activation of $I_{Cl(Ca)}$ is the development of feed-forward excitation. Membrane depolarization results in a rise in intracellular Ca^{2+}, which in turn activates $I_{Cl(Ca)}$, resulting in further depolarization and an additional opening of VDCCs. Feed-forward excitation is limited by Ca^{2+}-activated K^+ channels. The development of a depolarizing afterpotential following one or a few action potentials observed in some DRG neurons represents an example feed-forward excitation (Mayer 1985). Currently, there is no evidence that Ca^{2+} influx through a particular subtype of VDCC selectively activates $I_{Cl(Ca)}$.

5 Extracellular Calcium Sensor

It is well documented that increases in intracellular Ca^{2+} can excite or depress sensory neuronal excitability by activating different types of Ca^{2+}-dependent currents (see earlier). Changes in extracellular Ca^{2+} concentrations can also result in excitability changes in primary sensory neurons. A modest reduction in extracellular Ca^{2+} can induce an excitatory inward current in chick DRG neurons (Hablitz et al. 1986). In guinea pig vagal afferents, reducing extracellular Ca^{2+}selectively increases the excitability of airway nociceptors as manifested by a substantive increase in action potential discharge in response to mechanical stimulation.

Subsequent whole-cell patch recordings from airway-identified vagal primary afferent cell bodies revealed that extracellular Ca^{2+} can regulate a nonselective cation conductance (Undem et al. 2003). These studies indicate that some primary sensory neurons contain extracellular-Ca^{2+}-sensing receptors similar to those characterized in endocrine glands and other mammalian tissues (Conigrave et al. 2000). With normal concentrations of extracellular Ca^{2+}, the nonselective cation channels responsible for the inward current are tonically inhibited, but upon reduction in the concentration of extracellular Ca^{2+} this block is removed, leading to an inward cation current. It remains to be determined whether the increased afferent nerve excitability following a reduction in the concentrations of extracellular Ca^{2+} reflects a physiological or a pathophysiological process.

6 Calcium Regulation and Excitability

As described already, intracellular Ca^{2+} directly or indirectly activates several ionic conductances. It is therefore critical to understand the regulation of Ca^{2+} and the regulation of those proteins responsible for handling intracellular $Ca^{2+}$to fully appreciate the complexity of the role of Ca^{2+} in excitability. Changes in the cytosolic Ca^{2+} concentrations and the activities of Ca^{2+} regulatory proteins have been shown to lead directly to changes in primary sensory neuron ionic currents and excitability (Ayar et al. 1999; Usachev et al. 2002). Indeed, diseases that alter sensory neuronal excitability, such as in diabetes, have been correlated with abnormalities in the expression and/or function of Ca^{2+}-regulating proteins and organelles (Kostyuk et al. 1999; Kruglikov et al. 2004; Yusaf et al. 2001).

In sensory neurons, the baseline concentration of intracellular Ca^{2+} and the shape of the Ca^{2+} transients during electrical, chemical, thermal, or mechanical stimulation are controlled by numerous proteins and organelles. These include, on the plasma membrane, the plasma membrane calcium ATPase (PMCA) and the sodium–calcium exchanger (NCX); on the ER membrane, the ryanodine receptor (RyR), the IP_3 receptor (IP_3R), and the sarcoplasmic reticulum/ER calcium ATPase (SERCA); in the cytosol, various calcium binding proteins (CBP) and mitochondria. The overall effect these proteins and organelles will have on Ca^{2+} regulation is dependent on their location, density, and functional state.

Depolarization of the plasma membrane of nerves cells results in Ca^{2+} influx via the opening of numerous VDCCs. This Ca^{2+} influx raises the intracellular concentration of Ca^{2+} from its normal resting concentration of about 50 nM (Fig. 4; Gover et al. 2007a). In addition to Ca^{2+} influx across the plasma membrane, primary sensory neurons have effective mechanisms for amplifying Ca^{2+} signals, including calcium-induced calcium release (CICR) from intracellular stores through RyRs (Cohen et al. 1997; Hoesch et al. 2004). Ca^{2+} can also be released from intracellular stores through IP_3Rs (Thayer et al. 1988). CBPs act to transduce calcium signals

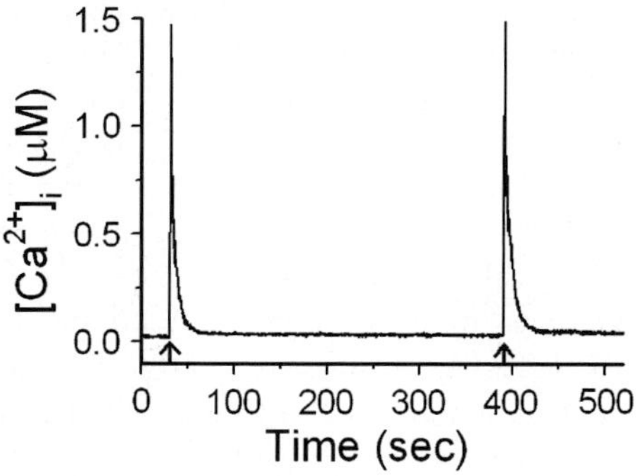

Fig. 4 Depolarization of the plasma membrane of sensory nerves cells results in reproducible Ca^{2+} influx via the opening of numerous VDCCs. The trace represents Ca^{2+} transients recorded from an acutely dissociated trigeminal ganglion cell that was stimulated by local (puffer) application of 50 mM KCl for 500 ms (*first arrow*). After 6-min superfusion with normal physiological solution, the cell was again stimulated with a 50 mM KCl puff (*second arrow*), producing a Ca^{2+} transient that was similar in amplitude ($p = 0.446$, $n = 18$) and time to decay ($p = 0.165$, $n = 18$) to the first transient

into molecular signaling pathways and to buffer intracellular Ca^{2+} in the cytosol (Bainbridge et al. 1992; Chard et al. 1993; Honda, 1995). To terminate Ca^{2+} transients, efficient Ca^{2+} clearance mechanisms must also exist. These include transport of Ca^{2+} across the plasma membrane by the PMCA, and by the NCX (Usachev et al. 2002; Verdru et al. 1997). Calcium may also be transported from the cytosol into Ca^{2+}-sequestering intracellular organelles, the most prominent of which are the ER and mitochondria (Fig. 5). Both of these organelles have been shown to take up Ca^{2+} from the cytoplasm of primary sensory neurons (Shishkin et al. 2002). The Ca^{2+} regulatory proteins are controlled by multiple signal tranduction pathways as well as transcriptional regulation. Unfortunately, currently there is a lack of data on the transcriptional regulation of these calcium regulatory proteins in primary sensory neurons.

6.1 Plasma Membrane Calcium ATPase

The PMCA is the predominant protein that moves Ca^{2+} across the plasma membrane in primary sensory neurons (Werth et al. 1996; Gover et al. 2007a). The PMCA uses the energy of ATP hydrolysis to remove Ca^{2+} ions across the plasma membrane from the cytosol. Four genes encode for the PMCAs (PMCA1–4). In addition, as a result of splice variants there are over 20 isoforms. The most dominant isoforms in sensory neurons are PMCA2a and PMCA4b, with only small amounts of PMCA1 present and no detectable PMCA3 (Usachev et al. 2002). CBPs, such as calmodulin, interact with PMCAs, regulating its activity. PMCA's affinity for Ca^{2+} increases over 30-fold (K_m of 30 to 1 μM) and its enzyme velocity increases over tenfold after binding to calmodulin (for a review see Carafoli 1991). Pottorf and Thayer (2002) demonstrated that previous Ca^{2+} transients would result

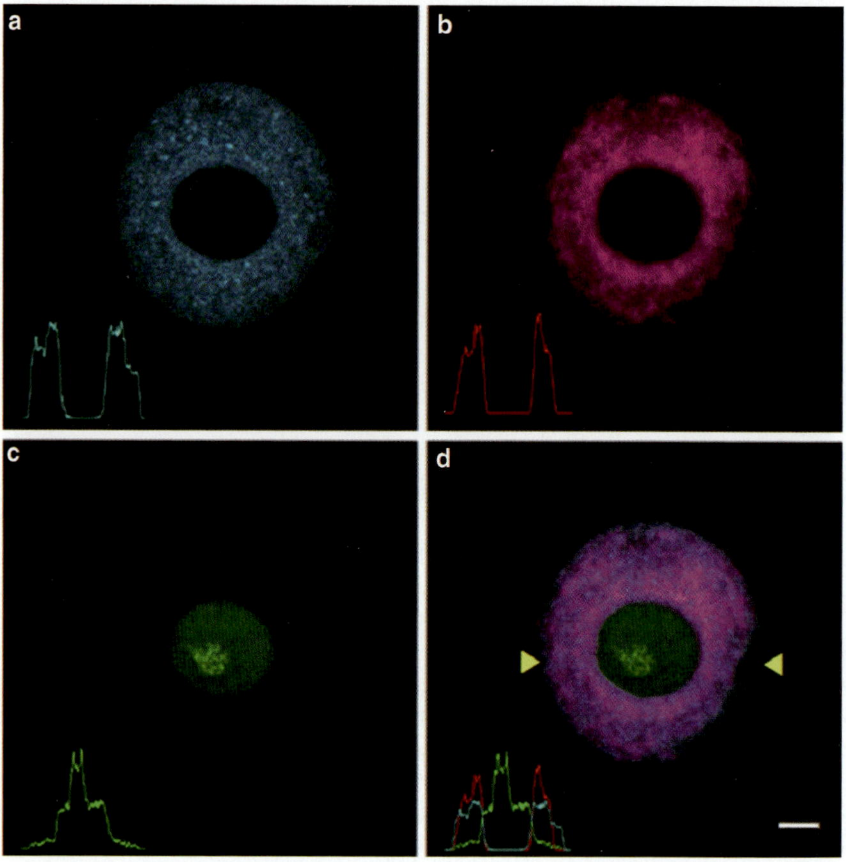

Fig. 5 Distribution of endoplasmic reticulum (ER) and mitochondria in trigeminal ganglion neurons (TGNs). **(a)** Confocal image showing the distribution of ER in a TGN as revealed by labeling with ERtracker Blue–White DPX (1 μM). **(b)** Distribution of mitochondria revealed by labeling with Mitotracker Deep Red (0.1 μM). **(c)** The nucleus, with its higher aqueous volume, was visualized by loading the TGN the cell permeable calcium indicator, fluo-3 acetoxymethyl ester (1 μM) a Ca^{2+}indicator dye. **(d)** Overlay of images from **(a–c)**: *Scale bar* 5 μm. *Yellow arrows* on the composite image represent the location where a 5-pixel-wide intensity profile was measured for each image. An intensity profile for each dye is shown in the *bottom-left corner* of each image. The neurons were incubated with the dyes for 1 h at room temperature

in increased PMCA Ca^{2+} extrusion activity for up to 1 h owing to the slow dissociation of calmodulin from the PMCA. The activity of the PMCA also depends on its state of phosphorylation.

Direct phosphorylation of the PMCA by protein kinase C (PKC) and protein kinase A (PKA) has been shown to increase the activity of PMCA (Zylinska et al. 1998). Tyrosine phosphorylation of the PMCA has been shown to be inhibitory (Dean et al. 1997). In DRG neurons, application of bradykinin and ATP leads to increased PKC activity. Subsequently, the PMCA's activity in DRG neurons is increased, resulting in shorter Ca^{2+} transients (Usachev et al. 2002). Usachev et al. (2002) demonstrated that increased PMCA activity leads to greater neuronal excitability owing to a decrease in Ca^{2+}-activated K^+ currents after an action potential.

6.2 *Sodium–Calcium Exchanger*

The NCX, like the PMCA, is a protein responsible for removing Ca^{2+} from the cytosol of neurons. The NCX uses the favorable electrochemical gradient of three Na^+ ions to remove a single Ca^{2+} ion. This exchanger is therefore electrogenic and its activity is dependent not only on the relative concentrations of Na^+ and Ca^{2+}ions but also on the neuron's membrane potential. Multiple regulatory domains have been identified on the NCX, including phosphorylation sites and Ca^{2+} binding domains (for a review see Philipson and Nicoll 2000). However, in sensory somata, peripheral axons, and sensory nerve terminals, blocking the NCX has little, if any, effect on evoked Ca^{2+} transients (Thayer and Miller 1990; Wächtler et al. 1998; Gover et al. 2007a, b; see, however, Verdru et al. 1997).

6.3 *Ryanodine Receptors*

Owing to the fact that Ca^{2+} concentrations in the ER are typically in the millimolar range and ER membranes have significantly larger surface area than plasma membranes, release of Ca^{2+} from the ER may result in substantial cytoplasmic Ca^{2+} transients. At least two Ca^{2+} release channels are responsible for ER Ca^{2+} release in peripheral sensory neurons: they are the IP_3R and the RyR. (Moore et al. 1998; Shmigol et al. 1995; Gover et al. 2007a). Most primary sensory neurons have robust CICR. CICR is mediated through the activation of RyRs residing on the membrane of the ER. There are three isoforms of the RyRs in mammals (RYR1–3) that form homomeric tetramers (for a review see McPherson and Campbell 1993). Primary sensory neurons possess RyR3 with no detectable levels of RyR1, and RaR2, as demonstrated through western blot analysis (Lokuta et al. 2002). RyRs are activated by Ca^{2+} between concentrations of 1 and 10 μM. At higher concentrations of Ca^{2+} (1–10 mM), the RyRs become inhibited. The RyRs have numerous regulatory domains, including phosphorylation sites for PKA, PKC, protein kinase G, Ca^{2+}/calmodulin-dependent protein kinase II, and protein tyrosine kinases, and sites for binding several regulatory proteins such as calmodulin, calsequestrin, and FK-506. Ooashi et al. (2005) demonstrated that the activation of PKA facilitates the RyR3 activation in DRG neurons. Activation of the RyR and CICR may lead to the direct activation of several different calcium-activated ionic conductances on the plasma membrane (see above). For example, both glutamate and bradykinin have been shown to excite DRG neurons by activation of Ca^{2+}-activated inward currents (McGuirk and Dolphin 1992; Crawford et al. 1997). Both of these inward currents were abolished by depletion of ER calcium stores or by the addition of the RyR antagonist ryanodine. In addition, CICR has been demonstrated to mediate the sAHP in nodose neurons that results in spike frequency accommodation (Moore et al. 1998; see Sect. 4.3). CICR has also been demonstrated to participate in the activation of depolarizing membrane potentials in injured NGNs and cultured DRG neurons (Ayar et al. 1999; Lancaster et al. 2002).

6.4 Inositol Triphosphate Receptor

Like the RyR, the IP_3R is a Ca^{2+} release channel that resides on the ER membrane. There are three isoforms of the IP_3R (IP_3R1–3). At least types 1 and 3 have been shown to be present in primary sensory neurons (Dent et al. 1996; Blackshaw et al. 2000). Activation of several metabotropic plasma membrane receptors can lead to the activation of phosphoinositide phospholipase C. Phospholipase C subsequently cleaves phosphatidylinositol bisphosphate producing diacylglycerol and IP_3. Diacylglycerol may than activate PKC and IP_3 may bind to and activate the IP_3R, releasing Ca^{2+} from ER stores. As with the RyR, there are numerous regulatory domains on the IP_3R. They include several binding domains for regulatory proteins such as calmodulin, FKBP12, and CBP1, and multiple phosphorylation sites and Ca^{2+} binding sites (for a review see Mikoshiba 2007). The physiological role of these regulatory domains in primary sensory neurons is not yet known. Hoesch et al. (2004) demonstrated using caged IP_3 that nodose ganglion neurones posses a K^+ current that is activated by Ca^{2+} released following activation of the IP_3R that is pharmacologically distinct from other Ca^{2+}-activated K^+ channels.

6.5 Sarcoplasmic/Endoplasmic Reticulum Calcium ATPase

ER Ca^{2+} stores in sensory cell bodies are replenished by the activity of SERCA. Vertebrates have three different genes that encode for SERCA (ATP2A1–3). With multiple splice variants, there are a total of nine different isoforms (for a review see Wuytack et al. 2002). The identity of the SERCA protein(s) present in primary sensory neurons has yet to be determined. SERCA uses the energy from the hydrolysis of a single ATP molecule for the removal of two Ca^{2+} ions from the cytosol to the ER (for a review see Wuytack et al. 2002). Pharmacological inhibition of SERCA has demonstrated that this protein has a role in removing Ca^{2+} from the cytosol of primary sensory neurons after a Ca^{2+} transient (Usachev et al. 2006; Gover et al. 2007a). This protein appears to be solely responsible for replenishing the ER Ca^{2+} store, as inhibition of SERCA results in a completely depleted Ca^{2+} pool (Cohen et al. 1997). SERCA interacts with several regulatory proteins, including phospholambam, sarcolipin, calreticulin, and calnexin (Wuytack et al. 2002). In addition, direct phosphorylation of SERCA may lead to an increase in its activity

(Xu et al. 1993). Indeed, Usachev et al. (2006) have demonstrated that the activity of SERCA in DRG neurons is increased after the activation of PKC. The increased activation of SERCA leads in these neurons to a more rapid decrease in cytoplasmic Ca^{2+} and possibly increases in excitability resulting from decreased Ca^{2+}-activated K^+ channels.

6.6 *Mitochondria*

In addition to the ER, the mitochondria play a significant role in Ca^{2+} regulation and sensory neuronal excitability. Calcium is passively transported down a favorable electrochemical gradient into the mitochondria through a calcium uniporter. Calcium leaves the mitochondria through a NCX. It has been demonstrated that mitochondria in DRG and TG neurons buffer Ca^{2+} transients under normal

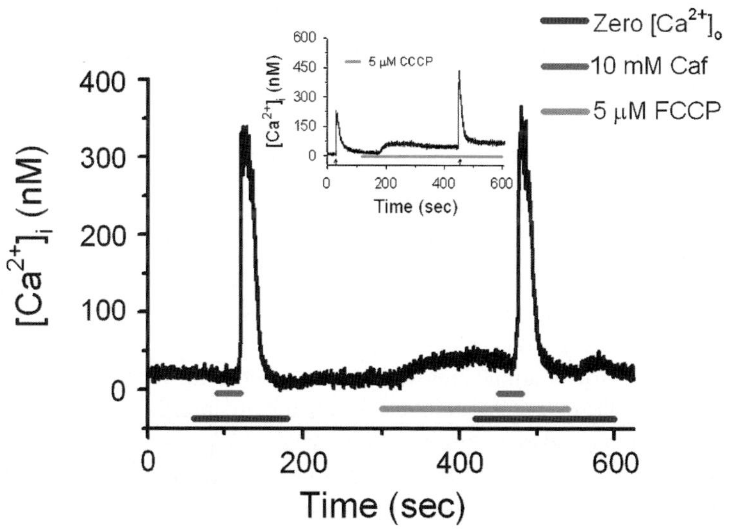

Fig. 6 Mitochondria buffer entry of extracellular Ca^{2+} but not release of Ca^{2+} from internal stores in TGNs. A 30-s application of 10 mM caffeine in a nominally free Ca^{2+} solution evoked a Ca^{2+} transient in an acutely dissociated TGN. After incubation with carbonyl cyanide p-(trifluoromethoxy) phenylhydrazone (FCCP; 5 μM), an uncoupler of mitochondrial oxidative phosphorylation, for 2.5 min, a second 30-s application of 10 mM caffeine evoked a Ca^{2+} transient that was not significantly different in amplitude relative to the control. *Inset:* A 500-ms pulse of 50 mM KCl (*first arrow*) evoked a Ca^{2+} transient in an acutely dissociated TGN. After incubation with the mitochondrial proton motive force inhibitor, carbonyl cyanide-m-chlorophenylhydrazone (CCCP; 5 μM) for 3 min, a KCl pulse (*second arrow*) evoked a Ca^{2+} transient that had a significantly larger amplitude relative to the control. Proton ionophores such as p-trifluoromethoxyphenylhydrazone (FCCP) or carbonyl cyanide 3-chloro-phenylhydrazone (CCCP) inhibit mitochondrial Ca^{2+} uptake

physiological conditions (Werth and Thayer 1994; Gover et al. 2007a). Indeed, the disruption of the ability of the mitochondria to buffer Ca^{2+} leads to the activation of Ca^{2+}-activated potassium conductances and possible quiescence of the neuron (Duchen 1990). Interestingly, mitochondria appear to preferentially take up Ca^{2+} entering the cell across the plasma membrane and not from intracellular Ca^{2+} release in DRG and TG sensory neurons (Svichar et al. 1997; unpublished observations; Fig. 6).

7 Altered Excitability and Ca^{2+} Regulation as a Result of Peripheral Neuropathies

There are numerous peripheral sensory neuronal diseases and neuropathies that alter sensory nerve excitability. Many of these conditions have been correlated with changes in Ca^{2+} regulation. Whether these Ca^{2+} alterations are the result of compensatory mechanisms associated with changes in excitability or whether the Ca^{2+} alterations directly change sensory nerve excitability requires more investigation. In the following sections a few examples of diseases and neuropathies that are associated with changes in the handling of sensory nerve Ca^{2+} are described.

7.1 Chemotherapy-Induced Neuropathies

Antineoplastic agents, particularly those derived from plant alkaloids, often produce severe peripheral neuropathic side effects, which become dose-limiting (Wiernik et al. 1987). Paclitaxel is one of the most commonly used chemotherapeutic agents for the treatment of ovarian, breast, and small-cell lung cancers. Neuropathies associated with the administration of paclitaxel are mostly sensory in nature, producing symptoms such as tingling, numbness, and burning pain usually manifesting first in the distal extremities (for a review see Mielke et al. 2006). Paclitaxel's antineoplastic effects are thought to be due to its ability to bind ß-tubulin and promote microtubule polymerization. There is evidence that paclitaxel (at clinically relevant doses) induced sensory neuropathies are not the result of microtubule disruption in sensory axons (Polomano et al. 2001). We would predict from several recent reports a disruption in Ca^{2+} signaling in sensory neurons after administration of paclitaxel (Wang et al. 2004; Boehmerle et al. 2006; Matsumoto et al. 2006). Disruption of Ca^{2+} signaling may lead to direct increases in sensory nerve excitability or changes in metabolic/enzymatic processes that ultimately would lead to increases in excitability. Matsumoto et al. (2006), for example, reported an increase in the expression of the $Ca\alpha_2\delta$-1 Ca^{2+} channel subunit in rat DRG after administration of a single clinically relevant dose of paclitaxel. The $Ca\alpha_2\delta$-1 subunit is an associated subunit of an L-type Ca^{2+} channel, the dominant voltage-operated Ca^{2+}

current contributor in sensory nerve terminals (Gover et al. 2003). In another study, Boehmerle et al. (2006) demonstrated that paclitaxel can directly bind to and activate the neuronal Ca^{2+} sensor-1, leading to Ca^{2+} oscillations via activation of the IP_3 pathway in human neuroblastoma cells. In addition, several in vivo studies have demonstrated that selective Ca^{2+} channel blockers, such as ethosuximide and gabapentin, and Ca^{2+} chelators reduce the neuropathic side effects of paclitaxel and vincristine (Siau et al. 2006; Flatters and Bennett 2004; Xiao et al. 2007). However, to date, no studies have examined Ca^{2+} homeostasis during neuropathies in peripheral sensory nerve terminals.

7.2 Diabetic-Induced Neuropathies

Diabetic-induced peripheral neuropathies are extremely complex. A common complicating symptom of diabetes is the onset of chronic pain (Boulton et al. 1985). Numerous studies implicate mishandling of Ca^{2+} as a major cause for changes in excitability in diabetic neuropathies. Ca^{2+} transients elicited in small DRG neurons (18–25 μm in diameter) by depolarization are significantly prolonged in mice with induced diabetes (Kostyuk et al. 1995). This prolongation of the Ca^{2+} transient may be the result of disruption of mitochondrial or ER Ca^{2+} uptake mechanisms (Svichar et al. 1998; Kruglikov et al. 2004). In addition, primary sensory neurons in animals with experimentally induced diabetes have altered VDCC expression (Yusaf et al. 2001). Jagodic et al. (2007) demonstrated that the T-type Ca^{2+} currents are upregulated in DRG neurons after induction of diabetes. This lead to more prominent ADP and lower action potential threshold for burst firing, making the DRG neurons from diabetic animals more excitable.

8 Nerve Injury

Traumatic peripheral nerve injury, such as axotomy, may produce chronic pain owing to increased nerve excitability (Devor et al. 1994; Nordin et al. 1984). Several ionic conductances have been reported to change after nerve injury (Lancaster et al. 2001). Both HVA and LVA Ca^{2+} currents are downregulated in DRG neurons after nerve ligation, resulting in reduced intracellular Ca^{2+} transients (Fuchs et al. 2007). Subsequently, AHPs are reduced, resulting in increased membrane excitability (McCallum et al. 2006). Surprisingly, in a subpopulation of NGNs, unlike DRG neurons, Ca^{2+} currents are increased after axotomy (Lancaster et al. 2002). In this same subpopulation, there is an appearance of an ADP not normally found in NGNs. However, unlike DRG neurons, all axotomized NGNs are less excitable than controls (Lancaster et al. 2001). In addition to ionic conductance changes, the expression of Ca^{2+} regulatory proteins is modified. PMCA4 is upregulated in DRG neurons after spinal ligation. While PMCA1-3 are downregulated

(Ogura et al. 2007). The effect of this modification in expression on excitability is not yet known.

Acknowledgements We would like to thank Jessica Swartz for her valuable input to this work and for her critique of an earlier version of this manuscript. This work was supported by NIH grants NS22069 (D.W.) and ST32-NS007375 (T.D.G.).

References

Adelman JP, Shen KZ, Kavanaugh MP, Warren RA, Wu YN, Lagrutta A, Bond CT, North RA (1992) Calcium-activated potassium channels expressed from cloned complementary DNAs. Neuron 9(2):209–216

Atkinson NS, Robertson GA, Ganetzky B (1992) A component of calcium-activated potassium channels encoded by the *Drosophila slo* locus. Science 253:551–555

Ayar A, Storer C, Tatham EL, Scott RH (1999) The effects of changing intracellular Ca^{2+} buffering on the excitability of cultured dorsal root ganglion neurones. Neurosci Lett 271(3): 171–174

Bader CR, Bertrand D, Schlichter R (1987) Calcium-activated chloride current in cultured sensory and parasympathetic quail neurones. J Physiol 394:125–148

Baimbridge K, Celio M, Rogers J (1992) Calcium-binding proteins in the nervous system. Trends Neuroscience 15:303–308

Belmonte C, Gallego R (1983) Membrane properties of cat sensory neurones with chemoreceptor and baroreceptor endings. J Physiol 342:603–614

Bird MM, Lieberman AR (1976) Microtubule fascicles in the stem processes of cultured sensory ganglion cells. Cell Tissue Res 169(1):41–47

Blackshaw S, Sawa A, Sharp AH, Ross CA, Snyder SH, Khan AA (2000) Type 3 inositol 1,4,5-trisphosphate receptor modulates cell death. FASEB J 14(10):1375–1379

Boehmerle W, Splittgerber U, Lazarus MB, McKenzie KM, Johnston DG, Austin DJ, Ehrlich BE (2006) Paclitaxel induces calcium oscillations via an inositol 1,4,5-trisphosphate receptor and neuronal calcium sensor 1-dependent mechanism. Proc Natl Acad Sci USA 103(48):18356–18361

Bond CT, Herson PS, Strassmaier T, Hammond R, Stackman R, Maylie J, Adelman JP (2004) Small conductance Ca^{2+}-activated K^+ channel knock-out mice reveal the identity of calcium-dependent afterhyperpolarization currents. J Neurosci 24(23):5301–5306

Boulton AJ, Knight G, Drury J, Ward JD (1985) The prevalence of symptomatic, diabetic neuropathy in an insulin-treated population. Diabetes Care 8(2):125–128

Carafoli E (1991) The calcium pumping ATPase of the plasma membrane. Annu Rev Physiol 53:531–547

Catterall WA, Striessnig J, Snutch TP, Perez-Reyes E (2005) International Union of Pharmacology. XL. Compendium of voltage-gated ion channels: calcium channels. Pharmacol Rev 55(4): 579–581

Chard PS, Bleakman D, Christakos S, Fullmer CS, Miller RJ (1993) Calcium buffering properties of calbindin D28k and parvalbumin in rat sensory neurones. J Physiol 472:341–357

Christian EP, Taylor GE, Weinreich D (1989) Serotonin increaes excitability of rabbit C-fiber neurons by two distinct mechanisms. J Applied Physiol 67:584–591

Christian EP, Togo J, Naper KE (1994) Guinea pig visceral C-fiber neurons are diverse with respect to the K^+ currents involved in action-potential repolarization. J Neurophysiol 71(2): 561–574

Cohen AC, Moore KA, Bangalore R, Jafri MS, Weinreich D, Kao JPY (1997) Ca^{2+}-induced Ca^{2+} release mediates Ca^{2+} transients evoked by single action potentials in rabbit vagal afferents. J Physiol 499:315–328

Conigrave AD, Quinn SJ, Brown EM (2000) Cooperative multi-modal sensing and therapeutic implications of the extracellular Ca^{2+} sensing receptor. Trends Pharmacol Sci 10:401–407

Cordoba-Rodriguez R, Moore KA, Kao JP, Weinreich D (1999) Calcium regulation of a slow post-spike hyperpolarization in vagal afferent neurons. Proc Natl Acad Sci USA 96(14):7650–7657

Crawford JH, Wootton JF, Seabrook GR, Scott RH (1997) Activation of Ca^{2+}-dependent currents in dorsal root ganglion neurons by metabotropic glutamate receptors and cyclic ADP-ribose precursors. J Neurophysiol 77(5):2573–2584

Currie KPM, Scott RH (1992) Calcium-activated currents in cultured neurones from rat dorsal root ganglia. Br J Pharmacol 106:593–602

Dean WL, Chen D, Brandt PC, Vanaman TC (1997) Regulation of platelet plasma membrane Ca^{2+}-ATPase by cAMP-dependent and tyrosine phosphorylation. J Biol Chem 272(24):15113–15119

Dent MA, Raisman G, Lai FA (1996) Expression of type 1 inositol 1,4,5-trisphosphate receptor during axogenesis and synaptic contact in the central and peripheral nervous system of developing rat. Development 122(3):1029–1039

Deschenes M, Feltz P, Lamour Y (1976) A model for the estimate of the ionic basis of presynaptic inhibition: an intracellular analysis of the GABA induced depolarization in rat dorsal root ganglia. Brain Res 18:486–493

Devor M, Jänig W, Michaelis M (1994) Modulation of activity in dorsal root ganglion neurons by sympathetic activation in nerve-injured rats. J Neurophysiol 71(1):38–47

Duchen MR (1990) Effects of metabolic inhibition on the membrane properties of isolated mouse primary sensory neurones. J Physiol 424:387–409

Ertel EA, Campbell KP, Harpold MM, Hofmann F, Mori Y, Perez-Reyes E, Schwartz A, Snutch TP, Tanabe T, Birnbaumer L et alet al (2000) Nomenclature of voltage gatedcalcium channels Neuron 25:533–535

Faber ES, Sah P (2003) Ca^{2+}-activated K^{+} (BK) channel inactivation contributes to spike broadening during repetitive firing in the rat lateral amygdala. J Physiol 552(2):483–497

Flatters SJ, Bennett GJ (2004) Ethosuximide reverses paclitaxel- and vincristine-induced painful peripheral neuropathy. Pain 109(1-2):150–161

Fowler JC, Greene R, Weinreich D (1985) Two calcium-sensitive spike after-hyperpolarizations in visceral sensory neurones of the rabbit. J Physiol (Lond) 365:59–75

Fox AJ, Barnes PJ, Venkatesan P, Belvisi MG (1997) Activation of large conductance potassium channels inhibits the afferent and efferent function of airway sensory nerves in the guinea pig. J Clin Invest 99:513–519

Frings S, Reuter D, Kleene SJ (2000) Neuronal Ca^{2+}-activated Cl^{-} channels – homing in on an elusive channel species. Prog Neurobiol 60(3):247–289

Fuchs A, Rigaud M, Sarantopoulos CD, Filip P, Hogan QH (2007) Contribution of calcium channel subtypes to the intracellular calcium signal in sensory neurons: the effect of injury. Anesthesiology 107(1):117–127

Gallagher JP, Higashi H, Nishi I (1978) Characterization and ionic basis of GABA-induced depolarizations recorded in vitro from cat primary afferent neurons. J Physiol 275:263–282

Gallego R, Eyzaguirre C (1978) Membrane and action potential characteristics of A and C nodose ganglion cells studied in whole ganglia and in tissue slices. J Neurophysiol 41 (5):1217–1232

Gold MS, Shuster MJ, Levine JD (1996) Role of a Ca^{2+}-dependent slow afterhyperpolarization in prostaglandin E2-induced sensitization of cultured rat sensory neurons. Neurosci Lett 205(3):161–164

Gover TD, Moreira TH, Kao JP, Weinreich D (2007a) Calcium homeostasis in trigeminal ganglion cell bodies. Cell Calcium 41(4):389–396

Gover TD, Moreira TH, Kao JP, Weinreich D (2007b) Calcium regulation in individual peripheral sensory nerve terminals of the rat. J Physiol 578(Pt 2):481–490

Gover TD, Kao JP, Weinreich D (2003). Calcium signaling in single peripheral sensory nerve terminals. J Neurosci 23;4793–4797

Hablitz JJ, Heinemann U, Lux HD Step reductions in extracellular Ca^{2+} activate a transient inward current in chick dorsal root ganglion cells. Biophys J 50:753–757

Hay M, Kunze DL (1994) An intermediate conductance calcium-activated potassium channel in rat visceral sensory afferent neurons. Neurosci Lett 167(1–2):179–182

Hartzell C, Putzier I, Arreola J (2005). Calcium-activated chloride channels. Ann Rev Physiol 67: 719–758

Hille B (2001) Ion channels of excitable membranes, 3d edn. Sinauer, Sunderland, MA

Hoesch RE, Yienger K, Weinreich D, Kao JP (2002) Coexistence of functional IP(3) and ryanodine receptors in vagal sensory neurons and their activation by ATP. J Neurophysiol 88(3):1212–1219

Honda CN (1995) Differential distribution of calbindin-D28K and parvalbumin in somatic and visceral sensory neurons. Neuro Science 68(3):883–892

Hoesch RE, Weinreich D, Kao JP (2004) Localized IP3-evoked Ca^{2+} release activates a K^+ current in primary vagal sensory neurons. J Neurophysiol 91(5):2344–2352

Ishii TM, Silvia C, Hirschberg B, Bond CT, Adelman JP (1997) A human intermediate conductance calcium-activated potassium channel. Proc Natl Acad Sci USA 94:11651–11656

Jafri MS, Moore KA, Taylor GE, Weinreich D (1997) Histamine H_1 receptor activation blocks two classes of potassium current, $IK_{(rest)}$ and I_{AHP}, to excite ferret vagal afferents. J Physiol 503.3:533–546

Jagodic MM, Pathirathna S, Nelson MT, Mancuso S, Joksovic PM, Rosenberg ER, Bayliss DA, Jevtovic-Todorovic V, Todorovic SM (2007) Cell-specific alterations of T-type calcium current in painful diabetic neuropathy enhance excitability of sensory neurons. J Neurosci 27 (12):3305–3316

Kostyuk E, Pronchuk N, Shmigol A (1995) Calcium signal prolongation in sensory neurones of mice with experimental diabetes. Neuroreport 6(7):1010–1012

Kostyuk E, Svichar N, Shishkin V, Kostyuk P (1999) Role of mitochondrial dysfunction in calcium signalling alterations in dorsal root ganglion neurons of mice with experimentally-induced diabetes. Neuroscience 90(2):535–541

Kruglikov I, Gryshchenko O, Shutov L, Kostyuk E, Kostyuk P, Voitenko N (2004) Diabetes-induced abnormalities in ER calcium mobilization in primary and secondary nociceptive neurons. Pflugers Arch 448(4):395–401

Lancaster E, Oh EJ, Weinreich D (2001) Vagotomy decreases excitability in primary vagal afferent somata. J Neurophysiol 85:247–253

Lancaster E, Oh EJ, Gover T, Weinreich D (2002) Calcium and calcium-activated currents in vagotomized rat primary vagal afferent neurons. J Physiol 540(Pt 2):543–556

Lee M-G, Kollarik M, Chaychoo B, Undem BJ (2004) Ionoteropic and metabotropic receptor mediated airway sensory nerve activation. Pulm Pharmacol Ther 17:355–360

Li W, Gao SB, Lv CX, Wu Y, Guo ZH, Ding JP, Xu T (2007) Characterization of voltage- and Ca^{2+}-activated K^+ channels in rat dorsal root ganglion neurons. J Cell Physiol 212(2): 348–357

Lokuta AJ, Komai H, McDowell TS, Valdivia HH (2002) Functional properties of ryanodine receptors from rat dorsal root ganglia. FEBS Lett 511(1–3):90–96

Marrion NV, Tavalin SJ (1998) Selective activation of Ca^{2+}-activated K^+ channels by co-localized Ca^{2+} channels in hippocampal neurons. Nature 395(6705):900–905

Matsuda Y, Yoshida S, Yonezawa T (1976) A Ca-dependent regenerative response in rodent dorsal root ganglion cells cultured in vitro. Brain Res 115(2):334–338

Matsumoto M, Inoue M, Hald A, Xie W, Ueda H (2006) Inhibition of paclitaxel-induced A-fiber hypersensitization by gabapentin. J Pharmacol Exp Ther 318(2):735–740

Mayer ML (1985) A calcium-activated chloride current generates the afterdepolarization of rat sensory neurones in culture. J Physiol 364:217–239

McCallum JB, Kwok WM, Sapunar D, Fuchs A, Hogan QH (2006) Painful peripheral nerve injury decreases calcium current in axotomized sensory neurons. Anesthesiology 105(1):160–168

McGuirk SM, Dolphin AC (1992) G-protein mediation in nociceptive signal transduction: an investigation into the excitatory action of bradykinin in a subpopulation of cultured rat sensory neurons. Neuroscience 49(1):117–128

McPherson PS, Campbell KP (1993) The ryanodine receptor/Ca^{2+} release channel. J Biol Chem 268(19):13765–13768

Mielke S, Sparreboom A, Mross K (2006) Peripheral neuropathy: a persisting challenge in paclitaxel-based regimes. Eur J Cancer 42(1):24–30

Mikoshiba K (2007) The IP3 receptor/Ca^{2+} channel and its cellular function. Biochem Soc Symp 74:9–22

Mongan LC, Hill MJ, Chen MX, Tate SN, Collins SD, Buckby L, Grubb BD (2005) The distribution of small and intermediate conductance calcium-activated potassium channels in the rat sensory nervous system. Neuroscience 131(1):161–175

Moore KA, Cohen AS, Kao JP, Weinreich D (1998) Ca^{2+}-induced Ca^{2+} release mediates a slow post-spike hyperpolarization in rabbit vagal afferent neurons. J Neurophysiol 79 (2):688–694

Neylon CB, Nurgali K, Hunne B, Robbins HL, Moore S, Chen MX, Furness JB (2004) Intermediate-conductance calcium-activated potassium channels in enteric neurones of the mouse: pharmacological, molecular and immunochemical evidence for their role in mediating the slow afterhyperpolarization. J Neurochem 90(6):1414–1422

Nordin M, Nyström B, Wallin U, Hagbarth KE (1984) Ectopic sensory discharges and paresthesiae in patients with disorders of peripheral nerves, dorsal roots and dorsal columns. Pain 20(3): 231–245

Ogura H, Tachibana T, Yamanaka H, Kobayashi K, Obata K, Dai Y, Yoshiya S, Noguchi K (2007) Axotomy increases plasma membrane Ca^{2+} pump isoform4 in primary afferent neurons. Neuroreport 18(1):17–22

Oh EJ, Weinreich D (2004) Bradykinin decreases K^+ and increases Cl^- conductances in vagal afferent neurones of the guinea pig. J Physiol 558(Pt 2):513–526

Ooashi N, Futatsugi A, Yoshihara F, Mikoshiba K, Kamiguchi H (2005) Cell adhesion molecules regulate Ca^{2+}-mediated steering of growth cones via cyclic AMP and ryanodine receptor type 3. J Cell Biol 170(7):1159–1167

Philipson KD, Nicoll DA (2000) Sodium-calcium exchange: a molecular perspective. Annu Rev Physiol 62:111–133

Polomano RC, Mannes AJ, Clark US, Bennett GJ (2001) A painful peripheral neuropathy in the rat produced by the chemotherapeutic drug, paclitaxel. Pain 94(3):293–304

Pottorf WJ, Thayer SA (2002) Transient rise in intracellular calcium produces a long-lasting increasein plasma membrane calcium pump activity in rat sensory neurons. J Neurochem 83(4):1002–1008

Ransom BR, Holz RW (1977) Ionic determinants of excitability in cultured mouse dorsal root ganglion and spinal cord cells. Brain Res 136(3):445–453

Ringer S, (1882a) Regarding the Action of Hydrate of Soda, Hydrate of Ammonia, and Hydrate of Postash on the Ventricle of the Frog's Heart. J Physiol 3:195–202

Ringer S, (1882b) Concerning the Influence exerted by each of the Constituents of the Blood on the Contraction of the Ventricle. J Physiol 3:380–393

Ringer S, (1883a) A further Contribution regarding the influence of the different Constituents of the Blood on the Contraction of the Heart. J Physiol 3:29–42

Ringer S, (1883b) A third contribution regarding the Influence of the Inorganic Constituents of the Blood on the Ventricular Contraction. J Physiol 3:222–225

Sah P, Faber ES (2002) Channels underlying neuronal calcium-activated potassium currents. Prog Neurobiol 66(5):345–353

Salkoff L, Butler A, Ferreira G, Santi C, Wei A (2006) High-conductance potassium channels of the SLO family. Nat Rev Neurosci 7(12):921–931

Schlichter R, Bader CR, Bertrand D, Dubois-Dauphin M, Bernheim L (1989) Expression of substance P and of a Ca^{2+}-activated Cl^- current in quail sensory trigeminal neurons. Neuroscience 30:585–594

Scott RH, McGuir SM, Dolphin AC (1988) Modulation of divalent cation-activated chloride ion currents. Br J Pharmacol 94:653–662

Scott RH, Sutton KG, Griffin A, Stapleton SR, Currie KP (1995) Aspects of calcium-activated chloride currents: a neuronal perspective. Pharmacol Ther 66:535–565

Scroggs RS, Fox AP (1992) Multiple Ca^{2+} currents elicited by action potential waveforms in acutely isolated adult rat dorsal root ganglion neurons. J Neurosci 12(5):1789–1801

Shah M, Haylett DG (2000) Ca^{2+} channels involved in the generation of the slow afterhyperpolarization in cultured rat hippocampal pyramidal neurons. J Neurophysiol 83(5):2554–2561

Shishkin V, Potapenko E, Kostyuk E, Girnyk O, Voitenko N, Kostyuk P (2002) Role of mitochondria in intracellular calcium signaling in primary and secondary sensory neurons of rats. Cell Calcium 32:121–130

Shmigol A, Verkhratsky A, Isenberg G (1995) Calcium-induced calcium release in rat sensory neurons. J Physiol 489 (Pt 3):627–636

Siau C, Xiao W, Bennett GJ (2006) Paclitaxel- and vincristine-evoked painful peripheral neuropathies: loss of epidermal innervation and activation of Langerhans cells. Exp Neurol 201(2):507–514

Sung KW, Kirby M, McDonald MP, Lovinger DM, Delpire E (2000) Abnormal GABAA receptor-mediated currents in dorsal root ganglion neurones isolated from Na-K-2CL cotransporter null mice. J Neurosci 20:7531–7538

Svichar N, Kostyuk P, Verkhratsky A (1997) Mitochondria buffer Ca^{2+} entry but not intracellular Ca^{2+} release in mouse DRG neurones. Neuroreport 8(18):3929–3932

Svichar N, Shishkin V, Kostyuk E, Voitenko N (1998) Changes in mitochondrial Ca^{2+} homeostasis in primary sensory neurons of diabetic mice. Neuroreport 9(6):1121–1125

Thayer SA, Miller RJ (1990) Regulation of the intracellular free calcium concentration in single rat dorsal root ganglion neurons in vitro. J Physiol (Lond) 425:85–115

Thayer SA, Perney TM, Miller RJ (1988) Regulation of calcium homeostasis in sensory neurons by bradykinin. J Neurosci 11:4089–4097

Thayer SA, Usachev YM, Pottorf WJ (2002) Modulating Ca^{2+} clearance from neurons. Front Biosci 7:d1255–d1279

Undem BJ, Hubbard W, Weinreich D (1993) Immunologically-induced neuromodulation of guinea pig nodose ganglion neurons. J Auton Nerv Syst 44:35–44

Undem BJ, Oh EO, Lancaster E, Weinreich D (2002) Effect of extracellular calcium on excitability of guinea pig airway vagal afferent nerves. J Neurophysiol 89:1196–1204

Undem BJ, Oh EJ, Lancaster E, Weinreich D (2003) Effect of extracellular calcium on excitability of guinea pig airway vagal afferent nerves. J Neurophysiol 89:1196–1204

Usachev YM, DeMarco SJ, Campbell C, Strehler EE, Thayer SA (2002) Bradykinin and ATP accelerates Ca^{2+} efflux from rat sensory neurons via protein kinase C and the plasma membrane Ca^{2+} pump isoform 4. Neuron 33:113–122

Usachev YM, Marsh AJ, Johanns TM, Lemke MM, Thayer SA (2006) Activation of protein kinase C in sensory neurons accelerates Ca^{2+} uptake into the endoplasmic reticulum. J Neurosci 26(1):311–318

Verdru P, De Greef C, Mertens L, Carmeliet E, Callewaert G (1997) Na^+–Ca^{2+} exchange in rat dorsal root ganglion neurons. J Neurophysiol 77:484–490

Vogalis F, Storm JF, Lancaster B (2003) SK channels and the varieties of slow after-hyperpolarizations in neurons. Eur J Neurosci 18:3155–3166

Wächtler J, Mayer C, Grafe P (1998) Activity-dependent intracellular Ca^{2+} transients in unmyelinated nerve fibres of the isolated adult rat vagus nerve. Pflűgers Arch 435:678–686

Wang MS, Davis AA, Culver DG, Wang Q, Powers JC, Glass JD (2004) Calpain inhibition protects against Taxol-induced sensory neuropathy. Brain 127(Pt 3):671–679

Weinreich D, Wonderlin WF (1987) Inhibition of calcium-dependent spike after-hyperpolarization increases excitability of rabbit visceral sensory neurones. J Physiol 394:415–427

Werth JL, Thayer SA (1994) Mitochondria buffer physiological calcium loads in cultured rat dorsal root ganglion neurons. J Neurosci 14:348–356

Werth JL, Usachev YM, Thayer SA (1996) Modulation of calcium efflux from cultured rat dorsal root ganglion neurons. J Neurosci 16(3):1008–1015

Wiernik PH, Schwartz EL, Strauman JJ, Dutcher JP, Lipton RB, Paietta E (1987) Phase I clinical and pharmacokinetic study of taxol. Cancer Res 47(9):2486–2493

Wuytack F, Raeymaekers L, Missiaen L (2002) Molecular physiology of the SERCA and SPCA pumps. Cell Calcium 32(5–6):279–305

Xiao W, Boroujerdi A, Bennett GJ, Luo ZD (2007) Chemotherapy-evoked painful peripheral neuropathy: analgesic effects of gabapentin and effects on expression of the alpha-2-delta type-1 calcium channel subunit. Neuroscience 144(2):714–720

Xu A, Hawkins C, Narayanan N (1993) Phosphorylation and activation of the Ca^{2+}-pumping ATPase of cardiac sarcoplasmic reticulum by Ca^{2+}/calmodulin-dependent protein kinase. J Biol Chem 268(12):8394–8397

Yusaf SP, Goodman J, Gonzalez IM, Bramwell S, Pinnock RD, Dixon AK, Lee K (2001) Streptozocin-induced neuropathy is associated with altered expression of voltage-gated calcium channel subunit mRNAs in rat dorsal root ganglion neurones. Biochem Biophys Res Commun 289(2):402–406

Zhang XF, Gopalakrishnan M, Shieh CC (2003) Modulation of action potential firing by iberiotoxin and NS1619 in rat dorsal root ganglion neurons. Neuroscience 122, 1003–1011

Zylinska L, Guerini D, Gromadzinska E, Lachowicz L (1998) Protein kinases A and C phosphorylate purified Ca^{2+}-ATPase from rat cortex, cerebellum and hippocampus. Biochim Biophys Acta 1448(1):99–108

Future Treatment Strategies for Neuropathic Pain

Fabien Marchand, Nicholas G. Jones, and Stephen B. McMahon

Contents

Abstract The prevalence of people suffering from chronic pain is extremely high and pain affects millions of people worldwide. As such, persistent pain represents a major health problem and an unmet clinical need. The reason for the high incidence of chronic pain patients is in a large part due to a paucity of effective pain control. An important reason for poor pain control is undoubtedly a deficit in our understanding of the underlying causes of chronic pain and as a consequence our arsenal of analgesic therapies is limited. However, there is considerable hope for the development of new classes of analgesic drugs by targeting novel processes contributing to clinically relevant pain. In this chapter we highlight a number of molecular species which are potential therapeutic targets for future neuropathic

S.B. McMahon (✉)
London Pain Consortium, King's College London, London SE1 1UL, UK
stephen.mcmahon@kcl.ac.uk

B.J. Canning and D. Spina (eds.), *Sensory Nerves*,
Handbook of Experimental Pharmacology 194, DOI: 10.1007/978-3-540-79090-7_17,

pain treatments. In particular, the roles of voltage-gated ion channels, neuroinflammation, protein kinases and neurotrophins are discussed in relation to the generation of neuropathic pain and how by targeting these molecules it may be possible to provide better pain control than is currently available.

Keywords Neuropathic pain, Sodium channels, Neuropeptides, Cannabinoids

1 Introduction

Neuropathic pain (NP), which the International Association for the Study of Pain defines as pain "initiated or caused by a primary lesion or dysfunction in the nervous system" (Treede et al. 2008), is estimated to afflict millions of people worldwide. It can be caused by either peripheral nervous system or central nervous system (CNS) injury (peripheral vs. central neuropathy) and while peripheral neuropathy is by far the more common, central neuropathy is probably the more difficult to treat. The underlying causes of NP are numerous and diverse and can be genetic in origin (Charcot–Marie–Tooth disease) or caused by injury to nerves either directly (amputation, spinal cord injury, nerve root avulsion) or indirectly by metabolic stress (diabetes mellitus type 1 or 2), inappropriate immune responses (Guillain–Barré syndrome) or iatrogenically (HIV neuropathy). NP is characterized by numerous different symptoms that include spontaneous pain, paraesthesia (such as burning pain or tingling), dysesthesia, and exaggerated responses to innocuous and noxious mechanical and/or thermal stimuli (allodynia and hyperalgesia, respectively), and although an individual with NP may exhibit only one of the above-mentioned symptoms, it is more common for NP patients to exhibit a combination of symptoms. Furthermore, although NP symptoms are common, it is unfortunate that current treatments of NP are still unsatisfactory, with only 40–60% of patients responding to treatment with mild pain relief (around 50% improvement) (Sindrup and Jensen 1999; McQuay et al. 1996). Therefore, it is of no surprise that NP represents a clear unmet clinical need. This was highlighted at a recent consensus meeting during which evidence-based recommendations of current therapies for pharmacological management of NP were proposed (Dworkin et al. 2007). At this meeting three different lines of treatment for NP were suggested. Tricyclic antidepressants, selective serotonin and norepinephrine reuptake inhibitors, gabapentin and in specific circumstances topically applied 5% lidocaine were all recommended as first-line treatments. Opioid analgesics, certain antiepileptics, *N*-methyl-D-aspartate (NMDA) antagonists and topically applied capsaicin were recommended as second- and third-line treatments. However, although all these have analgesic actions, with the first-line treatments having in general greater efficacy than second- and third-line treatments, it is accepted that their use is restricted by dose-limiting side effects and none of the medications to date successfully ameliorate all NP symptoms in all patients.

It is clear from the above discussion that despite there being a range of existing drugs to treat NP, they have limited efficacy at attenuating and preventing the debilitating symptoms that NP patients experience. This is highlighted by the limited numbers of patients responding to these therapies, a consequence of their limited therapeutic indices. It is also evident that there is an urgent need for new, more effective treatments for NP. In particular, novel treatments based on our knowledge of the underlying mechanisms of NP have the potential to provide NP patients with effective therapies which at present are desperately needed. In the following, a number of these potential future treatments are discussed.

2 Future Treatment Strategies for NP

2.1 Voltage-Gated Ion Channel Blockers

Evidence from preclinical NP studies indicates that ectopic activity in damaged/dysfunctional peripheral primary sensory neurons may play an active role in the generation and maintenance of NP. Therefore, modulation/attenuation of this ectopic activity seems an attractive strategy for future treatments of NP, especially as there are a number of molecular targets (which include sodium, potassium and calcium channels) which are already known to play a role in generating and propagating action potentials and thus control neuronal firing. In fact, some analgesics (such as lidocaine) that block these channels have already been shown to have appreciable clinical efficacy (Wood 2006). However, unfortunately many of these existing agents are likely to be of limited use owing to the intolerable side effects that are associated with their activity within the CNS.

Nevertheless, ion channels explicitly linked to neuronal activity are credible and exciting potential targets for future NP treatments, and sodium channels are one prime example. In particular, the voltage-gated sodium channels $Na_v1.3$, $Na_v1.7$ and $Na_v1.8$, have been shown to be involved in the manifestation of NP in several preclinical models as well as in humans (for a review see Cummins et al. 2007; Wood and Boorman 2005; Amir et al. 2006). Of these three channels, $Na_v1.7$ is probably the most exciting target as congenital mutation of this particular channel confers the inability to experience pain in humans (Cox et al. 2006; Ahmad et al. 2007). However, preclinical data from mice in which the $Na_v1.7$ gene was selectively knocked out in nociceptive dorsal root ganglia (DRG) neurons show that they develop mechanical allodynia after nerve injury similar to that developed by wild-type controls (Nassar et al. 2005), indicating at least in mice that $Na_v1.7$ may not be pivotally involved in the generation of NP. However, it is interesting to note that humans lacking functional $Na_v1.7$, while insensitive to pain, are generally healthy, while mice with a global $Na_v1.7$ gene knockout die just after birth, thus suggesting a different role for $Na_v1.7$ in mice than in humans, where its role may be exclusively pain related.

Unlike $Na_v1.7$, which is expressed in all unmyelinated axons, $Na_v1.3$ expression is limited in the adult DRG. However, this tetrodotoxin (TTX)-sensitive channel is markedly upregulated in peripheral sensory nerve fibres in several NP models, including axotomy, spinal nerve ligation, chronic constriction injury and diabetic neuropathy (Amir et al. 2006), where it is thought to contribute to neuronal hyperexcitability. In addition, treatment with glial cell line derived neurotrophic factor (GDNF), after initiation of NP, has been shown to normalize $Na_v1.3$ expression, reduce ectopic activity in A-fibres and also reduce pain, suggesting that $Na_v1.3$ maybe an important mediator in the expression of NP. Further preclinical studies using antisense and transgenic strategies to specifically downregulate functional $Na_v1.3$ channels have also achieved modest success in reducing pain behaviour (Hains et al. 2003, 2004; Lindia et al. 2005; Nassar et al. 2006). Thus, these observations suggest that $Na_v1.3$ could be an important contributor to neuronal hyperexcitability in NP. However, the role that $Na_v1.3$ plays in NP is still controversial and the benefits to NP patients of future pain therapies designed to antagonize $Na_v1.3$ function will not be clear until specific pharmacological agents that block $Na_v1.3$ are available.

$Na_v1.8$, unlike $Na_v1.3$ and 1.7, is a TTX-resistant voltage-gated sodium channel that is almost exclusively expressed in nociceptive neurons, a feature which makes it a plausible potential target for novel pain therapies. To test this hypothesis, a number of different strategies (including antisense and gene deletion studies) have previously been used to block functional $Na_v1.8$ activity and investigate an involvement of this channel in inflammatory pain and NP (Cummins et al. 2007). While a role for $Na_v1.8$ in inflammatory pain could clearly be assigned, an involvement of $Na_v1.8$ in NP could not be positively identified (Cummins et al. 2007). The reason for this ambiguity is not readily apparent. However, genetic manipulations such as those performed in these studies can induce compensatory changes in other related ion channels, and these compensatory changes could potentially confound the interpretation of the resulting data. Selective $Na_v1.8$ inhibitors have the potential to overcome these experimental drawbacks and to provide evidence that $Na_v1.8$ may play a role in NP. However, until recently, selective $Na_v1.8$ inhibitors have not been available. Fortunately, a μO-conotoxin peptide from marine cone snails has now been identified which has a sixfold to tenfold higher potency at blocking $Na_v1.8$ currents than neuronal TTX-sensitive currents and this peptide has been shown to attenuate NP behaviour when injected intrathecally in rats (Ekberg et al. 2006; Bulaj et al. 2006). Furthermore, a small-molecule inhibitor of $Na_v1.8$ channels, A-8033467, has also been recently identified and shows promising results in numerous pain models, including models of inflammatory pain and NP, whereby it exhibits a better therapeutic index than existing therapies (Jarvis et al. 2007). These latest data thus suggest that novel selective $Na_v1.8$ inhibitors have the potential to be efficacious treatments for NP and indicate that further research in selective $Na_v1.8$ inhibitors is a worthwhile avenue to pursue in the development of effective NP therapies.

Voltage-gated potassium channels, like voltage-gated sodium channels, are critical mediators of nerve impulse conduction. They provide inhibitory control of neuronal excitability and under normal conditions could be a major factor preventing ectopic activity. As such they are also potential NP therapy targets and numerous studies examining the role of potassium channels in NP have reported a reduction in the expression of specific potassium channels (including K_v1 and K_v2 family subunits) in DRG neurons after axotomy and/or peripheral nerve injury (Rasband et al. 2001; Chien et al. 2007). In particular, substantial evidence indicates that K_v7 (KCNQ) channels may be intimately involved in the generation and maintenance of NP (Munro and Dalby-Brown 2007). Importantly, they are expressed on various DRG cells, including small-diameter DRG cells, and by blocking these channels it is possible to reduce the threshold for action potential firing. Conversely, K_v7 openers hyperpolarize the resting membrane potential and thus make it less likely that action potentials are generated by increasing the threshold for firing in these neurons. Therefore, K_v7 openers through their ability to reduce neuronal excitability could be highly efficacious NP treatments. In fact, retigabine, a K_v7 opener, has already been shown to diminish pain hypersensitivity to mechanical and cold stimuli in chronic constriction injury and spared nerve injury models of NP. Importantly these antinociceptive affects can be reversed by the specific K_v7 inhibitor (linopirdine), indicating that the pain-relieving effects of retigabine are a consequence of its actions on K_v7 channels and not through some other non-specific actions (Blackburn-Munro and Jensen 2003; Dost et al. 2004). Unfortunately, like most other current efficacious pharmacological interventions, retigabine does have its drawbacks. In rats and mice it has a relatively poor neurotoxicity profile, while in humans it can evoke dose-limiting side effects including ataxia and somnolence, which probably reflect its activity at other ion channels. Therefore, while potassium channels are interesting novel targets for future NP treatments, development of new more selective pharmacological tools will be required before effective NP treatments targeting potassium channels are realized. Like the voltage-gated ion channels already mentioned, the importance of voltage-dependent calcium channels in the modulation and control of neuronal excitability has been known for some time and as such these channels have been extensively studied. The voltage dependent calcium channel family consists of a diverse array of ion channels which most likely reflects the diverse functions that calcium plays in normal cellular processes. In the nervous system in particular, voltage dependent calcium channels (and calcium influx) are intrinsically involved in mediating neurotransmitter release and the activation of intracellular cascades which, in turn, can modulate membrane excitability either directly or indirectly via the initiation of protein transcription. It is the ability of these channels to affect neuronal excitability so profoundly that makes them obvious targets for the development of novel NP treatments. Consequently, the role of voltage dependent calcium channels as therapeutic targets in NP has been succinctly documented in a timely review by Yaksh (2006). The diverse voltage dependent calcium channels have different structural subunit compositions (Ca_v1, Ca_v2, Ca_v3) and can be defined by their activation characteristics (they are either high or low voltage activated channels), or their pharmacological properties (voltage dependent calcium channels are classed as either L-, P/Q-, N-, R- or T-type). While a number of these channels seem to be expressed within the pain pathway, e.g. by putative nociceptors, it is the N-type channel in particular which looks the most promising molecular target for treating NP, in part because pharmacological block of the other voltage-dependent calcium channels does not seem to markedly attenuate NP behaviour in preclinical studies. Importantly, the N-type channel is also expressed in DRG cells and in the superficial dorsal horn as well. However, in direct contrast to the other voltage dependent calcium channels, blockers of the N-type channel attenuate pain behaviour in numerous NP models. Specifically, N-type-channel blockers (i.e. ω-conopeptides) exert a direct inhibitory effect on ectopic activity observed in injured fibres (Liu et al. 2001), and possibly owing to this effect intrathecal administration of specific N-type blockers have been shown to reverse NP behaviours in several animal models (Matthews and Dickenson 2001). Additionally, ziconotide, another specific N-type blocker, has been demonstrated to have antiallodynic effects in humans with diverse neuropathological conditions, but again only after spinal delivery (Cox 2000; Doggrell 2004). Interestingly, the structural subunits are not the only components of functional calcium channels which may play a role in NP. In fact, the auxiliary α2-δ1 subunit, which characterizes the L- and N-type channel, may be the most likely of all the Ca^{2+} channel family subunits to generate an efficacious new generation NP therapy. The reason for this is due to the fact that the regulation of this subunit is particularly responsive to NP conditions and is upregulated significantly after nerve injury in both the DRG and the spinal cord, where it facilitates the functional expression of α1 channels as well as enhancing the peak current amplitude. Blocking the activity of this subunit would therefore seem an effective means of treating NP and this does seem to be the case as this subunit is the putative target of gabapentin (and its congeners, e.g. pregabalin), which has wide-ranging antinociceptive activity in numerous NP models. While gabapentin is generally regarded as the current gold standard for NP treatment, it does have it limitations as its use is linked with unwanted side effects such as dizziness, fatigue and somnolence. Therefore, there has also been considerable interest in the use of other anticonvulsants, such as levitiracetam and lamotrigine, as NP treatments, as they can also inhibit calcium channels. However, they also present complex pharmacological profiles and as a consequence their use is also linked to dose-limiting side effects. Therefore, it seems clear that there is considerable potential for more specific antagonists of calcium channels being developed, and by particularly targeting the α2-δ1 subunit, they could offer promising new treatments of NP with an improved efficacy when compared with the present ones.

2.2 *Immune Cells and Their Released Factors in Neuropathic Pain*

During the last decade the "neurocentric" concept of NP has been challenged by several demonstrations of a critical role of the immune system in the generation and maintenance of NP (Watkins and Maier 2003: Marchand et al. 2005; Thacker et al.

2007). Here we consider the types of immune cells involved as well as the factors they release that contribute to NP.

2.2.1 Periphery

Several types of immune cells have been implicated in NP, but their relative contributions and the timing of their effects has not been fully elucidated. Here, we only focus on the pain-producing effects of peripheral immune cells; potential analgesic actions are discussed elsewhere (see the chapter by Stein and Zöllner, this volume). For example, following a partial ligation of the sciatic nerve, the resident population of mast cells are activated and release several proinflammatory mediators such as histamine, serotonin, cytokines and proteases (Galli et al. 2005; Zuo et al. 2003; Metcalfe et al. 1997). As neuronal histamine receptors are upregulated in specific NP states and treatment with antagonists of these receptors attenuates mechanical allodynia in neuropathic rats (Zuo et al. 2003; Kashiba et al. 1999), it seems plausible that peripheral antihistamine treatment could be an effective therapy for NP states where a peripheral component is evident. In fact, the antiallodynic effect of these agents was shown to be less efficacious than sodium cromoglycate treatment (a mast cell stabilizer), suggesting that other mast cell derived mediators may also be involved in the generation of NP either directly by acting on peripheral nociceptors or indirectly via the recruitment of other key immune cell types which in turn could generate pain by releasing other pronociceptive mediators.

The role of neutrophils in the production of inflammatory pain is well documented (Levine et al. 1985; Bennett et al. 1998b) and while neutrophils are almost absent in the intact nerve, significant infiltration of these cells has been observed at the site of injury in a number of rodent NP models (Zuo et al. 2003; Perry et al. 1987; Clatworthy et al. 1995). Interestingly, Perkins and Tracey (2000) demonstrated that pre-emptive rather than postlesional depletion of circulating neutrophils attenuated thermal hyperalgesia after partial transection of the sciatic nerve. Thus, neutrophils may be important during the early stages of NP development. However, this hypothesis is still controversial as several authors have reported an extremely limited neutrophil response which also seems to be rather transient following nerve injury. Nonetheless, neutrophils do release mediators such as chemokines that initiate macrophage infiltration and activation (Scapini et al. 2000) and there are now several lines of evidence showing the importance of macrophages in a variety of NP models (Myers et al. 1996; Sommer and Schafers 1998; Liu et al. 2000; Cui et al. 2000; Rutkowski et al. 2000). In particular, most of these studies have found a temporal correlation between resident macrophage activation and haematogenously derived macrophage invasion and development of allodynia/hyperalgesia. Some authors (Rutkowski et al. 2000; Heumann et al. 1987) have also reported a lack of thermal hyperalgesia in a neuropathic model in the Wld mouse which shows delayed recruitment of non-resident macrophages. Depletion of circulating monocytes/macrophages with intravenous administration of liposome-encapsulated clodronate was also shown to reduce the number of macrophages in the injured nerve, and alleviated thermal hyperalgesia following nerve injury (Liu et al. 2000). However, Rutkowski et al. (2000) failed to relieve mechanical allodynia after clodronate administration. These discrepancies may reflect differences in the role of macrophages in the mechanisms of hyperalgesia versus allodynia, or discrepancy between the study methods.

2.2.2 Central

Peripheral as well as central nerve injuries leading to NP states may cause not only changes at the periphery, but also centrally in the processing of sensory information at the spinal level. It is notable that these central changes also include alterations of immune cell function.

Two types of immune cells have been extensively studied in the context of NP: haematogenous leucocytes and resident microglia. The specific role of the infiltrating cells (macrophages and/or T cells) remains unclear; they could have either neuroprotective or hyperalgesic functions, or both (Rutkowski et al. 2004). In addition, it has also been recently suggested that the haematogenous macrophages could infiltrate the spinal cord and differentiate into activated microglia cells (Zhang et al. 2007). Microglia, the resident macrophages of the CNS, express surface markers identical to those expressed by macrophages/monocytes and are quiescent under normal circumstances. However, a number of events, including CNS injury, microbial invasion and some pain states, lead to their activation, with a concomitant release of inflammatory cytokines, chemokines and other potentially pain-producing substances (see the next section). A number of studies have shown that specific microglial inhibitors and/or modulators can block and sometimes reverse NP states (Meller et al. 1994; Milligan et al. 2000, 2003; Aumeerally et al. 2004; Raghavendra et al. 2003; Ledeboer et al. 2005). In particular, minocycline, a tetracyclic antibiotic, and the immunosuppressants propentofylline, methotrexate and thalidomide have all been found to be effective in alleviating NP syndromes (Sommer et al. 1998; Hashizume et al. 2000; George et al. 2000; Sweitzer et al. 2001). However, for most of these drugs, only pre-emptive treatment is reported to potently block development of NP after peripheral injury, suggesting that microglia might be important in the initial phase of peripheral NP. However, some recent studies have demonstrated a reversal effect of intrathecal treatment with minocycline on pain behaviours and neuronal hyperresponsiveness following thoracic spinal cord contusion injury. This suggests that activated microglia may also be involved in the maintenance of pain following spinal cord injury.

Owing to the evidence given above, it is now widely accepted that microglia activation is a crucial factor in the development of NP and that microglia may participate along with other cell types (e.g. astrocytes) in the maintenance of NP. However, how microglia are involved in generating pain and which mediators are responsible are still questions which have to be thoroughly elucidated and the current evidence is discussed in the following.

2.2.3 Which Factors Released from Immune Cells Modulate Pain Processing?

The factors that lead to spinal microglial activation in peripheral NP states have already been extensively reviewed (Marchand et al. 2005; Watkins and Maier 2003). As these factors supposedly act at early time points after injury, the effective time window to target them is rather narrow and thus the use of novel therapies that target these factors would be of limited practical use. Instead, it is envisaged that therapies which act to negate the effects of the factors released from activated microglia will be more clinically relevant. Here, we focus on recent evidence that indicates how factors released from immune cells and microglia can modulate the nociceptive system in NP states.

Among the family of proinflammatory cytokines tumour necrosis factor (TNF)-α and interleukin (IL)-1β have been studied the most and both are known to initiate a cascade of events including the activation and secretion of cytokines and growth factors. Several studies have demonstrated that intraneurial, epineurial and intrathecal injections of TNF-α or IL-1β can all elicit NP like behaviours (Reeve et al. 2000; Zelenka et al. 2005), and a correlation between increased TNF-α/IL-1β expression and TNF receptor 1 and 2 expression and the development of allodynia/hyperalgesia in different NP models has also been documented (Wagner and Myers 1996; Sommer and Schafers 1998; George et al. 1999; Schafers et al. 2003a–c; George et al. 2005). Furthermore, preventing the upregulation of TNFα/IL-1β after nerve injury significantly attenuates the resulting pain behaviour (Wagner et al. 1998; Lindenlaub et al. 2000; Sommer et al. 2001a, b; Schafers et al. 2001; Clark et al. 2006). However, only pre-emptive (but not delayed) treatment with etanercept (a TNF-α sequestering drug) or thalidomide inhibited mechanical allodynia in NP models, which suggests that TNF-α is particularly important in the initiation of NP (Schafers et al. 2003a–c; Sommer et al. 2001a, b).

Other studies have also reported an involvement of IL-6 and the chemokine CCL2 in NP (Flatters et al. 2004; Tanaka et al. 2004; White et al. 2005). CCL2 is upregulated within the nerve, DRG neurons and also the spinal cord; therefore, it has the potential to act at several levels of the pain pathway by attracting and activating macrophages and microglia and by also acting directly on DRG and spinal cord neurons. Furthermore, Abbadie et al. (2003) have demonstrated that NP behaviours fail to develop in null mutant CCR2 mice after partial nerve ligature, indicating that this chemokine is a key mediator and critically involved in the manifestation of NP in this model. Unfortunately, despite clear evidence of a role for CCL2 in the generation of NP, the therapeutic opportunities of blocking CCL2 are small as it seems to act only at the early stages of NP. Nevertheless, it is evident that cytokines can modulate pain processing in several ways and a selective upregulation of pronociceptive or proinflammatory cytokines would therefore be envisaged to cause a pain phenotype.

Interestingly, recent human studies have found that such a change in the balance between pro- and anti-inflammatory cytokines in NP patients may actually occur. They observed an increase of proinflammatory cytokines (IL-2, TNF-α) and a decrease of anti-inflammatory cytokines (IL-4 and IL-10) in patients with painful neuropathy compared with patients with painless neuropathy (Lindenlaub and Sommer 2003; Uceyler et al. 2007). Therefore, blocking proinflammatory cytokines and/or increasing or supplying anti-inflammatory cytokine could re-equilibrate the cytokine balance and may be a potential effective treatment for NP. In fact, some studies have already demonstrated that anti-inflammatory treatment, using mainly viral vectors overexpressing IL-10, could block NP (Milligan et al. 2005), indicating that this treatment regime could be of benefit to NP patients.

2.3 Protein Kinases

Protein kinases belong to a very large family of proteins (the human genome encodes some 518 protein kinases) involved in a plethora of intracellular mechanisms; therefore, it is perhaps not surprising that these proteins were not particularly favoured as targets for analgesics. However, recent studies have demonstrated that kinases play important roles in regulating neuronal plasticity and pain sensitization (for a review see Ji et al. 2007; Ji and Suter 2007; Ma and Quirion 2005; Velazquez et al. 2007). Previous studies have established a role for protein kinase C (PKC) and protein kinase A in central sensitization. Specifically, the PKC isoforms PKC-ε and PKC-α appear to be involved in peripheral nociception, while PKC-γ is important in central sensitization (Velazquez et al. 2007), and many more PKC isoforms as well as other kinase proteins may also be intimately involved in the generation of pain behaviours. Therefore, isoform-specific agents might be attractive candidates for analgesic drug development.

Among the many kinases, the mitogen-activated protein kinases (MAPKs), consisting of p38, extracellular-signal-regulated kinase (ERK) and c-Jun N-terminal kinase (JNK), seem the most promising (Ji et al. 2007; Ji and Suter 2007; Ma and Quirion 2007). They are downstream of many other kinases and can be activated by a variety of factors (e.g. growth factors and inflammatory mediators) and they are expressed in neurons as well as in glial cells.

In NP models, multiple studies have observed that p38 MAPK is specifically activated in hyperactive microglia in the spinal cord and also in DRG neurons (Kim et al. 2002; Schafers et al. 2003a–c; Jin et al. 2003; Tsuda et al. 2004; Sweitzer et al. 2004; Daulhac et al. 2006; Clark et al. 2007). Moreover, pretreatment and to a more limited extent posttreatment with inhibitors of p38 MAPK (SB203580, FR167653, SD-282 and CNI-1493) reduced NP behaviours in some of these studies. Together, these findings strongly suggest that p38 phosphorylation is a key intracellular signal, at least in microglia, that regulates their algogenic actions. However, the literature is not entirely consistent, most notably in the reported time course of p38 activation; for example, while some groups have found that in the DRG p38 is activated transiently hours after injury, others report a delayed (more than 3 days) activation of p38 after injury (Kim et al. 2002; Jin et al. 2003; Tsuda et al. 2004; Schafers et al. 2003a–c). The effects of p38 inhibitors are also somewhat difficult to interpret since p38 is activated at multiple sites in the pain pathway, e.g. in sensory neurons as well as microglia in the same NP models (Kim et al. 2002; Schafers et al. 2003a–c; Jin et al. 2003). It seems the simplest explanation for these findings is that peripheral nerve injuries associated with NP states lead to a p38-dependent activation of spinal microglia which is followed subsequently by p38 activation in DRG neurons. Furthermore, the activation of p38 in DRG neurons appears to be crucial for the full emergence of NP behaviour. As a result, the development of more specific p38 isoform inhibitors or the development of activation status specific inhibitors could offer some interesting and potentially therapeutic advances in NP therapies.

A similar case to p38 MAPK can be made for ERK. Zhuang et al. (2005) demonstrated sequential activation of ERK in neurons, followed by microglia and astrocytes. Inhibitors of ERK also block mechanical allodynia following peripheral nerve injury, suggesting that specific inhibitors of ERK could exhibit some efficacy in the treatment of NP. JNK also seems an emerging target for new and novel NP therapies; however, at present there is less evidence supporting a role for JNK in NP than for the other members of the protein kinase family previously mentioned (Zhuang et al. 2006).

Other protein kinases such as phosphatidylinositol 3-kinase (PI3K), protein kinase B/Akt and Src-family kinases have also recently emerged as potential targets for new NP drug treatments (Katsura et al. 2006; Xu et al. 2007). PI3K and protein kinase B/Akt kinases are upregulated in the DRG and the spinal cord in a model of spinal nerve ligation, but their expression peaked at 3 days, returning to basal levels at 7 and 14 days, respectively. In addition, only early treatment with inhibitors of these kinases following injury blocks pain behaviour, suggesting an involvement in the development rather than the maintenance of NP. In contrast, phospho-Src-family kinases are upregulated mainly in microglia in the spinal cord, up to 14 days following nerve injury, and a wide spectrum inhibitor, 4-amino-5-(4-chlorophenyl)-7-(t-butyl)pyrazolo[3,4-d]pyrimidine (PP2) of these kinases administered intrathecally reduced both the development and the maintenance of some NP behaviours (Katsura et al. 2006).

As we review here, protein kinases represent a number of potential therapeutic targets for the treatment of NP and a variety of kinase inhibitors are available or currently under development by various pharmaceutical companies. However, as protein kinases are integral components in many normal cellular functions, kinase inhibitors have the potential to cause a plethora of unwanted side effects. Therefore, development of more specific protein kinase inhibitors or activated-state-dependent inhibitors seems a more likely beneficial treatment strategy for the management of NP.

2.4 Gene Therapy

While pharmacological approaches are the conventional and probably first choice treatment strategy for NP and a wide-range of other diseases, they are not without their disadvantages. In particular, it is extremely difficult to target discrete organs and tissues (e.g. the DRG or a specific nerve) with drugs and as a result effective systemic doses are often associated with side effects. In contrast, in vivo gene therapy offers exciting opportunities to circumvent these issues (for a review see Goss 2007) by introducing and expressing therapeutic DNA or RNA sequences into specific tissues or cells of interest. This is achieved using two main delivery systems: viral and non-viral vectors. Non-viral vectors usually consist of DNA for genes of interest expressed in a plasmid and encapsulated in a liposome; however, while they are relatively simple to construct, getting them into the desired cell in sufficient amounts has proved problematic. Fortunately, conjugating the liposomes with specific targeting antibodies has been shown to be a particularly promising development. Furthermore, when this technique is employed, no inflammatory response is likely to occur because of the absence of viral proteins and the use of humanized targeting antibodies (Shi and Pardridge 2000). In fact, in a number of examples intramuscular gene transfer of vascular endothelial growth factor (VEGF)-expressing plasmids has been successfully used to treat ischaemia and prevent ischaemia-induced sensory nerve loss associated with diabetic neuropathy in animal models (Goss 2007). These experiments were so successful that the technique has recently been tested in phase I/II clinical trials. However, this particular method of gene therapy has one major disadvantage, which is that even though a number of techniques have been devised to maximize gene delivery it still is not very efficient. As a consequence, viral vectors may actually represent better future gene therapy strategies.

The reason for this is because by taking advantage of the innate ability of viruses to infect cells, viral vectors are able to efficiently incorporate their desired gene into the targeted cell. Several types of viral vectors are now known and all have advantages and disadvantages. For example, retroviral vectors are a group of viruses that reverse-transcribe their RNA into double-stranded DNA which is integrated into the genome of the host and is thus expressed relatively stably. However, worryingly, the incorporation of target genes into the host genome can potentially result in the development of malignancies as the DNA is inserted randomly; thus, other potential viral vectors have been explored. Lentiviral vectors have shown promise as like retroviruses they have the ability to integrate both dividing and non-dividing cells. It is also known that the transgenes can escape "gene silencing" and can remain stably expressed in the host genome for a long period of time in vivo. Another advantage of lentiviral vectors is that they can also accommodate transgenes up to about 9,000 bases (Blits and Bunge 2006), which is beneficial if your gene of interest is large. Adenoviral vectors, on the other hand, have the ability to express a transgene as soon as 24 h after the initial infection. This, of course, can be seen as a beneficial trait for potential viral vector therapies. However, unfortunately, expression typically declines dramatically after a few weeks. Prolonged expression of the transgene would be required for the viral vector to be an efficacious NP therapy (Blits and Bunge 2006). Finally, herpes simplex viral vectors are neurotropic double-stranded DNA viruses. They are particularly good potential therapeutic viral vectors as like adenoviruses they are capable of retrograde transport. Furthermore, they have the capability of permanently transducing cells when the vector is in a latent state (Glorioso and Fink 2004). Already, a number of these different viruses have been used in a variety of models of NP, mainly to overexpress neurotrophic factors such as nerve growth factor (NGF), neurotrophin-3, GDNF and VEGF, but also to block or overexpress pro- and anti-inflammatory cytokines, respectively (Goss 2007).

Most of the studies using neurotrophic factors expressing viruses have demonstrated electrophysiological improvements and some prevention of nerve fibre loss and/or regeneration. Importantly, some of these studies have also demonstrated an effect on pain behaviours and inhibition of some neurochemical markers of neuronal damage such as ATF3 (for a review see Goss 2007). Others studies have also used viral vectors to express endogenous opioids (enkephalins) and observed a sustained antiallodynic effect and an enhanced effect of morphine without tolerance (Wolfe et al. 2007). Finally, herpes simplex virus has been successfully used to block the proinflammatory cytokine TNF-α and reverse pain behaviour as well as p38 microglia activation in models of peripheral and central neuropathy (Peng et al. 2006; Hao et al. 2007). Alternatively, viruses can be utilized to supply anti-inflammatory cytokines (IL-4 or IL-10), for example, in the spinal cord after nerve injury, and injection of these viruses has been shown to prevent and reverse established pain behaviour (Hao et al. 2006; Milligan et al. 2005).

Owing to the points discussed above, non-viral and viral vectors appear attractive strategies to treat NP. However, questions remain regarding their potential immunogenicity, transduction efficiency, cellular targeting, long-term expression and, most importantly, their safety. All of these factors will have to be addressed before they become viable effective NP treatments.

2.5 Neurotrophic Factors

There is good preclinical evidence that two members of the neurotrophin family, NGF and brain-derived neurotrophic factor (BDNF), play important roles as peripheral and central mediators of pain, respectively. Blocking their biological activity may subsequently provide desperately needed analgesia for individuals with NP. In fact, for the former (NGF), clinical trials have commenced using a neutralizing antibody designed to prevent its bioavailability and positive phase II data in osteoarthritis pain have been reported. The evidence for these neurotrophins as pain mediators is presented in the following sections and their potential as novel NP therapies is discussed.

2.5.1 NGF as a Peripheral Pain Mediator

Administration of small doses of NGF to adult animals, including humans, can produce pain and hyperalgesia. In rodents, thermal hyperalgesia develops within tens of minutes of systemic NGF administration, and both thermal and mechanical hyperalgesia are apparent after a few hours. In humans, intravenous injections of very low doses of NGF produce widespread aching pains in deep tissues and hyperalgesia at the injection site (Petty et al. 1994). The rapid onset of some of these effects and their localization to the injection site strongly suggests that they arise at least in part from a local effect on the peripheral terminals of nociceptors, many of which express the high-affinity NGF receptor trkA. This has been substantiated by the observation that acute administration of NGF can sensitize nociceptive afferents to thermal and chemical stimuli (Rueff and Mendell 1996). Isolated DRG cells in culture and nociceptive terminals studied using a skin-nerve preparation have been shown to become sensitized following acute exposure to NGF (Shu and Mendell 1999). However, there is also evidence that some of the sensitizing effects of NGF may be indirect via mast cells, sympathetic efferent neurons and neutrophils (for a review see Bennett 2001). Cutaneous nociceptors chronically exposed to elevated NGF levels (in an NGF overexpressing mouse) show a marked heat sensitization (Stucky et al. 1999). Although the exact mechanism of sensitization is not known in this case, the data nonetheless demonstrate that persistent peripheral sensitization is possible. NGF is a potent regulator of gene expression in sensory neurons. Some sensory neuropeptides, which are released with activity from central nociceptors terminals, are strongly upregulated by NGF. These include calcitonin gene-regulated peptide (CGRP) and substance P (Lindsay and Harmar 1989). NGF has also been shown to produce a dramatic upregulation of BDNF in trkA-expressing DRG cells (Michael et al. 1997), and there is now growing evidence that BDNF may serve as a central regulator of excitability, as discussed later. NGF also regulates the expression of some of the receptors expressed by nociceptors. Capsaicin sensitivity is increased by NGF (Shu and Mendell 1999), which results from NGF regulation of the heat transducer TRPV1 and specific members of the acid-sensing ion channel family are also strongly regulated by NGF at a transcriptional level (Mamet et al. 2003). Finally, several ion channels such as $Na_v1.8$ are also regulated by NGF availability (Boucher et al. 2000).

The dramatic effects of exogenously administered NGF on pain signalling systems do not reveal the role of endogenous NGF. To ascertain if any of the "pharmacological" effects of NGF truly reflect those of endogenous NGF, one must perform experiments in which the biological actions of endogenous NGF are somehow blocked. This has been achieved by two major experimental approaches: targeted recombination in embryonic stem cells to selectively knock out either NGF or its receptor trkA and the administration of proteins that inhibit the bioactivity of NGF. Each of these techniques has advantages and disadvantages, but studies using them largely confirm an important role for endogenous NGF in regulating pain sensitivity. The knockout approach, in particular, has provided information regarding the developmental role of NGF, and has confirmed that essentially all spinal nociceptive afferents require this factor for survival in the perinatal period (Crowley et al. 1994). However, because mice with NGF or trkA deletions rarely survive past the first postnatal week, most of what we know about endogenous NGF function in the adult has been determined by the use of blocking agents. A number of studies have used a synthetic chimeric protein consisting of the extracellular domain of trkA fused to the Fc tail of human immunoglobulin G (trkA-IgG) to investigate the actions of endogenous NGF in nociception (Koltzenburg et al. 1999; Xu et al. 2001). Local infusion of trkA-IgG into the rat hind paw leads to thermal hypoalgesia and a decrease in CGRP content in DRG neurons projecting to the infused area (McMahon et al. 1995). These changes take several days to develop. In addition, there is a decrease in chemical sensitivity of nociceptors projecting to the area and a decrease in the epidermal innervation density (Bennett et al. 1998a, b). These results provide strong evidence that NGF continues to play an important role in regulating the function of the small peptidergic sensory neurons in the adult.

Finally, there is now compelling evidence that the biological actions of NGF described above are particularly important in many forms of inflammation and may also contribute to NP states (Woolf et al. 1994; Koltzenburg et al. 1999; Pezet and McMahon 2006 for review). NGF is found in many cell types in tissues subject to inflammatory insult, and a great deal of evidence now supports the hypothesis that upregulation of NGF levels is a common component of the inflammatory response that relates to hyperalgesia. Elevated NGF levels have been found in a variety of inflammatory states in both humans and animal models (for a review see McMahon and Bennett 1999) and there is now widespread agreement that blocking NGF bioactivity (either systemically or locally) blocks a large component of the effects of inflammation on sensory nerve function. For instance, intraplantar injection of carrageenan produces an acute inflammatory reaction, which is widely used in behavioural studies of pain mechanisms. When trkA-IgG was coadministered with carrageenan, it could largely prevent the development of thermal hyperalgesia and the sensitization of primary afferent nociceptors that normally develops (McMahon et al. 1995) and there are now many other similar examples, as reviewed in Pezet and McMahon (2006). Thus, from the above discussion it is clear that owing to the wide-ranging effects of NGF on the nociceptive system there is considerable promise for the development of anti-NGF drugs as novel therapeutic agents for the treatment of NP. Other neurotrophic factors may also be good targets for new NP therapies and the evidence for one in particular (BDNF) is discussed next.

2.5.2 BDNF as a Central Pain Mediator

Neurotrophic factors are best known for their roles as secreted factors both during development (as target-derived survival factors) and in the adult. But there is now a growing body of evidence that at least one of the neurotrophins, BDNF, may act as a neuromodulator (for a review see Pezet et al. 2002b). That is, in some neurons BDNF does not enter the secretory pathway, but instead is packaged in synaptic vesicles and is released with neuronal activity to modulate postsynaptic neurons. Such a role has been suggested in hippocampus, cortex, cerebellum and spinal cord (for reviews see McAllister et al. 1999; Malcangio and Lessmann 2003; Pezet and

McMahon 2006). Here we consider the role of BDNF in nociceptive processing. This protein is constitutively expressed in a significant minority of small and medium-sized sensory neurons of the DRG (Barakat-Walter 1996; Zhou and Rush 1996), where it is contained in dense-core vesicles. Moreover, it is dramatically upregulated in many small-diameter nociceptive sensory neurons in models of inflammatory pain and in larger neurons in some animal models of NP (Michael et al. 1997, 1999; Zhou et al. 1999; Ha et al. 2001). One important trigger for the increased synthesis of BDNF in nociceptive neurons is the peripheral increase in NGF availability that is a common feature of inflammation (see earlier). BDNF is known to be released from the central terminals of sensory neurons with activity, and in a frequency-dependent manner (Balkowiec and Katz 2000). In normal tissue, release is associated specifically with activity in nociceptors either induced by chemical algogens such as capsaicin, or by electrical stimulation of, specifically, small-diameter sensory neurons. Interestingly, the patterns of electrical activity necessary for BDNF release are different from those producing release of other sensory neuron transmitters such as glutamate and substance P (Lever et al. 2001).

High-affinity receptors for BDNF (the tyrosine kinase receptor trkB) are widely expressed on spinal neurons, including spinal projection neurons. We have previously shown that nociceptor activation in a variety of experimental preparations leads to activation (phosphorylation) of dorsal horn trkB receptors, indicating that BDNF can be released from nociceptors and activate postsynaptic neurons (Pezet et al. 2002a). We have also shown that intrathecally injected BDNF can also induce ERK phosphorylation in laminae I-II neurons of the spinal cord (Pezet et al. 2002a), and this kinase is known to be an important second messenger in mediating some changes in spinal nociceptive processing associated with persistent pain states (Ji et al. 1999). In other experiments we showed that endogenous BDNF release from nociceptors accounts for about a third of the activation of ERK (Pezet et al. 2002a). Thus, there is a body of biochemical evidence implicating BDNF as a pain-related central modulator. There are also functional studies demonstrating the neuromodulatory role of BDNF in the spinal cord. Exogenous BDNF selectively enhances sensory-neuron-evoked spinal reflex activity and NMDA-induced depolarization of in vitro preparation of rat spinal cord (Kerr et al. 1999; Thompson et al. 1999). BDNF null mutant mice have been shown to display a selective deficit in the ventral root potentials evoked by nociceptive primary afferents (Heppenstall and Lewin 2001). In adult rats, intrathecal injection of anti-BDNF antibodies or sequestering fusion molecule trkB-IgG prevented the development of thermal hyperalgesia associated with acute peripheral inflammation (Kerr et al. 1999) or NP (Fukuoka et al. 2001), respectively. It is not clear what the intracellular mechanism is of BDNF-induced modulation. One plausible mechanism is that synaptically released BDNF activates the MAPK ERK in second-order cells, and this second messenger produces a posttranslational change in NMDA receptor properties. Recently, however, Garraway et al. (2003) showed that the initial facilitation of lamina II neurons by BDNF depends critically on activation of phospholipase C (PLC) and PKC. Whatever the mechanism, there is a clearly documented pathway linking nociceptor activity with BDNF-mediated central modulation of sensory transmission. It is not clear at present when this pathway is active. The data so far suggest that it is one important mediator of central sensitization, and might therefore contribute to a variety of hyperalgesic states. BDNF, therefore, joins a list of promising new targets for analgesic drug development, although the relatively widespread expression of BDNF may indicate that CNS side effects might be a problem.

2.6 Neuropeptides

Since the discovery of substance P, there has been a lot of interest in the role that this and other neuropeptides play in the generation of pain. However, despite promising preclinical results (e.g. substance P deficient mice demonstrate attenuated responses to intense noxious stimuli), clinical trials using substance P antagonists have been very disappointing (Rice and Hill 2006). So much so that it is accepted that NK1 antagonists are not effective analgesics in humans. Another peptide, CGRP, is also abundant in primary afferent fibres, plays an important role in pain transmission and may be a better therapeutic target. Several antagonists of CGRP receptors are now available and one in particular, BIBN4096BS, was effective as an acute abortive treatment of migraine headache (Olesen et al. 2004) and may also be effective in NP states (Ma and Quirion 2006). However, the most promising anti-CGRP NP therapy to date may be cizolirtine, which has antinociceptive effects in a variety of animal pain models, probably owing to an inhibition of the spinal release of CGRP and substance P (Ballet et al. 2001). Furthermore, results in NP patients suggest that it may attenuate allodynia, albeit at high doses (Shembalkar et al. 2001).

As well as substance P and CGRP, other peptides and their receptors are also good candidate therapeutic targets and one specific example is cholecystokinin. The reason for this is because NP patients are often resistant to morphine treatment; therefore, enhancement of morphine analgesia could be an effective treatment strategy and the endogenous opioid system is known to be negatively modulated by cholecystokinin. Antagonists of CCK_1 and CCK_2 have been developed and have demonstrated marked success at enhancing morphine analgesia. Specifically, CCK_1 selective blockers (e.g. MK-329 or devazepide) have been shown to enhance the effects of morphine in persistent pain patients (McCleane 1998). Consequently, it is feasible that they could be at least used as an adjunct in the treatment of NP by opioids.

2.7 Cannabinoids

Cannabis has been used for medical purposes, including pain relief for millennia. However, the identification of the two cannabinoid receptors (CB1 expressed on neurons and CB2 expressed on immune cells) and several endogenous ligands has only recently (within the last two decades) been ascertained and subsequently renewed interest in the therapeutic potential of cannabinoids (Lever and Rice

2007). This renewed interest has led to a number of synthetic cannabinoids and inhibitors of endogenous cannabinoid metabolism being developed. Unfortunately, despite these recent advances, data from randomized clinical trails examining the efficacy of cannabinoids in NP treatment has been quite disappointing, with relatively modest analgesic effects being demonstrated with cannabinoid treatment. Better results have been observed in trials examining the analgesic effects of cannabinoids in multiple sclerosis patients; however, all current cannabinoid treatments seem limited by acute side effects associated with cannabinoid exposure. More worrying still is the fact that recent epidemiological studies suggest that even a modest use of cannabis by young people can lead to increased risk of serious mental illness in later life, especially in individuals with pre-existing risk factors for psychosis. These adverse events could potentially be avoided by targeting CB2 receptors or peripheral CB1 receptors only or by using non-psychotropic cannabinomimetics (e.g. palmitoylethanolamide or CT-3). The use of inhibitors of the metabolism of endogenous cannabinoids could also be a useful treatment strategy and a combination of the two approaches may yield an effective future cannabinoid-based NP treatment.

2.8 *Neurostimulation*

Despite concerted efforts to develop effective drug treatments for NP, pharmacological relief is often insufficient, with around 50% of patients being pharmacoresistant. Therefore, electrical neurostimulation could be an effective alternative solution capable of addressing the analgesic needs of these NP patients. Currently, there are several techniques which have demonstrable analgesic affects, including transcutaneous electrical nerve stimulation (TENS), spinal cord stimulation, motor cortex stimulation (MCS) and deep brain stimulation (Cruccu et al. 2007; Garcia-Larrea and Peyron 2007).

TENS is probably the most popular and widespread neurostimulation technique and involves using high-frequency and low-intensity electric stimuli to evoke strong activation of Aβ fibres; however, the inhibition is strictly homotopic and pain relief rapidly declines after the stimulation stops. Consequently, the stimulation is usually repeated several times during the day and its efficacy for attenuating pain is still to be demonstrated conclusively (Cruccu et al. 2007).

Spinal cord stimulation consists of implanting electrodes into the epidural space ipsilateral to the pain and at the appropriate spinal cord level. Using this technique, there is good evidence for pain relief in failed back surgery syndrome and complex regional syndrome and some evidence for pain relief in diabetic and peripheral nerve injury (Cruccu et al. 2007). While it seems to be a more efficacious pain therapy than TENS, it is of course a more invasive procedure and is subsequently poorly tolerated by a subset of patients. Likewise, deep brain stimulation is also an invasive procedure using electrical stimuli to target a variety of brain areas, including the ventral posterior thalamus and periventricular grey matter. While it has been shown to alleviate chronic pain, its mechanisms of action are mostly unknown and like spinal cord stimulation this analgesic technique can be poorly tolerated, making the selection of patients a challenging task.

For to the reasons mentioned above, the relatively new treatment strategy, MCS, is probably the most promising tool among the current neurostimulation techniques to treat NP (Garcia-Larrea and Peyron 2007). MCS consists of electrically stimulating the motor cortex, representing the painful body area in question, using implanted electrodes. While the exact mechanism of action of MCS is unknown, it is hypothesized that MCS can alter the intensity of pain by the activation of descending pain control pathways and possibly most interestingly by blunting the emotional aspect of pain via activation of orbitofrontal-perigenual cingulate brain areas. Furthermore, the delayed and long-lasting activation of several brain areas after MCS discontinuation confers to MCS an effect that can last hours to days.

The techniques described above are all interesting options for NP treatment in pharmacologically resistant patients. However, at present our current knowledge of their mechanisms of action is generally inadequate. While the need to understand the underlying modes of action of these techniques is evident, doing so could also lead to a better understanding of supraspinal processing of NP and may thus have an additional benefit of revealing other as yet unidentified drug targets for the treatment of NP.

3 Conclusions

Despite the existence of numerous pharmacological and non-pharmacological therapies to treat NP, their efficacy is overall unsatisfactory. It seems a better understanding of the underlying mechanisms responsible for the clinical manifestation of NP in patients is required if more effective pain therapies are to be developed. As reviewed here, this strategy does seem to offer new hope for patients struggling to manage debilitating NP symptoms and the number of new treatments being tested in clinical trials is testament to this fact.

However, it should also be noted that while new treatments have the potential to provide better pain relief, it is also much more likely that combination therapies will prove to be more efficacious at providing pain relief than any one treatment alone. Furthermore, it also seems likely that in the future personalized pain management using pharmacogenetics, as well as targeted drug delivery (i.e. using viral and non-viral vectors), will also play a significant role in targeting and preventing the incidence of NP.

References

Abbadie C, Lindia JA, Cumiskey AM, Peterson LB, Mudgett JS, Bayne EK, DeMartino JA, MacIntyre DE, Forrest MJ (2003) Impaired neuropathic pain responses in mice lacking the chemokine receptor CCR2. Proc Natl Acad Sci USA 100:7947–7952

Ahmad S, Dahllund L, Eriksson AB, Hellgren D, Karlsson U, Lund PE, Meijer IA, Meury L, Mills T, Moody A, Morinville A, Morten J, O'Donnell D, Raynoschek C, Salter H, Rouleau GA, Krupp JJ (2007) A stop codon mutation in SCN9A causes lack of pain sensation. Hum Mol Genet 16:2114–2121

Amir R, Argoff CE, Bennett GJ, Cummins TR (2006) The role of sodium channels in chronic inflammatory and neuropathic pain. J Pain 7:S1–S29

Aumeerally N, Allen G, Sawynok J (2004) Glutamate-evoked release of adenosine and regulation of peripheral nociception. Neuroscience 127:1–11

Balkowiec A, Katz DM (2000) Activity-dependent release of endogenous brain-derived neurotrophic factor from primary sensory neurons detected by ELISA in situ. J Neurosci 20: 7417–7423

Ballet S, Aubel B, Mauborgne A, Polienor H, Farre A, Cesselin F, Hamon M, Bourgoin AS (2001) The novel analgesic, cizolirtine, inhibits the spinal release of substance P and CGRP in rats. Neuropharmacology 40:578–589

Barakat-Walter I (1996) Brain-derived neurotrophic factor-like immunoreactivity is localized mainly in small sensory neurons of rat dorsal root ganglia. J Neurosci Methods 68:281–288

Bennett DL, Koltzenburg M, Priestley JV, Shelton DL, McMahon SB (1998a) Endogenous nerve growth factor regulates the sensitivity of nociceptors in the adult rat. Eur J Neurosci 10:1282–1291

Bennett G, al-Rashed S, Hoult JRS, Brain SD (1998b) Nerve growth factor induced hyperalgesia in the rat hind paw is dependent on circulating neutrophils. Pain 77:315–322

Bennett DL (2001) Neurotrophic factors; important regulators of nociceptive function. Neuroscientist 7:13–17

Blackburn-Munro G, Jensen BS (2003) The anticonvulsant retigabine attenuates nociceptive behaviours in rat models of persistent and neuropathic pain. Eur J Pharmacol 460:109–116

Blits B, Bunge MB (2006) Direct gene therapy for repair of the spinal cord. J Neurotrauma 23:508–520

Boucher TJ, Okuse K, Bennett DL, Munson JB, Wood JN, McMahon SB (2000) Potent analgesic effects of GDNF in neuropathic pain states. Science 290:124–127

Bulaj G, Zhang MM, Green BR, Fiedler B, Layer RT, Wei S, Nielsen JS, Low SJ, Klein BD, Wagstaff JD, Chicoine L, Harty TP, Terlau H, Yoshikami D, Olivera BM (2006) Synthetic mu O-conotoxin MrVIB blocks TTX-resistant sodium channel $Na_v1.8$ and has a long-lasting analgesic activity. Biochemistry 45:7404–7414

Chien LY, Cheng JK, Chu DC, Cheng CF, Tsaur ML (2007) Reduced expression of A-type potassium channels in primary sensory neurons induces mechanical hypersensitivity. J Neurosci 27:9855–9865

Clark AK, D'Aquisto F, Gentry C, Marchand F, McMahon SB, Malcangio M (2006) Rapid co-release of interleukin 1beta and caspase 1 in spinal cord inflammation. J Neurochem 99:868–880

Clark AK, Yip PK, Grist J, Gentry C, Staniland AA, Marchand F, Dehvari M, Wotherspoon G, Winter J, Ullah J, Bevan S, Malcangio M (2007) Inhibition of spinal microglial cathepsin S for the reversal of neuropathic pain. Proc Natl Acad Sci USA 104:10655–10660

Clatworthy AL, Illich PA, Castro GA, Walters ET (1995) Role of peri-axonal inflammation in the development of thermal hyperalgesia and guarding behavior in a rat model of neuropathic pain. Neurosci Lett 184:5–8

Cox B (2000) Calcium channel blockers and pain therapy. Curr Rev Pain 4:488–498

Cox JJ, Reimann F, Nicholas AK, Thornton G, Roberts E, Springell K, Karbani G, Jafri H, Mannan J, Raashid Y, Al Gazali L, Hamamy H, Valente EM, Gorman S, Williams R, Mchale DP, Wood JN, Gribble FM, Woods CG (2006) An SCN9A channelopathy causes congenital inability to experience pain. Nature 444:894–898

Crowley C, Spencer SD, Nishimura MC, Chen KS, Pitts-Meek S, Armanini MP, Ling LH, McMahon SB, Shelton DL, Levinson AD (1994) Mice lacking nerve growth factor display perinatal loss of sensory and sympathetic neurons yet develop basal forebrain cholinergic neurons. Cell 76:1001–1011

Cruccu G, Aziz TZ, Garcia-Larrea L, Hansson P, Jensen TS, Lefaucheur JP, Simpson BA, Taylor RS (2007) EFNS guidelines on neurostimulation therapy for neuropathic pain. Eur J Neurol 14:952–970

Cui JG, Holmin S, Mathiesen T, Meyerson BA, Linderoth B (2000) Possible role of inflammatory mediators in tactile hypersensitivity in rat models of mononeuropathy. Pain 88:239–248

Cummins TR, Sheets PL, Waxman SG (2007) The roles of sodium channels in nociception: implications for mechanisms of pain. Pain 131:243–257

Daulhac L, Mallet C, Courteix C, Etienne M, Duroux E, Privat AM, Eschalier A, Fialip J (2006) Diabetes-induced mechanical hyperalgesia involves spinal mitogen-activated protein kinase activation in neurons and microglia via *N*-methyl-≻d-aspartate-dependent mechanisms. Mol Pharmacol 70:1246–1254

Doggrell SA (2004) Intrathecal ziconotide for refractory pain. Expert Opin Investig Drugs 13:875–877

Dost R, Rostock A, Rundfeldt C (2004) The anti-hyperalgesic activity of retigabine is mediated by KCNQ potassium channel activation. Naunyn Schmiedebergs Arch Pharmacol 369: 382–390

Dworkin RH, O'Connor AB, Backonja M, Farrar JT, Finnerup NB, Jensen TS, Kalso EA, Loeser JD, Miaskowski C, Nurmikko TJ, Portenoy RK, Rice ASC, Stacey BR, Treede RD, Turk DC, Wallace MS (2007) Pharmacologic management of neuropathic pain: evidence-based recommendations. Pain 132:237–251

Ekberg J, Jayamanne A, Vaughan CW, Aslan S, Thomas L, Mouldt J, Drinkwater R, Baker MD, Abrahamsen B, Wood JN, Adams DJ, Christie MJ, Lewis RJ (2006) mu O-conotoxin MrVIB selectively blocks Na_v1.8 sensory neuron specific sodium channels and chronic pain behavior without motor deficits. Proc Natl Acad Sci USA 103:17030–17035

Flatters SJ, Fox AJ, Dickenson AH (2004) Nerve injury alters the effects of interleukin-6 on nociceptive transmission in peripheral afferents. Eur J Pharmacol 484:183–191

Fukuoka T, Kondo E, Dai Y, Hashimoto N, Noguchi K (2001) Brain-derived neurotrophic factor increases in the uninjured dorsal root ganglion neurons in selective spinal nerve ligation model. J Neurosci 21:4891–4900

Galli SJ, Nakae S, Tsai M (2005) Mast cells in the development of adaptive immune responses. Nat Immunol 6:135–142

Garcia-Larrea L, Peyron R (2007) Motor cortex stimulation for neuropathic pain: from phenomenology to mechanisms. Neuroimage 37(Suppl 1):S71–S79

Garraway SM, Petruska JC, Mendell LM (2003) BDNF sensitizes the response of lamina II neurons to high threshold primary afferent inputs. Eur J Neurosci 18:2467–2476

George A, Schmidt C, Weishaupt A, Toyka KV, Sommer C (1999) Serial determination of tumor necrosis factor-alpha content in rat sciatic nerve after chronic constriction injury. Exp Neurol 160:124–132

George A, Marziniak M, Schafers M, Toyka KV, Sommer C (2000) Thalidomide treatment in chronic constrictive neuropathy decreases endoneurial tumor necrosis factor-alpha, increases interleukin-10 and has long-term effects on spinal cord dorsal horn met-enkephalin. Pain 88:267–275

George A, Buehl A, Sommer C (2005) Tumor necrosis factor receptor 1 and 2 proteins are differentially regulated during Wallerian degeneration of mouse sciatic nerve. Exp Neurol 192:163–166

Glorioso JC, Fink DJ (2004) Herpes vector-mediated gene transfer in treatment of diseases of the nervous system. Annu Rev Microbiol 58:253–271

Goss JR (2007) The therapeutic potential of gene transfer for the treatment of peripheral neuropathies. Expert Rev Mol Med 9:1–20

Ha SO, Kim JK, Hong HS, Kim DS, Cho HJ (2001) Expression of brain-derived neurotrophic factor in rat dorsal root ganglia, spinal cord and gracile nuclei in experimental models of neuropathic pain. Neuroscience 107:301–309

Hains BC, Klein JP, Saab CY, Craner MJ, Black JA, Waxman SG (2003) Upregulation of sodium channel $Na_v1.3$ and functional involvement in neuronal hyperexcitability associated with central neuropathic pain after spinal cord injury. J Neurosci 23:8881–8892

Hains BC, Saab CY, Klein JP, Craner MJ, Waxman SG (2004) Altered sodium channel expression in second-order spinal sensory neurons contributes to pain after peripheral nerve injury. J Neurosci 24:4832–4839

Hao S, Mata M, Glorioso JC, Fink DJ (2006) HSV-mediated expression of interleukin-4 in dorsal root ganglion neurons reduces neuropathic pain. Mol Pain 2:6

Hao S, Mata M, Glorioso JC, Fink DJ (2007) Gene transfer to interfere with TNFalpha signaling in neuropathic pain. Gene Ther 14:1010–1016

Hashizume H, Rutkowski MD, Weinstein JN, Deleo JA (2000) Central administration of methotrexate reduces mechanical allodynia in an animal model of radiculopathy/sciatica. Pain 87:159–169

Heppenstall PA, Lewin GR (2001) BDNF but not NT-4 is required for normal flexion reflex plasticity and function. Proc Natl Acad Sci USA 98:8107–8112

Heumann R, Lindholm D, Bandtlow C, Meyer M, Radeke MJ, Misko TP, Shooter E, Thoenen H (1987) Differential regulation of mRNA encoding nerve growth factor and its receptor in rat sciatic nerve during development, degeneration, and regeneration: role of macrophages. Proc Natl Acad Sci USA 84:8735–8739

Jarvis MF, Honore P, Shieh CC, Chapman M, Joshi S, Zhang XF, Kort M, Carroll W, Marron B, Atkinson R, Thomas J, Liu D, Krambis M, Liu Y, McGaraughty S, Chu K, Roeloffs R, Zhong CM, Mikusa JP, Hernandez G, Gauvin D, Wade C, Zhu C, Pai M, Scanio M, Shi L, Drizin I, Gregg R, Matulenko M, Hakeem A, Grosst M, Johnson M, Marsh K, Wagoner PK, Sullivan JP, Faltynek CR, Krafte DS (2007) A-803467, a potent and selective $Na_v1.8$ sodium channel blocker, attenuates neuropathic and inflammatory pain in the rat. Proc Natl Acad Sci USA 104:8520–8525

Ji RR, Suter MR (2007) p38 MAPK, microglial signaling, and neuropathic pain. Mol Pain 3:33

Ji RR, Baba H, Brenner GJ, Woolf CJ (1999) Nociceptive-specific activation of ERK in spinal neurons contributes to pain hypersensitivity. Nat Neurosci 2:1114–1119

Ji RR, Kawasaki Y, Zhuang ZY, Wen YR, Zhang YQ (2007) Protein kinases as potential targets for the treatment of pathological pain. Handb Exp Pharmacol 359–389

Jin SX, Zhuang ZY, Woolf CJ, Ji RR (2003) p38 Mitogen-activated protein kinase is activated after a spinal nerve ligation in spinal cord microglia and dorsal root ganglion neurons and contributes to the generation of neuropathic pain. J Neurosci 23:4017–4022

Kashiba H, Fukui H, Morikawa Y, Senba E (1999) Gene expression of histamine H1 receptor in guinea pig primary sensory neurons: a relationship between H1 receptor mRNA-expressing neurons and peptidergic neurons. Mol Brain Res 66:24–34

Katsura H, Obata K, Mizushima T, Sakurai J, Kobayashi K, Yamanaka H, Dai Y, Fukuoka T, Sakagami M, Noguchi K (2006) Activation of Src-family kinases in spinal microglia contributes to mechanical hypersensitivity after nerve injury. J Neurosci 26:8680–8690

Kerr BJ, Bradbury EJ, Bennett DL, Trivedi PM, Dassan P, French J, Shelton DB, McMahon SB, Thompson SW (1999) Brain-derived neurotrophic factor modulates nociceptive sensory inputs and NMDA-evoked responses in the rat spinal cord. J Neurosci 19:5138–5148

Kim SY, Bae JC, Kim JY, Lee HL, Lee KM, Kim DS, Cho HJ (2002) Activation of p38 MAP kinase in the rat dorsal root ganglia and spinal cord following peripheral inflammation and nerve injury. Neuroreport 13:2483–2486

Koltzenburg M, Bennett DL, Shelton DL, McMahon SB (1999) Neutralization of endogenous NGF prevents the sensitization of nociceptors supplying inflamed skin. Eur J Neurosci 11: 1698–1704

Ledeboer A, Sloane EM, Milligan ED, Frank MG, Mahony JH, Maier SF, Watkins LR (2005) Minocycline attenuates mechanical allodynia and proinflammatory cytokine expression in rat models of pain facilitation. Pain 115:71–83

Lever IJ, Bradbury EJ, Cunningham JR, Adelson DW, Jones MG, McMahon SB, Marvizon JC, Malcangio M (2001) Brain-derived neurotrophic factor is released in the dorsal horn by distinctive patterns of afferent fiber stimulation. J Neurosci 21:4469–4477

Lever IJ, Rice AS (2007) Cannabinoids and pain. Hadb Exp Pharmacol 177:265–306

Levine JD, Gooding J, Donatoni P, Borden L, Goetzl EJ (1985) The role of the polymorphonuclear leukocyte in hyperalgesia. J Neurosci 5:3025–3029

Lindenlaub T, Sommer C (2003) Cytokines in sural nerve biopsies from inflammatory and non-inflammatory neuropathies. Acta Neuropathol 105:593–602

Lindenlaub T, Teuteberg P, Hartung T, Sommer C (2000) Effects of neutralizing antibodies to TNF-alpha on pain-related behavior and nerve regeneration in mice with chronic constriction injury. Brain Res 866:15–22

Lindia JA, Kohler MG, Martin WJ, Abbadie C (2005) Relationship between sodium channel $Na_v1.3$ expression and neuropathic pain behavior in rats. Pain 117:145–153

Lindsay RM, Harmar AJ (1989) Nerve growth factor regulates expression of neuropeptide genes in adult sensory neurons. Nature 337:362–364

Liu T, van Rooijen N, Tracey DJ (2000) Depletion of macrophages reduces axonal egeneration and hyperalgesia following nerve injury. Pain 86:25–32

Liu XZ, Zhou JL, Chung KS, Chung JM (2001) Ion channels associated with the ectopic discharges generated after segmental spinal nerve injury in the rat. Brain Res 900: 119–127

Ma W, Quirion R (2005) The ERK/MAPK pathway, as a target for the treatment of neuropathic pain. Expert Opin Ther Targets 9:699–713

Ma W, Quirion R (2006) Increased calcitonin gene-related peptide in neuroma and invading macrophages is involved in the up-regulation of interleukin-6 and thermal hyperalgesia in a rat model of mononeuropathy. J Neurochem 98:180–192

Ma W, Quirion R (2007) Inflammatory mediators modulating the transient receptor potential vanilloid 1 receptor: therapeutic targets to treat inflammatory and neuropathic pain. Expert Opin Ther Targets 11:307–320

Malcangio M, Lessmann V (2003) A common thread for pain and memory synapses? Brain-derived neurotrophic factor and trkB receptors. Trends Pharmacol Sci 24:116–121

Mamet J, Lazdunski M, Voilley N (2003) How nerve growth factor drives physiological and inflammatory expressions of acid-sensing ion channel 3 in sensory neurons. J Biol Chem 278:48907–48913

Marchand F, Perretti M, McMahon SB (2005) Role of the immune system in chronic pain. Nat Rev Neurosci 6:521–532

Matthews EA, Dickenson AH (2001) Effects of spinally delivered N- and P-type voltage-dependent calcium channel antagonists on dorsal horn neuronal responses in a rat model of neuropathy. Pain 92:235–246

McAllister AK, Katz LC, Lo DC (1999) Neurotrophins and synaptic plasticity. Annu Rev Neurosci 22:295–318

McCleane GJ (1998) The cholecystokinin antagonist proglumide enhances the analgesic efficacy of morphine in humans with chronic benign pain. Anesth Analg 87:1117–1120

McMahon SB, Bennett DL, Priestley JV, Shelton DL (1995) The biological effects of endogenous nerve growth factor on adult sensory neurons revealed by a trkA-IgG fusion molecule. Nat Med 1:774–780

McQuay HJ, Tramer M, Nye BA, Carroll D, Wiffen PJ, Moore RA (1996) Systematic review of antidepressants in neuropathic pain. Pain 68:217–227

Meller ST, Dykstra C, Grzybycki D, Murphy S, Gebhart GF (1994) The possible role of glia in nociceptive processing and hyperalgesia in the spinal cord of the rat. Neuropharmacology 33:1471–1478

Metcalfe DD, Baram D, Mekori YA (1997) Mast cells. Physiol Rev 77:1033–1079

Michael GJ, Averill S, Nitkunan A, Rattray M, Bennett DL, Yan Q, Priestley JV (1997) Nerve growth factor treatment increases brain-derived neurotrophic factor selectively in TrkA-expressing dorsal root ganglion cells and in their central terminations within the spinal cord. J Neurosci 17:8476–8490

Michael GJ, Averill S, Shortland PJ, Yan Q, Priestley JV (1999) Axotomy results in major changes in BDNF expression by dorsal root ganglion cells: BDNF expression in large trkB and trkC cells, in pericellular baskets, and in projections to deep dorsal horn and dorsal column nuclei. Eur J Neurosci 11:3539–3551

Milligan ED, Mehmert KK, Hinde JL, Harvey LO, Martin D, Tracey KJ, Maier SF, Watkins LR (2000) Thermal hyperalgesia and mechanical allodynia produced by intrathecal administration of the human immunodeficiency virus-1 (HIV-1) envelope glycoprotein, gp120. Brain Res 861:105–116

Milligan ED, Twining C, Chacur M, Biedenkapp J, O'Connor K, Poole S, Tracey K, Martin D, Maier SF, Watkins LR (2003) Spinal glia and proinflammatory cytokines mediate mirror-image neuropathic pain in rats. J Neurosci 23:1026–1040

Milligan ED, Langer SJ, Sloane EM, He L, Wieseler-Frank J, O'Connor K, Martin D, Forsayeth JR, Maier SF, Johnson K, Chavez RA, Leinwand LA, Watkins LR (2005) Controlling pathological pain by adenovirally driven spinal production of the anti-inflammatory cytokine, interleukin-10. Eur J Neurosci 21:2136–2148

Munro G, Dalby-Brown W (2007) K_v7 (KCNQ) channel modulators and neuropathic pain. J Med Chem 50:2576–2582

Myers RR, Heckman HM, Rodriguez M (1996) Reduced hyperalgesia in nerve-injured WLD mice: relationship to nerve fiber phagocytosis, axonal degeneration, and regeneration in normal mice. Exp Neurol 141:94–101

Nassar MA, Levato A, Stirling LC, Wood JN (2005) Neuropathic pain develops normally in mice lacking both $Na_v1.7$ and $Na_v1.8$. Molecular Pain 1:24

Nassar MA, Baker MD, Levato A, Ingram R, Mallucci G, McMahon SB, Wood JN (2006) Nerve injury induces robust allodynia and ectopic discharges in $Na_v1.3$ null mutant mice. Mol Pain 2:33

Olesen J, Diener HC, Husstedt IW, Goadsby PJ, Hall D, Meier U, Pollentier S, Lesko LM (2004) Calcitonin gene-related peptide receptor antagonist BIBN 4096 BS for the acute treatment of migraine. N Engl J Med 350:1104–1110

Peng XM, Zhou ZG, Glorioso JC, Fink DJ, Mata M (2006) Tumor necrosis factor-alpha contributes to below-level neuropathic pain after spinal cord injury. Ann Neurol 59:843–851

Perkins NM, Tracey DJ (2000) Hyperalgesia due to nerve injury: role of neutrophils. Neuroscience 101:745–757

Perry VH, Brown MC, Gordon S (1987) The macrophage response to central and peripheral nerve injury. A possible role for macrophages in regeneration. J Exp Med 165:1218–1223

Petty BG, Cornblath DR, Adornato BT, Chaudhry V, Flexner C, Wachsman M, Sinicropi D, Burton LE, Peroutka SJ (1994) The effect of systemically administered recombinant human nerve growth factor in healthy human subjects. Ann Neurol 36:244–246

Pezet S, McMahon SB (2006) Neurotrophins: mediators and modulators of pain. Annu Rev Neurosci 29:507–538

Pezet S, Malcangio M, McMahon SB (2002b) BDNF: a neuromodulator in nociceptive pathways? Brain Res Brain Res Rev 40:240–249

Pezet S, Malcangio M, Lever IJ, Perkinton MS, Thompson SW, Williams RJ, McMahon SB (2002a) Noxious stimulation induces Trk receptor and downstream ERK phosphorylation in spinal dorsal horn. Mol Cell Neurosci 21:684–695

Raghavendra V, Tanga F, DeLeo JA (2003) Inhibition of microglial activation attenuates the development but not existing hypersensitivity in a rat model of neuropathy. J Pharmacol Exp Ther 306:624–630

Rasband MN, Park EW, Vanderah TW, Lai J, Porreca F, Trimmer JS (2001) Distinct potassium channels on pain-sensing neurons. Proc Natl Acad Sci USA 98:13373–13378

Reeve AJ, Patel S, Fox A, Walker K, Urban L (2000) Intrathecally administered endotoxin or cytokines produce allodynia, hyperalgesia and changes in spinal cord neuronal responses to nociceptive stimuli in the rat. Eur J Pain 4:247–257

Rice AS, Hill RG (2006) New treatments for neuropathic pain. Annu Rev Med 57:535–551

Rueff A, Mendell LM (1996) Nerve growth factor NT-5 induce increased thermal sensitivity of cutaneous nociceptors in vitro. J Neurophysiol 76:3593–3596

Rutkowski MD, Pahl JL, Sweitzer S, van Rooijen N, DeLeo JA (2000) Limited role of macrophages in generation of nerve injury-induced mechanical allodynia. Physiol Behav 71:225–235

Rutkowski MD, Lambert F, Raghavendra V, Deleo JA (2004) Presence of spinal B7.2 (CD86) but not B7.1 (CD80) co-stimulatory molecules following peripheral nerve injury: role of nondestructive immunity in neuropathic pain. J Neuroimmunol 146:94–98

Scapini P, Lapinet-Vera JA, Gasperini S, Calzetti F, Bazzoni F, Cassatella MA (2000) The neutrophil as a cellular source of chemokines. Immunol Rev 177:195–203

Schafers M, Brinkhoff J, Neukirchen S, Marziniak M, Sommer C (2001) Combined epineurial therapy with neutralizing antibodies to tumor necrosis factor-alpha and interleukin-1 receptor has an additive effect in reducing neuropathic pain in mice. Neurosci Lett 310:113–116

Schafers M, Geis C, Svensson CI, Luo ZD, Sommer C (2003a) Selective increase of tumour necrosis factor-alpha in injured and spared myelinated primary afferents after chronic constrictive injury of rat sciatic nerve. Eur J Neurosci 17:791–804

Schafers M, Lee DH, Brors D, Yaksh TL, Sorkin LS (2003b) Increased sensitivity of injured and adjacent uninjured rat primary sensory neurons to exogenous tumor necrosis factor-alpha after spinal nerve ligation. J Neurosci 23:3028–3038

Schafers M, Svensson CI, Sommer C, Sorkin LS (2003c) Tumor necrosis factor-alpha induces mechanical allodynia after spinal nerve ligation by activation of p38 MAPK in primary sensory neurons. J Neurosci 23:2517–2521

Shembalkar P, Taubel J, Abadias M, Arezina R, Hammond K, Anand P (2001) Cizolirtine citrate (E-4018) in the treatment of chronic neuropathic pain. Curr Med Res Opin 17:262–266

Shi N, Pardridge WM (2000) Noninvasive gene targeting to the brain. Proc Natl Acad Sci USA 97:7567–7572

Shu X, Mendell LM (1999) Nerve growth factor acutely sensitizes the response of adult rat sensory neurons to capsaicin. Neurosci Lett 274:159–162

Sindrup SH, Jensen TS (1999) Efficacy of pharmacological treatments of neuropathic pain: an update and effect related to mechanism of drug action. Pain 83:389–400

Sommer C, Schafers M (1998) Painful mononeuropathy in C57BL/Wld mice with delayed Wallerian degeneration: differential effects of cytokine production and nerve regeneration on thermal and mechanical hypersensitivity. Brain Res 784:154–162

Sommer C, Marziniak M, Myers RR (1998) The effect of thalidomide treatment on vascular pathology and hyperalgesia caused by chronic constriction injury of rat nerve. Pain 74:83–91

Sommer C, Lindenlaub T, Teuteberg P, Schafers M, Hartung T, Toyka KV (2001a) Anti-TNF-neutralizing antibodies reduce pain-related behavior in two different mouse models of painful mononeuropathy. Brain Res 913:86–89

Sommer C, Schafers M, Marziniak M, Toyka KV (2001b) Etanercept reduces hyperalgesia in experimental painful neuropathy. J Peripher Nerv Syst 6:67–72

Stucky CL, Koltzenburg M, Schneider M, Engle MG, Albers KM, Davis BM (1999) Overexpression of nerve growth factor in skin selectively affects the survival and functional properties of nociceptors. J Neurosci 19:8509–8516

Sweitzer SM, Schubert P, Deleo JA (2001) Propentofylline, a glial modulating agent, exhibits antiallodynic properties in a rat model of neuropathic pain. J Pharmacol Exp Ther 297: 1210–1217

Sweitzer SM, Peters MC, Ma JY, Kerr I, Mangadu R, Chakravarty S, Dugar S, Medicherla S, Protter AA, Yeomans DC (2004) Peripheral and central p38 MAPK mediates capsaicin-induced hyperalgesia. Pain 111:278–285

Tanaka T, Minami M, Nakagawa T, Satoh M (2004) Enhanced production of monocyte chemoattractant protein-1 in the dorsal root ganglia in a rat model of neuropathic pain: possible involvement in the development of neuropathic pain. Neurosci Res 48:463–469

Thacker MA, Clark AK, Marchand F, McMahon SB (2007) Pathophysiology of peripheral neuropathic pain: immune cells and molecules. Anesth Analg 105:838–847

Thompson SW, Bennett DL, Kerr BJ, Bradbury EJ, McMahon SB (1999) Brain-derived neurotrophic factor is an endogenous modulator of nociceptive responses in the spinal cord. Proc Natl Acad Sci USA 96:7714–7718

Treede RD, Jensen TS, Campbell JN, Cruccu G, Dostrovsky JO, Griffin JW, Hansson P, Hughes R, Nurmikko T, Serra J (2008) Neuropathic pain: redefinition and a grading system for clinical and research purposes. Neurology 70:1630–1635

Tsuda M, Mizokoshi A, Shigemoto-Mogami Y, Koizumi S, Inoue K (2004) Activation of p38 mitogen-activated protein kinase in spinal hyperactive microglia contributes to pain hypersensitivity following peripheral nerve injury. Glia 45:89–95

Uceyler N, Rogausch JP, Toyka KV, Sommer C (2007) Differential expression of cytokines in painful and painless neuropathies. Neurology 69:42–49

Velazquez KT, Mohammad H, Sweitzer SM (2007) Protein kinase C in pain: involvement of multiple isoforms. Pharmacol Res 55:578–589

Wagner R, Myers RR (1996) Endoneurial injection of TNF-alpha produces neuropathic pain behaviors. Neuroreport 7:2897–2901

Wagner R, Myers RR, O'Brien JS (1998) Prosaptide prevents hyperalgesia and reduces peripheral TNFR1 expression following TNF-alpha nerve injection. Neuroreport 9:2827–2831

Watkins LR, Maier SF (2003) Glia: a novel drug discovery target for clinical pain. Nat Rev Drug Discov 2 973–985

White FA, Sun J, Waters SM, Ma C, Ren D, Ripsch M, Steflik J, Cortright DN, LaMotte RH, Miller RJ (2005) Excitatory monocyte chemoattractant protein-1 signaling is up-regulated in sensory neurons after chronic compression of the dorsal root ganglion. Proc Natl Acad Sci USA 102:14092–14097

Wolfe D, Hao S, Hu J, Srinivasan R, Goss J, Mata M, Fink DJ, Glorioso JC (2007) Engineering an endomorphin-2 gene for use in neuropathic pain therapy. Pain 133:29–38

Wood JN (2006) Molecular mechanisms of nociception and pain. Handb Clin Neurol 81:49–59

Wood JN, Boorman J (2005) Voltage-gated sodium channel blockers: target validation and therapeutic potential. Curr Top Med Chem 5:529–537

Woolf CJ, Safieh-Garabedian B, Ma QP, Crilly P, Winter J (1994) Nerve growth factor contributes to the generation of inflammatory sensory hypersensitivity. Neuroscience 62:327–331

Xu J, Gingras KM, Bengston L, Di Marco A, Forger NG (2001) Blockade of endogenous neurotrophic factors prevents the androgenic rescue of rat spinal motoneurons. J Neurosci 21:4366–4372

Xu JT, Tu HY, Xin WJ, Liu XG, Zhang GH, Zhai CH (2007) Activation of phosphatidylinositol 3-kinase and protein kinase B/Akt in dorsal root ganglia and spinal cord contributes to the neuropathic pain induced by spinal nerve ligation in rats. Exp Neurol 206:269–279

Yaksh TL (2006) Calcium channels as therapeutic targets in neuropathic pain. J Pain 7:S13–S30

Zelenka M, Schafers M, Sommer C (2005) Intraneural injection of interleukin-1[beta] and tumor necrosis factor-alpha into rat sciatic nerve at physiological doses induces signs of neuropathic pain. Pain 116:257–263

Zhang J, Shi XQ, Echeverry S, Mogil JS, De Koninck Y, Rivest S (2007) Expression of CCR2 in both resident and bone marrow-derived microglia plays a critical role in neuropathic pain. J Neurosci 27:12396–12406

Zhou XF, Rush RA (1996) Endogenous brain-derived neurotrophic factor is anterogradely transported in primary sensory neurons. Neuroscience 74:945–953

Zhou XF, Chie ET, Deng YS, Zhong JH, Xue Q, Rush RA, Xian CJ (1999) Injured primary sensory neurons switch phenotype for brain-derived neurotrophic factor in the rat. Neuroscience 92:841–853

Zhuang ZY, Gerner P, Woolf CJ, Ji RR (2005) ERK is sequentially activated in neurons, microglia, and astrocytes by spinal nerve ligation and contributes to mechanical allodynia in this neuropathic pain model. Pain 114:149–159

Zhuang ZY, Wen YR, Zhang DR, Borsello T, Bonny C, Strichartz GR, Decosterd I, Ji RR (2006) A peptide c-Jun N-terminal kinase (JNK) inhibitor blocks mechanical allodynia after spinal nerve ligation: respective roles of JNK activation in primary sensory neurons and spinal astrocytes for neuropathic pain development and maintenance. J Neurosci 26:3551–3560

Zuo Y, Perkins NM, Tracey DJ, Geczy CL (2003) Inflammation and hyperalgesia induced by nerve injury in the rat: a key role of mast cells. Pain 105:467–479

Index